Life
Extension

A Practical
Scientific Approach

Life Extension

A Practical Scientific Approach

DURK PEARSON AND SANDY SHAW

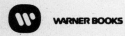 WARNER BOOKS

A Warner Communications Company

All royalties from this book are payable directly to the Laboratory for the Advancement of Bio-Medical Research, a non-profit research foundation for Life Extension.

Warner Books, Inc., 666 Fifth Avenue, New York, NY 10103

W A Warner Communications Company

Printed in the United States of America

First Warner Books Printing: June 1983
10 9 8 7 6

Library of Congress Cataloging in Publication Data

Pearson, Durk, and Shaw, Sandy.
    Life extension.

    Includes index.
    1. Health.   2. Longevity.   I. Shaw, Sandy, joint
author.   II. Title. [DNLM: 1. Health.   2. Longevity—
Popular works.   3. Nutrition—Popular works.   WT 120
P361L]
RA776.5.P34   613   80-27589
ISBN 0-446-38-503-4 (U.S.A.)   AACR1
ISBN 0-446-38-504-2 (Canada)

Book design: H. Roberts Design

DEDICATION

This book is dedicated to Dr. Denham Harman, originator of the free radical theory of aging, whose papers first interested us in this field

and

to Dr. Albert Hofmann, a visionary pharmaceutical chemist who invented Hydergine® and a host of other modern wonder drugs

and

to James Watson and Francis Crick, Nobel Prize winners, discoverers of the structure (secret) of life.

I hate death.

—Bernard Strehler, eminent gerontologist

... Leave the dreams of yesterday, take the torch of knowledge, and build the dreams of the future.

—Marie Curie (on the 25th anniversary of the discovery of radium)

Contents

Part II: Life Extension Theory and Practice   61

**Part III: Improving the Quality of Life—
            In Sickness and Health   159**

Part V: Your Personalized Life
Extension Program   427

Part VI: Appendices, Chapter Notes, and
Literature References   529

Foreword

This popularly written medical science book serves two major sectors of the reading public: 1) physicians and their allied health professionals, and 2) lay people concerned with health maintenance. The numerous references and scientific presentations of the information will serve the first group well, while the stepwise structure of the book, ready explanations, good humor, and Glossary will help the general public. For both groups, this book offers two things:

- First, it represents a cohesive "clearinghouse" of information that, to date, had previously been scattered in diverse sources ranging from medical books to media headlines. The book reveals the medical scientific bases for preventing the major lethal disorders, stressing, for example, the molecular level reasons why it may be possible to prevent or delay 80% of all cancers. Moreover this data, rather than being presented in a "dry" encyclopedic form, is brought to life literally and figuratively, so that it serves as both a reference work and as an educational tool. Instead of dealing solely with nutrient supplements, the book is concerned primarily with the molecular biochemical pathology that underlies the major human disorders and the effects of various nutrients upon them.
- The second thing provided by this book, to both sectors, is partly controversial and deals with what actions may be taken by physicians and the general public, based on the information provided. In other words, now that we have begun to understand the origin and progression of

the major human disorders, what, if anything, can we do about them *now,* rather than wait until further research provides more information and better guidance? Is there, in fact, enough known to launch some type of action at this time? The answer provided by the authors is yes, and it is substantiated by considerable research that has been recently reported. For example, carotenoids and retinoids (see the Glossary for these orange and yellow plant compounds that are chemically related to vitamin A) appear to offer important cancer prevention properties during the twenty-to-thirty-year lag phase in the development of human cancer, even *after* exposures have occurred (e.g. Japanese epidemiologists have shown that cigarette smokers who eat green and yellow vegetables have 30% less lung cancer, compared to appropriately matched controls who do not eat these retinoid- and carotenoid-containing vegetables). The nutrient supplements discussed by the authors for prevention involve relatively large doses, and the cautions noted throughout their book are to be taken seriously. A physician's supervision is advised, together with periodic laboratory examinations. A prudent diet that is low in fats and high in fresh fruit and vegetables is also desirable, as is moderation of disease-provoking habits such as smoking and alcoholism.

For many physicians and related personnel, the area of nutrient supplements (vitamins, amino acids, minerals, and other purported health aids) is not adequately covered during their schooling to the extent that the general public is currently using these materials. Whether we as physicians approve or disapprove of the use of these supplements in large doses is perhaps moot; the startling fact is that millions of people in the USA are using them at ever escalating rates and ever increasing doses and combinations. Many of these nutrient supplements are powerful chemicals and, when taken in "megadoses," can have profound effects, some of which are the subject of active research. (For example, cancer patients undergoing radiation treatments and/or chemotherapy may unknowingly influence the outcome of their treatments, for better or for worse, by the use of large doses of nutrient supplements that have antioxidant properties; this may be particularly true when such substances as ascorbic acid, ascorbyl palmitate, BHT/BHA, alpha tocopherol, cysteine, and others are taken together in megadoses. Antioxidants can act as "antidotes" to radiation, which is not necessarily desirable, since they may diminish the antitumor effect of radiation if used concomitantly with radiation. However, the administration of antioxidant mixtures at some time *after* treatment with radiation, or following therapy with drugs such as Adriamycin, may ameliorate some of the damage to normal tissues that can be caused by these cancer treatments. Research is under way now to explore such beneficial programs in a time frame and dosage regimen that will not affect the desirable antitumor effects of radiation and drugs. In accordance with these possibilities, it may become helpful to include in the personal history part of treatment protocols a specific section for noting in some detail whether the patient is self-administering megadoses of nutrient supplements.)

The potential problem of drug–drug interactions also appears to be real for other situations that do not involve cancer. For example, Parkinson patients on L-DOPA are routinely instructed not to use pyridoxine (vitamin B_6), since it counteracts L-DOPA. The use of para-amino benzoic acid (PABA) is also contraindicated if an infection is being treated with sulfa antibiotic groups. Ascorbic acid can interfere with the performance of certain clinical laboratory tests. Other over-the-counter drugs that are used as health aids, such as aspirin, can apparently block the effects of interferons (substances being developed and tested for their relatively nontoxic property of inhibiting tumor growth).

Because of the diverse chemical properties of the nutrient supplements and other health aids—a few of which appear to be helpful in slowing the development of some diseases (chronic, low doses of aspirin are widely used to inhibit occlusive atheroscleroris)—and because people are in fact "megadosing" now, this book may be a necessity for many physicians and their co-workers.

The term *life extension* deserves explanation, for not only is it the title of this book, but it is the goal of all medical practice. Life extension is, simply, the potential increase in one's life expectancy through the modification of certain behavioral and environmental factors. The latter does *not* refer to general air pollution.* (See end of foreword.)

Life extension is not a new concept. Pioneers such as Semmelweis, who advocated that doctors wash their hands before examining pregnant women in labor (to control the deadly bacterial infection called puerperal fever); sanitation engineers; and other public-health officials around the turn of the century extended life substantially by preventing communicable diseases through antisepsis, immunizations, sewage control, and sanitary food and water processing.

Some people may feel that taking megadoses of nutrient supplements is not "natural" and that we should derive what we need through food. Such "naturalistic" concepts may have some validity; however, vaccination against smallpox and immunization against polio, diphtheria, tetanus, measles, and hepatitis require growing vast amounts of bacteria and viruses and administering to billions of people. This is not natural; nor are enclosed sewers, sewage treatment plants, reservoirs for clean water, refrigeration, antibiotics, coronary-care units, modern surgery, and other practices that have increased our life expectancy.

The immense basic science support provided by the National Institute of Health has made possible the development of cautious proposals for the prevention or delay of major human disorders. The information is not yet complete, and considerably more basic research is absolutely needed. However, attempting to harvest some of the new information is entirely reasonable and is in the best traditions of medical scientific progress; such attempts often have a positive feedback to the basic research and may provide insights for the "bench" scientists. Further, some such applications must be tried, especially with regard to the aging process. As Dr. Marvin Kuschner, the dean of the State University of New York Medical School at Stony Brook, has asked, what do "we," as physician-scientists, offer to government and societal planners as an option to the tripling of the number of people over the age of sixty-five that will occur between now and the year 2,000? Do we advise them to build *three times* the number of nursing homes and *triple* the projections for Medicare outlays (in which case planning must start now to secure the land, plan the buildings, and obtain the enormous sums of money this will require)? Or do we try something that is more humane, less expensive, and possibly capable of producing "old-timers" whose health has been maintained?

In the future the role science plays in society is destined to increase. Presently many millions of Americans are megadosing on vitamins, minerals, amino acids, nucleic acids, and other substances without medical advice and without understanding the possible risks or the possible benefits. Medicare is projected to be bankrupt by 1990; 100,000 coronary by-passes are performed yearly at an average cost of $50,000 each ($5 billion); and 1,000 United States citizens die *every day* of cancer. Medical care costs (after you become sick) are pacing inflation, and in view of these facts Richard Schweicker, Secretary of Health and Human Resources, and Senator Alan Cranston have noted that prevention and more rational approaches to diseases and aging are mandatory. In this book some prudent orientation for these areas has been provided for physicians, the general public, and those officials whose constitutional mandate it is to "safeguard the general welfare."

Harry B. Demopoulos, M.D.,
New York City

*See Demopoulos and Gutman, "Cancer in New Jersey and Other Complex Urban/Industrial Areas," pp. 219–236, and Demopoulos et al, "The Possible Role of Free Radical Reactions," pp. 273–304, and Cimino and Demopoulos, "Introduction: Determinants of Cancer Relevant to Prevention, in the War on Cancer," pp. 1–10 and several other outstanding papers in the special issue of the *Journal of Environmental Pathology and Toxicology*, Vol. 3, No. 4, March 1980, edited by H.B. Demopoulos and M.A. Mehlman (published by Pathotox Publishers, Inc., 2405 Bond St., Park Forest South, IL 60466)

The Engraved Invitation; or, What This Book Will Do for You

Until late in this century, the dream of lengthening the human life span was purely a matter of science fiction. Nothing could be done about it. Many, nevertheless, tried. Five hundred years ago, Leonardo da Vinci dissected many corpses in an attempt to discover the secrets of life and death. But there was inadequate basic biological knowledge for him to draw upon in his studies. Benjamin Franklin even wrote in a letter that he regretted that he could not be preserved in a wine cask, to be revived after a hundred years or so!

We are both research scientists who have been involved in aging and biomedical research for many years. We both enjoy life tremendously and want to stay young and live as long as possible. Sandy is a biochemist, a graduate of UCLA in 1966. Durk is a physicist, a graduate of MIT in 1965. We began working together on aging research in 1968. Throughout this time, we have applied our ideas about anti-aging treatments to ourselves and have had hundreds of clinical tests done on ourselves to monitor for possible negative as well as positive effects. When, in 1978, Warner Books approached us with the idea of writing about aging and what can be done about it, we were delighted. Writing this book has given us the opportunity to inform the lay public about this new and exciting area of research, to communicate our ideas to other scientists and to physicians, and to generate private funds so that we and others can do even more sophisticated and ambitious aging research!

How successful have we been in slowing or reversing our

own aging? We don't really know how long we might live because tests capable of providing this information have not yet been devised. Until people have an opportunity to live to advanced ages such as 150 years and more, animal experiments will provide the best evidence for the possibility of extended life spans. What we can say is that, on the basis of the clinical tests we've taken, we do not seem to have harmed ourselves. We both have extremely low cholesterol levels although our diets contain plenty of fats (butter, milk, meats, etc.) We both have hard muscular bodies although both of us are "middle-aged" and almost 100 percent sedentary. We think that, in many ways, our physical and mental performances have improved. For more details, see Part V, Chapter 7, describing our nutrient and prescription drug supplements and our case histories in Appendix L. We believe that anyone can benefit from at least some of the ideas in this book.

In any new field of endeavor, the progress taking place is hardly ever widely known at first. Scientific research results may be overlooked for years before their practical applications are recognized. The future arrives sooner or later for all of us, but we can reap benefits from developing technologies sooner if we are prepared. The rapid development of modern aging research began in the late 1950s with Dr. Denham Harman's free radical theory of aging. **We are still in a period when self-experimentation with anti-aging therapies is pioneering. Therefore, we include in this book precautions you should take seriously if you want to lengthen rather than shorten your life span.**

There is no single expert who knows everything about life extension and can tell each of us when new technologies are available for our own personal use. In order to benefit early from the new science and technology of life extension, you have to learn some basic biological facts about your body and how scientists perform and interpret experiments. With this basic knowledge, you can deal with the myriad theories and data in circulation. You will then be better prepared to make use of our detailed how-to-do-it-yourself instructions so that you can start lengthening your healthy active life span right now!

That is what this book can do for you. It is our belief that a reader with above average intelligence, but not necessarily a college graduate, interested in extending and improving his or her life span will be able to understand and profit from our book. It is an invitation to a personal adventure that may lead to a longer and more vigorous lifetime, an adventure we ourselves have been researching and living for over twelve years!

DISCLAIMER

The worldview expressed in this book is our own. Although we have drawn heavily on the research work of many other scientists, we alone are responsible for our interpretations and uses of their ideas. This is a book which, in the final analysis, is about us and our values, as much as it is about scientific data and ideas.

<u>This set of comments is usually called a disclaimer, that is, our attempt to provide certain principles which govern what we consider reasonable use of our book. This is not a mere formality. We really mean what we say here.</u>

<u>Don't be careless with new knowledge. As you read this book, it is important to keep these factors in mind:</u>

1. We are research scientists, not physicians.

2. We are not infallible. Certainly there will be some errors in the book, even though we and a few scientific colleagues have carefully proofread it.

3. You are responsible for planning your own nutritional regimen. Everyone is biochemically distinct from other people. Take your time in considering these ideas and acting on them. Remember that one definition of a pioneer is a guy with an arrow in his back!

4. We do not provide "The Answer" to aging in our book. There is no such thing. We provide a number of options which you can choose among, based on *your* values, not ours.

5. We have no financial involvement with any of the suppliers listed here. No one is paying us to recommend any of the discussed nutrients or prescription drugs. We own no stock in pharmaceutical, nutrition, or health firms.

6. We are definitely not interested in being cult leaders. We want people to think for themselves and check our sources, not to be true believers who worship our ideas as a religion.

7. The use of prescription drugs and large doses of nutrients for the improvement of health in normal people is still experimental. Some applications of scientific findings we report are based on results in a small number of people. Be sure

to have regular clinical laboratory tests if you plan to experiment with any of these substances yourself. (See Part V, Chapter 4 for clinical laboratory tests.)

8. The experimental nutrient and prescription drug formulas discussed herein are **_not_ for children, pregnant women, or careless persons.** If you are a daredevil who enjoys risking his or her life, please go buy someone else's book.

9. None of the nutrients and prescription drugs we use are FDA-approved as a therapy for life extension. There is no such category of approval. (See Appendix E, "What Is the Government Doing About Aging Research?")

10. You should consult your physician about megadose vitamins. There are serious illnesses that may be aggravated by megadose vitamins. Here are three examples, and there are more:

(a) If you have an ulcer of your esophagus, stomach, or duodenum, large doses of acidic vitamins, taken on an empty stomach, can make the ulcer worse. It might even perforate or bleed seriously.

(b) If you have high blood pressure, heart disease, or kidney trouble, vitamin preparations that contain sodium may worsen your condition.

(c) If you have Parkinson's disease and are on treatment with L-Dopa, taking vitamin B-6 will counteract the L-Dopa and worsen your condition.

11. Your laboratory results must be sent to your doctor. A good clinical pathology laboratory will not send you the results, but will insist, for the sake of safety, that the lab tests go to your doctor first.

12. Do *not* imagine that any of our suggestions can substitute for your doctor's treatments of serious disorders such as heart disease, high blood pressure, cancer, kidney disease, and the like. So do *not* stop your prescribed medications, and make sure you consult with your doctor about adding our suggestions!

Caveat: Don't be fooled by the large amount of information in this book into thinking that we know just about all there is to know about aging. Far from it. We know only a small fraction of what there is to discover about aging. We and other scientists will continue our efforts to find out how aging occurs and how to slow it, put a stop to it, and even partially reverse it. We hope that reasonable funding—from both public and private sources—will be made available so that this important research can go forward.

Live Long and Prosper,

Durk Pearson

Sandy Shaw

April 22, 1981
Los Angeles

How to Use This Book

If all else fails, read the instructions.

> —from a tag on new scientific equipment

Nothing will ever be attempted if all possible objections
must first be overcome.

> —Samuel Johnson

*Whether you want to live forever or just a healthy active three
score and ten, this book is for you. We have written it so that
people of above average intelligence, but without special education, and with widely varying life extension goals will be
able to choose from a large selection of techniques that retard
some aspects of aging and foster youth. You don't have to follow any special order for reading the chapters. If you like,
you can read the book from cover to cover. Or, feel free to
browse! The following suggestions will help you decide how
to read our book to satisfy your own goals and interests. If
you do browse, or read chapters selectively, you should make
certain to read the Disclaimers in our "Engraved Invitation,"
particularly in regard to having your physician's consultation and clinical laboratory tests done periodically.*

Aging involves many different mechanisms. You can now
slow and even partially reverse some of these different mechanisms of aging. We wrote this book to tell you how different
factors in aging work and how you may be able to slow or par-

tially reverse most of them. You can apply many of these anti-aging, pro-youth techniques right now. You do not have to wait another ten years. You can promptly benefit from life extension research. You can improve your health within a few weeks while at the same time slowing some of the detrimental processes that contribute to the aging process. Some moderation of lifestyle and decreases in dietary fat intake may be needed, together with a little exercise. Many excellent books have been written on these areas and we recommend that you read them (see the general reading list and references in Appendix A and the specific references and Chapter notes in Appendix K). When we talk about life extension, we are talking about extending the active pleasurable portion of one's life, not extending the time one survives in a hospital bed. Both of us were born in 1943; we are youthful, enjoy life very much, and plan to go on enjoying it to the hilt for many more decades. Whether you are young, middle-aged, or old, this book can be very valuable to you. If you are old, not only can your life span be extended but, especially, the quality of that life span can be greatly improved by your own actions right now. If you are middle-aged, this book will tell you how you can partially regain some aspects of your youth, dramatically improve the quality of your life, and increase your life span. If you are a young adult, the immediate improvement in the quality of your life will naturally be less dramatic, but the duration of your youthfulness should be dramatically increased.

Scientific reports have been published in which current life extension techniques as much as double the life spans of experimental animals. Almost all this prolongation occurs in the healthy active portions of life; the decrepit elderly portion of the life span is extended relatively little. We have been applying some of these techniques to ourselves for the past twelve years, and we think that you will be fascinated by what we have done and what you can do yourself. Although we have encountered pitfalls, we believe that it is possible to avoid them, provided you do not go off on your own and utilize these substances recklessly. If you continue to follow scientific evidence as it emerges, further pitfalls can be minimized.

Different people are looking for different types of life extension information. Perhaps you have had a heart attack. Naturally you are most interested in preventing a second attack and partially reversing the underlying cardiovascular disease; you may not have the time or the interest to read about preventing or curing cancer or arthritis or senility. People are individuals with different problems and interests. We wrote this book so that it could be used to find ways—usually several different ways—to prevent, slow, or partially reverse some aspects of the aging problem or problems of greatest concern to you.

This is not a textbook. A textbook is designed to be read from the start, one chapter after another until the end. If you wish, you can use this book as a text, reading it from cover to cover. Read this way, we think that it is the most comprehensive book ever written for the intelligent lay person on biological gerontology, the science of youth and aging, and the technology for extending youth and reversing some of the ravages of age.

Most likely, however, you are very interested in one type of aging problem, a little interested in a few others, and not at all interested in the remainder. For those of you who feel you have other things to do with your time than studying an entire book to understand the portion of interest to you, this book is designed so that you don't have to read all of it to find what you want. It contains many chapters, each on a different topic. Most of them are quite short and begin with an italicized paragraph, summarizing the contents, so that you can quickly scan the book for chapters of particular interest. Look over the chapter titles, find the one that is most interesting to you, turn to that page, and start reading. If you read the book this way, you may come across an unfamiliar scientific word. We have often put the lay term in parentheses following the scientific term, for example: "Lipids (fats) are damaged by oxygen." It is much easier to learn new words this way than it is to memorize them. (We wrote this book so that you don't have to try to memorize anything. If you read something interesting that is repeated often enough, you will eventually remember it effortlessly.) Once in a while, you will see an unfamiliar scientific word which doesn't have a lay definition right with it. Don't despair. There is a glossary at the end of the book with easy-to-understand definitions. We have done our best, however, to make sure that you won't need to refer to it very often. If you read the book from the start, you will rarely need to consult the glossary. If you jump right into a chapter in the middle of the book, it's nice to know that the glossary is there to help you whenever you need it.

The index at the end of the book is also very helpful in

coping with scientific terms. Definitions of words are hard to remember. Children do not learn new words by memorizing their definitions; they expand their vocabulary by hearing new words used. After using the glossary to find a lay translation of a scientific term, you can use the page references in the index to see how that term is used, and in this way you can "absorb" the new word rather than working hard to "memorize" it.

Aging involves many different mechanisms. Because of this diversity, slowing and partially reversing aging may be accomplished in many different ways. There is no single royal road to life extension.

You have different medical concerns from your neighbor; perhaps you would like to be as lusty as you were in your early twenties, whereas your neighbor would like to be as slim as she was when a teenager. First, look over the chapter titles and read the obviously pertinent chapters. In many cases, that chapter or chapters will direct you to other closely related chapters. Next, look the topic up in the index. In most cases, you will find several other chapters containing some information on your principal interest. **Be sure to read the indexed cautions, precautions, and warnings (under those heads and in boldface type under other index entries) before** administering any substance to yourself. When you use the book this way, you won't be bored by information that is not yet interesting to you. As you track down the information trails leading from the chapters of greatest interest to you, your knowledge will gradually and painlessly expand. In fact, you may suddenly discover that you have read the entire book— but in a very different order from that in which we wrote it, and also very different from the order in which your neighbor is reading it.

Our book is individualized for you in yet another way. Even if you have exactly the same type of interests in life extension as your neighbor, both of you will have differing personal values. Because of these differences in personal values, the best life extension approach for you will not be the best for your neighbor, even if you are concerned about the same medical condition. Once the fundamental biochemical mechanisms of a problem have been discovered, it is almost always possible to achieve the desired results by many different methods. You will prefer some of these methods; the next person will prefer others. This is why we offer many alternative ways of getting the effects you want so that you can choose a way *you* like. For example, if you smoke but would like to reduce your risk of lung cancer, other competing health books have one prescription: Stop smoking. Our book is totally different. We assume that you like some of the effects of smoking or you wouldn't be doing it. We will tell you many different ways that you can reduce your risk by a factor of two to ten—or even more—*without* giving up the pleasures of smoking. We tell you the benefits, limitations, and costs of each of these several roads to better health. You will make the final decision as to which method or combination of methods is best for you, based on your (not our) own personal values and lifestyles.

This is a practical how-to-do-it-yourself book on life extension. Unlike the authors of most other health books, we have consistently kept in mind that our readers are individuals with a combination of desires, problems, personal values, and lifestyles of their own, so we have provided maps of many roads to many different goals. We have provided enough information so that you can select those routes and goals that may be best for you. In doing this, we have been careful to provide references to the original scientific research reports, so you do not have to accept what we say on faith. How do we know we are on the right track? Just read Chapter 13 in Part I, "How Do You Know Who's Right?", which will provide you with our criteria for distinguishing information based on sound scientific research from the fanciful panaceas offered by faddists.

How would we read a book like this? We have been involved in life extension research for more than a dozen years, so we would read it from start to finish. Since you don't have this background, we recommend that you read Part I first, for an introductory overview of life extension, prolonging youth, aging, and reversing aging. Then read a few of the chapters of greatest interest to you, after which you can go back and fill in the theory presented in Part II, which, though more difficult to digest than other sections, will now seem much more relevant to you. Finally, we hope you will be so captivated by the immense prospect that life extension offers that you will read on to the end. We have been practicing life extension techniques on ourselves for a dozen years, but it shouldn't take more than a few weeks of your using some of them before you notice some differences in yourself. Vive la différence!

Acknowledgments

The following items appearing in this book have been provided by courtesy of the sources credited and are reprinted here with their consent. Items are listed in the order of their appearance in the book or, in the case of multiple items credited to the same source, in order of appearance of the first item from that source.

page 10— Graphs from "Molecular Clocks, Molecular Profiles, and Optimum Diets: Three Approaches to the Problem of Aging" by Arthur B. Robinson, *Mechanisms of Aging and Development* 9 (1979), page 226. Reprinted by permission of Elsevier Sequoia S.A. and Arthur B. Robinson.

page 16— Photograph © 1980 by Sue Houle. All rights reserved.

pages 21, 48, 84, 173, 188, 248, 287, 294, 329, 372, 439, 456, 496, 565, 609— Cartoons by Sidney Harris from *Chicken Soup and Other Medical Matters,* Los Altos, California: William Kaufmann. Copyright © 1979 by Sidney Harris.

page 27— "How to Figure the Cost of Living a Longer Life" is provided by courtesy of General Motors Research Laboratories.

pages 28,   Cartoons reprinted from *The Calbiovinquinquen-*
65, 327,   *nial* and used by courtesy of Calbiochem, San Di-
389,   ego, California.
463—

page 32—   Epigraph lines provided by kind permission of
             Gemrod Music, Inc.

page 34—   Epigraph lines credited to Dylan Thomas are re-
             printed from *The Poems* of Dylan Thomas, J. M.
             Dent, Publishers (London) and New Directions
             Publishing Corporation (New York), by permis-
             sion of the Trustees for the copyright for the late
             Dylan Thomas and by permission of New Direc-
             tions Publishing Corporation. Copyright © 1952
             by Dylan Thomas.

page 35—   Art by Joe Pearson, from the collection of the au-
             thors.

pages 50,   Cartoons by Sidney Harris from *What's So Funny*
57, 58,   *About Science?* Los Altos, California: William
141, 183,   Kaufmann. Copyright © 1977 by Sidney Harris.
262, 365,
383, 472,
507—

pages 52,   Epigraph lines from "Eat Starch Mom" copyright
375—   © 1967 by Mole Music/Fishscent Music. Reprint-
             ed by permission.

page 73—   Graph reprinted from "The Impaired Capability
             for Biochemical Adaptation During Aging" by
             Richard C. Adelman and Gary W. Britton, *Bio-
             Science* 25-10 (October 1975), page 639, with per-
             mission of the authors and the American Institute
             of Biological Sciences.

page 76—   Diagram reprinted from "A DNA Operator-Re-
             pressor System" by Tom Maniatis and Mark
             Ptashne, *Scientific American* 234-1 (January
             1976). Copyright © 1975 by Scientific American.
             All rights reserved.

page 77—   Cartoon by Casserine Toussaint reprinted by per-
             mission of Casserine Toussaint and *Technology
             Review*. Copyright © 1979 by the Alumni Associ-

ation of the Massachusetts Institute of Technology.

page 88— Photograph from *Essential Immunology* by Ivan Roitt, page 52. Copyright © 1971 by Blackwell Scientific Publications, Oxford.

page 105— Graphs reprinted by courtesy of the National Institute on Aging.

page 109— Cartoons by R. J. Gryglewski from *Trends in Pharmacological Sciences,* February 1980. Copyright © 1979. Reprinted by permission of Elsevier/North-Holland Biomedical Press and R. J. Gryglewski.

pages 113– 117— Advertisement reprinted by courtesy of Monsanto.

page 122— Illustrations reprinted by permission from *Aging,* Volume 1 (*Clinical, Morphologic, and Neurochemical Aspects in the Aging Nervous System,*) H. Brody, D. Harman, and J. Mark Ordy, editors. Copyright © 1975 by Raven Press Books, Ltd.

page 123— Graph reprinted from Mann and Yates, "Lipoprotein Pigments: Their Relationship to Aging in the Human Nervous System" in *Brain* 97 (1974) by permission of Oxford University Press.

pages 130, 131— Diagrams reprinted with permission of Van Nostrand Reinhold Company from *Psychopharmacology: A Biochemical and Behavioral Approach* by Lewis S. Seiden and Linda A. Dykstra. Copyright © 1977 by Litton Educational Publishing, Inc.

page 145— Graphs by Arthur Schwartz reprinted from *Experimental Cell Research* 94 (1975) and 109 (1977) respectively by permission of the Fels Research Institute, Temple University Health Sciences Center, Philadelphia, Pennsylvania.

page 147— Graph reprinted by permission from "Correlation Between DNA Excision-Repair and Lifespan in a Number of Mammalian Species" by Hart and Setlow in *Proceedings of the National Academy of Sciences, U.S.A.* 71 (1974), page 2172.

page 151— "Firm Hopes to Market Bone-Growth Device" reprinted by permission of *The Wall Street Journal*, copyright © Dow Jones and Company, Inc., 1979.

page 185— Cartoon by Ed V. Shea, M.D. Reprinted by permission of Creative Computing and Ed V. Shea.

pages 191, 346, 443, 552— Cartoons by Aaron Bacall, copyright © 1981. Reprinted by permission of Aaron Bacall.

pages 198, 292, 596— Cartoons by Alexis A. Gilliland from *The Iron Law of Bureaucracy*, Mason, Michigan: Loompanics Unlimited, 1979. Reprinted by permission.

page 203— Graph by Christopher Tietze reprinted with permission from *Family Planning Perspectives* 9-2 (1977).

page 205— Cartoon by Sidney Harris. Copyright © 1975 by Playboy.

page 216— Cartoon by Sidney Harris. Copyright © 1979 by Playboy.

page 245— Chart reprinted from the booklet *Good News for Smokers,* copyright © 1980 by Durk Pearson and Sandy Shaw, published by Donsbach University.

page 253— Cartoon by T. W. Stone. Reprinted from *Trends in Pharmacological Sciences* (July 1980) by permission of Elsevier/North-Holland Biomedical Press.

page 280— Chart reprinted from the booklet *What You Always Wanted to Know About Alcohol,* copyright © 1980 by Durk Pearson and Sandy Shaw, published by Donsbach University.

pages 309–311— Photographs courtesy of Harry B. Demopoulos, M.D., New York University Medical Center.

page 326— Photograph courtesy of Sanders T. Frank, M.D., and reprinted by permission of *The New England Journal of Medicine* from volume 289 (1973), page 328.

page 335— Cartoon by Sidney Harris. Copyright © 1980 by Sidney Harris and *American Scientist* magazine.

page 344—	Epigraph lines from "Alexander the Medium" copyright © god tunes 1972. Reprinted by permission of the publisher.
page 353—	Chart © 1977 by the American Heart Association and reprinted with their permission.
page 355—	Adaptation of a poster by the New York City Department of Health.
pages 358– 360—	Immunization schedules reprinted from *Parents Guide to Childhood Immunization,* a pamphlet prepared by the United States Department of Health, Education and Welfare.
pages 379, 380—	Charts reprinted by courtesy of Eastman Chemical Products, Inc.
page 381—	Chart reprinted from "Antioxidant Activity of Tocopherols, Ascorbyl Palmitate, and Ascorbic Acid and Their Mode of Action" by W. M. Cort, *Journal of the American Oil Chemists' Society* 51-7 (July 1974), page 322, by permission of W. M. Cort and the American Oil Chemists' Society. Copyright © 1974 American Oil Chemists' Society.
page 433—	Epigraph lines copyright © 1929 by Universal Pictures, a Division of Universal City Studios, Inc. Reprinted by courtesy of MCA Publishing, a Division of MCA, Inc.
page 444—	Cartoon by Sandy Dean, reprinted by courtesy of Sandy Dean and with permission of Creative Computing.
page 445—	Advertisement reprinted by courtesy of JS&A Products That Think®.
page 480—	Cartoon by Sidney Harris. Copyright © 1974 by Sidney Harris and *American Scientist* magazine.
pages 512, 513, 523—	Cartoons by Leonard Todd. Reprinted by courtesy of Leonard Todd and with permission of Creative Computing.
page 517—	Cartoon by Sidney Harris. Copyright © 1981 by Sidney Harris and *American Scientist* magazine.
page 541—	Cartoon reprinted from *Chemtech,* April 1975, page 197. Copyright © 1975 by the American

Chemical Society and reprinted by permission of the copyright owner.

pages 545–547— List of Regional Medical Libraries and MEDLARS Centers reprinted from *Remington's Pharmaceutical Sciences*, 15th edition, pages 1767–1769, 1970, by permission of the Philadelphia College of Pharmacy and Science.

pages 548–549— Bibliographic Search Request provided by courtesy of UCLA Biomedical Library.

page 553— Cartoon reprinted from *Chemtech*, March 1975, page 137. Copyright © 1975 by the American Chemical Society and reprinted by permission of the copyright owner.

page 568— Cartoon reprinted from *Chemtech*, August 1975, page 473. Copyright © 1975 by the American Chemical Society and reprinted by permission of the copyright owner.

page 577— "Barking Cats" by Milton Friedman. Copyright © 1973 by Newsweek, Inc. All rights reserved. Reprinted by permission.

page 578— The Brozen comment is excerpted by permission from Peltzman, *Regulation of Pharmaceutical Innovation*, Washington, D.C.: American Enterprise Institute, 1974. Copyright © 1974 by American Enterprise Institute.

page 579— The Telser comment is excerpted from Lester G. Telser, "The Legal and Economic Effects of Drug Regulatory Policies," pages 213–225 in *Regulating New Drugs*, Richard Landau, editor, Chicago: University of Chicago Press, 1973.

pages 581–589, 594— The Peltzman comments are excerpted by permission from Peltzman, *Regulation of Pharmaceutical Innovation*, Washington, D.C.: American Enterprise Institute, 1974. Copyright © 1974 by American Enterprise Institute.

pages 599–603— Cartoon panels are drawn by Roberta Gregory, with story lines by Durk Pearson and Sandy Shaw. Copyright © 1981.

pages 604– 607—	Cartoons by Randall Hylkema, 1368 Sydney Drive, Sunnyvale, California 94087. Copyright © by Durk Pearson and Sandy Shaw.
page 707—	Drawing courtesy of Worthington Diagnostics.
page 710—	Diagram and caption reprinted from "Clocked Cell Cycle Clocks" by L. N. Edmunds and K. J. Adams, *Science* 211-4486 (March 6, 1981), page 1010. Copyright © 1981 by the American Association for the Advancement of Science.
page 776—	Cartoon copyright © 1981 Punch/Rothco.

PART I
ADDING YEARS TO YOUR LIFE
AND LIFE TO YOUR YEARS

I
The Psychology of Life Extension

The easiest thing in the world to do is to figure out an excuse not to do something.

—Dr. Jack Wheeler, *The Adventurer's Guide*

The firm determination to submit to experiment is not enough; there are still dangerous hypotheses; first, and above all, those which are tacit and unconscious. Since we make them without knowing it, we are powerless to abandon them.

—Henri Poincaré

The slowing down and partial reversal of aging involves much more than knowledge of life extension techniques. Without the right attitude, you won't be able to implement that knowledge, no matter how much you know. You may be immobilized by a number of myths about aging that you believe without even realizing it. Find out in this chapter whether you are really mentally prepared to extend your life span and improve its quality. Don't let obsolete assumptions and misconceptions drive you prematurely to your grave.

It takes action on your part to extend your life span. Nothing is free. You have to decide that you want to extend your life, then you must study various techniques for doing so, and finally you actually have to apply one or more of these methods. Many difficulties may stand in the way of your accomplishing one or all of these steps. Probably the most significant roadblock to overcome is that of identifying the many misconceptions you have—conscious or unconscious—that cause you to doubt the validity of life extension and your ability to prolong your own life. These false beliefs may undermine your resolve and prevent you from acting.

Below is a list of prevalent misconceptions about life extension. You may find some of these statements ridiculous. But to the extent that any of them still exist in your mind, it will be more difficult for you to take advantage of your full potential for life extension. We were born into a society in which aging has always been taken for granted. Such a long-standing belief is not easy to discard. By reading and thinking about the following misconceptions, you may be able to liberate yourself from them:

MYTHS AND MISCONCEPTIONS ABOUT LIFE EXTENSION

• Nothing can be done about aging.

• If most doctors don't know about life extension therapy, it can't really be effective.

• If lots of other people don't know about it, it can't be true.

• If the government says it can't be done, it can't be done.

• Only natural processes, those that take place without human intervention, are beneficial to health and life span.

• The knowledge required to take actions to extend my own life span are too difficult for me to grasp.

• Methods for extending life span are so expensive that only the wealthy can afford them.

• Anti-aging therapies will only benefit me in some distant future; there are no immediate benefits.

• Life extension will be available for my grandchildren, but not for me.

Comment: If you really believe that, that is just what will happen.

• Life extension only means a longer period of doddering old age and suffering.

• If you just wait a little while, anti-aging drugs will be available at drugstores.

Comment: The Food and Drug Administration approves drugs only for the prevention, alleviation, or cure of disease. The FDA considers aging to be a natural development (which it is), not a disease. The FDA does not approve drugs for life extension, and it may take decades to change their approach. In addition, many of the anti-aging drugs and nutrient supplements can be purchased now in drugstores and health-food shops.

• If you want to live longer, you have to give up all your favorite habits completely, including smoking, drinking, and late-night partying, and restrict yourself to an unenjoyable low-calorie health-food regimen.

Comment: Reasonable decreases in fat intake, increases in moderate exercise, and sensible decreases in the use of excess salt, high-tar cigarettes, and excessive quantities of alcohol do not mean the end of all of our pleasures—only moderation. In later chapters, we will tell you ways to reduce the damage caused by your favorite vices so that moderation won't be nearly as bad as it sounds.

• Restoring youth with life extension techniques is not as good as "actually" being young.

Comment: Aging is a multifaceted process of biochemical degradation. If damage can be slowed, prevented, or repaired, you actually are younger than you would have otherwise been.

• Life extension is only for the old.

• Life extension is possible only if you start young.

You can be thoroughly familiar with the theories of aging and still be victimized unconsciously by beliefs such as these that prevent you from applying your knowledge to lengthening your own life span.

Prepare your mind for life extension. The beliefs of the subconscious have a tremendous effect upon what we are able to do with our lives. The slowing, prevention, and partial reversal of aging is a new phenomenon, one that we are not prepared for by the general culture around us. The following ideas may help you to alter your own attitudes toward life extension.

SOME FACTS ABOUT LIFE EXTENSION

• The general population does not know the true nature of aging, which is usually considered a single, time-related process. Actually, aging refers to a naturally occurring progressive deterioration of various biochemical and cellular functions.

There are several aging mechanisms that attack different functions of the body at different rates, leading to impaired health and a decreased probability of surviving as the years progress.

• The activities of the general population are not good indications of when and how you can extend your life and at what cost.

• An increased risk with age of degenerative diseases like cancer and heart disease for the general population does not have to mean that *you* are at risk for these conditions. You can lower your risks greatly by appropriate actions, regardless of whether most other people do so.

• It is wise to take advantage of life extension techniques now rather than waiting for some indefinite time in the future—when everyone is using such methods. Such a time may come, but don't bet your life on it. When more effective techniques come along, you will be better able to take advantage of them if you have kept yourself in good condition. Life extension methods can improve health now, not just in the distant future.

• Life extension does not happen without serious effort. It would be nice if it were free, but natural aging processes occur whether we like it or not unless we do something about them. Reducing the damage of aging processes requires your purposeful action. You'll have to decide what you want to do and how to do it. This book will help you.

• Your desire for life extension does not imply an ability to choose between no life extension and immortality. There are different degrees of actions possible, and what you do depends upon your resources and values; for example, how much you wish to change your habits, and what you are willing to spend in time, effort, and money.

• You will not suddenly become immortal. At best, you will have to creep up on it, a step at a time, by inhibiting aging and the age-associated disorders of cancer and occlusive atherosclerosis. There is no final answer. You may never reach immortality, but you can live much longer and in far better health than you expected.

• Your present life expectancy is probably far from what you could achieve with your present resources and possible range of actions. Your approach to this optimum must be discovered by careful planning and investigation. You do not have automatic knowledge of this subject, and living the same life as that of the general populace will get you roughly the same life span.

• The Food and Drug Administration (FDA) does not approve drugs specifically for life extension, and the approval of a new drug for conventional anti-disease purposes takes eight to twelve years, on the average. The scientific information upon which the drugs have been based will generally be known many years before any practical applications may be offered in the American marketplace. See Part IV, Chapter 5, and Appendix E, on the FDA.

• Life extension does not begin by stopping all aging mechanisms at once; you start by slowing down one and then another, and so on.

• Anyone now attempting life extension is a pioneer. It will be many years before life extension intervention is a routine part of most people's lives. Before taking any life extension drugs, carefully read and reread our cautions. Remember that one description of a pioneer is a guy with an arrow in his back, so think before acting, and don't try to develop your own life extension program overnight. Life extension is a lifelong activity, so wade in prudently and gradually, rather than jumping in over your head.

2
It's a New Age

> "I mean," she [Alice] said, "that one can't help growing older."
>
> "*One* can't, perhaps," said Humpty Dumpty, "but *two* can. With proper assistance, you might have left off at seven."
>
> —Lewis Carroll, *Alice in Wonderland*

Although conceptions of aging differ among lay persons and even among scientists, we all know that aging accelerates as time progresses. But aging is more than just the passage of time. It is a number of different processes taking place in our bodies, the totality of which is what we mean by aging (lack of strength and endurance; loss of ability to resist disease, including cardiovascular disease and cancer; wrinkling and sagging of skin; loss of hair and teeth; and other familiar aging signs). Before we can do anything about aging, we have to know what we mean when we refer to "aging." The most important factor in solving a difficult problem is often defining exactly what problem you wish to solve. Here is what we mean by "aging" when we discuss how it is possible to slow and even partially reverse important aspects of the aging process.

A reasonable definition of aging is the increased likelihood of dying from almost any adverse situation; that is, a minor infection, uncomplicated surgery, etc. Aging is a progressive impairment of physiological functions that reduces the individual's chances of continued vitality and survival. But there is more to it than that. Aging means different things to different people, even to different scientists. To the very young, aging is something that will not happen for a long time. To the elderly, functional decrements are a way of life and accepted as a result of the passage of years. In the minds of most people, aging is a process associated with the clock. Time passes and we age and die. An English insurance actuary, Benjamin Gompertz, formulated in 1832 a simple mathematical rule describing the increasing probability of dying with time. The Gompertz law states that the probability of dying roughly doubles every eight years after puberty.

The rate of aging depends on the relationship between the destruction and repair of tissues, cells, and molecules within the body. As destruction and repair take place in the body even before birth, aging is a process occurring not only in the old but continuously throughout our lifetime. As time progresses, the repair/destruction ratio declines because older individuals are less able to repair the accumulated damage of the years and because the unrepaired damage promotes more damage. Physiological functions decline and we perceive that aging is proceeding. A good analogy is the way your car ages. When your car finally collapses, you cannot ascribe its demise to just a single factor. Many functions decline over the years and, even toward the end, the car may run well in easy circumstances (such as on a level road) but be hard pressed in a difficult one (such as climbing a steep hill). Eventually, a final load placed on the weakened car's system ends its useful life. The final stress may be one that, in youth, the car could have handled easily.

Aging increases in rate as time passes. This is graphically shown in Figure 1, depicting a survival curve as a function of time. Note that functions can degrade over a long period of time before survival is threatened. We are all familiar with the fact that some people at the age of sixty are not as healthy or as able to perform various physical tasks as other sixty-year-olds. Aging proceeds at different rates in different people.

The traditional Western attitude toward aging—to deny it as long as possible and then resign yourself to the old folk's home and the cemetery—was pretty sensible until recently. This attitude can now cost you many years of productive and healthy life. As a result of scientific life extension research, we

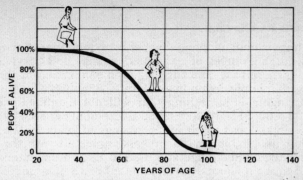

Figure 1. Aging curve for a human population comprised of American males. The curved line was calculated from the 1974 life expectancy compilations of the U.S. Public Health Service. Individuals who suffered accidental death or homicide were omitted from the calculation. (Females were excluded, so that sexual differences would not affect the profiling experiment in which this curve was used.)

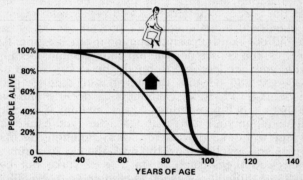

Figure 2. Example of a change in the human aging curve through improvements in nutrition and other living conditions, but with no change in intrinsic life span.

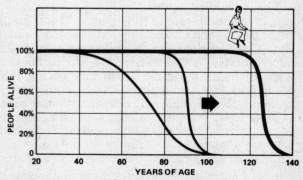

Figure 3. Example of a change in the human aging curve through improvements in nutrition and other living conditions and through an increase in intrinsic life span.

no longer have to accept passively the unpleasant consequences of aging. Scientific data exist demonstrating that some aspects of aging can be slowed down and even reversed. We now know that aging is not a single process, and that different systems age at different rates within the same individual. Often the limiting factor for survival is a single faulty system—as is the case when relatively young persons die of heart attacks. Although the average rate of physiological decline is about 1 percent per year, some body systems age faster than others. In subsequent chapters we will discuss what can be done to slow or reverse aging in particular systems.

Scientists, as well as the lay public, have differing views of the problems of aging. Most scientists specializing in gerontology study old people and their behavior. Only about 10 percent of American gerontologists funded by the government are engaged in research on biological aging processes. This proportion represents a fundamental division in this science. Funds used for social and psychiatric studies of old people cannot be used to study the biology of aging. At present, only a small percentage of public funds earmarked for "aging" are actually used for biological studies.

Scientists who are involved in gerontology can be further divided into groups designated as meliorists, incrementalists, and immortalists. The meliorists are social gerontologists who aim to make old age as comfortable and pleasant as possible. Incrementalists are biologists and clinicians who hope to eliminate the degenerative diseases of old age, thus expanding the healthy life span to its maximum natural genetic potential (around 110 years). This approach is sometimes called "squaring the curve," because if all these diseases were eliminated, people would tend to die suddenly at the end of their lives without a prolonged period of decline, indicated by the curve of survival in Figure 2. The immortalists are scientists who would like to increase healthy human life span beyond 110 years of age. The survival curve which reflects an increase in maximum human life span would look like Figure 3.

The authors of this book belong to both the incrementalist and immortalist categories of gerontologists. The multidimensional nature of aging—and the consequent difficulty in developing an overall picture of aging—has greatly hindered the development of the science of gerontology. You have to be able to define a goal in order to be able to pursue it rationally. To solve a difficult problem like aging, it is necessary to break the problem down into smaller parts. We do not have to solve all these smaller problems at once in order to benefit from research that has been achieved in some of them. As we shall see in later chapters, there are many practical ways now available that will enable you to slow or even partially reverse many of your aging processes.

3
Your Responsibility for Your Own Life Span

Planning is bringing the future into the present so that you can do something about it now.

> —Alan Lakein,
> *How to Get Control of Your Time and Your Life*

No one can make you do anything about the quality or quantity of your life span—except you. Your actions can be as simple as avoiding the negative effects on your life span of such activities as smoking and drinking alcohol in excess. Or you can study life extension literature and decide to use a broad spectrum of anti-aging and youth-promoting nutrients, drugs, and techniques. This book presents many different roads to life extension. The choice among them is definitely up to you.

Your life span is a "very personal matter." No one can make you practice life extension except yourself. Techniques for extending life exist. You have to decide how much life extension is worth to you and how much effort you are willing to put into it. Each person's decision will be based upon his or her own scale of values, and therefore no two people will have an identical evaluation of life extension.

You can ask an expert for a technical opinion of a complex scientific subject, but only you can answer the central question of how much the results are worth to you. Only you know yourself well enough to recognize your resources, interests, and ability to act. You will have to determine what aspects of life extension technology you want for your own life (of course, you are somewhat limited by the unavailability of some life extension drugs, which do not have FDA approval for this purpose). Whatever you choose to do about your life span, you will reap the benefits (and costs) of your own actions.

Taking responsibility for your own life span may mean cutting down on smoking or alcohol. Or it may mean increasing your vitamin C intake. It involves reading widely about life extension techniques and then actually using some of them. Responsibility means having the courage to act on your own judgment, even when others may not understand. Responsibility means seeking facts, not uncritically accepting other people's fallacious and wishful thinking. Responsibility means proceeding slowly and methodically while keeping both eyes open for danger. Responsibility means recognizing that no one can increase your life span for you, that you have to be willing to take actions on your own informed initiative, and with proper medical consultation.

You have taken the first step by purchasing this book. It does take courage to face the issue of personal aging and to explore the unfamiliar new technology of life extension. It is an extremely exciting personal adventure that we have been researching and living for more than a dozen years. Join us in this adventure. Live Long and Prosper!

4
Aging Isn't Beautiful

There are many virtues to growing old. [*long pause*] I am
just trying to think what they are.

— Somerset Maugham at the age of eighty

As much as we may wish otherwise, old age is an unpleasant
and unattractive affliction. Some people, it is true, have been
active and productive into very old age—among them Picasso,
George Bernard Shaw, Ludwig von Mises, Artur Rubinstein,
and Helena Rubinstein. But such people are exceptions. And
we don't think anybody will argue that they were as vigorous
in old age as in their youth. Here we take a hard look at the
basic reason why we ourselves have devoted so much of our
time and energy to the scientific investigation of aging: be-
cause old age without intervention really isn't beautiful. The
best that can be said for aging is that it is better than being
dead.

Most people believe that there is nothing they can do
about aging. Their strategy for facing this unpleasant prospect
is first, to deny their own decline into old age and, then, to
resign themselves to the progressive deterioration of mental
and physical capacities. Finally, as joy in life fades away, many
old people even welcome death. This tragic scenario need not
be exactly like this for you, if you take action to change it.

We must face the facts of aging in the absence of intervention. Your body's muscles become weak, your senses lose

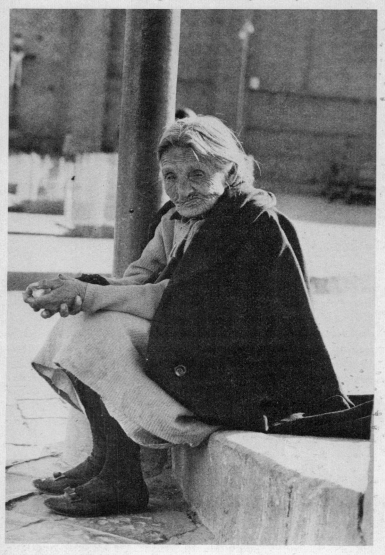

A decrepit elderly woman

acuity, your mental faculties lose clarity and slow down, your skin wrinkles and sags, and your desire for life may be lost. The sight of very old people struggling to walk or talk, their limbs trembling, is pathetic. Social consequences for the old, with their deteriorating minds and bodies, include rejection of them and disinterest among the younger and more vigorous. The very old are thought of as living on borrowed time and are not considered for future plans. Obviously the old do not have much of a future.

The philosophical among the old point out that there are some folks like Bertrand Russell who have been productive even into very old age. But Bertrand Russell himself points out that he was a mathematician early in life and then became a philosopher. Because of aging, he explained, he could no longer handle the complexities of mathematics and so switched to the less intellectually rigorous (to him) occupation of philosopher.

We are indeed fortunate to live in a time when the traditional horror story of old age is not necessarily inevitable. The practice of life extension requires effort, but with the technology that has been demonstrated in some laboratories, scientists have succeeded in doubling the life span of various animal species. Evidence shows that the aging mechanisms acting in humans are basically like those in other animals. With the help of this book, you can start planning now for your future of a longer life span and a greatly extended period of youth. For you, "old" age may be young and beautiful.

5
The Evolution of Aging

We have to deal with Man as a product of Evolution; with
Society as a product of Evolution; and with moral
phenomena as products of Evolution.

—Herbert Spencer, *Principles of Ethics*

*We did not always live as long as we do now. A few million
years ago, human forebears lived only to about half our current life span. Modern chimpanzees, very close relatives to
man, live only 45 or 50 years, about half man's present maximum life span. How did we develop into such a long-lived
creature? How can we use this knowledge to live even longer?*

In this chapter, we tell you about some current thinking
on the role evolution plays in the determination of a species'
maximum natural life span. We are looking for evolutionary
reasons why animal species live to a particular life span. Why
not more—or less?

Evolution is the sum of the genetic changes that occur
over time as species adapt to their changing environments.
The animals best adapted to an environment tend to be more
successful than their competitors in producing offspring,
eventually displacing those competitors. Evolution is concerned with the stuff of heredity, the genes, which carry the
DNA, the genetic blueprints. A gene is successful, in evolutionary terms, if it increases the number of existing copies of
itself.

People concerned about the limited life span of auto-
mobiles sometimes refer to "planned obsolescence" without

realizing that extending automobile life span is costly. In fact, the goal of maximizing auto life span is different from the goal of producing the most cost-effective auto (the most transportation service per dollar). A Rolls-Royce lasts far longer than a Volkswagen bug, but its cost per mile is far higher than that of the bug, too. To engineer self-repair capabilities and to use long-lived components is generally more expensive than to use shorter-lived, disposable units. This is why deep space probes such as Viking, Pioneer, and Voyager are so astronomically expensive. In a similar fashion, biological systems do not feature perfect repair mechanisms. They must have repair systems adequate to ensure survival to adulthood, reproduction, and, in higher animals, the rearing of young to adulthood at a rate at least equal to the death rate, or the species will quickly die out under natural conditions. Complex repair mechanisms able to preserve human life for hundreds of years would (we presume) be a less cost-effective means of making gene copies than our present limited life span. Scientist Thomas Kirkwood looks at it this way: The body is a disposable package carrying the genes. The package is "designed" (evolves) to facilitate the genes' making copies of themselves. A short-lived disposable package is a more efficient use of scarce resources for gene reproduction than a longer-lived package. The interests of the package (you, the individual carrying the genes) can be quite different from the interests of the genes, which is to make copies of themselves. Birth control is an explicit recognition of this fact. Another example: The temperatures yielding the longest life spans in fruit flies and nematodes (roundworms) are not the same as the temperatures resulting in the optimal production of offspring (gene copies). The temperature yielding the maximum life span gives about half the number of viable offspring as the optimum reproductive temperature. Here is another case of the "selfish gene" in action; what is best for making a lot of gene copies (offspring) is not necessarily best for the individual. See *The Selfish Gene* by Richard Dawkins (Oxford University Press, 1976) for a fascinating discussion of this type of conflict.

Dr. Gerald P. Hirsch, a mathematical biologist, has shown, for a species reproducing to the end of its life span—as most do in the wild—that the life span increases to just that point where the reproductive advantage of additional life span is just offset by the reproduction disadvantage of the increased reproductive mutation level. In human females, menopause occurs after a period of steadily increasing probability of defective reproduction (the chances of a woman bearing a Down's Syndrome baby, for example, increases sharply after age thirty-five). The shutdown of reproduction in humans does not mean the end of life, however. Evolutionary factors which may have resulted in this extended life span include the long dependency period of human children and the survival value to human groups of at least a few older experienced persons.

A small number of genes may be responsible for the evolution of our increased life span. The genetic differences between man and chimpanzee, according to Dr. Richard Cutler, is only about 1 percent. Yet people live twice as long as chimps. This large life span difference is thought to have evolved in a relatively short period, only in the last few million years or so. Cutler calculated that an average increase in the maximum life span potential (MLS) of approximately two-fold occurred during the past 3 million years or so along the human evolutionary pathway (people live twice as long as the longest-lived other primates). Between 100,000 and 200,000 years ago, the aging rate was decreasing by about 12.5 percent and MLS increasing on the average by about ten years. (The MLS was predicted by using Sacher's formulation wherein maximum life span is correlated with brain weight and body weight. This formula gives an MLS for all living animal species accurate to about 25 percent.)

From known average rates of change in genetic and amino acid sequences over time, Cutler calculates that this increase in longevity has occurred with relatively few genetic changes. He concludes that both intelligence and longevity may be controlled by a few genes. As Cutler suggests, "An interesting prediction of these results is that the mutation rate, acting as a primary aging process, may have actually decreased during the evolution of the primates." Such a decrease could be due to the evolution of more effective DNA repair mechanisms. It is definitely true that longer-lived species have better DNA-repair mechanisms than shorter-lived species—it is perhaps ironic that this success should slow further natural evolution of human beings.

The evolutionary reason we live as long as we do now (up to 110 years or so) may very well be that there are no genetic pressures (no reproductive advantage to genes) to increase that life span. However, this limit can be overcome by learn-

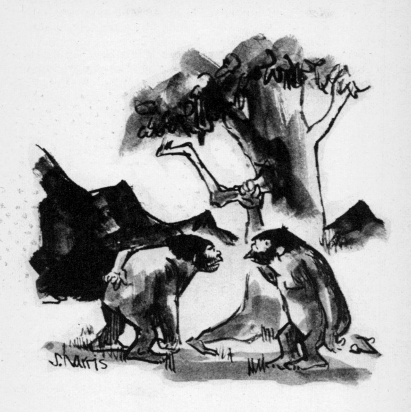

"Since we got up off all fours I've been having these low back pains."

ing which genes control for life span and how to intervene in this control system. The complete sequencing of human DNA will most likely be achieved in ten years or so, thus opening the door to research dealing with the direct manipulation of basic genetic clocks to increase life span.

Genetic engineering has already given laboratory mice a functioning gene which they were not born with. This work was performed on adult mice at UCLA by Dr. Martin J. Cline and his co-workers. Preliminary studies are already under way to use these techniques to correct genetic (inherited) metabolic defects in humans. These same techniques might be usable within a decade or two for adding more and better age-control genes to ourselves.

See "Turning Back Aging Clocks" (Part II, Chapter 10) for further discussion of life extension by intervention in aging clocks.

6
Alternate Pathways to a Longer Life Span

"Cheshire Puss," she [Alice] began . . . "would you tell me, please, which way I ought to walk from here?"
"That depends a good deal on where you want to get to," said the Cat.

—Lewis Carroll, *Alice in Wonderland*

There isn't just one aging process, and there isn't just one way to retard aging and promote youthfulness. Modern aging research has uncovered considerable information about how aging happens and about a number of different pathways of aging damage. We can intervene in many places along these pathways to slow or partially reverse aging. Unlike most health books, which claim a single cure for all ills, this book provides detailed instructions for an extraordinarily wide range of methods for partially controlling many of the ravages of age. Which of these different alternatives you choose for yourself depends on your goals and the resources (such as time and energy) that you wish to devote to achieving a longer and healthier life span.

As we have described, aging is a multidimensional process involving several different aging mechanisms. As a result, there are many effective and yet different ways to go about increasing your life span. Some techniques are as simple as avoiding some activities that shorten your life span, such as smoking, heavy drinking, or overeating to obesity. Others involve taking certain inexpensive nutrients, such as calcium pantothenate, that have been shown to have life-extending capabilities. (Large doses of calcium pantothenate—vitamin B-5—have extended the life span of mice by 20 percent.)

If you do not wish to alter your lifestyle or your habits, this need not preclude your taking effective steps to extend your life span. Many people enjoy drinking and will not be willing to stop doing so. However, it is possible to reduce the amount of damage done by the toxic compound acetalde-hyde, formed in the liver from the alcohol, by taking appro-priate dosages of vitamins C and B-1 and the amino acid cysteine (more about the effects of these nutrients in Part III, Chapter 12). If you do not want to stop eating fat-rich foods or decrease your intake of them (we ourselves eat lots of but-ter, whole milk, eggs, and meat), you can take vitamins C and E, niacin, and other nutrients to keep down the level of se-rum lipids (fats and oils in the bloodstream) and help to retard formation of harmful uncontrolled oxidation products of the lipids called organic peroxides. These organic peroxides are mutagens (causing damage to your cells' DNA, the blueprint for each cell's structure and activities) and also carcinogens (cancer-causing substances) and do other types of damage. (See Part II, Chapter 7 for more information on peroxide damage.)

The choice is yours. No one will be interested in using ev-ery possible available technique. What you choose to do will depend on the extent of your interest, knowledge, funds, and willingness to act. Some people are more conservative than others. They will obviously have different choices than less conservative individuals. There is no single "answer" that fits the needs and desires of everyone.

Although there are a good many alternative therapies that will probably result in life-span increases, we do not yet have the choice of entirely stopping aging or entirely revers-ing aging damage. Such an eventuality is not out of the realm of possibility (at least there seems to be no physical law which precludes it). What is required for an indefinite life span (death caused only by accidents, murder, and suicide) is that the life span be increased by at least one year for every year lived. This does not seem to be inherently impossible. In fact, we personally believe that our own life extension research ap-plications of the last twelve years have extended our life ex-pectancy by well over twelve years.

How do you decide between different ways of increasing life span? That depends on benefits versus costs, or, improved health now and probable increase in life span vs. risks and costs (including both physiological and financial). Only you can decide what level of risk you are willing to take—and what costs you are willing to pay—for what level of increased life span. Remember, too, that life extension does not just benefit you at the tail end of life. Techniques that increase life span improve the quality of life now as well. For example, you can look more youthful, reduce aches and pains, increase muscular strength, improve resistance to diseases and stress, and even increase sexual and mental performance, including memory and learning capabilities. It is also possible to alter and control your own moods with the appropriate nutrients.

Even if you are in your eighties, it is not too late to do something about your own aging processes. In laboratory experiments with old mice (the rough equivalent in age to eighty years for a human), their remaining life span was increased by 50 percent by giving them a drug that is readily available by prescription for human use (see Part III, Chapter 2). Another FDA-approved (for another purpose) prescription drug has reduced the chances of a second or subsequent fatal heart attack by 74 percent for patients who have already had a heart attack (see Part III, Chapter 18). Still another drug, commonly prescribed for elderly patients, has been found to restore the swimming capability of old rats (the rough equivalent of eighty years old) to that of the young-adult animals (see Part III, Chapter 2).

1
Benefits Versus Costs of Aging Intervention

Some people try to achieve immortality through their offspring or their works. I prefer to achieve immortality by not dying.

—Woody Allen

In order to decide intelligently between different possible life extension methods, you require knowledge of the benefits and the costs of a range of life extension choices. Benefit-versus-cost information is ultimately judged in the context of primary data, such as your own values and desires, the resources (time and money) you are willing to invest in this project, and the risks you are willing to take to achieve your goals. Nothing is risk-free, but it is possible to have reasonably good information on levels of risk versus levels of benefits for many life extension therapies. You can choose the levels of risk and benefit you are willing to accept.

In any decision-making process, there are two basic kinds of errors you can make: (1) You take action which does not yield the benefits you expected, and (2) You do not take action even though you would have benefited if you had acted. Depending upon your beliefs, you can make errors of commission (acting in error) or omission (not acting).

Generally, in an area of rapidly increasing knowledge (such as life extension technology), most people prefer to wait for other people (the least conservative ones) to be the guinea

What's the fairest way of allocating the nation's limited funds to reduce various risks to human life and health? A loaded question, to be sure.

One way of evaluating a given risk-reduction program is to compare estimated costs with expected benefits, both measured in dollars. But this kind of analysis is controversial. For one thing, it requires placing a price on life itself.

Here at the General Motors Research Laboratories, societal analysts have developed a method which avoids that problem completely. It focuses on longevity and rests on the simple logic that since all life inevitably ends, no amount of risk reduction can *save* lives . . . only *lengthen* them.

The method involves using the extensive data for all categories of mortality risks and determining the effect on longevity of each category independently. The results can be summarized for each risk by the equation: Average Years Of Longer Life = 0.2 x Annual Deaths Per Million Population.

This equation serves two purposes. First, it provides a perspective of days or years gained from risk-reduction programs. Second, combined with cost estimates, it helps rate the effectiveness of those programs

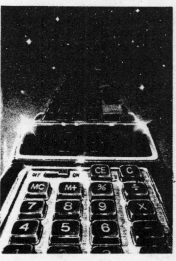

How to figure
the cost of living
...a longer life.

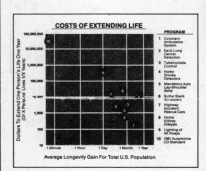

To illustrate its utility, we performed a study to compare the cost-effectiveness of several medical, environmental, and safety programs presently under serious consideration. The chart above shows the extreme variation in the costs of extending life by implementing those options.

Through such unbiased comparisons, policy-makers can obtain a clearer picture of which programs offer the greatest potential gain for a fixed budget and, thereby, have a better basis for decision.

 **General Motors
Research Laboratories**
Warren, Michigan 48090

How to figure the cost of living a longer life. This is an example of costs versus benefits for some conventional techniques for increasing average human life span. It is based on a paper prepared by Richard C. Schwing of General Motors Research Laboratories. Courtesy General Motors Research Laboratories.

pigs, wait for the reports of results, and then decide. This is possible in life extension therapies for evaluating the possible side effects of treatments, as well as seeing the more immediate benefits. But the actual amount of human life span increase cannot be known precisely in advance; it can only be roughly estimated based on the results of animal experiments and the effects of the therapies on known human aging mechanisms. The final figure for life extension benefits, the actual increase in life span, will not be known until people have attained these greatly advanced ages. That is why short-lived animals have been used in life extension experiments; we don't want to have to wait many decades for the end of the experiment.

Because of the inherent uncertainty of the actual number of years of increased human life span, people will probably tend to undervalue the benefits of life extension therapies. However, as we have discussed, life extension is not just a way of increasing numbers of years at the end of life but of improving the quality of life now. For example, by choosing to take large doses of vitamin E (a few hundred to 2,000 IU per day), you improve your immune system's ability to fight bacterial and viral infections and cancer. It isn't difficult to realize that something which can increase your life span must be improving your present physiological functions as well, either by increasing present capabilities or by decreasing the rate of their decline with time.

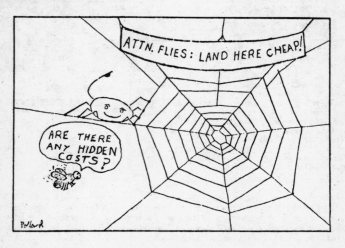

What are some specific benefits and costs to consider? Benefits include: (1) improved appearance, vitality, health, and abilities now, and (2) a possibly longer overall life span. In the following chapters, we'll show you how you can improve your resistance to infections, look younger, increase your muscular strength and stamina, and even be more intelligent and sexually capable with the use of proper nutrients (such as certain vitamins) and, in a few cases, of prescription drugs. Costs include (1) possible drug toxicities (individual variations must be considered), (2) expenses of materials involved, (3) time spent learning about life extension, (4) foregone opportunities (time and money spent on life extension can't be spent on your other values), (5) expenses for clinical laboratory tests, and (6) fees to your doctor for his or her consultations.

In subsequent chapters, we shall provide information on various life extension techniques including data on drug toxicities, availability and some sources of materials involved, improvements in function to watch and test for periodically, and research data on experiments in which the life spans of animals have been increased and on other experiments in which aging mechanisms in animals (also present in humans) have been slowed or reversed. Plug this information into your own benefits vs. costs accounting sheet.

8
Quality of Life Versus Quantity of Life

Longevity is only desirable if it increases the duration of youth, and not that of old age. The lengthening of the senescent period would be a calamity.

—Alexis Carrel, *Man the Unknown* (1935)

Nothing is too wonderful to be true.

—Michael Faraday

Many people fear that an extended life span would mean even more time spent in the decrepit, bedridden, barely alive tail end of life. But this fear is unrealistic. Life-extended animals spend more time in the youthful and healthy middle-aged parts of life, not in old age. Life extension techniques can improve both the quality and quantity of our lives.

Many people want to know why they should spend any time, effort, and money to extend their lives when they have no guarantee of ever reaching an extended life span. Even if your judgment in choosing life extension methods is perfect, you might get run over by a truck tomorrow! Our reply to this objection is that you have no guarantee of achieving an especially long life span, but your chances can be increased over your present chances by acting now, without excessive expense. In addition, as we have mentioned before, life extension techniques will improve the quality of your present life as well as the quality and quantity of your life in the future. Perhaps you will survive that serious truck accident if you are taking megadoses of vitamin C (ten grams a day, for example).

Laboratory experiments have shown that anesthetized guinea pigs, given an injection of at least 100 milligrams of vitamin C per kilogram (2.2 pounds) of body weight after receiving crushing injuries to their legs, always survived the injury even when all untreated guinea pigs (not given extra vitamin C after injury) died. Do you live in a smoggy area? When rats were exposed continuously to a toxic level of one part per million of ozone, vitamin E (dl-alpha-tocopherol acetate) added to the diets of one group of the rats, at a level of 100 milligrams E to each kilogram of food daily, extended their lives to an average of 2.3 times that of the untreated rats.

What about the effects of pollution and toxic chemicals in your food? Again, you can protect yourself from damage by using substances which may have life-extending capabilities. Vitamin C, for example, can block formation of carcinogenic (cancer-causing) nitrosamines formed from nitrites or nitrates and amines found in foods. In fact, many food manufacturers who use nitrites or nitrates as inhibitors of botulism and afla-toxin organisms in bacon and other meats have been also adding ascorbate (another name for vitamin C).

Are you under a great deal of stress? Pantothenic acid, or another form of this vitamin called calcium pantothenate, can greatly increase resistance to stress, in both humans and experimental animals. This same vitamin (B-5) has been found to increase mouse life span by 20 percent when fed in a quantity of 12 milligrams per kilogram of body weight per day (comparable to about one gram per day for an adult human).

You do not have to choose between quality and quantity of life. If you're smart, you can choose both!

9
Doubling Time for Knowledge

... high as a kite, if you want to
faster than light, if you want to
Speeding through the universe
thinking is the best way to travel.

—Mike Pinder, The Moody Blues,
"The Best Way to Travel"

*We have good reasons for believing that the near future holds
even more rapid progress in the prevention and reversal of
aging than we have experienced in the past decade. The
amount of information we have about aging and other biological sciences is doubling every five to ten years, meaning
that what we know now is only a small fraction (between
1/16 and 1/4) of what we will know by the year 2000! Each
year that you extend your life with present methods will increase your chances of receiving even greater benefits in the
future. If we can keep ourselves in good condition, we will
have the opportunity in the years to come to help ourselves
with ever more safe and effective methods.*

Our present techniques for life extension are limited. We
cannot entirely stop or entirely reverse aging processes. We
can significantly slow many aging mechanisms and can even
partially reverse some of them. But research into better understanding of aging and its control is needed for the complete elimination of aging.

Do we have any reasons to believe that such an ultimate
solution will ever be forthcoming? Yes, we do. The doubling

time for knowledge in biological sciences—that is, the amount of time it takes to roughly double the amount of information that we now have—is somewhere between five and ten years. This means that in ten years or less we will know twice as much as we know now about the biology of aging. In another ten years or so we'll know twice as much as we knew ten years from now, or about four times what we know now. And so on, as with compound interest. In a reasonably short period of time, the amount of knowledge available to life extension scientists will be staggering and will make today's knowledge seem minute in comparison. Considering the advances that have already been made in the control of aging mechanisms and in extending experimental animals' life spans, we have good reason to be optimistic.

It is not necessary to solve completely all aging systems problems at once. If we can increase our life expectancy by at least one year for every year we live, we will have an indefinite life span.

Many of the people who are doing productive research on biological aging are themselves personally interested in the elimination of aging. There are private foundations involved in supporting these researches whose directors are looking for answers to their own aging problems. Much private research will continue despite vagaries of government funding. (More on the government's role in aging research in Appendix E.) Such men and women, scientists and lay persons, have the most powerful motivations driving them—a thirst for knowledge, and a fight for their very lives. Much has been done already, but there is far more to come.

10
An Appointment with Death; or, Why Some People Prefer to Die

How ironic, that writers often refer to people being 'freed' by death!—when in fact death is the complete, the absolute absence of freedom, since both power and will are reduced to nil.

—R.C.W. Ettinger, *Man into Superman*

Do not go gentle into that good night,
Old age should burn and rave at close of day;
Rage, rage against the dying of the light.

—Dylan Thomas

Every now and then you may wonder, "Why isn't everybody interested in increasing the length and quality of life?" But of course not everybody is. And there are many reasons for this lack of interest. Here we've put together a little list of reasons why some people will not try to cancel their appointment with death—or will wait until it's too late.

Why people might want to die on schedule (the traditional three score and ten years):
1. They are in physical or mental pain.
2. They're bored or depressed.
3. They "believe" in death (it's part of a traditional worldview, such as "If it's natural, it must be good").
4. They aren't having any fun.
5. They're resigned because "nothing can be done about it."

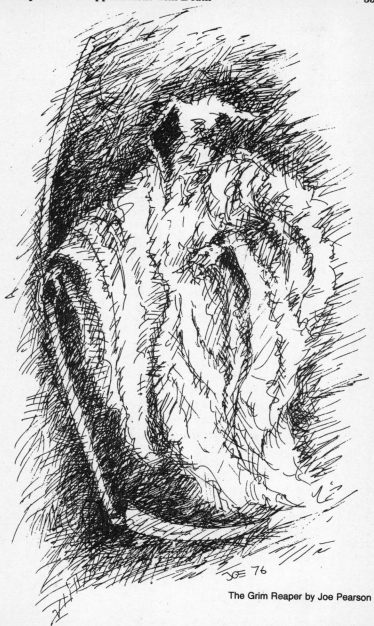

The Grim Reaper by Joe Pearson

6. Science frightens them, à la Frankenstein.

7. They believe in reincarnation or other "life after death."

8. They have a big investment in planning their lives by assuming death at a certain point.

9. They may find it less unpleasant to know approximately when they will die than not to know.

10. They may be crazy.

11. They wonder what it's like.

12. All their friends want to.

II
Common Fears About Life Extension

All men dream, but not equally. Those who dream by night in the dusty recesses of their minds wake in the day to find that it was vanity; but the dreamers of the day are dangerous men, for they may act their dreams with open eyes, to make it possible.

—T. E. Lawrence, *The Seven Pillars of Wisdom*

A greatly extended human life span will bring about many changes in our society. It is wise to be prepared for these changes by anticipating as many as we can. This chapter explores some of the possible negative consequences of life extension which people have expressed to us.

• If people lived a lot longer, we would have a severe population explosion. The birth rate would be much higher than the death rate and remain that way, owing to constantly improving life extension technology. This would lead to a food and energy shortage of terrible proportions.

There would be an increase in population only if people reproduced at a higher rate than the reduced death rate. At the present time in the United States, the birth rate is below that required for replacement. Our birth rate is now lower than during the Great Depression, and the rapid growth of vocational opportunities for women is apt to keep it this way. In addition, there is every reason to suppose that the future populations of this and other nations will not be limited only to the planet Earth. The practicability of large space colonies, capable of holding many billions of persons, has been demonstrated with calculations based on present principles of engineering. It seems likely that such colonies will be a reality within the next fifty years. Energy from thermonuclear fusion and space solar satellites holds the key to adequate power for a much larger population than lives now on earth, and these generators, too, are possible using near-term technological principles. Most important, people's lives will be extended in the productive part of life, not in the decrepit dependent part of life. Thus, most of the extended-life-span population will be increasing wealth, rather than merely consuming it. As with other food and energy crises throughout history, technological solutions can prevent disaster.

• Life extension will encourage selfishness.

Life extension encourages concern with oneself in much the same way as any type of self-improvement (memory and learning drugs, psychological self-exploration, or training for a new job). Selfishness is a necessary part of life. There is no guarantee that, now or in the future, individuals with an extended life span will show more wisdom in their actions than those living the traditional three score and ten years.

• Widespread life extension will result in a large population of old people who are set in their ways and hence become obstacles to new thinking. Our society will stagnate.

This scenario would be a serious problem if life extension prolonged mainly the old-age part of life. However, life extension methods described in this book extend the vigorous productive part of life and can improve mental, as well as physical, functions. Life extension causes people to live longer because their bodies and brains are better able to repair and prevent aging damage. When a person's ability to cope with this damage reaches a minimal point, death becomes very likely. In life extension experiments on laboratory animals, the animals with extended life spans do not have prolonged periods of decline. In fact, in some experiments the animals are vigorous and, to all outward appearances, youthful until just a few hours before death, when they succumb suddenly. In our society, there may be a problem in those organizations where seniority is very important, such as corporations, unions, philanthropic organizations, and governments, allowing officeholders to hold power for many decades before dying. In industry, if the old life-extended executives do not adapt to new situations, their companies will eventually go out of business because of competition from young, innovative companies. In government, which allows no competition, the problem may well be more serious. The seniors on Capitol Hill may uphold older thinking, in opposition to younger constituencies. Structural reforms may alleviate the difficulties (such as less power for seniority and more frequent turnover of elected congressmen). Biochemical reform to increase the imagination and creativity of congressional seniors may also be possible. Or government as we now know it may simply become less important as a source of leadership—the most likely alternative, in our opinion.

• What about the survival of social institutions in a society of long-lived people? Can marriage still be meaningful when people are living two or three times longer than at present? What about family structure? Will great-great-great-great-great-great-grandparents still be concerned about their descendants?

These are difficult questions to answer, involving entirely novel situations. We can't perform experiments to let us know what will happen to these human institutions. It seems reasonable to suppose that family and marriage will continue to exist in varied and modified forms because they are basic parts of our genetic heritage. We can count on the development of new social institutions to replace older ones that no longer function well. People will continue to care about one another and to have social groups. A long-lived individual will still seek friends and other social relationships. People will certainly continue to want offspring, though the timing of childbearing may be altered.

• Life extension will destroy society because the people who extend their lives will be opposed by other people who disapprove of life extension.

In many science-fiction stories, life extension techniques were generally available only to a few rich, politically powerful, or genetically fortunate individuals, thus creating envy in the rest of the population. But today's life extension technology is available to all who have the desire to make use of it and the willingness to acquire the necessary knowledge. Neither power nor riches nor genetic luck are necessary in an effective life extension plan. Government programs which transfer wealth from young to old—particularly Social Security—have a very real potential for creating serious class friction, and irresponsible politicians often thrive on worsening class polarization.

• Life will become boring.

If you're bored now, you'll probably be bored in the future. But you'll have more time to find out how to stop being bored. If you're not bored now, there is no reason to suppose that you'll be bored later, especially since the rates of social, scientific, and technological change will continue to accelerate.

• If a person lives long enough, he or she will use up all the brains's memory storage capacity and be unable to absorb any new experiences.

This is a problem that may occur with regularity in the declining years of an ordinary life span. Neurochemicals required for memory and data processing decline in concentration in the brain of aging individuals, making it more and more difficult for these people to acquire new memories and to learn. However, biochemical therapies now exist for some of these problems. Memory may be improved by a variety of nutrients and other chemicals, and there are also a variety of creativity-increasing substances that have been developed (but these are not yet widely available, due to the Food and Drug Administration regulations; see Part III, Chapter 2, "Revitalizing Your Brain Power").

12
Some Social Consequences of Life Extension

Death, be not proud, though some have called thee
Mighty and dreadful; for thou art not so. . . .
And Death shall be no more: Death,
thou shalt die!

—John Donne (1573–1631)

The consequences to ourselves and our society of greatly ex-
tended human life span are sure to be far reaching. An ex-
tended life span does not mean that we simply go on living
as we have except that we go on a lot longer. The quality of
our life changes as well as its length.

As with all rapid technological change, some people will
find the pace or the type of change not to their liking. Many
people do not want to live an indefinite life span. Some people may want to but lack the courage to try it and resent those
who do. Other people want the power to determine when
and by what means other people extend their lives. This includes power seekers within government and in the medical
profession. For example, the Food and Drug Administration
(FDA) and the Congress have been retarding some applications of life extension research by greatly hindering the introduction of new drugs into the marketplace. The FDA and the
FTC (Federal Trade Commission) have prevented vitamin,
nutrient, and pharmaceutical manufacturers from making scientifically valid health claims for their products. We surmise
that the government's concern about where they will get

funds to cover their welfare and funds-transfer programs for the aged underlies some of their reluctance to fund biological aging research. Dr. Alexander Leaf, former head of the President's Commission on Aging, has said that it would be irresponsible to spend resources on extending human life span until after funding is found to support the increased number of older people. As we mentioned before, only about 10 percent of the funds dispensed by the National Institute of Aging actually goes into basic research on biological aging. (And none of these funds are specifically aimed at extending human life span.) An extended human life span, if it happens "too fast," will create serious problems for the government's vast income-transfer schemes (from young to old) that include Social Security. For further information, see Appendix E. The Social Security system is in trouble, life extension or no life extension. Life extension didn't create Social Security's problems, but it may accelerate Social Security's collapse. If people live 20 percent longer, for example, they might collect Social Security for twenty-two years instead of the present average of about eight years. This could require Social Security taxes to increase from 14 percent of pre-tax income to 40 percent, severely reducing your take-home pay.

Such problems, however, will not happen overnight. At present, only a relatively small percentage of the population is seriously involved in personal life extension, perhaps because most people do not feel adequate to decide how to go about it. We hope to help remedy this situation.

How will your life change? The most important change you will notice as you become more confident of your ability to extend your life span is a realization of how much more time there is to do the things you want to do. You can afford to spend more time learning new skills or enjoying leisure activities because there is more time available. At any moment in your life, you can expect that more time remains than you would have had in the absence of intervention. The reproductive period will take up a smaller percentage of most people's extended lifetimes, thus leaving more of their lives available for other activities. People will have time available as never before to explore different ways to enjoy life.

The promise of increased time does not, of course, guarantee happiness. The use of the extra time is up to each person. Some will use it wisely, others won't. Because of the potential for a greatly increased life span, the planning that most people do today for their post-retirement life (assuming retirement at sixty-five and living for about an additional ten years) will be inadequate. With life extension, planning should consider the possibility of living at least twenty or thirty years beyond retirement at age sixty-five.

Society will have to deal with the existence of a new class of persons—the life extenders—and reconcile this with the non-life extenders who (as in many science-fiction stories) may oppose or resent extended life spans for others as well as for themselves.

13
How Do You Know Who's Right?

Don't ever confuse hard work with hard thinking.

—James Watson, Nobel laureate

One famous doctor says, "Eat mostly starches and little fats or protein." Another famous doctor claims, with equal vigor, "Eat mostly protein, little starches or fats." A third doctor argues against both of them by citing a research study indicating that Eskimos on a traditional diet high in saturated fats don't get cardiovascular disease. Who is right? And what should you eat?

In aging and nutrition, as in every area of life, we find many different views, even among scientists. To make sensible use of life-extending techniques, we must be able to sift the seeds of truth from the chaff. This takes us back to the basic science called epistemology, the study of the sources of knowledge. Using the techniques we discuss here, you'll be much better able to decide between many competing claims for theories of aging and products for rejuvenation. Epistemology can help you to tell who's right.

Epistemology is the study of the origins of knowledge; in other words, how you know what is right. With the many theories of health, nutrition, and aging being actively espoused today, it is easy to become confused and be unable to separate the useful from the absurd. Proper investigation of the sources of information is an essential step toward this goal.

The scientific method is an important and indispensable

element in scientific epistemology. This tool is a procedure that allows scientists to distinguish facts from hypotheses, actualities from wishes and hopes. The basic ideas of the scientific method are these:

• Science begins with observation and description. Wherever possible, observations are recorded using numerical (quantitative) data for description. It is important to be aware of biases and preconceptions, since no scientist is entirely free of them. In fact, it is not possible to be bias-free, because in order to know what to observe, it is necessary to begin with some ideas (a hypothesis) concerning the phenomena being observed.

• Isolation of particular observations of interest requires that some parts of a phenomenon are neglected, while others are focused upon. Some problems are so complex (such as aging) that they must be analyzed; i.e., separated into a number of parts. Upon detailed study of the various parts, it may be possible at some point to synthesize, or put together, a model that includes the various parts.

• After collecting data, a scientist creates a hypothesis or tentative model of the phenomenon. The basic business of science is to dispassionately test the hypothesis, not to "prove it." An ideal scientist would be just as happy to find no support for a hypothesis as to find support for it. In the first case a new hypothesis or a modification of the old one is needed. Hypothesis formation also occurs before and during data collection. As more data are collected, hypotheses can be modified to reflect reality more accurately. A powerful tool in science is known as Occam's Razor (first formulated by William of Occam in the fourteenth century). This rule of thumb states that if two hypotheses fit the facts and one requires fewer assumptions than the other, the former hypothesis is more likely to be a true description of events. This guide has been proven mathematically in information theory. The creation of hypotheses depends upon inductive reasoning, which is the process of drawing inferences about a class of observations based on a sample of data points.

• As E. Bright Wilson points out in *An Introduction to Scientific Research*, logic, or deductive reasoning, does not enter the picture until a hypothesis has been formulated. Various consequences of a hypothesis may be generated by logical thought processes. These logical consequences are then tested in the next step of the scientific method.

• Successful prediction by a hypothesis is considered strong evidence in support of its validity. Thus, tests for various logical consequences of a hypothesis are devised. For example, Einstein's general theory of relativity required that a ray of light passing a massive object (such as a star) would be bent by the gravitational field of that object. This prediction was not tested until years after the theory was first published, and its verification then provided strong support for the theory. Most scientists wouldn't claim that a hypothesis represents reality exactly, but is an approximation of it.

There are primary, secondary, and lay sources for information about life extension. Primary literature consists of scientific papers, which are usually published in refereed journals. Refereed journals are those which have a panel of scientists who review papers before publication to judge whether they have an adequate experimental design, whether the description of methods and materials is adequate for other scientists to replicate the experiment, and whether adequate data are presented to justify the conclusions reached. The refereed journals, because of this peer review, are sometimes reluctant to publish papers with unorthodox findings. Secondary sources of information are magazines that report on scientific papers published in primary journals or presented at scientific conferences. The excellent publications *Science News* and *Scientific American* are two good examples of secondary sources. In the main, lay sources of information are unsatisfactory, as in our experience, they may contain over 50 percent incorrect statements. Lay sources include newspapers and popular magazines. In our recommended publications list, in Appendix A, we do include some books and magazines written for the lay public. But we do *not* recommend the most popular nutrition magazines because of a high content of misinformation.

In a survey of several hundred college students conducted by Barry Singer and Victor A. Benassi, " . . . we were surprised to find that 'scientific media' was also listed as a source of occult beliefs—more frequently than popular media, personal experience, personal faith, or logical arguments. When the students were asked afterwards to list examples of the scientific media in question, however, not one mentioned even a single genuinely scientific source. Instead, *Reader's Digest* and the *National Enquirer* were occasionally cited as 'scientific media,' as were such films as *The Exorcist* and *Star Wars* (i.e. 'the Force'). Television 'documentaries' were also frequently mentioned, with the documentary 'Chariots of the Gods?' being the single most frequently cited 'scientific' source."

It has long been known that the expectations of people involved in an experiment can influence or even determine the results. For example, if patients in pain are given a sugar pill and told it is morphine, 40 percent of those receiving the sugar pill will experience relief or reduction of pain, at least temporarily. Because of such subjective reactions, well-designed human experiments are done in what is called a double-blind fashion. That is, the treatments and placebos (nonactive ersatz treatments like the sugar pills) are coded by one group of researchers, administered by another group (who don't know which are the "real" treatments and which are placebos), and the results are analyzed by a third group of researchers who do not know which subject received a placebo and which received the treatment being tested. In this way, an experimenter's and patient's desires and expectations are kept apart from actual drug performance. Experiments which are not done in the double-blind fashion are always subject to question because of human biases.

Dr. Andrew Weil has pointed out that the placebo effect can be a legitimate form of therapy. About 40 percent of the population is a strong placebo, responder (showing significant initial improvement with a placebo). Clinical patient's expectations of pain relief can provide some relief, at least temporarily. After a week of regular placebo medication, only about 10 percent of test subjects still show the positive placebo response.

A form of evidence often cited in lay health and nutrition magazines is what is called anecdotal evidence. Anecdotal evidence consists of individual case histories which are used to support a particular treatment. It is important to realize that these individual cases can never be proof of anything because of individual-to-individual biochemical variation. Usually such treatments are not administered double-blind, and therefore the results are strongly subject to biases. When people expect something to happen (like pain relief with a drug that is really a sugar pill), it often does. But this is not evidence for the efficacy of a treatment. On the basis of individual cases, you can find people claiming therapeutic benefits from almost any imaginable substance. In Appendix L, we provide some case

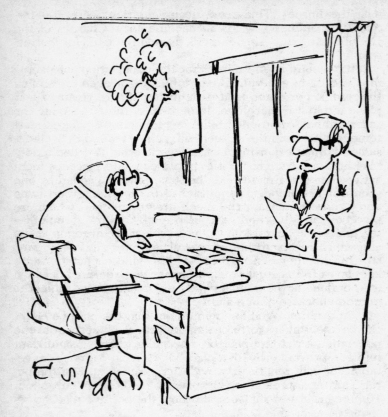

"It was more of a *triple*-blind' test. The patients didn't know which ones were getting the real drug, the doctors didn't know, and, I'm afraid nobody knew."

histories of people who have used some of the nutritional concepts presented in this book. We want you to be aware that, by themselves, these case histories do not prove that our nutritional thinking is correct. We present experimental evidence throughout the book that we believe supports our ideas. Consider the case histories as supplements to these experiments.

In scientifically sound studies, researchers allow for variations by using a device called controls. Controls are experimental subjects who are exposed to exactly the same conditions as the test subjects—those receiving treatment—except that they do not receive the treatment being tested. Ideally, this should be the only variable between control and experimental groups. Controls may or may not receive a placebo. Controls are compared to test subjects afterward to evaluate the results seen in the test subjects. So, if 40 percent of the test subjects receiving a new painkiller are relieved of their pain, and 40 percent of the controls receiving a placebo are also relieved of their pain, we know that it is very unlikely that the proposed painkiller is more effective than the placebo (inactive material). The next time you hear someone touting any form of therapy and citing a study in which x percent of the subjects received benefits, ask about the controls in the study. If none are mentioned, there probably weren't any, in which case it was a poorly designed study and should usually be ignored.

An important source of information about nutrition and life extension comes from popular "experts" we hear on radio and see on TV. Which ones should we be listening to? Many such nutrition "experts" are actually cult leaders, men and women who assume the position of guru or fount of knowledge in an organization and whose ambition is to "spread the word" (their own word, of course) and possibly to make a great deal of money. You can usually recognize cult leaders by these characteristics:

• They use emotion-laden words.
• They scorn all other methods employed in their area of specialty.
• They cite studies favorable to their beliefs which are either heavily anecdotal in nature, were not done double-blind, or had no controls.
• They tend to sound like evangelists, high on "pep talk" but low on technical evidence.
• They will not cooperate with attempts of outsiders to determine experimentally what are the effects of their treatments and what are their mechanisms of action. Such attempts are considered a threat to their monopoly on their particular intellectual "territory."
• They attempt to limit their clients' access to data about competitive or alternative methods. In a field as large as gerontology, no one person can know more than a small fraction of the available useful information. Cult leaders are not al-

ways entirely wrong, but it is reasonable to think that at best they are only partially correct.

· They have a bad case of the "not invented here" syndrome.

· They collect acolytes who preach "the word."

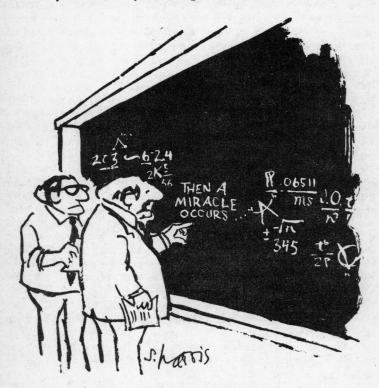

"I think you should be more explicit here in step two."

Among the examples of cultist "experts" are many health-food advocates who are heavily biased against anything "chemical," even though all food, vitamins, nutrients, and, in fact, all the substances of life are chemicals. The scientific selection of the many foods available in nature can enhance the intake of beneficial chemicals such as antioxidants (which retard chemical processes that lead to aging) and vitamins, but such choices must be based on science. An example of a non-cultist popular expert is Dr. Roger Williams, the discoverer of Vitamin B-5 and its life-span–extending effects.

Statistics is a factor to consider in the interpretation of experimental results because it is possible for scientists to honestly disagree on the basis of using different statistical models. In most instances, however, such sophisticated knowledge is not necessary for the type of information you are most likely to be seeking. Elementary statistics texts are numerous and the subject matter is not difficult to learn, if you wish to pursue it (see some recommended texts in Appendix K). A knowledge of statistics is definitely not necessary to the understanding of the material in this book. However, some familiarity with statistics is required to interpret original scientific papers.

When you shop for books on life extension and nutrition, the most important single indicator of a book's probable scientific validity is the bibliography. Take a good look at it before you buy. If the book contains references primarily from respected and reputable scientific journals, such as some of those listed in Appendix J, it is much more likely to be scientifically sound and of value to you than if references are primarily cited from unscientific sources such as popular lay nutrition magazines and newspapers, especially of the tabloid variety. Do not assume that if a book is written by a doctor or even a scientist that the data it contains are correct. Check out its bibliography and reference notes and see Appendix B, "How to Find Research References."

14
The Synthetic Versus Natural Controversy

You say nothing's right but natural things . . . you fool.
Poison oak is a natural plant—why don't you put some in
    your food?
I don't care if there's chemicals in it, as long as my lettuce
    is crisp!
Preservatives might just be preserving you,
I think that's something you missed!

        —"Eat Starch Mom," lyrics by Grace Slick

"Natural is best! Buy our 100 percent natural vitamins," the magazine advertisement says. But is it true that these vitamins are best? A controversy has been raging for years about the relative virtues of synthetic versus natural nutrients. Is natural vitamin C really better for you than synthetic C? Is a molecule of vitamin C produced by a natural biological factory like an orange or a bell pepper different from a molecule of vitamin C synthesized in a man-made chemical factory? This question has been answered by an experiment we report here. You may be surprised by the answer.

A heated debate has been going on for years in the lay nutrition literature over the issue of which is better, synthetic or natural. Many self-styled nutrition experts claim that "natural" vitamins and "natural" food and "natural" everything are better for your health than man-made (synthetic) vitamins, nutrients, and foods. For example, in the booklet "The Prevention System for Better Health," written in 1975 by J.I.

Rodale (founder of *Prevention* magazine) and Robert Rodale (the publisher of *Prevention*), we find (on page 8): "... the very idea of swallowing chemicals manufactured in a laboratory as dietary supplements is abhorrent. Such products may seem to the chemist to be identical twins to nature's own nutrients. But their biological activity is different from that of nature's products—the body's ability to absorb and use them is less than when getting its nutrition from natural food—and synthetic vitamins can produce side effects, sometimes dangerous ones, as is seldom or never the case with natural foods." To some degree, most popular nutrition publications share these myths.

A basic fact is that all foods, vitamins, and nutrients, and all the other substances of life, are chemicals. Though you wouldn't normally refer to common biological substances by their chemical names, some of them have extremely complex names and structures. For example, if you had scrambled eggs for breakfast, you ate (among other things) ovalbumin, conalbumin, ovomucoid, mucin, globulins, cysteine (an amino acid), lipovitellin, livetin, cholesterol, lecithin, lipids, butyric acid, acetic acid, lutein, zeaxanthin, phosphates, and carotene. (If you didn't know that these compounds were naturally found in a chicken's body, you might think they came from a chemical plant.) An example of a compound produced in your own body is the sodium salt of 2-pyrrolidone-5-carboxylic acid (Na-PCA), which is the primary natural moisturizer in your skin. By holding water in your skin, Na-PCA keeps it soft and supple. If your own body isn't making enough, you can add some externally, as Na-PCA is an ingredient in some premium moisturizing cosmetics; thus Na-PCA can be manufactured in the laboratory independently of the human body's capacity to produce it. It may be cheaper to make it in a tank than in your body (the body can then use the requisite starting materials for something else).

"A vitamin C is a vitamin C is a vitamin C." A synthetic (made by a chemical factory) molecule of vitamin C is exactly the same as a natural (made by a plant's biochemical factory) molecule of vitamin C. It is argued that there may be nutritional cofactors (some possibly unidentified) accompanying natural vitamins. It is true that there are known cofactors in natural vitamins, such as the bioflavonoids found with vitamin C. Bioflavonoids may be purchased separately from C, and if you wish to take significant quantities you'll have to buy bio-

NATURAL VITAMIN C   SYNTHETIC VITAMIN C

NATURAL VITAMIN B-5   SYNTHETIC VITAMIN B-5

flavonoid supplements because the bioflavonoid content of natural C extracts is low. As for unidentified nutritional factors, why assume that such substances in natural vitamin extracts must necessarily be beneficial? We now know that impurities in some natural vitamin extracts have undesirable properties. For example, some people are allergic to pollen impurities in natural C. There is no pollen in synthetic C. Vitamin E extracted from cold-pressed wheat germ oil often contains enough natural estrogens (female sex hormones) that, when this type of E is taken in high doses, it can cause testicular degeneration and loss of sex drive in some male animals and men. Megadoses of natural vitamin E of this type represents a vastly larger estrogen intake than that from eating beef raised on feed with DES (diethylstilbesterol) added to it. (A slice of natural whole-wheat bread contains more estrogens than a pound of DES-treated calves liver!) Yet you don't hear loud outcries against this type of natural vitamin E. Natural vitamin E that is produced by vacuum distillation does not contain these undesirable estrogens. However, it is now so pure that there can be no advantage from any accompanying unknown cofactors, since they have been removed. The choice between this type of natural E and synthetic E should be made strictly on the basis of price. Potatoes contain solanine, a natural poison. You probably eat enough solanine in a year to kill a horse if it ingested that amount all at once. Hence, megadoses of solanine containing natural potato extract should be avoided!

Just because vitamin-producing plants co-exist with us on the same planet doesn't mean that the plants make the vitamins for our sakes. They have their own uses for the vitamins they make. Vitamins E and C, for example, in many seeds serve as lipid and membrane antioxidants (prevent damage by uncontrolled reactions of oils and fats with oxygen). See Part II, Chapter 7 for more information on antioxidants. The more oxidized the seed's lipids and membranes, the less likely it is to germinate. And the estrogens in wheat are an evolutionary mechanism for limiting the reproduction of those animal species which eat wheat and the cereal grasses from which wheat was derived.

A wide variety of antioxidants are made by plants (many vitamins belong to this chemical class, including A, C, E, B-1, B-5 [pantothenate], B-6, and PABA). These antioxidants have chemical names as long and complex as those of synthetic antioxidants. They function similarly, too. Using a wide variety of metabolic tests, Monsanto's synthetic antioxidant ethoxyquin—which is not an exact copy of any known natural antioxidant—is able to replace dietary vitamin E in poultry (though not in people).

Synthetic vitamins are usually much less expensive than natural vitamins. If you are interested in taking large doses of certain vitamins and nutrients, you'll find the cost differential very significant. In one study on the biological availability of synthetic versus natural vitamin C, synthetic C was found to be slightly more biologically usable by the body than natural C, which has membrane-binding factors to hold it in position for use by the plant from which it is extracted. Before you can make use of the plant's vitamin C, you have to break down these structures binding the C.

Don't worry about the reduced bioavailability of the "natural" or "organic" vitamin C you may have been purchasing. The "natural" or "organic" vitamin C that you purchase in a health food store is really over 99 percent synthetic vitamin C. There is so little vitamin C in rose hips, acerola berries, and other "natural" sources that C extracted from plants would cost over $1,000 per kilogram to manufacture. So why pay a lot of extra money for a minute trace of C extracted from plants mixed with synthetic vitamin C?

A final word: There is nothing natural about taking five or ten grams of vitamin C a day, whether it's natural or synthetic. You couldn't possibly get that much C in a natural diet, even if you ate only fruit. Gorillas on a natural diet get only about three grams per day of vitamin C. In order to practice life extension, you have to free yourself from the myth that nature is always good. Sometimes it is good. And sometimes it just makes you grow old.

15
Prolonging Life in the Laboratory; or, Why Animal Experiments Are Relevant to Humans

The most beautiful thing we can experience is the
mysterious. It is the source of all true art and all science.
He to whom this emotion is a stranger, who can no longer
pause to wonder and stand rapt in awe, is as good as dead:
his eyes are closed.

—Albert Einstein

*Most biological experiments are done with animals other than
humans, including rats, mice, guinea pigs, and frogs. None of
these animal species is exactly like people. How can life extension data derived from animal studies be applied to humans?*

Animal studies can be considered relevant to people
when (1) the experiment affects a system in the animal that
is like a similar system in humans, and (2) the method of
bringing about these changes in the animal involve a biochemical pathway (a chain of chemical reactions) found in
both the animal and humans.

In order to make such sophisticated interpretations, a
certain amount of biochemical understanding of the physiological systems involved is required. That is the function of aging theories. They provide a framework within which data
can be interpreted. Sometimes the data cannot be fitted into
a pre-existing theoretical structure. Then scientists must decide whether there were experimental errors or whether the
theory should be modified or even abandoned.

It is not necessary for all aging mechanisms to be identi-

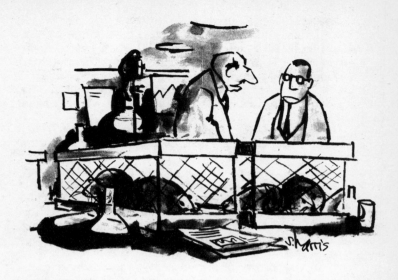

"You don't seem to understand, Prescott. We're not trying to cure diseases occurring *only* in guinea pigs."

fied and biochemically understood in order to get useful information from animal experiments. Experiments designed to study the aging immune system in rats may not reveal anything about aging caused by damage to other systems, but they can give us useful ideas about what happens in aging human immune systems. (Your immune system is made up of your white blood cells, antibodies, interferon, complement, and other large disease-fighting molecules, lymph nodes, spleen, and thymus gland. It recognizes disease-causing agents, such as viruses, bacteria, and cancer cells, as distinct from "you" and attacks them. Your immune system is your body's police force.)

There are two measures of life span commonly used in animal experiments. The *mean* life span is the average life span of the specified group of animals. The *maximum* life span is the longest life span achieved by any animal of the specified group. In humans, the maximum life span is about 110–120 years, while the mean life span is about 73 years (in technologically advanced areas). Increasing the maximum species life span, which involves inherited aging clocks (see Part II, Chapter 10, "Turning Back Aging Clocks"), has proved difficult. Although maximum life span has been increased in some animal studies with certain nutrients and prescription drugs, the mean life span has been far easier to increase by interfering with mechanisms of aging that involve random damage (see Part II, Chapter 1, "The Many Mechanisms of Aging").

In the interpretation of animal studies, we have to make allowances for known differences in metabolic biochemistry. For example, animals metabolize drugs at greatly varying rates. It may take a mouse 12 minutes to inactivate 50 percent of a drug dose, while people may take 12 hours to do so, or vice versa! The more information available in a particular area of metabolic studies concerning animal-human differences, the more understanding scientists will have of the significance of their experimental results and the more sure they can be of successful human applications.

Early in the history of gerontology—only a few decades ago—progress was very slow because scientists were seeking an overall definition of aging. We still do not have enough

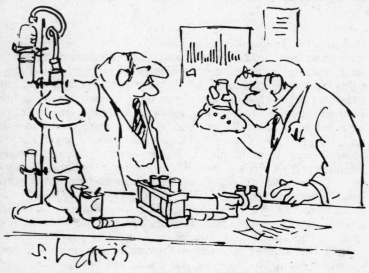

"It may very well bring about immortality, but it will take forever to test it."

knowledge to define aging completely as an overall process. However, various *aspects* of aging are rapidly coming to be fairly well understood, as, for example, the immune system. We can much more easily compare one system at a time of other animals to that of humans than the whole range of physiological aging processes between them.

The experimental animals used for life span studies are short-lived species, such as rats, mice, guinea pigs, and so on. They are all subject to the same aging mechanisms as humans, though not to the same degree. We could use primates like monkeys for life-span studies, but these animals live a fairly long time (see Appendix H, "How Long Do Humans and Animals Really Live?"). We don't want to have to wait for many years, perhaps decades, to find out the results of life extension methods. For one thing, such longitudinal experiments are very expensive. A life-span study using two-year-old rats cost $800 per rat per year as of a few years ago. Larger animals are far more expensive. It is reasonable to suppose that some methods that extend life span in rats or mice can extend human life span too, since biochemical studies have shown that the chemistry of aging is very similar in all species.

In Part II, we shall introduce you to some of the reasonable theories on mechanisms of aging now being tested and refined in both animal and human studies. These theories have already led to significant slowing of several aging processes and equally significant increases in life span with a markedly decreased incidence of cancer and cardiovascular disease. And we will show you how to apply this type of knowledge to your own life.

PART II
LIFE EXTENSION THEORY AND PRACTICE

I
The Blind Men and the Elephant; or, The Many Mechanisms of Aging

"The Parable of the Blind Men and the Elephant"

It was six men of Indostan
  To learning much inclined,
Who went to see the Elephant
  (Though all of them were blind),
That each by observation
  Might satisfy his mind.

The First approached the Elephant
  And, happening to fall
Against his broad and sturdy side,
  At once began to bawl:
"God bless me, but the Elephant
  Is very like a wall!"

The Second, feeling the tusk,
  Cried, "Ho! what have we here
So very round and smooth and sharp?
  To me 'tis very clear
This wonder of an Elephant
  Is very like a spear!"

The Third approached the animal
  And, happening to take
The squirming trunk within his hands,
  Thus boldly up he spake:
"I see," quoth he, "The Elephant
  Is very like a snake!"

The Fourth reached out an eager hand,
  And felt about the knee:
"What most the wondrous beast is like
  Is very plain," quoth he;

" 'Tis clear enough the Elephant
    Is very like a tree!"

The Fifth, who chanced to touch the ear,
    Said, "E'en the blindest man
Can tell what this resembles most;
    Deny the fact who can:
This marvel of an Elephant
    Is very like a fan!"

The Sixth no sooner had begun
    About the beast to grope
Than, seizing on the swinging tail
    That fell within his scope,
"I see," quoth he, "the Elephant
    Is very like a rope!"

And so these men of Indostan
    Disputed loud and long,
Each in his own opinion
    Exceeding stiff and strong.
Though each was partly in the right,
    They all were in the wrong!

                                    —John Godfrey Saxe

What can a bunch of blind men tell us about aging? In this chapter, some blind men show us that we can disagree about what we mean by aging if we refer to different aspects of aging. This is because aging comes about, not as a single process, but as a number of different processes. This is a great discovery of modern aging research, because it gives us the opportunity of conquering aging a bit at a time, rather than requiring that we understand everything at once.

People tend to think of aging as one degenerative process which develops over time. This is not at all the case. In the parable of the blind men and the elephant, all the blind men were right, yet none of their individual answers was a complete description of an elephant. There are at least seven mechanisms of aging known today which have been chemically characterized to some extent. Partially successful methods of slowing all of them have already been developed. None of these aging mechanisms entirely explains aging. Even all of them put together cannot yet entirely explain aging. Aging is a multidimensional process in which different repair and destruction mechanisms in the body are turned on and off at different times and different rates in a single individual. These changes may vary widely between individuals.

Although there are wide differences between people in aging rates, the maximum human life span (in the absence of effective intervention) seems to be around 110 or perhaps 120 years—no claims much beyond this have been proved. (See Appendix H for comments on alleged extreme longevity among the people of Vilcabamba, Ecuador; Hunza, Kashmir; and the Russian Caucasus.) Most biologists studying aging believe that there are internal clocks which turn on certain types of aging in animals, including humans. Examples of such clocks are male pattern baldness and female menopause. Scientists have begun to find ways of successfully intervening in some of these aging clocks. By resetting the proper clocks in the correct order, we can now prevent some of this programmed aging. To quote Bernard Strehler, an eminent gerontologist, "Aging and death do seem to be what Nature has planned for us. But what if we have other plans?" Other plans are what this book is all about!

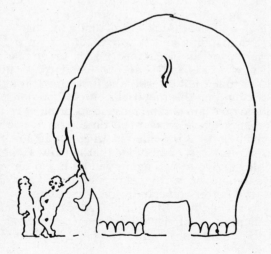

"I just got tired of guinea pigs, guinea pigs, guinea pigs."

Progress in control of aging was very slow in the early years of gerontological research, a few decades ago. Researchers did not understand *why* various procedures (such as dietary restriction in young rats) or substances (like RNA) prolonged animal life spans. The discoveries of several mechanisms of aging have vastly accelerated the rate of progress. Now it is possible to predict beforehand, with more success than earlier researchers could, materials that might prolong life span by intervening in a particular mechanism. It is the knowledge of the biochemical "map" of different biological aging mechanisms that allows scientists to have some success in predicting newer and better ways to control each aging mechanism. Mechanism by mechanism, aging is becoming defined and partially controllable, rather than mysterious and inevitable.

Several sections to follow explain how the major known mechanisms of aging are thought to work in your body and what types of aging damage occur as a result of each one. This information, while not *essential* to your taking actions to slow your own aging, will prepare you to make far better decisions in that regard. For example, if your family tends to get atherosclerosis, which is largely a result of free radical peroxidative (abnormal oxidation of fats) damage and immune failure (two major aging mechanisms), you'll want to take actions in particular against these mechanisms of aging.

You may find the discussions of aging mechanisms somewhat more demanding and slower reading than the preceding material. After all, biochemistry is an unfamiliar field for you, with new words and concepts. Don't try to memorize any of this or to learn it entirely the first time through. Don't make understanding this material a chore. You don't have to. There will be no exam and no judgments pronounced on you. You can spend as little or as much time on it as you wish (an auxiliary reading list is provided in an appendix for the really ambitious reader). Just remember that whatever choices you make for slowing your own aging will be based on your own knowledge, whatever your level of understanding. The more you know, the better you can decide what to do.

Before proceeding with more detailed discussions of each aging mechanism, we'll give a brief overview-introduction to the most important ones and to the basic biochemical structure of your body.

2
Overview of Some Theories of Aging

We cannot retard senescence or reverse its direction, unless we know the nature of the mechanisms which are the substratum of duration [basis of longevity].

—Alexis Carrel, *Man the Unknown*, 1935

In this chapter, we take an overall view of what we are up against in the way of aging mechanisms. There are two basic types of aging: One is caused by random damage brought about by a large variety of dangerous substances found both outside of our bodies and made in our bodies. The other type of damage is nature's "planned obsolescence," wherein we are subject to natural programs which eventually turn us off. Successful life extensions in experimental animals indicate that animals are subject to these same types of aging damage. So far, most of the life extension successes have involved interfering with the random damage aging, but progress is being made in understanding and intervening in "planned" aging, as well. In humans, random aging damage is usually the most important up to about 110 years of age, with programmed "planned obsolescence" becoming very important thereafter.

There are two basic types of aging events: (1) random (accident), and (2) planned, as in nature's "planned obsolescence." The planned events of aging involve aging clocks, which cause a programmed sequence of alterations and shut-

downs to various body systems, resulting in physiological decline as time passes. The reasons for these clock-directed
changes are not well understood, although promising theories
exist (see Part I, Chapter 5, "The Evolution of Aging," and
Part II, Chapter 10, "Turning Back Aging Clocks"). Well-
known examples of aging clocks include menopause and male
pattern baldness.

Random aging events result in a cumulative damage
which occurs in a sporadic fashion, such as damage caused by
ultraviolet light, X-rays, free radicals (chemically reactive entities produced in the body, particularly by the abnormal oxidation of fats, and also encountered in the environment),
aldehydes (a common class of often nasty compounds found
both inside and outside of the body), etc. The body has repair
mechanisms for damage caused by such entities to DNA (your
genetic master blueprint), cell membranes, and other structures. However, these repair systems are not perfect. The rate
of repair declines relative to the rate of damage, partly because of planned events (aging clocks) and partly because
damage is not perfectly repaired, leading to further damage,
etc. Since the rate of physiological decline with age is only
about 1 percent per year, on the average, a small improvement in the ratio of repair to damage can have a significant
impact on average species life span (the age most species
members live to) and, perhaps, on maximum species life span
(the longest life span reached by a member of a species). Here
is a simple hypothetical example: Suppose that one of your vital life support systems is randomly damaged at a rate of 10
percent per year, while your damage repair rate for that system is 9 percent per year. That system will degrade—age—
at 10 percent − 9 percent = 1 percent per year. Now suppose that you use life extension technologies which slow the
damage rate by only 1 part in 10 and speed up the repair by
only 1 part in 10. Your damage rate is now about 9 percent
per year, but your repair rate is now about 10 percent per
year. You are now repairing your damaged system by 1 percent per year faster than it is being damaged. Each year, that
vital life support system of yours will in some ways be 1 percent *better* instead of the normal 1 percent worse. Each year,
parts of your system become a bit younger rather than a bit
older! Note that this remarkable feat has been accomplished
by a very small decrease in the damage rate plus a very small
increase in the repair rate.

Experiments in animals have shown that it is possible to successfully intervene to reduce damage rates by interfering with the reactions of particular classes of damaging chemicals and to increase activity levels of protective and repair systems. It is even possible to alter the effects of some aging clocks, so that animals' life spans are extended.

The same aging mechanisms seem to be operating in all animals. The differences between animals' life spans are due to different relative contributions of all these aging mechanisms. Different species of animals have different levels of and types of protective mechanisms and different time sequences on their aging clocks. Understanding biochemical differences between long- and short-lived species is one way to find out what enables longer lived animals, such as man, to live such relatively long lives, and to improve our techniques for increasing our life span.

3
How Aging Kills

Old age must be resisted
and its deficiencies supplied.

—Cicero

We know that as we grow older, our chances of continued survival decline. How does aging kill us? The answers to this question lead directly to the big payoff—how to slow or partially reverse these deadly processes.

The accumulated result of the unrepaired or imperfectly repaired damage done by all the different aging mechanisms is what we call aging. The probability of dying doubles about every eight years after puberty (the Gompertz law). Although we know a fair amount about a number of aging mechanisms, we don't yet know how much each mechanism contributes to the final result: the individual aging rate of each person. Research is now being done by us and many others which we hope will be able to shed some light on this problem.

There are two basic classes of aging mechanisms, random damage and genetically programmed obsolescence. Most people die of random age-related damage, such as cancer escaping control by a deteriorating immune system or a coronary thrombosis from an arterial blood clot caused by inhibition of the formation of your natural clot-preventing hormone PGI_2 (also called prostacyclin) by organic peroxides produced by free radicals. (These things are explained in later chapters.) If these random damage events were eliminated or perfectly repaired, you could live a healthy life to the end of your genetically determined life span, probably around 110 to 120 years. At this time, it is thought that aging clocks, particularly those located in the brain, would rather suddenly shut off some of your vital systems. We know more about the causes and "cures" for random aging damage than for the programmed aging. Maximum possible life span seems to be determined by the programmed aging, whereas average life span is determined by random aging damage. Nevertheless, if we could remain healthy and active until 110 or 120 years of age, that would be a tremendous improvement over our present pattern of aging, which is dominated by random damage and progressive loss of functions.

There is some evidence that there are programmed aging clocks in the testes, ovaries, pituitary, and hypothalamus which measure accumulated random damage and are triggered when this damage reaches a critical level. Perhaps this is how antioxidants, which are effective against many random damage mechanisms, have been able to increase measurably the maximum life span of a few species. In any case, the time that you "buy" by reducing the rate of random damage is time which scientists are using to attack the problem of genetically programmed aging. Remember that the difference between the average human life span of 73 years and the maximum potential life span (limited by genetic programs) of 110 to 120 years is 40 years. Forty years ago, we did not know what DNA—the program blueprints—did or how it worked. Since knowledge in this area is doubling every 5 to 10 years, this potential for at least an extra 40 years gained from the control of random damage means a knowledge increase of 16 to 256 times over what we know now. Fortunately, when you are buying time, you don't have to buy it all at once.

A phenomenon characteristic of aging populations is the reduced speed or degree of the body's biochemical adaptation in response to changes in the environment. This problem has been extensively studied by Dr. Richard D. Adelman. An older animal's greatly increased risk of death may be largely explainable in terms of this particular physiological change due to aging. For example, following administration of glucose to two-month-old Sprague-Dawley rats after a 72-hour-fast there is an increase of activity of hepatic glucokinase (a sugar-processing liver enzyme) by several fold. The time required for aged rats (24 months old) to increase this enzyme's activity to the same level is three times as long.

Life is a state of dynamic equilibrium (movement and change combined with balance), rather like walking a tightrope. Your continued life requires that your body manufacture tens of thousands of chemicals in the right amounts, at the right places, and at appropriate times. Accumulated damage at the cellular level (regardless of cause) will interfere with this balancing act. Finally a stress comes along (an infection, a mutation causing cancer, or simply exertion from shoveling snow) that you could have handled easily in your youth—but now it pushes you too far from your living dynamic equilibrium, and you fall off the tightrope of life into your grave.

The response of enzyme systems in different tissues of several animal species to environmental stimuli have been studied by Adelman. He found that there are four basic types of responses (as depicted in the graphs):

1. The old animal is slower in altering its enzyme level, but eventually this reaches a young adult level.

2. The old animal increases its enzyme activity at the same rate as the young adult animal, but the old animal's enzyme level cannot reach the high final level of the young animal.

3. The old animal's enzyme activity responds more slowly *and* cannot reach the high level of the young adult.

4. The time course and level of activity of both old and young are very similar. (Only in this case has the enzyme system been little affected by aging.)

Enzyme activity levels depend on a large number of control systems. Delayed enzymatic adaptation could, for example, be due to impairment of regulation of enzyme synthesis. And this, in turn, could be due to several factors. One of the mechanisms of impaired liver enzyme adaptation during aging, as suggested by Adelman, is changes in availability and/or potency of one or more hormones involved. Adelman has found in old rats that seven slightly different versions of insulin were produced, only one of which had the pharmacological activity of the young rat insulin, but all of which could take up chemical sites normally occupied by the single correct insulin molecule. The common clinical laboratory hormone-measuring tests cannot distinguish between closely related but not equally functional molecules.

The production of slightly different versions of enzymes and hormones might also lead to autoimmune disease, since

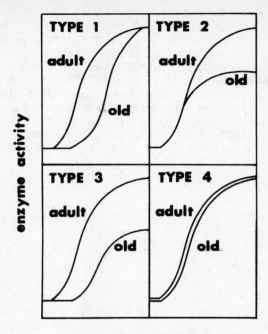

Patterns of enzyme adaptation during aging. The four general effects of aging on time course and magnitude of a hypothetical adaptive increase in enzyme activity are illustrated. For the sake of convenience, identical basal levels of activity are indicated for each age; changes in magnitude are presented as decreases; and changes in time course are presented as delays.

the immune system might identify some of these versions as foreign proteins and subsequently launch a self-destructive attack on the body's own cells which produce them. Dr. W. Donner Denckla thinks that part of the death genes' process is the production in older animals of "fake" versions of growth hormone and thyroid hormone (and perhaps others) by the pituitary gland. In his experiments, old rats (but not young rats) with their pituitaries removed show a greater physiological response to administered growth or thyroid hormones than when they still have their pituitary gland. This supports his notion that the old pituitary gland decreases the effectiveness of the mentioned hormones. (For more information on Dr.

Denckla's death-hormone theory, see Part II, Chapter 10, "Turning Back Aging Clocks.")

The degenerative diseases of aging (such as heart disease, cancer, stroke, and arthritis) reflect the fact that various systems in our bodies age at different rates, so that we may be in pretty good condition in general but be in serious trouble due to one particularly degraded system. All the body's systems are subject to aging damage via each of the different mechanisms of aging, but the resulting overall aging rates may vary markedly due to differences in structure, repair and protective capabilities, and exposure to sources of damage.

4
Molecules of Life and Life Extension: An Introduction to the Cast

. . . all diseases may by sure means be prevented or cured, not excepting that of old age, and our lives lengthened at pleasure even beyond the antediluvian standard.

—Benjamin Franklin, in a letter to English chemist Joseph Priestley

The same molecules that serve us well by keeping us alive and healthy can, if they fail to do their proper jobs, lead us to our graves. The story of these molecules is an important part of the story of our lives, how we age, and how we can slow and even partially reverse aging. It would take a complete book to provide an overall view of the major molecules of human biochemistry. Hence, in this short chapter, we provide only a brief mention of several particularly important classes of biochemicals which form the basis of our physiological structures and functions as living organisms. (See Appendix K for some general works on biochemistry for lay persons and for medical professionals.) The most important thing to remember from this chapter is that all life is made of chemical molecules, and that a chemical's structure, not its source, determines its function.

The purpose of this chapter is to lay some basic groundwork for what is to come, and to introduce you to some key chemicals that participate in your living and aging.

The master molecule of all bodily functions is DNA, deoxyribonucleic acid. This complex material contains the

blueprints that specify the way your body is built and repaired, your height, eye, hair, and skin color, blood and tissue
type, and susceptibilities to many diseases and aging mechanisms. Damage to DNA is now accepted as a major cause of
aging.

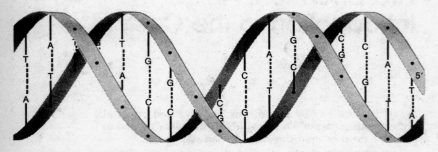

Double helix of DNA encodes the genetic information of all cellular organisms and
most viruses. (In some viruses the genetic material is RNA.) The genetic code is
written in the particular sequences of nitrogenous bases that connect the two strands
of the DNA molecule. The bases are of four kinds: adenine (*A*), thymine (*T*), guanine
(*G*), and cytosine (*C*). *A* always pairs with *T* and *G* always pairs with *C*. The hair of the
double helix consist of alternating subunits of phosphate and ribose, a five-carbon
sugar. From "A DNA Operator-Repressor System" by Tom Maniatis and Mark
Ptashne. Copyright © 1975 by Scientific American, Inc. All rights reserved.

The DNA blueprints specify the variety of ways your
body can interact with the environment. Man possesses a
wide degree of flexibility in these responses. RNA, ribonucleic
acid, is a closely related molecule made from a master plan
DNA for copying pieces of the DNA instructions which are
used to make proteins (enzymes and structural molecules and
polypeptide hormones). Some proteins (including enzymes)
are like little machines, often with moving parts. The different pieces of the protein molecule may swing into place to
bring other chemicals into proper position for metabolic reactions or serve as supporting structures like the steel framework of a building. Polypeptides are small proteins like
hormones (chemical messengers in the blood).

Proteins, in turn, are composed of amino acids. Some of
these are the essential amino acids, which means that we do
not have the chemical machinery in our bodies to manufacture them (some plants and animals can). We have to get a

supply of these essential amino acids from our environment in order to survive.

Other building materials supplied by our diet or by taking supplements include:

Carbohydrates are simple sugars, or sugars linked together to form starches, an important source of energy.

Lipids, fats and oils, are another source of energy and also of essential fatty acids. Fats differ from oils in that they are solid at body temperature, while oils are liquids at that temperature.

Vitamins are molecules required in relatively small amounts for normal metabolism. We can manufacture some of them in our bodies (except for persons with genetic defects); these are called the nonessential vitamins, because we do not need to get them in our diet. Of course, we may not be able to manufacture enough for maximum protection, as is the case with the B vitamin PABA. Other vitamins, such as C and A, are called essential and must be obtained from our environment for survival. There are two basic classes of vitamins, the water soluble and the fat soluble. Most vitamins are

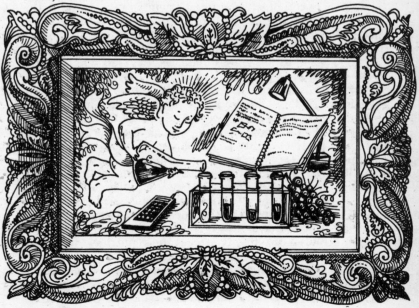

Casserine Toussaint

soluble in either the watery or the fatty tissues of our bodies, but not in both. Vitamins C and B are water soluble; vitamins A, E, D, and K are fat soluble. Both types of vitamins are necessary for health and long life.

We have different storage capacities for different vitamins. For example, if we received no vitamin C in our diet, we would die within a few months. With a diet containing no vitamin B-12, we would live years before dying of B-12 deficiency. Vitamin E can be stored in the body for only a few days to weeks, depending on intake, but it takes many years to die of vitamin E deficiency, since the damage caused by E deficiency is slow but progressive (the damage causes more damage) and cumulative.

Amino acids are the building blocks of proteins and peptides. There are about twenty-six common amino acids (eight of which we require for normal metabolism because we cannot synthesize these in our bodies).

Minerals are compounds containing metals, such as iron, copper, zinc, and selenium, which often function as parts of enzymes. For example, four atoms of selenium are part of every molecule of your protective anti-aging enzyme glutathione peroxidase (see the subject index for more about this), and zinc or manganese and copper are found in the protective anti-aging enzyme superoxide dismutase (see index).

ATP, adenosine triphosphate, is the substance which stores energy that is created when the body burns carbohydrates and fats in the citric acid cycle (see below). When energy is needed by the body (as, for example, in muscular contraction), ATP is broken down to release the stored energy. ATP is the universal energy molecule for your body in the same way that electricity is the universal energy source for a computer.

Although we have the capacity to manufacture certain nutrients, such as the vitamin PABA, it is still an advantage in some cases to take supplementary amounts. These materials cannot be manufactured in the body without expending raw materials and scarce bodily resources like enzymes. Sometimes it is more cost-effective to get these nutrients from supplements. For example, rats manufacture their own vitamin C, an important chemical in withstanding stress. Experiments have shown that giving the rats vitamin C supplements enables them to survive greater stresses than if they have to rely only on their own internally manufactured supplies. There is

Diagram of the citric acid (Krebs) cycle

no difference between a synthetic molecule of a vitamin or other nutrient and a natural molecule of the same chemical. One comes from a biological factory and the other from a glass and stainless steel factory, but the sources of the chemical's characteristics come from its structure, not from where it is made.

5
Aging and the Immune System

... just as the pigment of the hair is destroyed by phagocytes, so also the atrophy of other organs of the body, in old age, is very frequently due to the action of devouring cells which I have called macrophages.

—Elie Metchnikoff, *The Prolongation of Life* (1908)

Instead of preventing diseases only by protecting the individual against their agents, we must, by artificially increasing the efficiency of his adaptive functions, render each man capable of protecting himself.

—Alexis Carrel, *Man the Unknown* (1935)

Your immune system is what protects you from the enemies all around and within you: bacteria, viruses, and even cancer and atherosclerotic plaques. Without your immune system, you would have to live in a plastic bubble like some children do because the slightest exposure to bacteria or viruses would quickly lead to a deadly infection. As we age, our immune system's ability to protect us deteriorates seriously. In fact, most of us die because our immune system fails to protect us from cancer, atherosclerosis, or infectious disease. Few of us ever reach the maximum genetic potential life span of our species, 110 to 120 years. Using the right nutrients, we can improve the performance of our immune system whatever our age.

Microbes are everywhere!

If your doctor took a scraping from the inside of your mouth or from the skin covering your body and then looked at it under a powerful microscope, he would see dangerous microorganisms lurking among harmless ones. Every normal, healthy human being has deadly bacteria and viruses both inside and outside the body. So why aren't we all sick?

The reason you aren't always sick is that your body has a powerful self-defense force known as the immune system. The immune system is the police force that protects you from bacteria, viruses, and even from cancer cells and atherosclerotic plaque cells. The immune system is made up of the thymus gland (located behind your breastbone), several types of white blood cells (these identify, attack, kill, and eat deadly invaders, as well as make substances like antibodies), bone marrow (which makes some of these white blood cells), the spleen, lymph nodes and ducts, and a variety of protein and polypeptide chemical weapons such as antibodies, complement, and interferon.

After puberty, the thymus gland shrivels up and ceases to function at the high level of activity that it had in the youthful years before puberty. The thymus is very important in the function of the immune system. It "instructs" certain white blood cells (called T-cells) what to attack and when. Some of the T-cells, in turn, control other white cells that make certain antibodies. Without the thymus's instructions, the T-cells may fail to attack enemies like bacteria, viruses, and cancer cells, or they may even mistake some of your own cells for an enemy and attack you. This vital function of the thymus gland was not recognized until within the past fifteen years or so. Many doctors still do not know about this.

Scientists have discovered that it is possible to increase the size of the thymus gland and its functional capacity with several nutrients. These nutrients include vitamins A, C, E, the amino acid cysteine, and the minerals zinc and selenium. There are others. Vitamin E in doses of 200 I.U. (International Units) to 2,000 I.U. per kilogram (2.2 lbs.) of food fed to barnyard animals (chickens, turkeys, lambs) led to a greatly increased ability of the animals to survive inoculations of bacteria, viruses, and even live cancer cells. Vitamin A alone is able to double the size of the thymus gland. Vitamin C increases the activity of certain white blood cells, making them more vigorous in seeking out and killing undesirable invaders, and stimulates other cells to make more interferon, a powerful natural anti-viral and anti-cancer biochemical.

Arthritis is believed to be a disease stemming from an attack of our own T-cells on our joint membranes and fluids. The T-cells make deadly free radicals to use in attacking enemies like bacteria, viruses, and cancer cells. But when the T-cells make mistakes and attack our own cells, they use the damaging free radicals on us. In arthritis, the chemically reactive free radicals damage the joint membranes and lubricants, resulting in the pain and limited mobility of arthritis. Nutrients which improve immune system function can often provide dramatic relief of arthritis symptoms both by improving the ability of the T-cells to tell us from enemies and also by reacting with the free radicals directly to stop the chain reaction of damage (a free radical is a substance with an unpaired electron in an outer orbital; it has magnetic properties and unusually great and promiscuous chemical reactivity).

As we grow older, we become less and less able to handle all types of diseases. The diseases of age most likely to kill or disable us, such as atherosclerosis, cancer, arthritis, etc., can all be prevented by a well-functioning immune system. Scientists have been able to take aging rats (the equivalent of 80 years old for a human) and improve their immune system functions back to a young adult level. You can rejuvenate your own immune system to a certain extent with the proper nutritional supplements, available at any health food store and a rapidly growing number of drugstores.

If you were to maintain the physiological condition you have in very early adulthood, you might reach a life span of over 800 years. The immune system is very important in determining your physiological condition. Together, the components of your immune system patrol your body to watch for undesired invaders like bacteria and viruses or defective cells of your own body, such as cancer cells. These dangerous entities are detected, located, and killed by a competent immune system. It is because of immune system errors and failures that we get the flu or cancer or even atherosclerotic plaques (a type of tumor in which fats like cholesterol can penetrate and further damage artery walls). But if the immune system makes a mistake by identifying some of your own cells (which are not defective) as an enemy and attacking them, this error can be extremely serious, even fatal, and causes what is known as an autoimmune disease (your own

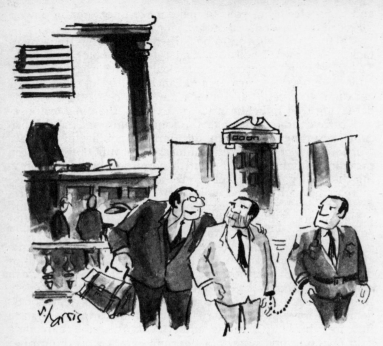

"Don't worry. Soon there'll be drugs that'll keep you alive far beyond 99 years and a day."

immune system attacks you). Examples are multiple sclerosis, rheumatic diseases such as arthritis, and, possibly, adult-onset diabetes. One of the earliest pioneers of aging research, Elie Metchnikoff, wrote in his book *The Prolongation of Life* (1908): ". . . the atrophy of . . . organs of the body, in old age, is very frequently due to the action of devouring cells which I have called macrophages." He also noticed that some of these macrophages attacked nerve cells in old age. Curiously, women are far more likely to contract autoimmune diseases than men are. This may be because the two X chromosomes that women have give them a more active immune system than men, who have only one X chromosome along with the Y chromosome that makes them male. The X chromosome carries plans for part of the immune system, but the much smaller Y chromosome does not.

What are the parts of your immune system? It consists of about a trillion (1,000,000,000,000) lymphocytes (white blood cells) and about 100 million trillion (100,000,000,000, 000,000,000) antibody molecules, other chemical weapons such as interferon, as well as the tissues of the bone marrow, the spleen, the thymus (a small organ located behind the breastbone), and lymph nodes.

Special white blood cells called T-cells (which make up about half the lymphocyte population and are manufactured in the thymus) kill hazardous bacteria, viruses, and cancer cells when they recognize them. The reason we become sick sometimes is that the T-cells sometimes fail to recognize these enemy cells. Or some of the T-cells may mistakenly attack your own cells, as in autoimmune disorders. Usually programmed by your T-cells, other lymphocytes called B-cells (made in the bone marrow) can produce antibody molecules to kill or disable dangerous invaders. Only B-cells make antibodies, usually under orders from the T-cells. Both B- and T-cells are necessary to a properly functioning immune system.

The B-cell antibody system can make errors too. Sometimes they fail to make antibodies to invaders in the body. They may receive faulty instructions from the T-cell system. And sometimes the B-cells make antibodies to parts of your own body—these antibodies are called autoantibodies and are found with much greater frequency in older animals, including people, than in the young. The presence of antibodies against their own neurons in the serum of old mice suggests a possible cause of neuronal degeneration in aging. These autoantibodies are not found in young mice. Such conditions as multiple sclerosis, myasthenia gravis, and arthritis may be due to autoantibodies attacking one's own body.

Medical men used to believe (and unfortunately many still do) that the thymus gland serves no important function and its functional decline in adulthood is harmless and normal. We now know that the thymus is essential to the proper function of the T-cell lymphocytes. The thymus "instructs" the T-cells how to mature, whether to be a detective, a helper, or a killer, and what to kill and what not to kill. The shrinking of the thymus in adulthood is part of immune system failure that accelerates as one ages. Old people's immune systems are far more likely to fail to kill bacteria, viruses, and cancer cells than younger people's. And older people's immune systems are far more likely to attack their own cells, that is, to develop an autoimmune disease like arthritis.

One of the most important factors leading to immune system decline is the greatly reduced rate of release of growth hormone by the brain as we age. This hormone, produced by the pituitary gland, begins to fall off in quantity after your teens. Since the thymus gland requires growth hormone to function properly, this decrease in growth hormone output is a severe blow to the immune system. Growth hormone is normally released in response to sleep, exercise, and fasting. In fact, the old wives' tale that you should starve a fever has a ring of truth because the growth hormone released as a result of fasting (but not starvation) stimulates the immune system! (For more on growth hormone, see the index.)

Can we improve the function of our immune system and slow its rate of aging? Yes, to some extent we can. In fact, it is now possible to slow and even partially reverse aging changes in the immune systems of aged animals. This has been done in animals *and in humans* using newly discovered techniques, the most important being nutrients like vitamins A, C, E, the minerals zinc and selenium, drugs like mercaptoethanol, hormones like thymosin, and complex techniques such as T-cell cloning. You can take advantage of some of the simpler techniques now; still others are in the experimental stage and not likely to be released by the FDA for wider-range use in the near future.

Here are examples of methods you can use to improve function of your own immune system, including supplementation of your diet with particular vitamins, minerals, and amino acids:

1. Vitamin E acetate was found by Dr. Cheryl F. Nockels of the University of Colorado to stimulate the immune system of a number of animals, including chickens, lambs, turkeys, and rats. The control animals (which did not receive a vitamin E mega-supplement) did receive in their diet what agricultural nutritionists consider to be adequate vitamin E (40 to 60 I.U. in each kilogram of food. This ordinary feed level is already several times as much E as most Americans get in their diet and 4 or 5 times the FDA Recommended Dietary Allowance for humans), and all were old enough to have adult immune capabilities. The experimental (but not the control!) animals were given in addition to the same diet as the controls a supplement of 200 to 2,000 I.U. of E in each kilogram of food. These dosages were effective in causing the treated animals' immune systems to respond much more strongly (a

tenfold increase in the performance of B-cells, and three to five times improvement in activity of T-cells) to the presence of bacteria, viruses, and cancer cells than the immune systems of the animals supplemented with E at lower levels.

2. Vitamin A can prevent the decrease in thymus weight and numbers of thymic lymphocytes that occur in injuries. Vitamin A has a stimulatory effect on the immune system and can protect animals from developing tumors in the presence of some chemical carcinogens (cancer-causing agents). Excess doses of vitamin A, however, can cause serious harm and even foster the development of some cancers.

3. Arginine and ornithine, both amino acids, were able to block formation of tumors in mice inoculated with MSV (a cancer-causing virus). A 1 percent arginine or ornithine supplement to mouse chow increased the animals' thymus weights and lymphocytes in both MSV and non-MSV injected mice and markedly extended survival time in the animals receiving the cancer virus inoculation.

4. Proteases (enzymes which split protein molecules), such as trypsin, bromelain (found in raw pineapple), and papain (found in papaya) stimulate formation of blast cells (an early developmental immune system cell) in rat thymocytes, a type of white blood cell derived from the thymus gland.

5. Zinc deficiency can cause severe thymus shrinkage, which can be reversed with zinc. The results of animal experiments suggest that many humans may be zinc deficient, that is, receive less than the optimum amount.

6. Some thiol compounds (these contain a sulfur-hydrogen link called a sulfhydryl bond) can greatly stimulate the immune system. However, some of these compounds in high doses can damage organs such as the kidneys. A road map through the many available chemicals and nutrients is necessary to select effective and yet relatively safe substances. This book provides this road map to a substantial extent. Mercaptoethanol is one thiol that has been used beneficially in old mice, restoring antibody response to the foreign test "invaders" (sheep red blood cells) to that of young adult mice. However, mercaptoethanol is not available to the public for this use, nor is enough known at this time to justify its long-term use in humans. Cysteine, another thiol compound, which is a nutrient and an amino acid, is also an effective immune system stimulant, available at some health food stores. Vitamin B-1 (thiamine) is a thiol as well, and although it has not been

tested in this regard, it is another possibly effective immune stimulant having low toxicity.

7. Selenium, a mineral, is an important trace element in immune system function. It has been found in experimental animals to act as an anti-carcinogen and anti-mutagen (can prevent DNA mutations—undesired alterations of your DNA master blueprint in the presence of some mutagenic agents). Selenium is an essential part of your enzyme called glutathione peroxidase, which is important in preventing damage by peroxides like those formed by the abnormal (free radical) oxidation of body fats and oils. Peroxidized fats are immune system suppressants, mutagens, carcinogens, cross-linkers; and compounds like hydrogen peroxide, which have a -O-O-H chemical group, are implicated as sources of damage that contribute to aging. Macrophages, a type of white blood cell, are inhibited in the presence of peroxidized fats from attacking, killing, and eating harmful bacteria and other enemies. Preventing or slowing the creation of peroxidized fats helps our immune system function more effectively.

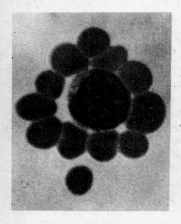

Mouse spleen cell forming a rosette with sheep red blood cells which are bound by the specific surface receptors. Cytocentrifuged preparation. This is a test of immune function; the more sheep red blood cells bound, the greater the immune response.

8. Vitamin C is a demonstrated immune stimulant, although its mechanisms of action are not well understood. We do know that Vitamin C increases the activity of certain white blood cells which patrol the body for invaders like bacteria, viruses, and cancer cells. Vitamin C also increases the quantity of interferon, a chemotherapeutic substance made in the lymphocytes (white cells) and fibroblasts (connective tissue

cells) and used against these invaders. Vitamin C in supplements of 10 grams per day has been reported to extend life spans of terminal cancer patients who had not undergone immune-suppressing chemotherapy by an average of over four times. Vitamin C has produced beneficial effects in the aortas of rabbits fed a high-cholesterol diet followed by a diet containing both high cholesterol and vitamin C. The dose used was 100 milligrams of vitamin C per kilogram of body weight of the rabbits. Note that rabbits, unlike humans, can manufacture their own vitamin C in their liver, yet additional vitamin C supplements were very useful in the very high-cholesterol diet.

Many of the materials used in these experiments are readily available and safe for use in humans at the proper dosage, especially vitamins E, A, and C, and the minerals zinc and selenium. The amino acids arginine, ornithine, and cysteine and the enzymes trypsin, bromelain, and papain may be less easy to find, but all are nutrients which can occasionally be found in health food stores.

Scientists are working on an even more extraordinary improvement in immune system functions. Dr. Takashi Makinodan was able to revitalize the immune functions of old mice to levels approaching those of young adult mice by injecting them with young mouse stem cells (the multi-purpose immune cells which can be matured into T-cells according to thymus gland instructions) and grafting young thymus tissues. It seems a future practical possibility that people could store some of their own antifreeze-protected stem cells and thymic tissue in liquid nitrogen while they are young, then utilize these materials later when their immune systems have declined, to restore immune capacities. Use of such frozen tissues and cells is not presently feasible for humans, however, and more research is needed. The hormone thymosin that biochemist Allan L. Goldstein extracted from thymus gland material (from calves in meat-packing plants) can improve the immune system in many sick or old animals and people. It has produced benefits in people suffering from a wide range of diseases resulting from immune incompetence, including cancer, systemic lupus erythematosus, primary immunodeficiency, leukemia, and allergy. Scientists have succeeded in synthesizing thymosin, and procedures for its manufacture have been developed. FDA restrictions are the final block to its wider use and availability.

How do you know that you have stimulated your own immune system and by how much? This is an extremely important question. After all, no one responds exactly like anyone else. You can find out by having *specific clinical laboratory tests* done on yourself before and after you use supplements for immune system stimulation. You can find out more about your immune system by using only one new supplement at a time (you'll know where the changes are coming from). However, the tests are well worth doing even if you take several new supplements at once.

There are several possible choices of tests, ranging in price and in the particular aspect of the immune system to be tested. (See "Clinical Laboratory Tests," Part V, Chapter 4.)

6
Cross-linked Molecules and Aging in Skin, Arteries, and Other Tissues

Empiricism may serve to accumulate facts, but it will never build science. The experimenter who does not know what he is looking for will not understand what he finds.

—Claude Bernard, 1813–1878

When your skin wrinkles, or arteries or bread harden, or rubber becomes brittle, or old Jell-O® stiffens, we are seeing examples of the same aging process, called cross-linking. As we age, many tissues are cross-linked, so that our proteins lose their flexibility and our biochemical blueprints (DNA and RNA) give faulty instructions to our cells. Cross-linking increases our risks of cancer and atherosclerosis and makes us grow stiff with age. Many everyday substances found naturally in our bodies, as well as in cigarette smoke, and formed in the body during alcohol use, and exposure of skin to sunlight, can cause undesirable cross-linking. By taking certain nutrients, we can reduce this unwanted cross-linking in our bodies as well as gradually undo some of the pathological cross-linking that has already taken place, thereby restoring some of our youthful flexibility.

What do tanned leather, old hard bread, brittle windshield wipers, wrinkled skin, cracked plastic lawn furniture, and hardened arteries have in common? They have all been cross-linked, a process in which some undesirable chemical

91

bonds interconnect molecules in the food, leather, rubber, skin, plastic, or arteries. The result is a loss of flexibility and an increased tendency to tear. Cross-linked arteries are hard, inflexible, and can no longer pulse normally as the blood is pumped by the heart. Such arteries contribute to high blood pressure and can even "blow out," resulting in internal bleeding (hemorrhage). Wrinkled skin is a reflection of cross-linking that happens in other body tissues, as well as that caused by skin's exposure to ultraviolet light in sunlight, a damage source not affecting internal body systems. The nutrient PABA (a B vitamin), particularly in the form of its esters, is a very effective sun block which helps protect the skin from cross-linking by exposure to ultraviolet light.

Cross-linking is the progressive formation of chemical bonds as bridges between large molecules such as proteins (your structural framework and metabolic machinery) and nucleic acids (your blueprints).

Some carefully controlled cross-linked bonds are necessary for life; however, undesirable cross-linking damage builds up over time. Many agents in our environment and others made in our bodies as part of normal metabolism can cause this cross-linking damage. Acetaldehyde is a chemical found in cigarette smoke and smog. It is also made in the liver from the alcohol people drink and also from the alcohol we all naturally make in our own bodies. Acetaldehyde is a potent cross-linker. Dr. Herbert Sprince and his co-workers discovered a combination of nutrients which provide 100 percent survival in rats given a dose of acetaldehyde large enough to kill 90 percent of unprotected rats. This combination is vitamin C, vitamin B-1, and the amino acid cysteine (found in eggs and occasionally at health food stores or drugstores).

A very common source of cross-linking damage is due to free radicals, chemically reactive entities created by radiation, from breakdown of rancid fats in the body, and as part of normal metabolism, as well as other sources.

Nucleic acids, DNA and RNA, are the master and working copies of your cell's blueprints (which determine how your cells are constructed and how they operate). These molecules can be cross-linked too, and when they are, they may not function properly, leading to abnormal cells. Cancer can even result. It is thought that damage to DNA is a principal cause of aging.

As you grow older, your body becomes stiffer, less elastic, and less agile. This is due to cross-linking at a molecular level. You become stiffer for the same reason that old rubber becomes brittle and stiff—your large structural molecules such as collagen (an important protein in connective tissues) are welded together by cross-links. This process starts early; babies are so flexible that they can suck their toes, but an Olympic gymnast ends her competitive career before the age of 20 due to progressive loss of flexibility. We sadly watched Mikhail Baryshnikov, the superb ballet dancer, as he talked on television about the end of his dancing career, which he will reach before the age of 35, he says, because of loss of flexibility. It is possible, using the right nutrients, to greatly slow the cross-linking process. We hope Misha will learn of this so that he can continue on being beautiful and flexible.

You can roughly measure the cross-linking in your skin and in the skin of your friends without any equipment at all. Place the wrist and hand palm down on a flat surface with the fingers stretched as widely as possible (Figure 1). Take a pinch of skin on the back of the hand between your thumb and forefinger and pull it up as far as you comfortably can. Hold the pinched skin for five seconds and suddenly release it. (See Figure 2). The skin will snap back very rapidly in a healthy teenager. In an 80-year-old, the pinched skin may still form a visible ridge five minutes later. (See Figures 3, 4, and 5, each taken at a slightly later moment. Figure 5 was taken roughly $\frac{1}{4}$ second after the pinched skin was released. A quick eye can see that our skin snaps back slightly slower than that of a teenager.) The faster the skin snaps back, the less the undesirable cross-linking. We are both 37 years old, but our skin snapback is roughly like that of someone in their early 20s. If you slow the rate of cross-linking damage, your tissues can slowly—over a period of years—eliminate a considerable amount of the damage previously done. It takes a long time, however, because structural tissues like collagen are replaced very slowly, and cross-linking slows this natural repair even further.

Many safe nutrients can slow cross-link formation, including cysteine (a sulfur-containing amino acid); vitamins A, B-1, B-5, B-6, C, E, and PABA; the minerals zinc and selenium; and others, but the proper doses must be used: Too high an intake of cysteine, A, or selenium can be harmful, whereas insufficient amounts of these substances will be ineffective.

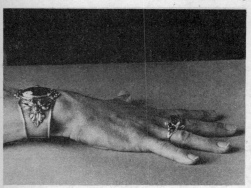

Figure 1.

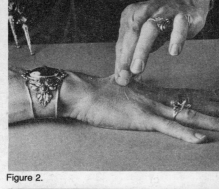

Figure 2.

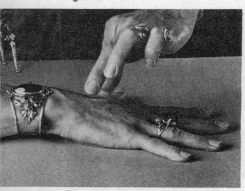

Figure 3

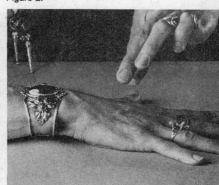

Figure 4

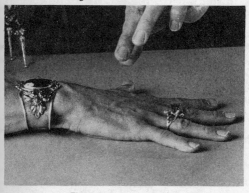

Figure 5.

The skin pinch snap-back test for cross-linking.

Proteins are complex molecules, made up of amino acids, which perform a wide variety of functions in the human body, from chemical reaction-controlling enzymes, to structural molecules like collagen, to necessary components in human memory. In order to function properly, proteins must assume a correct three-dimensional configuration. In their proper shape, some proteins act as little machines, some with moving parts, which serve to position other molecules for various metabolic reactions. Collagen is made of protein and is the major structural molecule of the body (comprising 30 percent of total body protein). Collagen provides the principal supporting tissue in most connective tissue, muscles, blood vessels, etc. As we age, there is a progressive increase in cross-linking of these important body constituents.

Some proteins contain sulfur, which is an important site for oxidation (losing an electron) and reduction (gaining an electron) reactions. As the body ages, the components of the body tend to become more oxidized. When the sulfur-hydrogen bonds (sulfhydryl) in proteins are oxidized, they can react with another sulfhydryl group in the same or another protein molecule to form a disulfide (sulfur to sulfur) bond. This is how rubber is vulcanized, turning soft latex into hard rubber combs. Scientists call these attachments cross-links. There are also oxygen- and nitrogen-based cross-links which behave in a similar manner. These bonds hold the proteins in rigid structural relation to each other. A certain number of these disulfide bonds are necessary to keep proteins in their proper shape and proper position with respect to each other. However, beyond this requirement, cross-links interfere with proper protein function and movement. Skin eventually becomes tough, hard, inelastic, brittle, and wrinkled. Collagen shrinks and loses flexibility. A good example of cross-linking is the tanning of soft cattle skin into hard, tough leather. Shakespeare wrote of tanning (a cross-link process) in *Hamlet* (Act V, Scene I):

HAMLET: "How long will a man lie i' the earth ere he rot?"

GRAVEDIGGER: "I' faith, if he be not rotten before he die—as we have many pocky corses now-a-days, that will scarce hold the laying in—he will last you some eight year or nine year: a tanner will last you nine year."

HAMLET: "Why he more than another?"

GRAVEDIGGER: "Why, sir, his hide is so tanned with his trade, that he will keep out water a great while; and your water is a sore decayer of your whoreson dead body."

The reason the tanner's body took longer to rot than others is that cross-linked proteins dissolve less easily and are more difficult for microorganisms to digest. In older animals, collagen is less soluble, has lower water absorption swelling capacity, and is digested more slowly by enzymes.

Cross-linking of arteries causes them to lose flexibility and become hard, contributing to susceptibility to cerebral blowouts (hemorrhages). This is exactly what happens to the radiator hoses in your car as they age, becoming progressively more cross-linked and brittle until they leak or burst.

When arterial walls have been hardened to a degree by excess cross-linking, there is a reduced ability of these arteries to pulsate with blood flow. As a result of this rigidity, the endothelium (inner lining) of the arteries is damaged and increases in permeability to the plasma (liquid part of blood). Plasma elements then diffuse into the arterial wall. This damage is greatest at the points of greatest stress—the bends and branch points of the arteries.

Many agents found in the body are cross-linkers. Ketones, found in the blood of diabetics, are potent cross-linkers. Many metal ions are cross-linkers, including cadmium, aluminum, copper, and titanium. Aldehydes (found in smog, cigarette smoke, and formed in the liver from alcohol), ultraviolet light, radiation, and free radicals are very potent cross-linkers. The actual chemical processes of forming the pathologic crosslinks generally require free radical intermediates. Ketones and aldehydes, for example, cross-link unsaturated fats via free radical reactions.

The loss of ability of aging tissue to hold bound water can be duplicated outside the body by adding cross-linking agents to a gel. Note that as jelled desserts, such as Jell-O®, become stiffer, they lose the ability to hold water (they "weep"). Such desserts would last longer if the water used in making them were treated so that metal ions are removed (as in soft water). Chelating agents, such as EDTA, have been effective in treating humans who have ingested heavy metals like lead, which can promote cross-linking reactions. The combination of EDTA and vitamin C has been found to be particularly effective in removing lead from the brain, where it does the most harm. Rotifers, multicellular microscopic organisms, lived longer in experiments where they were given regular brief immersions in solutions of one of the following chelating agents: sodium citrate (found in citrus fruits), sodium tartrate (found in wine), EDTA (a food additive), and EGTA. The treatments removed significant quantities of calcium, the levels of which increased throughout the life span of the animals. Chelation with EDTA has also been used in atherosclerotic patients with abnormally high plasma lipids. Some patients' lipid levels were reduced to a normal or near normal range by this treatment. Levels rose again after the discontinuation of EDTA therapy, but fell again when it was reinitiated. In atherosclerotic patients with normal plasma lipid levels, there was little or no plaque reduction with EDTA.

Skin is a visible organ which suffers cross-linking damage. However, unlike other tissues, skin is exposed to considerable ultraviolet light (UV) energy from sunlight. Ultraviolet light is a major cause of skin cross-linking. This type of damage can be prevented or retarded by staying out of sunlight or using sun-block preparations containing esters of PABA (p-amino-benzoic acid, a B vitamin). PABA and its esters absorb this UV energy, keeping it from injuring other skin cell components. Beta carotene (the yellow coloring matter in carrot juice, a nontoxic pro-vitamin A, converted to vitamin A on demand in the body) is also an effective protector of skin against UV damage. In fact, beta carotene is available as a prescription drug in this country for people who are especially sensitive to sunlight (photosensitive).

What do you do if you want a suntan but don't want UV damage to your skin? One solution we've found is to take canthaxanthin, available in Canada as a prescription drug, Orobronze®. It is a red pigment found in certain edible mushrooms, shellfish, and in flamingo feathers. Canthaxanthin is a carotenoid like beta carotene and is without harmful (toxic) effects. (Acute overdose results in gastrointestinal discomfort. Chronic overdose colors one orange or red, but this fades to a tan within one to three weeks.) It is used in some foods as a red coloring agent. Canthaxanthin, taken over a period of time, will yield a beautiful bronze color to the skin that looks like a suntan. In fact, it is being sold in Canadian drugstores now for just this purpose. Not only does it give a "tan" without UV, the canthaxanthin even provides protection to the skin against UV damage! Durk is using about 60 milligrams a day of the Canadian Orobronze® with splendid results. Although not yet approved for this use by the FDA (though it is approved as a food coloring agent), this approach to a "sun" tan is much safer than the use of either the real sun or a UV-A tanning booth. Since the FDA can do nothing to stop people from suntanning themselves in a conventional manner (causing unquestionable cross-linking skin damage as well as being the *principal* source of human skin cancer), their delay in the approval of canthaxanthin for this purpose can only injure the health of more Americans. Laws such as the FDA Kefauver Amendment of 1962 must be repealed, because while politically popular, the cost to good health is far greater than the benefits. This law attempted to eliminate all hazards of drug use by requiring greatly increased safety testing as well as proof of efficacy. The result has been far fewer drugs introduced in the American marketplace.

The nucleic acids DNA and RNA, which are the master and working copies of your blueprints respectively, are also subject to cross-linking. In older animals, cross-linked DNA is less easily degraded by heat—it becomes more stable. However, this increased stability in DNA molecules may interfere with decoding the genetic information and transcribing it to RNA, leading to errors or even failure of the cell to reproduce.

There are several methods which control the rate of cross-linking. In rats in which the pituitary has been removed from the brain, cross-links are greatly reduced. Limiting food intake in rats (which is capable of extending their life span) also resulted in a far lower rate of cross-linking. These methods may work because they slow down a biological death clock (programmed death) in the pituitary, a hypothesis formulated by Dr. W. Donner Denckla. The dietary restriction may slow the death clock by withholding nutrients necessary to run it. Removal of the pituitary would eliminate a death clock located there. These methods are, as yet, impractical as means of life extension in humans. A point made by Dr. Denckla, however, shows how it may be possible to accelerate what seems like "far-out" research into practical use; if an inhibitor can be found to block the releasing factor of this postulated "death hormone," the pituitary gland need not be removed.

As we mentioned earlier, some nutrients effective to a degree in slowing cross-linking include cysteine (a sulfur-containing amino acid, which helps maintain sulfur in proteins in the reduced state); vitamins A, B-1, B-5, B-6, C, E; the mineral selenium; and other antioxidants. Removal of calcium and heavy metals from collagen by chelating agents may be able to reverse some cross-linking.

Dr. Johan Bjorksten first formulated the cross-linking theory of aging (he was originally studying the process of tanning!). He discovered a microbial enzyme, micro-protease (made by a mutant strain of *Bacillus cereus*), which can de-tan skin, that is, reverse cross-links. This enzyme is still in the process of scientific development. Commercial development has been terminated, however, due to the extremely high cost in time and money (currently averaging about $56,000,000 and eight to twelve years) to obtain FDA approval.

Raw pineapple and raw papaya also contain large amounts of the proteolytic (protein-digesting) enzymes bromelain and papain respectively. When these foods are eaten fresh, significant quantities of these protein-dissolving de-cross-linking enzymes are found in the blood. While not as specific for cross-links as micro-protease, they are readily available right now in any supermarket. Some cross-linked and some non-cross-linked protein will be dissolved by these enzymes. The body will soon replace the non-cross-linked protein. Perhaps raw pineapple and papaya play a part in the relatively smooth, youthful skin enjoyed by many Polynesians in spite of long hours spent in the harsh tropical sun.

As with most things, you can go too far. When your mouth becomes sore and tender (especially at the corners of your lips), you are eating too much raw pineapple and papaya. Don't eat either of these foods if you have an ulcer—the speeded-up rate of protein digestion will slow healing. These raw foods can also be applied topically to the skin, thereby slowly dissolving the old highly cross-linked collagen protein so that it can be replaced with new young collagen (the new collagen made by even very old people is chemically identical to new collagen made by young people). You do have natural repair mechanisms which slowly replace cross-link damaged molecules. By using anti-cross-link nutrients, you can slow your rate of cross-link damage and give your overworked repair mechanisms a chance to catch up. This is a slow process, however, and requires plenty of patience. The time normally required to replace half the collagen in your body is several years. Don't expect to remove a half century of cross-linked tissue in a few months.

7
Our Subversive Free Radicals

... spontaneous mutations, cancer, and aging can be
looked upon as a result of continuous "internal radiation"
while these same processes produced by external radiation
are largely the result of an increment in the amount of
total "radiation" to which the organism is exposed.

—Dr. Denham Harman, originator of the free radical
theory of aging

Free radical pathology is as important an advance in
medicine as Pasteur's germ theory of disease.

—Dr. Harry Demopoulos

*Everyone knows that high-energy radiation is dangerous. It
can cause mutations, cancer, atherosclerosis, cross-linking
(loss of tissue elasticity), brain damage, immune system damage, etc. In fact, this is also a list of damage caused by aging.
The similarity is not coincidental. Nearly all high-energy radiation causes its damage by creating dangerous, highly reactive chemicals called free radicals. Unfortunately, we
cannot escape free radical damage by avoiding radiation, because chemical reactions in our bodies create free radicals too.
Some of these are normal and necessary, but others are pathologic and cause damage. In fact, the people downwind of the
Three Mile Island nuclear reactor accident were damaged*

more by their own natural biochemically produced free radicals than by free radicals from the escaping radiation. Ordinary air on a sunny day contains about 1,000,000,000 (one billion) hydroxyl free radicals (the most dangerous type of free radical) per quart of air. That's the bad news. The good news is that certain nutrients are very effective in destroying pathologic free radicals—in fact, that seems to be the only function of vitamin E. Here is how to control your own free radicals, thereby protecting yourself from both radiation (internal and external) and aging, at the same time!

The tiniest killer isn't a virus. It is a type of promiscuously reactive molecule or molecular fragment called a free radical. Since your life depends on very careful control of the chemical reactions within you, free radicals can be deadly.

Free radicals are chemically reactive molecules your body has to handle every day. Some free radicals are necessary participants in certain normal metabolic reactions. Here, your body supplies enzymes which control the free radicals so that they don't escape to do damage elsewhere. The enzymes superoxide dismutase (SOD) and glutathione peroxidase are two of these free radical control substances made in your body. Without these enzymes, you would quickly die. In fact, all air-breathing life on our planet must have such enzymes to survive.

High-energy radiation kills by generating free radicals in living organisms. In our bodies, the most important sources of free radicals which cause aging damage include the abnormal oxidation and breakdown of fats in your body, the breakdown of hydrogen peroxide produced in your body, and free radicals which escape from normal metabolism. They are almost everywhere.

Uncontrolled, these free radicals can damage proteins, fats, and nucleic acids (DNA and RNA, the master and working copies of your genetic blueprints) in your body. We have control systems for free radicals which include enzymes and also natural free radical scavengers like vitamins C and E. But these cannot control the free radicals perfectly. Some of them do escape and cause damage, which accumulates over the years. Mutations to your DNA caused by free radicals are a major cause of cancer. Free radicals can make blood clot abnormally in our arteries by destroying our body's ability to make PGI_2 (prostacyclin), a natural anti-clot hormone found in healthy arteries. Free radicals are also implicated in arthritis. Most of the brain damage caused by insufficient oxygen is due to free radicals. (The free radicals are partially controlled by oxygen but get out of control when oxygen is too low or too high.) Free radicals are also a major cause of cross-linking, which makes your tissues stiff and brittle, leading to loss of flexibility, emphysema of the lungs, and cerebral hemorrhage. Free radicals cause age pigment accumulation that slowly chokes brain cells to death and results in brownish "age spots" in your skin.

It is possible to prevent much of this damage by taking supplements of nutrients which provide protection against free radicals. Many of these nutrients have even extended the life spans of experimental animals. These anti-free-radical nutrients (also called antioxidants) include vitamins A, C, E, B-1, B-5, B-6, the amino acid cysteine (found in eggs and sometimes in health food stores), the triamino acid cysteine-containing compound glutathione, phenolic and catecholic amino acids like tyrosine and L-Dopa, catechols as found in bananas and potatoes, phenolics (compounds chemically similar to BHT) found in grapes and other fruits, the minerals zinc and selenium, bioflavonoids, and synthetic antioxidants such as BHT and BHA.

Oxygen is a poison, as well as a necessity, for most animals and plants. Organisms exposed to excessive oxygen can suffer severe damage or even die. Even in the course of normal metabolism involving ordinary amounts of oxygen, extremely promiscuous and reactive chemical compounds or atoms with unpaired electrons are sometimes created. Called free radicals, these are formed not only in normal metabolism, but also in the breakdown of peroxidized lipids (rancid fats), by radiation, and by white cells (free radicals generated by hydrogen peroxide are a major weapon they use to kill bacteria and viruses). Free radical damage plays a prominent role in the breakdown of plastics, rubber, paper, petroleum, food, and living tissues.

Hydroxyl radicals, the most potent oxidant known, can

attack any organic substance found in cells. They account for a large part of the damage done by radiation and are thought to be the principal damaging agent involved in arthritis. The enzyme xanthine oxidase catalyzes (stimulates) the production of both superoxide radicals and hydrogen peroxide, which react together to form hydroxyl radicals. These free radicals, along with crystals of uric acid and sodium hydrogen urate, cause the joint pain and tissue destruction of gout, both directly and by destabilizing the lysosomal membranes. Free radical reactions have been investigated as possible factors in the aging process since the late 1950s, when Dr. Denham Harman first formulated the free radical theory of aging.

Regarding the free radical theory, Dr. Harman says, ". . . spontaneous mutations, cancer, and aging can be looked upon as a result of continuous 'internal radiation,' while these same processes produced by external radiation are largely the result of an increment in the amount of total 'radiation' to which the organism is exposed." A great deal of evidence supports Dr. Harman's conception that free radical damage is a major factor causing aging as well as of many other disease conditions, such as cancer and cardiovascular disease. Free radicals have been measured in living organisms and increase in concentration with increasing metabolic rate. Changes due to free radicals include: (1) accumulative, undesirable oxidative alterations in collagen (the connective tissue which constitutes about 30 percent of body protein) and elastin (an elastic protein found, for example, in artery walls) and in genetic material, DNA and RNA, (2) breakdown of the large carbohydrate molecules that make up mucus (used as lubricant in your joints, for example) through oxidative degradation, (3) accumulation of age pigments such as lipofuscin and ceroid through oxidative polymerization (linking together) involving lipids (especially unsaturated fats) and proteins, (4) lipid membrane peroxidation, and (5) narrowing or closing of small arteries and capillaries due to toxic peroxidation products of serum, the formation of vessel wall irritants, and suppression of the synthesis of PGI_2 (prostacyclin, a natural hormone that helps prevent formation of abnormal blood clots).

Free radicals are intermediates in many normal and necessary metabolic reactions. Thus, all oxygen-using organisms have had to evolve defensive mechanisms against free radicals: The enzymes catalase and peroxidase break down hydrogen peroxide and other peroxides, superoxide dismutase (called SOD) controls the superoxide free radical, and glutathione peroxidase also controls peroxides. Antioxidants such as vitamins C, E, and the minerals zinc and selenium also help control free radicals. For example, each molecule of your enzyme glutathione peroxidase *must* contain four atoms of selenium. Protection is not perfect, however, and free radical damage proceeds throughout life. Occasionally, a genetic defect results in an individual missing part of his or her enzymatic free radical control system. One result may be a family of conditions called progeria, which is distinguished by extremely rapid aging, with victims dying at an early age (typically, before puberty), and showing many signs of old age: wrinkled and sagging skin, bald head, bent and frail body, advanced cardiovascular diseases, arthritis, etc. Dr. Armstrong found that he could control one type of progeria by giving a young male patient doses of the enzyme horseradish peroxidase, extracted from horseradish. This patient is now older than his brother was when he died (at 8) and shows none of the signs of old age, in spite of the progeria syndrome's appearance just before the start of therapy.

Superoxide radicals have been shown to degrade hyaluronate (the major lubricant in joint fluid), to degrade collagen (the most common protein in the body), to inactivate enzymes, to oxidize polyunsaturated fats, to damage DNA, and to kill viruses, bacteria, and mammalian cells.

Mammals can produce additional SOD (superoxide dismutase, an enzyme which destroys superoxide radicals) as a response to the presence of increased superoxide radicals. For example, rats can adapt to survive in an 85 percent oxygen atmosphere, which then allows them to survive in a 100 percent oxygen atmosphere, which they could not initially withstand. Increased levels of SOD are found in the lungs of these animals. Increased amounts of SOD and other protective antioxidant enzymes produced in the body in response to air pollutants may explain, at least in part, why cities with lots of air pollution (such as Birmingham, Alabama; Pittsburgh, Pennsylvania; Cleveland, Ohio; Detroit, Michigan; Los Angeles, California; and Newark, New Jersey) do not have higher cancer rates (adjusted for differences in population age distribution) than cities with relatively clean air (such as San Francisco, California).

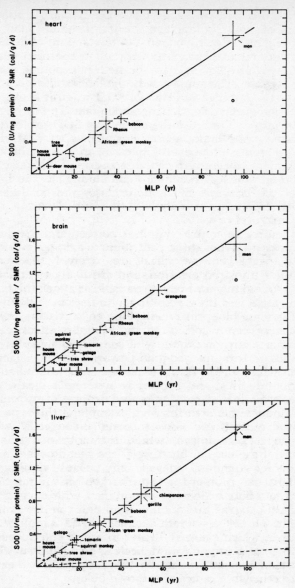

MLP is Maximum Lifespan Potential

In a study by the gerontologist Dr. Richard Cutler, the life spans of many mammalian species, including man, were found to be directly proportional to the amount of SOD they contain and inversely proportional to their specific metabolic rate (the number of calories burned per pound of body weight per day). The animals with the longest life spans, such as man, have the highest levels of SOD when it is expressed as a function of the oxidative metabolic rate. The three charts on the prior page indicate the amount of SOD protection in three tissue types (brain, heart, liver) versus MLP (Maximum Lifespan Potential) for several mammalian species, including man. There is a bacterium called radiodurans which actually thrives inside nuclear reactors! Radiodurans has the highest levels of the enzymes SOD, peroxidase, and catalase ever measured. It almost certainly has other antioxidant (anti-free radical) enzymes as well.

Of course, no control system is perfect, and the damage free radicals do is thought to contribute to aging. How do they do this damage? The free radicals are extremely reactive, owing to their unpaired electron, and are likely to attack any molecule found in your body. Free radicals attack the genetic material, DNA and RNA, resulting in mutations and other defects. If genetic blueprints controlling cell divisions are damaged, cancer can result. Free radicals also attack cellular membranes, damaging them with sometimes drastic results. Lysosomes, for example, contain powerful enzymes (acid hydrolases) which break down tissue constituents. When lysosomal membranes are ruptured by free radicals, these enzymes are released, causing severe damage to surrounding tissues. Rheumatoid arthritis is an example of this type of attack. Free radicals can also cause red blood cells to burst (hemolyze) by breaking their cellular membranes. The measurement of the ease of bursting of red blood cells is a common assay for vitamin E bioavailability because vitamin E, an antioxidant, can protect the red blood cell membranes. Peroxidized fats (fats which have combined with oxygen via a free radical catalyzed reaction, a condition you have smelled in rancidity) break down into malonaldehyde, a mutagen and cross-linker, which oxidizes further to create more free radicals. The great ability of free radicals to damage tissues is due to the chain reactions in which they engage. Free radicals generate other free radicals, as shown below:

OXIDATION OF ORGANIC COMPOUNDS BY MOLECULAR OXYGEN

$$\text{Fe or Cu catalyst}$$

INITIATION $RH + O_2 \longrightarrow R^* + HO_2^*$

PROPAGATION $R^* + O_2 \longrightarrow RO_2^*$

                $RO_2^* + RH \longrightarrow R^* + ROOH$

TERMINATION $R^* + R^* \longrightarrow R : R$

                $R^* + HO_2^* \longrightarrow ROOH$

where:
R is an organic molecule
ROOH is an organic peroxide
R:R are two organic molecules which have been cross-linked together
O_2 is oxygen
Cu is copper, Fe is iron
* is the unpaired electron
H is a hydrogen atom
HO_2^* is a superoxide free radical
RO_2^* and R^* are organic free radicals

Note that two free radicals can terminate their own chain reaction by combining. The resulting combination is stable, not a free radical, because the two electrons are paired.

Compounds that can help terminate the chain of free radical reactions are called free radical quenchers or scavengers. Antioxidants such as vitamins A, E, and C, the sulfur-containing amino acid cysteine, the cysteine-containing triamino acid glutathione, the phenolic and catecholic amino acids such as tyrosine and L-Dopa, the mineral selenium, and synthetic antioxidants such as BHT, BHA, and ethoxyquin are effective free radical quenchers. Aging is due, in part, to the decrease in blood and tissue levels of antioxidants that occurs in aging.

Since free radicals are able to cause genetic mutations, they have been implicated in the genesis of atherosclerotic plaques (a type of tumor) and cancer. Free radical quenchers such as C, E, BHA, BHT, selenium, and cysteine have been shown in experimental animals to prevent the development of some types of cancer. Peroxidized fats, the most common type of organic peroxide, are a source of free radicals (they also inhibit macrophages, white cells of the immune system, so that they do not attack and eat foreign invaders such as bacteria and cancer cells). Overweight individuals, who contain a larger amount of peroxidized fats in their body, are more likely to develop cancer and atherosclerosis than people of normal weight.

Peroxidized fats—found plentifully in atherosclerotic plaques—inhibit the production of PGI_2. PGI_2 was discovered by Vane and Moncada, for which they received the prestigious Lasker research award. PGI_2 (also called prostacyclin) is the natural hormone which prevents abnormal blood clots. If there is not enough PGI_2, a clot forms on the artery wall. Iron and copper leak from the hemolyzing red blood cells in the clot and promote the free radical peroxidation of still more fats, further decreasing PGI_2, and so the clot grows. After a while, part of the clot may break off. If it lodges in your coronary artery, you have a heart attack—coronary thrombosis. If it lodges in your brain, you have a stroke and suffer brain damage. In his clinical practice, Dr. Wilfred E. Shute has been using megadoses of vitamin E in humans for forty years to prevent abnormal clots, heart attacks, and strokes. Now that it is understood how the E works (it helps prevent the formation of the peroxidized fats), it will probably become used much more widely for these purposes.

Figures 1a and 1b illustrate the delicate balance between the formation of blood clots and their prevention. In Figure 1a we see an endothelial cell (lining an artery), with the enzyme prostacyclin synthetase manufacturing prostacyclin (PGI_2) to prevent blood from clotting inside the artery. A platelet in the bloodstream is shown making thromboxane, which causes blood to clot. In Figure 1b we see that a lipid (fat) peroxide has knocked out the prostacyclin synthetase, resulting in a drastic reduction in prostacyclin manufacture. In the meantime, the platelet increases production of thromboxane, resulting in abnormal blood clots which can cause heart attack or stroke.

BHT has extended the life spans of mice in experiments by Dr. Denham Harman. In some species which have a naturally short life span and tend to die of cancer, the BHT's life extending effects probably stemmed from its suppression of cancer development. Harman has also demonstrated an increase in average life span with BHT in long-lived mouse strains in which incidence of tumors is normally low.

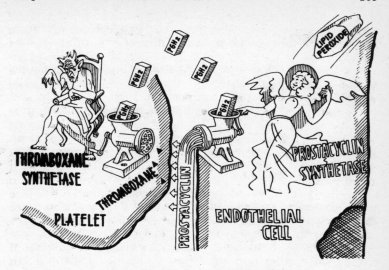

Figure 1a. Physiological balance between platelet and arterial endothelial cell

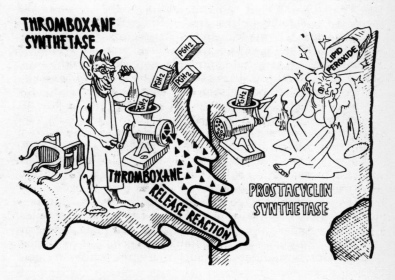

Figure 1b. How atherosclerosis may be initiated

Dr. Harman, who developed the free radical theory of aging (1956), suggests three methods of experimentally reducing free radical damage in the bodies of experimental animals:

1. Reduce calories in the diet to reduce the production of free radicals in metabolism.

2. Minimize dietary components such as copper and polyunsaturated fats which tend to increase free radical production.

3. Add to the diet one or more free radical quenchers, such as vitamins E, C, A, B-1, B-5, B-6, zinc, selenium, BHT, and cysteine.

A large number of studies with experimental animals found that some tested antioxidants can increase average and even, in some cases, maximum life span (in rats, mice, fruit flies, and nematodes, a type of worm); inhibit or regress cancer; stimulate the immune system; protect against radiation; and produce other desirable effects. The fact that the death rate in America from stomach cancer is declining while it is increasing in many other developed countries (such as Japan) seems to be associated with the addition of antioxidants such as BHT and BHA to breakfast cereals and other foods since about 1947 in the United States, and possibly because of the increased availability of fresh fruits and vegetables which contain antioxidants. A typical United States citizen gets an average of about 2 milligrams per day of BHT in food. While the cardiovascular disease rate had been increasing in the United States up to about ten years ago, it had been accompanied by a 37 percent rise in polyunsaturated fat consumption and only a 7 percent increase in saturated fat consumption. In the past several years, this death rate has declined by 20 percent, possibly due to increased health consciousness on the part of Americans and factors such as greater intake of vitamins C, E, and other antioxidant dietary supplements, dieting, moderate exercise, increased use of low doses of aspirin (another antioxidant) in the elderly, widespread use of beta-blocker drugs such as propranolol to control high blood pressure, and perhaps the increased availability of *fresh* fruits and vegetables. (It is interesting to note, however, that total per capita consumption of all fruits and vegetables is declining.) We know that polyunsaturated fats are much more susceptible to oxidation and the subsequent generation of free radicals. Since there is a high content in the brain of the very highly polyunsaturated fatty acid docosahexanoic acid (the precursor of which is dietary linolenic acid, also polyunsaturated), it is likely that a major part of brain aging is due to free radicals generated during the abnormal, inadequately controlled oxidation of these fatty acids. Possibly the decline in sensory perception associated with age may be due at least in part to free radical damage in the brain. Sensory nerves involving vision, hearing, taste, and smell all contain large amounts of very easily peroxidized docosahexanoic acid. There is experimental evidence to support these ideas. Sprague-Dawley rats fed semi-synthetic diets (which did not significantly affect the death rate) made more errors on a maze test when larger amounts of polyunsaturated fats were fed in place of saturated fats. In another experiment, rats fed safflower oil (polyunsaturated) plus 20 milligrams of vitamin E acetate per 100 grams of food performed better on a discrimination test than rats fed the safflower oil without E. Moreover, zinc (required for a common type of SOD) has a reputation of helping to restore lost taste and smell in some individuals.

Vitamin C plays an essential role in protecting these important polyunsaturated lipids in the brain and spinal cord from free radical attacks, to which they are very susceptible. There is a selective membrane surrounding the brain and spinal cord called the blood-brain barrier. This membrane contains pumps which require valuable energy to operate, but which move vitamin C from your bloodstream, across the membrane, and into the cerebral-spinal fluid (CSF) that bathes the brain and spinal cord (the central nervous system, CNS). These pumps concentrate vitamin C so that the CSF has about ten times the vitamin C concentration as your blood. Each nerve cell has its own membrane which contains more vitamin C pumps, so that the interior of each nerve cell contains about ten times the vitamin C concentration as the CSF—a total of 100 times the vitamin C concentration in your blood. This is a vivid illustration of the lengths to which a healthy body must go to protect the brain lipids from damaging autoxidation.

Hydergine® (made by Sandoz), a prescription drug, can prevent a considerable amount of the damage caused by free radicals in the brain. It is a very powerful antioxidant. It is useful in older persons who have a degree of cerebral hypoxia (insufficient oxygen), in preventing birth defects resulting from inadequate oxygen to the fetal brain (the usual cause of cerebral palsy), in accident victims who have suffered periods of inadequate oxygen (as in drownings), in stroke which involves extensive hypoxic free radical damage, and in normal persons, who have been shown to develop increased intelligence by using Hydergine®. In one study involving normal volunteers, 12 milligrams of Hydergine® per day for two weeks resulted in improved alertness and cognitive functions, including the ability to conceptually abstract (to identify patterns in a series of line drawings). See also subject index for more on the ability of Hydergine® to prevent free radical damage to brain and liver.

Free radical quenchers can improve the immune defense responses of both T-cells (manager and killer white cells) and B-cells (antibody-making cells, which usually receive their instructions from the T-cells). Effective tested antioxidant compounds include vitamin A, the food antioxidant BHT, the amino acid cysteine, 2-MEA, vitamin E, selenium, and zinc.

Lipofuscin aging pigment, which accumulates in nerve cells (neurons) in the brain and in skin, appears to contain peroxidized fats and cross-linked breakdown products, as well as proteinaceous material. The accumulation of age pigments probably causes brain damage, and Hydergine® can reduce the rate of age pigment accumulation in neurons by a factor of about four! See Part II, Chapter 8, for more on age pigments.

A rather unexpected finding has been that feeding antioxidants to pregnant mice resulted in an increased offspring life span. Swiss female mice were placed on a semi-synthetic diet to which was added either nothing (controls), Santoquin® brand ethoxyquin (a synthetic antioxidant), 2-MEA (2-mercaptoethylamine), vitamin E acetate, sodium hypophosphite (another food additive antioxidant), or ethoxyquin plus sodium hypophosphite. The mice were mated after one month on the diet. At weaning, the offspring were placed on a commercial diet. In male offspring, 2-MEA and sodium hypophosphite were most effective in extending life span. Ethoxyquin and 2-MEA were most effective in extending life span of female offspring. These fascinating results may be due to the reduction of free radical damage to the eggs and embryos by the antioxidants.

MONSANTO REPORT NO. 6 ON CURRENT TECHNOLOGY

Santoquin® Antioxidant
(ethoxyquin)
can it actually slow the process of aging?

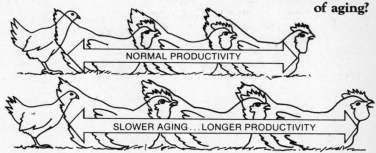

It's a question that could hardly have arisen at a busier time for the molecular biology group of Monsanto's Research Dept. For one thing, a pressing series of studies are afoot on the company's Polaris®, a higher sugar-producing treatment for ripening cane. The studies are trying to unravel the exact biochemical mechanism of *why* the compound can promote up to 15% more sucrose in the harvest. Is it the effect on invertase level? Why is there less response when ripening conditions approach the ideal?

In the middle of it, this intriguing aging question has arisen, too important to be set aside.

Is it possible that the company's well-established and long-commercialized Santoquin® feed antioxidant has this unexplored effect? The ability to *slow* the aging process in living bodies would include poultry, and that could perhaps be a way to prolong the producing life of chick breeders and laying hens. The same age-delaying mechanism might extend the siring virility of top-of-breed horses, bulls and boars and stretch out the milk-giving period of dairy cows. It might give pet dogs and cats a longer lease on life.

The published studies to date on slowing the aging process with antioxidant ingestion are scarcely definitive. There's too little data to show that it will, but too much to say that it won't. Yet the research programs necessary to check all this out will take a long, long time.

Nevertheless, in the struggle to produce more food, no byway can be left unexplored.

SO DIFFERENT, SO ALIKE

Santoquin antioxidant, more familar as a commonly-used feed ingredient by its generic nickname of ethoxyquin, is feed-grade: 6-ethoxy-1,2-dihydro-2,2,4 - trimethylquinoline. The structural formula looks like this:

One of the most familiar (and perhaps important) antioxidants that Mother Nature provides living bodies is Vitamin E. Its most potent isomer, -tocopherol looks like this:

There's no resemblance at all.

Yet despite this difference in structure, Santoquin antioxidant acts *like Vitamin E in all known metabolic functions!* One of its most pronounced effects is to inhibit the formation of peroxides during the process of digestion and metabolism.

The evidence which has been accumulating that ethoxyquin may slow down aging does not come from the highly enthused "mega" vitamin sector. It comes from published papers that report some solid research by eminent biochemists, biologists, chemists and gerontologists.

Monsanto's own research with feeding tests has also provided some supportive evidence, but purely from *chemical* and *feed-response* standpoints. Sadly, in all the work done to date, none has been focused on delving into this potential "aging inhibition" property.

But the chemical evidence plus the *in vivo* studies that have surfaced from various sources are too suggestive to shrug off.

TANTALIZING EVIDENCE

In a most erudite paper, *Aging At The Cellular Level,* Dr. B. L. Strehler cited twenty-three research models compiled by the Association for The Advancement of Aging Research. Of the physiological enigmas listed, a preponderence of the biochemical changes associated with aging *could* be triggered by or be the direct cause of *oxidation* in body tissues.

A number of eminent researchers—Drs. Denham Harman, William A. Pryor, and Johan Bjorksten among them—have offered evidence that the existence of free radicals in the body and cross-linking of various biomolecules are a significant factor in the aging process. Bjorksten, in over a quarter century of study, has reported comprehensively in books and papers on the subject. Pryor, too, has deeply investigated free radical propagation reactions and defined five types. The mode of occurrence of two of these and their possible biochemical effects was reported in *Chemical & Engineering News,* Special Feature Article, published June 7, 1971. This paper also examined the possible role of chemically-made antioxidants and Vitamin E in the aging process.

In a talk on the subject of "Free Radical Theory of Aging" at the 19th Annual Meeting of the Gerontological Society, Dr. Denham Harman symbolized the free radical reaction of oxygen with biomolecules in this fashion:

$$
\begin{array}{lllll}
 & & & \text{Cu} & \\
\text{Initiation:} & RH & + \ O_2 & \longrightarrow R\cdot & + & HO_2\cdot \\
\text{Propagation:} & R\cdot & \cdot \ O_2 & \longrightarrow RO_2\cdot & & \\
 & RO_2\cdot & + \ RH & \longrightarrow R\cdot & + & ROOH \\
\text{Termination:} & R\cdot & + \ R\cdot & \longrightarrow R{:}R & & \\
 & R\cdot & + \ HO_2\cdot & \longrightarrow ROOH & &
\end{array}
$$

He pointed out that the rate of reaction of propagation and ultimate chain-length of cross-linking depend on the number of times the propagation step is repeated, i.e. the incidences of free radical promoters and amounts of available oxidants, which would include peroxides.

ONE CLUE—HIGHLY SPECIFIC

In another talk at the 4th Annual Meeting of the American Aging Association, Sept. 1974, Eddy and Harman demonstrated the inhibiting effect of antioxidants in the diet on a specific phenomenon of aging: the formation of amyloid, a constituent of senile plaques—frequently referred to as aging pigments. In this report, it was stated that casein-induced amyloidosis in mice subjects was reduced from 65% to almost zero by diets containing 0.25% of two different synthetic antioxidants, with Santoquin (as one) having the somewhat greater effect.

Although the work was directed at amyloid formation, data was also cited that showed the pronounced beneficial effect on the mice's mortality rate by adding Santoquin antioxidant to the diet. Without the antioxidant in the diet, 20% survived to $18\frac{1}{2}$ months; on diets with 0.2% Santoquin, 20% survived for 23 months.

This was not the first intimation of increased longevity by any means. As early as 1966 and again in 1970, Dr. Harman demonstrated that by feeding weaned mice on diets containing 0.5–1% antioxidants the life span was increased 30–45%. He reported that in human terms this equated to a life expectancy of about 100 years.

ARE FREE RADICALS
THE CHIEF CULPRITS?

There has come to light a ponderous amount of data that shows (a) that free radical scavengers can have a critical role in slowing aging, (b) that inhibiting systemic oxidation DOES counteract certain effects of aging, and (c) that Santoquin antioxidant is highly effective in countering this kind of biochemistry.

Monsanto's research (and others as well) has amply proved that Santoquin antioxidant decreases the uptake of oxygen by unsaturated fats and prevents formation of organic peroxides in the bird and animal body. As a consequence, the recommended 125 ppm level of Santoquin in poultry feeds delays the breakdown of nutrients (vitamins, amino acids, pigment formers) in the diets and thereafter protects against loss throughout digestion and metabolism. This protection against free radical degradation thereby enables the animal to get more good out of the feed. In brief, there is no question that Santoquin does indeed scavenge free radicals in the animal system. As does Vitamin E. This was demonstrated early by feeding studies that showed Santoquin could fully protect poultry from the onset of encephalomalacia, an E-deficiency syndrome, even on diets from which all natural Vitamin E had been removed.

NO QUICK ANSWERS

What's Step One? Free radicals have already been shown to have a causative relation with the aging process. Santoquin antioxidant has been shown to scavenge free radicals, to inhibit formation of peroxides and its presence definitely slows down the oxidation of unsaturated oils and lipids. How can this effect be checked out against chickens, pigs, milk cows and pets?

In a small group-think session, one of Monsanto's cellular biology specialists pointed out a basic approach that would provide the first clue. When normal living cells are taken from an animal embryo and raised in a culture medium—they replicate a specific number of times, then die. The life span of the cell culture and number of replications are *species specific* and correlate with that animal's life span. If the presence of ethoxyquin in the culture lengthens the life span or increases the number of perfect replications. . .?

But that would be only a clue. It would still have to be checked out on whole living animals.

Breeding swine normally live 12–15 years; milk cows produce for 7–10 years; a stud horse is still going strong at 30! Rats and mice who give up the ghost at 2–3 years can't help; their metabolism of nutrients is radically different and pretty much their own. Any way you look at it—the final check-out—is going to take a long, long time.

It looks most logical from a pragmatic standpoint to start with laying hens. Their productive life is shorter, a mere 2–3 years. And egg laying drops off as they age. But any effect here would at least mean more eggs per hen!

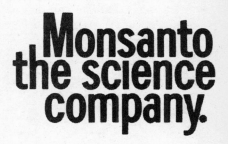

**Monsanto
the science
company.**

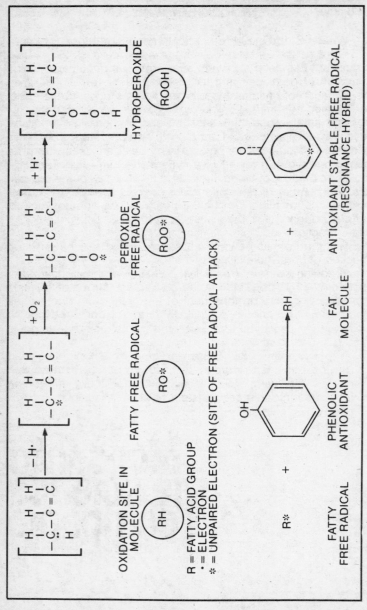

Free radical reactions with fats

Because of the toxicity of high concentrations of oxygen (via free radical mechanisms), hyperbaric oxygen (higher than normal atmospheric pressure) should be used with great caution. In very short repeated exposures it is possible that free radical destroying enzymes, such as SOD, may be induced to higher levels, thus increasing the patient's overall ability to handle free radicals. However, excessively long exposures would cause damage by creating conditions for massive peroxidations, especially in patients with a low level of antioxidants in their bodies. Both too high and too low levels of oxygen lead to increased radical activity. As Dr. Harry Demopoulos and others have shown, oxygen gas (O_2) can quench free radicals. He has found that the principal destructive consequence of hypoxia (oxygen deficiency) in tissues is due to free radicals produced under the hypoxic condition. When the amount of oxygen drops below about half of normal, the free radical generating ability of oxygen reacting with fats is almost as great as at full oxygen supply, but the free radical inhibiting activity of oxygen is mostly lost. This is why brain damage normally occurs within minutes after stoppage of breathing or brain blood circulation. Hydergine® can extend this safe period very substantially.

8
Accumulated Wastes: Those Telltale Brown Spots

With accurate experiment and observation to work upon, imagination becomes the architect of physical theory.

—John Tyndall

If you didn't carry out the garbage, you would soon be buried in waste. If you were only able to dispose of some of your garbage, it would take longer, but eventually you would suffer the same fate. Do our cells accumulate waste products of metabolism over the years—wastes that eventually poison us? Unfortunately, they do. One of the most noticeable wastes is yellowish-brown stuff that builds up in our skin and brain cells. These "age spots" contain the age pigment lipofuscin. Many scientists believe that lipofuscin damages our brain cells by clogging them so that vital nutrients cannot flow freely in the cells. By using the right nutrients and, optionally, certain prescription drugs, we can slow the rate of accumulation of lipofuscin and also speed up its removal. We can see ugly brown age spots in the skin disappear, over a period of several months, and stay away. Evidence indicates that similar events take place with regard to the accumulated age pigments in our brain cells.

Some scientists propose that aging (or at least parts of it) can be explained by the accumulation with age of toxic by-products of metabolism. There are, in fact, several materials which accumulate with age that seem to be associated with random aging damage.

Dr. A. L. Tappel points out that it doesn't matter whether you're a man, a mouse, a fruit fly, or even a cup of coffee or a slice of toast, you will still accumulate certain fluorescent pigments as you age. (Even foods are subject to aging via the same free radical reactions which cause human skin and nerve cells to accumulate lipofuscin pigment.)

When lipofuscin deposits appear in the skin, they are often called "age spots" or "liver spots," and are yellow-brown or brown spots which are not freckles, birthmarks, or scars. Lipofuscin pigment accumulates in nerve cells (neurons) in the brain too, more in some areas than in others. It is a pigment that can be made to fluoresce yellowish to yellow-green, orange, or yellow-brown under ultraviolet light. Measurement of this fluorescence is how the amount of pigment present is determined. Lipofuscin is found, in addition to neurons, in heart muscle, skeletal muscle, voluntary muscle, liver, adrenals, and other organs and tissues, particularly fatty tissues.

Drs. Chio and A. L. Tappel found that lipofuscin has a fluorescence spectra identical to compounds made from malonaldehyde (an aldehyde breakdown product of peroxidized fats) and amino compounds such as proteins. It is now widely accepted that both lipofuscin and ceroid (another type of age pigment) form as a result of peroxidative reactions in structures within cells, especially membranes, which often contain unsaturated fats. It is thought that the cellular lysosomes (packets of tissue-dissolving enzymes found in cells) engulf these damaged membranes, and the material that the lysosomes cannot digest remains as lipofuscin or ceroid debris.

It is not yet fully understood how lipofuscin and other age pigments might damage these tissues. In 1974, Drs. D. M. A. Mann and P. O. Yates found that, as the amount of lipofuscin in a cell increased, there was a corresponding decrease in the cellular RNA content. Other researchers believe that the pigments stored as wastes in cells do not interfere with cellular metabolism until they reach a critical volume. It is known that such deposits can interfere with diffusion-dependent biochemical reactions and could also lead to cell failure by blocking cytoplasm flow. The tissues of aged fruit flies contain lipopigments (lipid-derived age pigments like lipofuscin) which sometimes fill up to 50 percent of the cell volume. The fluorescence spectrum for fruit fly lipopigments is similar to that of aged mouse lipofuscin.

Lipofuscin pigment appears very early in life. It has been observed by some scientists in fetal nerve cells, though others have not found it in children under 10. In the cerebral cortex of rats, Dr. Kenneth R. Brizzee and his co-workers found a ten-fold increase in the amount of pigment in aged rats compared to that in young adults. In humans, lipofuscin may accumulate in neurons up to 70 percent of cellular volume before killing them. Figure 1 shows the progressive deterioration of brain cells getting clogged with lipofuscin age pigment. The pigment accumulates at the apex of the nerve cell, blocking the flow of vital nutrients to the long processes extending from the apex. Eventually, the fine nerve cell fibers die, followed by the death of the nerve cell itself. Without the fine interconnecting fibers, nerve cells cannot communicate with each other. Mental functions deteriorate. Figure 2 shows how the lipofuscin content of cells in a particular area of the human brain builds up over the years.

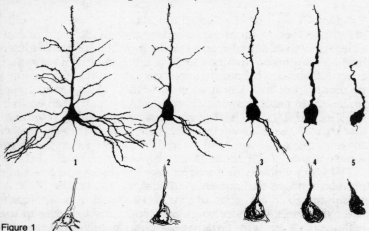

Figure 1

Reprinted from *Aging*, Vol. 1 *(Clinical, Morphologic, and Neuro-chemical Aspects in the Aging Nervous System)*, H. Brody, D. Harman, and J. Mark Ordy, editors. Copyright © 1975 by Raven Press Books, Ltd.

Similar to but not identical with lipofuscin, the age pigment ceroid is commonly found in vitamin E-deficient animals. In humans, ceroid is reportedly associated with liver and intestinal diseases which impair vitamin E absorption and utilization. In laboratory mammals, ceroid deposits can accumulate rapidly, becoming visible in only a few days to months under appropriate conditions.

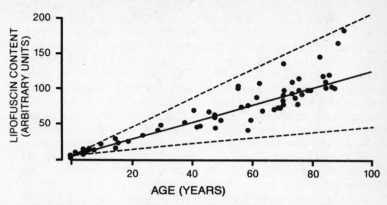

Figure 2. Graph of mean lipofuscin content plotted against age for nerve cells of inferior olivary nucleus of 67 human cases of age range 11 days to 91 years.

Yet another accumulated pigment, amyloid, is found in the nervous tissue of patients with various disease conditions and in old age. Whereas lipofuscin is composed of lipids (50 percent), proteins (30 percent), and residues, amyloid is made of perhaps three different proteins, including, in one type of amyloid, the immunological proteins from an autoimmune attack. It is thought that amyloid damages nervous tissues by compression and infiltration, blocking cytoplasmic flow and interfering with diffusion, movement, and reaction of vital biochemicals within the cell.

The accumulation of these aging pigments can be prevented or slowed by some prescription drugs. Drs. G. H. Bourne and Kalidas Nandy found that lipofuscin can be removed from cells by a drug called centrophenoxine or meclofenoxate (trade name, Lucidril®), used widely in several European countries. The molecule is made up of dimethylaminoethanol attached to p-chlorophenoxyacetic acid. The former compound is in Deaner®, and is closely related to the diethylaminoethanol in GH-3. The latter compound is half of auxin, a plant growth hormone. In spider monkeys, centrophenoxine greatly reduced lipofuscin from brain cells but did not reduce it in the heart or other organs. It also decreased this pigment in the nerve cells of guinea pigs and other rodents. Deaner® (Riker) is the p-acetamidobenzoate salt of dimethylaminoethanol and has many effects similar to those of centrophenoxine. Deaner® is a prescription drug which is available in the United States. We have personally observed 300 milligrams per day of Deaner® remove all visible lipofuscin age pigment (liver spots) from the skin of a man in his mid-60s. After a few months, his age spots had faded appreciably and were completely gone in about two years. Normal suntanning was not inhibited, and freckles (which are melanin) were unaffected. Since skin cells (keratinocytes) are biochemically similar to neurons, and indeed, both are derived from the same fetal tissue, it is plausible that Deaner® would also be effective in removing lipofuscin from nerve cells.

Hydergine® (made by Sandoz), the prescription drug mentioned earlier, has been proved to slow the rate of lipofuscin accumulation in the brain cells of mammals by a factor of 4. This impressive effect is probably related to its ability to protect the brain from free radical damage resulting from normal metabolism, lipid autoxidation, and hypoxia (insufficient oxygen). Hypoxia can be caused by heart attack, stroke, narrowed cerebral arteries, massive blood loss, etc. Since both hypoxic brain damage and lipofuscin accumulation are caused by undesired free radical reactions, it shouldn't be surprising that Hydergine® is very effective in preventing both types of damage. What is a bit surprising is that this safe and effective prescription drug has been available for a quarter century, is the fifth largest selling prescription drug in the world, but is almost unknown in the United States for either of these purposes, due to FDA restrictions on what its manufacturer may tell physicians. (Pharmaceutical manufacturers are not legally permitted to inform your physician of a new use for an already FDA-approved drug until they obtain FDA permission to do so. The process of obtaining this permission is often almost as time-consuming and expensive as obtaining FDA approval for a completely new drug.)

9
The Decline of Your Brain's Chemical Messengers

In senile degeneration the nerve-cells are surrounded by neuronophages which absorb their contents and bring about more or less complete atrophy.

—Elie Metchnikoff, *The Prolongation of Life* (1908)

Mind, mind alone,
Is light, and hope, and life, and power!

—Ebenezer Elliott (1833)

Your brain works because your nerves talk to each other with chemicals called neurotransmitters that they make out of certain nutrients in the food you eat. Aging damages your brain in several different ways. For example, you make less of these neurotransmitters and become less sensitive to their effects. The proper nutritional supplements can significantly slow aging in your brain. In fact, by taking more of the nutrients that your brain needs to make the neurotransmitters, you can restore your brain's vital messengers to more youthful levels. Most surprising of all, the right nutritional supplements can measurably improve brain function in normal, young, healthy people.

More people are concerned about senility (senile dementia, in medical terms) than about any other problem of aging. The prospect of mental degeneration to the point where you can hardly remember or learn anything, or taste, smell, hear, or see, or care whether you're alive or dead is almost as dismaying as death. We have all seen aging friends or relations to whom this has happened. Wouldn't it be wonderful if senility could be prevented?

A lot can be done to prevent aging in the brain and even to partially reverse senility if this sad state has already happened to somebody you know. Recently, a great deal of understanding has been achieved in the ways that the brain performs its various functions and how aging decreases the brain's ability to do what is easy when we are young. Although there is still a great deal to be discovered, we now know several ways to keep our brains more youthful.

Scientists have discovered that the brain cells (neurons) communicate with each other via special chemicals called neurotransmitters, made by the brain cells. All learning, remembering, moving your body, sleeping, and emotions you feel depend upon the ability of your brain cells to produce and deliver neurotransmitters to other brain cells as well as to respond to chemical messages from other brain cells. As your brain ages, the ability of your brain to make and respond to some of these vital messenger chemicals drops off. In some cases, we can increase the amounts of the deficient neurotransmitters, thus bringing function in aging brains up to young or near young adult levels.

Neurotransmitters are made by the brain from nutrient substances you eat in your food. For example, acetylcholine is a neurotransmitter which is important in the parts of the brain affecting primitive emotions like sex and the degree of responsiveness to outside stimuli (as in alertness versus sleep), and also plays a very important role in memory, learning, and long-term planning. The brain makes acetylcholine from choline you get in your diet (in fish, for instance) and from lecithin, which also contains choline (as phosphatidyl choline). In one study, MIT students taking 3 grams of choline a day had an improved memory and ability to learn a list of words. In another study, 80 grams of lecithin a day produced similar results. Deaner® (Riker) is a prescription drug which the brain can also use to increase its supply of acetylcholine. Deaner® has been used with some success in the treatment of senility.

Norepinephrine (NE) is another of the brain's arsenal of neurotransmitters, important in primitive drives and emotions like sex and in memory and learning. When the level of NE in the brain is too low, people become depressed and their immune systems do not function normally. (That's because NE can cause the brain to release growth hormone, which is essential to proper immune system function.) The brain uses phenylalanine and tyrosine, amino acids found in meat, eggs, and cheese (for example), to make NE. Both amino acids have been used successfully to treat people for depression arising from a variety of causes. Effective dosage of phenylalanine in one study was 100 to 500 milligrams a day for two weeks. For best results, the phenylalanine should be taken on an empty stomach at night just before going to bed or immediately after awakening in the morning. Some health food stores now offer phenylalanine. **WARNING:** see warning on page 136.

Another important neurotransmitter is dopamine, which affects sex and other drives, locomotion, tissue growth and repair, the immune system, and mood. The dopaminergic system is one of the systems which declines most in the aging brain. Lipofuscin age pigment (containing the same material as age spots in skin) forms especially rapidly in the dopamine-dependent tracts in the brain with age. Parkinsonism (tremors) is caused by damage to these dopamine-dependent brain areas. L-Dopa, an amino acid the brain uses to make dopamine, can increase the life span of experimental animals by up to 50 percent. The ability of old rats to swim has been improved to the level of young rats by L-Dopa treatment. Some patients on L-Dopa have experienced an increase in sex drive. L-Dopa is an excellent antioxidant because it is a catechol and has been used to protect against exposure to high-energy radiation. It should be used in conjunction with other nutrient antioxidants. (**Warning: Using L-Dopa, phenylalinine, or tyrosine in large quantities, however, may cause a preexisting pigmented malignant melanoma [a serious form of cancer] to grow faster.**)

Hydergine® (Sandoz) is a prescription drug which can help older persons with low to moderate levels of symptoms of senility (confusion, dizziness, apathy, lack of self-care, forgetfulness) to recover brain function. At 12 milligrams per day for only two weeks, Hydergine® improved both simple alertness and high-level cognitive function in normal volunteers. Hydergine® is the fifth most popular prescription drug in the world and the number-one favorite in France. It provides a lift like caffeine, but without the letdown or jittery aftereffects of caffeine. And Hydergine® stimulates the brain to grow neurites, the connections between nerve cells which are necessary for learning. One reason you can't teach an old dog new tricks is that he can no longer grow enough new neurites. Hydergine® is able to promote neurite growth like the natural hormone nerve growth factor, which you have less and less of as you age. We know of three cases of partial recovery of impaired sensory function with Hydergine® (two cases of hearing loss and one case of a person born without a sense of smell). See the Case Histories in Appendix L for details. Hydergine® is not just for old folks, though. We ourselves take large doses: 20 milligrams of Hydergine® per day, both for its ability to increase intelligence and for its ability to slow lipofuscin age pigment accumulation in brain cells by a factor of 4. For more about how lipofuscin waste accumulation damages the brain, see Part II, Chapter 8.

In this brief introduction to the major neurochemicals, we want to mention the important hormone, vasopressin. The prescription drug Diapid® (vasopressin, made by Sandoz) increased both memory and learning abilities in men in their 50s and 60s in one study. The men also experienced faster sensory-motor reactions. The dose used was 16 I.U. per day. No side effects occurred at this dose. Vasopressin is made in the brain and may slightly affect blood pressure and controls urine volume, and is also a memory and learning chemical. When a person has an accident that is a close call, he sometimes sees "his life flash before his eyes." That effect may possibly come from massive vasopressin release. In another study, vasopressin enabled people who had suffered amnesia in accidents (sometimes involving periods of amnesia as long as months) to recover their memories. The recovery of memory by the amnesiacs took from several hours to a few days in the studies so far published. Our own observations show that restoration by Diapid® of an amnesiac's memory can sometimes occur almost instantly. See Case Histories in Appendix L.

Dopamine, norepinephrine, and acetylcholine are three of the most important neurotransmitters in the brain. (See diagram of synaptic junction below.) Called catecholamines, dopamine and norepinephrine, though separate chemicals with different functions, are very closely related chemically. In fact, each can be chemically converted to the other in the brain. Acetylcholine has a different structure and, in most cases, different functions from the catecholamine neurotransmitters.

Catecholamines are responsible for a number of different effects in normal humans. They are involved in control of locomotor (moving about) behavior, aggressive behavior, sexual behavior, food intake, and behavior dependent upon positive (reward) and negative (punishment) reinforcement. Acetylcholine controls muscle tone and motor activity and has a role in memory, learning, and long-term planning, as well as in primitive emotions and drives.

Stimulants of the dopaminergic system (nerve cells using dopamine as the neurotransmitter) can cause the release of the pituitary gland's growth hormone, which is needed for growth and healing and also for proper functioning of the immune system. As humans age, the brain levels of dopamine and norepinephrine fall off. Without adequate quantities of these neurotransmitters, motivation is lost—people become apathetic and don't care about living any more. (This process may even be triggered by an aging clock in the brain. The dopaminergic system might be turned off, leading to loss of sexual interest and of the will to live, resulting in death shortly thereafter.) The release of growth hormone also falls off sharply with age, which accounts in part for the deficits that develop in the immune system's ability to resist infectious and autoimmune diseases, cancer, and atherosclerotic plaques (a type of tumor) in older people. Depression due to inadequate levels of neurotransmitters is also very common in the elderly.

As Metchnikoff observed in the early 1900s, attacks by white blood cells upon the body's own nerve cells become increasingly common with advancing age. Many degenerative nervous disorders are believed due to this type of attack, including multiple sclerosis, Creutzfeldt-Jakob disease, kuru (triggered by a viral attack), and perhaps Alzheimer's disease (a type of senility). These attacks on nerve cells by immune system cells results from defective control of the immune system. For more about this failure to distinguish the body's normal cells from disease-producing entities, see Part II, Chapter 5, on the age-related decline of the immune system.

Acetylcholine causes the release of the hormone vasopressin, a memory and learning chemical as well as a regulator of urine volume and, to a slight extent, blood pressure. In the mid-1960s, Dr. Friedman and his co-workers obtained life extensions in aging rats with whole posterior pituitary extract, which contains vasopressin and a closely related hormone,

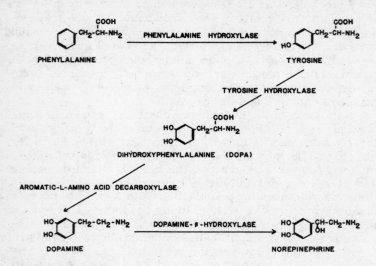

Catecholamine synthesis

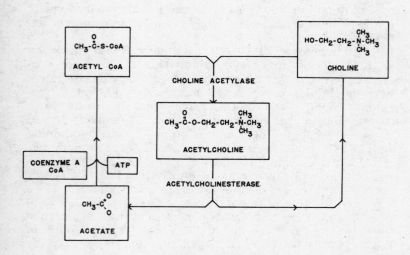

Acetylcholine synthesis and degradation. Choline acetylase is more formally called choline-acetyl transferase. ATP: adenosine triphosphate.

Pathway for synthesis and metabolism of serotonin.

oxytocin. In similar studies in rats, life extension was produced by giving oxytocin alone. Low acetylcholine levels contribute to the forgetfulness and lack of ability to concentrate which often occurs in old age. The cholinergic nervous system also controls the sensory input; too little acetylcholine and you are easily distracted by stimuli in your environment, whether you are trying to think (loss of concentration) or sleep (awakening too easily). In addition, too low acetylcholine levels cannot support normal motor (muscular activity) control, and coordination and motor response falter. The cholinergic nervous system in the body keeps mucous membranes lubricated and moist; without adequate acetylcholine levels in body tissues, the mucous membranes become dry, more easily irritated, infected, and damaged. Finally, acetylcholine is an important motivational chemical, along with the catecholamines.

The limbic or primitive part of the brain (the so-called "reptile brain") uses all three neurotransmitters mentioned above. Here is where the primitive drives and emotions, such as sex, are controlled. A too-low level of any of these neurotransmitters leads to loss of sex interest. It is thought that the catecholamines are involved in regulation of the release of the aphrodisiac polypeptide hormone LHRH by the hypothalamus (a master gland in the brain).

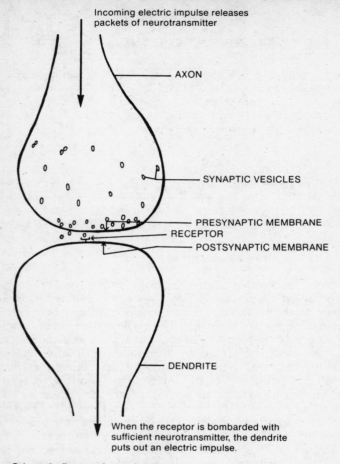

Incoming electric impulse releases
packets of neurotransmitter

AXON

SYNAPTIC VESICLES

PRESYNAPTIC MEMBRANE
RECEPTOR
POSTSYNAPTIC MEMBRANE

DENDRITE

When the receptor is bombarded with
sufficient neurotransmitter, the dendrite
puts out an electric impulse.

Schematic diagram of nerve junction

An example of a dopaminergic deficiency disease is Parkinsonism, where inadequate dopamine (or insensitivity of receptors to available dopamine) results in loss of fine motor control, with symptoms such as uncontrollable tremor, especially of the limbs. L-Dopa, which can be chemically converted by the brain into dopamine and norepinephrine, is an effective treatment for Parkinsonism in most cases. Bromocriptine (Parlodel®, Sandoz), another dopaminergic stimulant, is also effective, particularly when used in conjunction with L-Dopa. (L-Dopa and its metabolic product, dopamine, are subject to autoxidation. We think it likely that Parkinson's disease is caused by dopamine autoxidation damage to the dopaminergic nerves, perhaps initiated by a peroxidative autoimmune attack. Parkinson patients often gradually deteriorate; we suspect that this deterioration could be prevented or reduced with adequate antioxidants. We think it very unwise to take L-Dopa without a dietary supplement of antioxidants.) Bromocriptine plus about half of the usual dose of L-Dopa in Parkinson patients seems to frequently result in less long-term degeneration, and sometimes seems to lead to repairs of such damage. Bromocriptine is closely chemically related to Hydergine® and may be a potent antioxidant too. Vitamin C has been shown to prevent the autoxidation of L-Dopa.

A very dramatic story about the effects of L-Dopa on twenty patients with severe Parkinson's disease is contained in Oliver W. Sack's book *Awakenings*. Between 1916 and 1927, nearly five million people fell victim to encephalitis lethargica (sleeping sickness). A third of those affected died either in a coma or in a profound state of sleeplessness which could not be alleviated even with sedatives. Patients who survived were often in a condition of being conscious and aware but not fully awake. They were unmotivated and seemed like zombies. They commonly developed such symptoms of Parkinson's disease as tremor, rigidity, compulsive movements, and profound states of nonmovement. When, in 1967, it was realized that L-Dopa is an effective treatment for Parkinson's disease, Dr. Sacks treated twenty of these sleeping sickness victims (who were then quite old and had been zombies for nearly their entire lifetime). The book is a moving description of their awakenings with L-Dopa and subsequent developments, some of which were tragic. The poor results with L-Dopa, as experienced by some of these patients, is probably due to the autoxidation of L-Dopa, resulting in the production of 6-hydroxy-dopamine. The latter autoxidizes, producing free radicals and hydrogen peroxide, which damage dopaminergic nerve cell receptors. This problem could probably have been avoided, or at least mitigated, by giving the patients large doses of antioxidants (such as vitamins E, C, B-1, B-5, zinc, selenium and Hydergine®) along with the L-Dopa.

Warning: People who are taking L-Dopa for Parkinson's disease should not take vitamin B-6 supplements unless advised to do so by their physician. Vitamin B-6 helps convert the amino acid L-Dopa to the neurotransmitter dopamine in the brain where such conversion is desired, but it also helps to convert L-Dopa to dopamine peripherally (outside of the brain) in the remainder of the body. If a Parkinson's patient takes large doses of B-6, so much L-Dopa may be converted peripherally that there may be undesired peripheral side effects while, at the same time, not enough L-Dopa may be available to adequately elevate dopamine levels in the brain. (L-Dopa crosses the blood-brain barrier, the selective membrane surrounding the brain and spinal cord, but dopamine does not.) This can result in a temporary worsening of Parkinsonism symptoms.

Most of the persons we know who are currently participating in life extension experiments do not have Parkinson's disease, and many of these non-Parkinsonism patients have had a good response to $\frac{1}{4}$ to $\frac{1}{2}$ gram of L-Dopa at bedtime (as indicated by the fat loss and muscle buildup resulting from L-Dopa's stimulation of growth hormone release by the pituitary gland), even though they were also taking large doses of vitamin B-6 at the same time as they were taking L-Dopa.

Schizophrenia is thought by many researchers to involve errors in dopamine metabolism. The phenothiazines (most of which are antioxidants), used widely as treatment for schizophrenia, prevent excessive sensitivity in response to dopamine by blocking the dopamine receptors. Sometimes in long-term use of phenothiazines, uncontrollable movements in the jaw, tongue, and face (a disorder known as tardive dyskinesia) develop due to inadequate cholinergic stimulation. Recently, choline has been used successfully to treat tardive dyskinesia. Other cholinergics (such as Deaner® or lecithin) might also be effective therapy for this disorder.

In a recent study, old rats (the age equivalent of a human 80 years old) given L-Dopa regained the swimming abilities of healthy young rats. Swiss male mice fed L-Dopa in the lifespan study of Dr. George C. Cotzias had significant life extensions. (Dr. Cotzias developed L-Dopa therapy for Parkinson's disease.) However, in these mice there was a high initial mortality among the mice given the highest dose of L-Dopa (they were not given gradually increasing doses).

Old people often suffer from a deficiency of serotonin, an important inhibitory neurotransmitter that initiates sleep. Inhibitory neurotransmitters *reduce* neuron activity, in contrast to the above-mentioned neurotransmitters, which usually increase activity. Sleep disorders are common in old age, including difficulties in falling and staying asleep. Irritability and bedtime flights of ideas may occur. Tryptophan, an amino acid, is the natural substance used by the brain to make serotonin. Milk and bananas contain relatively large amounts (hot milk before bedtime really does help you sleep). Some vitamin stores sell tryptophan tablets. Possible side effects are headaches, sinus congestion, constipation, or intestinal cramping, resulting from the contraction of smooth muscle caused by serotonin. Tryptophan may help relieve migraine headaches due to serotonin's effect on smooth muscle in blood vessels.

The physical restlessness that may occur at night (or during the day) often responds to cholinergic stimulation, such as Deaner® (Riker), choline, or lecithin. Hyperkinetic children are often helped by Deaner® and should also respond to other cholinergics, such as choline or lecithin. Choline bitartrate, the most common type of choline sold at health food stores, can cause diarrhea. If you use it, begin at a low dose and slowly work your dose up. You may be able to avoid diarrhea. Choline chloride (properly called choline hydrochloride) does not have this side effect, but is very hygroscopic (absorbs moisture from the air), so that it cannot be readily used in tablets; we use a 50 percent solution in water.

One likely reason for the decline of the dopaminergic system in the brain is the high susceptibility of dopamine to autoxidation (the molecule oxidizes itself with molecular oxygen). In this process, dopamine is oxidized to 6-hydroxy-dopamine, producing hydrogen peroxide and hydroxyl radicals which damage the dopamine receptors. In the so-called burnt-out schizophrenics, there is abnormally low response to dopaminergic stimulation. These people are catatonic, with no desires and no pleasures. We think that this may be due to destruction of their dopaminergic receptors on the neurons by the hydrogen peroxide and associated free radicals. Since this damage is an oxidative process, antioxidants such as Hydergine® and vitamins C, E, B-1, B-5, B-6, and zinc and selenium should be able to provide a degree of protection to the receptors. Experiments by Drs. R. Poser and H. Demopoulos have clearly shown that vitamin C will prevent autoxidation of L-Dopa.

Hydergine® normalizes brain EEG energies under a variety of adverse conditions (such as low oxygen, old age, and alcohol intoxication). It reduces excess sensitivity to norepinephrine, too much of which can lead to irritability and rage, without tranquilizing effects. Bromocriptine (Parlodel® by Sandoz), a related compound, is another dopaminergic stimulant. It normalizes growth hormone output, when it is either too low (as in dwarfism) or too high (as in acromegaly). Bromocriptine also seems to reset some of the brain's aging clocks (natural programmed obsolescence), and it reinstates menstrual cycling in some postmenopausal women and in aging female experimental animals.

Depression due to inadequate levels of catecholamines can be safely treated with the amino acid phenylalanine. Phenylalanine is converted in the brain to dopamine and norepinephrine. It has been used in the treatment of depressed patients with great success at doses of 100 to 500 milligrams per day for two weeks. It was twice as effective as imipramine, the current prescription "drug of choice" for depression. D-phenylalanine has recently been found to be an effective treatment for severe pain in some people (See also Part III, Chapter 3, "Depression, Helplessness, and Aging," for dosage and precautions information.) **Warning: Phenylalanine supplements should be used with caution and under the supervision of a physician in cases of high blood pressure to make sure that the hypertension is not worsened. Phenylalanine supplements should not be used in patients with PKU (phenylketonuria) or with pre-existing pigmented melanoma, a particular type of cancer.**

10
Turning Back Aging Clocks

Everyone is familiar with the so-called "annual" plants which live only a few months, from the time when they sprout, until, after the production of seed, death comes to them naturally. . . . Natural death can be postponed if the plant be prevented from seeding.

—Elie Metchnikoff, *The Prolongation of Life* (1908)

Do DNA genetic clocks ticking away inside our brains turn off our vital functions so that we grow old and die? Unfortunately, this can occur. Menopause and male pattern baldness are examples. Salmon die soon after spawning as a result of damage triggered by a pituitary gland aging clock in their brains. If the pituitary gland is removed before spawning, the salmon don't spawn and they live for many years. The human aging clocks seem to be what limit man to a maximum life span of 110 or so years. We are just beginning to understand how these clocks work.

Some aging events are not random but may be "planned" parts of a genetic (DNA) program. Such events may be under the control of an aging clock or clocks located in the DNA. Clocks exist both at the cellular level and at higher levels (for example, under hormone control). Some possible reasons why aging clocks may have evolved are considered in Part I, Chapter 5, "The Evolution of Aging."

In 1965, Dr. Leonard Hayflick reported that cultured human WI-38 fibroblasts (fetal connective tissue cells grown at the Wistar Institute) would divide only about 50 times and then discontinue dividing, dying soon afterwards. He postulated that there is a genetic clock in cells which limits their number of divisions, thus supporting the theory of a cellular aging clock. Fibroblasts from young humans would divide more times than those from older ones; however, they still divided only about 50 times before discontinuing division. For several years, it was thought that this was an ultimate limit for cell division and that life span was correlated with cell-doubling capacity. However, recently it has been found at MIT that the keratinocytes (a type of skin cell) can divide 150 times and more if they are supplied with a natural polypeptide hormone called epidermal growth factor (EGF). This hormone is very similar to nerve growth factor, NGF. It was also found that the original WI-38 fibroblasts used by Hayflick and others in cell division experiments inadvertently came from a family with a high incidence of diabetes; it is now known that cells derived from diabetics seem to have a more limited life span than cells from normal individuals. Only the diabetic-derived cells seem to divide just 50 times. Moreover, mouse tongue epithelium divided 565 times in one study, even though mice have a far shorter life span than humans. Drs. Halliday and Tarrant are investigating the possibility that there is a small population of cells which can divide indefinitely, but that in cell culture techniques these "immortals" are diluted to a very low level approaching zero by the serial dilution culture techniques usually used. Such indefinitely dividing cells would be used as a store of cells for later differentiation for specific functions and would not be needed in large numbers.

Some familiar higher-level aging clocks are menopause and balding. Note that in women approaching menopause, the incidence of genetic defects in offspring increases rapidly. Such reproductive errors are caused by altered DNA in egg cells in the ovaries, degenerative changes that we believe are monitored by a clock or clocks that eventually, at a certain level of damage, turn off reproduction. There is some evidence that repair mechanisms which sustain life may also be turned off by this aging clock mechanism to inhibit reproduction. In rats, it has been found that lipofuscin builds up in the Leydig cells of the testis, where testosterone is produced and released to stimulate mating behavior. On the other hand, no lipofuscin is found in the spermatagonia cells of the rat testis, where the DNA-containing sperm is produced. This may indicate that the sperm-making tract has considerable protection against oxidative processes which would otherwise cause lipofuscin buildup, but that the testosterone-producing cells do not have such good protection. Such a process would assure that the clock monitoring mutations will turn off the testosterone (and, as a result, mating behavior) *before* a high level of damage is found in the sperm genetic (DNA) material.

Although male pattern balding is not necessarily tied to old age, it is very definitely due to a clock. If you transplant hairs from the balding area onto another part of the head, these hairs fall out right on schedule with the others remaining in the balding area. If you transplant hairs from nonbalding areas to the balding area, the hairs will keep right on growing, even while the hairs around them are falling out. (See Part III, Chapter 7, for recent research into methods for preventing or reversing balding.) Common male pattern balding seems to involve hormonal messages sent to the internal cellular clocks in the hair follicles in specific areas, such as the top of the head. Balding can be halted by castrating the balding male individual, thereby interrupting th hormone clock run signal. Therefore we know that balding depends to a degree on male hormones, and to some measure on the anatomic site. Testosterone causes hair to grow in other areas, such as the beard and moustache zones. We know that dihydrotestosterone, produced by the action of the enzyme testosterone-5-alpha-reductase on testosterone, causes some hair follicles to go into the resting (non-growing) phase. Only those cells which have a genetic susceptibility will be affected. These follicles are not usually immediately killed in the process, even though they no longer grow hairs large enough to be easily visible to the naked eye.

It is possible to reinstate menstrual cycling in most non-cycling older female rodents and in some human females with the drug bromocriptine (Parlodel®, made by Sandoz). Bromocriptine is a stimulant of the dopaminergic nervous system in the brain, which in turn stimulates the release by the pituitary gland of hormone-releasing factors (necessary for sex hormone production) and growth hormone (necessary for proper immune system function). The dopaminergic tract is one of the brain's systems showing the sharpest decline in activity with age—it is especially vulnerable to oxidative damage and accumulates lipofuscin throughout life. It is not yet understood just how bromocriptine reinstates menstrual cycling—resetting the clock—but it apparently involves increasing the level of dopaminergic stimulation to the hypothalamus and pituitary to the higher levels found in youth.

A clock, the one that programs the developmental stages of life, appears to be responsible for the finding that rats and mice can live much longer life spans if their caloric intake is restricted early in life. In rodents, reproduction can be delayed if conditions, especially the availability of food, are not supportive. It seems likely that the extended life span is due to putting the animals "on hold" by retarding development and delaying reproduction until food becomes more available. If food is fed ad lib (at the animal's chosen level) to these calorie-restricted animals, they rapidly mature and reproduce. In effect, the restricted food supply stalls the animals at an immature level of their development—and hence their reproduction—until more food becomes available. If severe caloric restriction during development is attempted with higher animals such as monkeys, which take several years to reach reproductive maturity, brain damage occurs and the animals do not live extended life spans.

It is possible to greatly extend the life spans of some insects by depriving their developing larvae of food and water. The larvae then become smaller in size and regress to an earlier larval development stage, failing to develop into adult insects. Given food and water again, the larvae proceed to develop normally. If deprived once again, the larvae again retrogress. Manipulating the maturation of the beetle *Trogoderma glabrum* in this manner, Drs. Beck and Bharadwaj (1972) produced larvae that lived over two years. The insect's normal life span (from egg to death of the adult) is only eight weeks. By two years of age, very extensive genetic damage had accumulated in these incredibly long-lived insect larvae, since they did not possess the quantities of protective and repair enzymes found in animals that normally live two years.

Aging clocks can turn off protective mechanisms essential to maintaining an animal's life. After spawning, salmon rapidly peroxidize and die. Major protective mechanisms that they have against peroxidation before spawning cease to function afterwards, leaving them defenseless against the release by the adrenal glands of massive amounts of pro-oxidant hormones. The "turning off" is thought to be due to a hyperactivity of the adrenals triggered by the spawning. If you

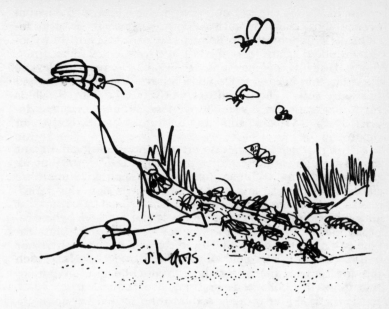

"If we ever intend to take over the world, one thing we'll *have* to do is synchronize our biological clocks."

prevent the fish from spawning by castration, by removal of the pituitary, or by hormone treatments, they live for many more years, whereas the spawning salmon die in hours. A similar phenomenon occurs with eels. This clock mechanism is an example where the interests of the genes (to make copies of themselves) conflicts with the interests of the individual animal. Yet another example: Female octopuses die soon after they hatch their young. But if you remove the preoptic gland (their version of the pituitary), they won't mate and will live on for years.

As mentioned earlier, Dr. W. Donner Denckla thinks he has discovered a death clock in the pituitary gland of the brain. If he removes this gland from mice and supplies them with the pituitary's growth hormone and thyroid hormone (which would normally be produced and released in response to pituitary hormonal messages), the animals live a somewhat longer average life span than intact animals. They appear young in all respects, sometimes up to only a few hours before their deaths. Denckla has isolated a hormone from cattle pituitaries which depresses the response of young rats (in which the pituitary has been removed) to thyroxine, a thyroid hormone. He calls this hormone DECO for Decreasing Oxygen Consumption hormone. Denckla believes that the pituitary is the source of a killing hormone, perhaps DECO itself, which turns down an animal's responsiveness to other hormones, especially to thyroxine and growth hormones, leading to its death.

If our own hypothesis is correct that at least some aging clocks monitor mutations, then improving DNA repair and inhibiting mutations with antioxidants and such enzymes as superoxide dismutase and peroxidases should slow down such clocks. This is an area where much more research is required. It is interesting to note that three of the methods which increase a species' maximum life span—that is, which slow age clocks—involve reducing free radical damage and mutations. Antioxidants directly control undesired free radicals. Underfeeding reduces the free radical production rate. Hypothermia (lowering body temperature) also reduces free radical production. While there are purely hormonal aging clocks, monitoring free radical mutation and other damage seems to be the modus operandi of at least some clocks involving growth- and sex-hormone output and sperm and egg production. From an evolutionary point of view, aging clocks involving reproduction are expected to play an important part in nature's "planned obsolescence" of our bodies. We, however, have our own plans!

11
Factors Which Correlate with Natural Longevity

Some years before birth, advertise for a couple of parents belonging to long-lived families.

—Oliver Wendell Holmes, Sr.

There is great variation in the longevity we see among people. We are all aware that a small percentage of people live to be over 100 years old, living much longer than the vast majority of us. This longevity, taking place in the absence of deliberate actions, is a result of natural functions in these long-lived people. Scientists have learned about some of the natural factors which allow such people to live so long. This understanding can help us to live a longer, healthier, and more active life.

This chapter lists eight of the more interesting factors which correlate with the natural life span of several mammalian species, including man.

1. Brain weight: In general, the greater the brain weight, the longer the life span. The higher the ratio of brain to body weight, the longer the species' average life span.

2. Body weight: There is not as good a correlation as with brain weight. A greater *species'* body weight does correlate with longer life span, but a lower *individual* body weight as compared to the species average usually seems to increase individual life span, probably due to reduced specific metabolic rate (see point 3 below).

3. Specific metabolic rate (SMR)—(food burned per day per unit of animal body weight). In general, the higher the SMR, the shorter the life span. Reduced caloric intake means a lower SMR for the individual. In many short-lived animals, caloric restriction (lowered SMR) dramatically increases life span. SMR is an index of how hard the metabolic equipment in a gram of tissue must work.

4. Body temperature: The higher the species' normal natural body temperature, the greater in general the life span. (A lower individual body temperature as compared to the *species'* average seems to increase that individual's life expectancy in cold-blooded species.) Reduction in body temperature results in a lower SMR. Species with higher normal average body temperatures seem to have more and/or better protective and repair enzymes.

5. The capacity to activate DMBA (an environmental pollutant, one of the very common class of carcinogens called polynuclear aromatic hydrocarbons, PAH, found in tobacco and other combustion tars) to a mutagenic form: DMBA and many other pollutants, especially the PAH, are not carcinogens in themselves but must be activated, particularly in the liver, to the metabolites which are carcinogenic. The longer the life span of the animal, the less the capacity to convert the pollutants to the carcinogenic form. In other words, in order to live longer, the damage that would be done to DNA by such carcinogens as activated PAH must be prevented or blocked. Blocking of attachment of these carcinogens to DNA is done more effectively by longer-lived species too. Even in their metabolized carcinogenic form, these molecules cannot cause cancer or atherosclerosis unless they bind to the DNA. In Figure 1, we see the DMBA-induced mutation rate (scale marked 0 to 700) versus the DMBA concentration. The fibroblast cells of rats suffer a much higher rate of DMBA-induced mutations than longer-lived animals. Humans, who live longest of all species in this study, show the lowest induced mutation rate. Figure 2 shows the amount of DMBA binding to DNA (on a scale of 0 to 120) versus time for a number of mammalian species, including man. You can easily see that the longer-lived animals bind the least amount of DMBA. Nature seems to be saying that it is necessary (but not sufficient) for your species to have half the PAH to DNA binding as another species if your species is to live twice as long as another species. BHT, BHA, selenium, and many other antioxidants

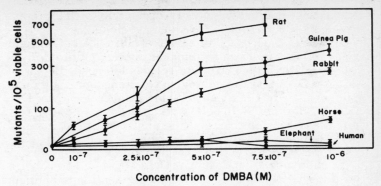

Figure 1. Higher concentrations (increasing from left to right) of the mutagen and carcinogen precursor DMBA cause increasingly more mutations in tissue cultures, but very long-lived species, such as humans and elephants, are much more resistant to this genetic damage than are short-lived species.

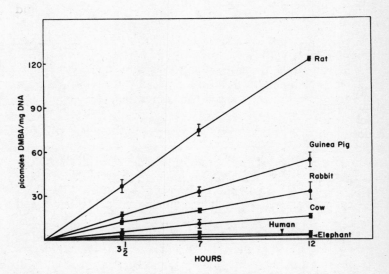

Figure 2. The activated form of the mutagen and carcinogen precursor DMBA first binds to DNA and then damages it. The longer the DNA is exposed to DMBA, the greater the quantity of DMBA that is bound, and the greater the damage to the DNA. Long-lived species, such as humans and elephants, bind much less DMBA and bind it much more slowly and, consequently, they are much more resistant to this genetic (DNA) damage.

interfere with PAH activation and/or binding to DNA, thereby reducing the amount of DNA damage done.

6. Rate and accuracy of repair of ultraviolet (UV) light damage to DNA in seven mammalian species' cultured fibroblasts correlates with maximum species life span. Repair of damage to DNA plays a vital role in retarding aging, although the importance of UV repair to aging is not yet known. Drs. Ronald W. Hart and R. B. Setlow demonstrated a positive correlation between life span and the ability of various species' fibroblasts (including man's) to repair UV damage to their DNA. It is interesting to note that humans live about twice as long as chimpanzees and human DNA repair is about twice as good as that of chimps. Xeroderma pigmentosa is a human genetic (inherited) disease caused by faulty ultraviolet light damage repair. It is a type of progeria (premature aging), not merely a strongly increased tendency to sunburn or contract skin cancer. Figure 3 shows the DNA repair capacity of fibroblasts exposed to ultraviolet light versus life span for a number of mammals, including humans. Man's much greater ability to repair DNA correlates with man's longer life span. The life span increasing effect of a greater DNA repair rate can probably be obtained by a comparable decrease in the DNA damage rate. Our self-administered experimental antioxidant mixture dramatically decreases the damage rate for both ultraviolet light and X-ray damage. In experiments on ourselves, we exhibit a three times greater resistance to both ultraviolet light and X-ray damage as measured by the amount of radiation required for skin erythema (reddening and burning).

7. Superoxide dismutase levels: SOD is an important enzyme which protects the body from the serious damage that would otherwise be caused by superoxide free radicals. These oxygen radicals are constantly being produced by normal processes. Life spans of several mammalian species, including man, have been shown to be directly related to their levels of SOD protection. This tends to lend support to the free radical theory of aging (see Part II, Chapter 7). This also applies to the other antioxidant enzymes so far studied, such as glutathione peroxidase. SOD is the fifth most abundant protein in our bodies, after collagen, albumin, globulin, and hemoglobin.

Surprisingly, people who live in cities with high levels of air pollution (such as Pittsburgh, Pennsylvania; Birmingham, Alabama; Newark, New Jersey; Detroit, Michigan; Los Angeles, California; and Cleveland, Ohio) do not have higher rates of cancer than people living in relatively clean cities, such as San Francisco, California. We and other scientists think that this is so, at least in part, because the presence of the air pollutants (such as ozone, nitrogen oxides, peroxyacetylnitrile, acetaldehyde, etc.) stimulates the body to produce more of protective enzymes, particularly superoxide dismutase.

8. The higher the rate of mutation in reproductive cells (egg and sperm forming), the lower the life span for several species. This supports the aging clock theory, in which the clock monitors and counts mutations in reproductive cells and turns the animal off when the damage becomes so high that it could no longer make a net positive contribution to the existing numbers of its viable (from the standpoint of being reasonably genetically accurate) offspring.

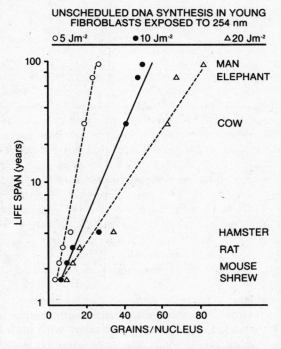

Figure 3. A correlation between the amount of unscheduled DNA synthesis measured at 13 hr after exposure to several UV fluences and the estimated life span of the species

12
Regeneration: Born-Again Limbs and Organs

Jupiter had Prometheus chained to a rock on Mount
Caucasus, where a vulture preyed on his liver, which was
renewed as fast as devoured.

—Greek mythology

*The blueprints for every part of our body are stored on our
DNA. We each developed from a fertilized egg that slowly
unfolded to the complex beings we now are. The program for
this development is still latent in the DNA of our cells. If we
knew how to fully access this program, we could regrow a leg
or any other body part. Regeneration, or the growth of new
cells, tissues, organs, or limbs upon loss of the old ones, is an
ability scientists have recently been learning a lot about. Scientists can now bring about partial regeneration of lost limbs
in adult rats. Using the same principles in humans, they can
make broken bones heal in 80 percent of fractures that have
resisted all other attempts at healing for months or even
years. These techniques will be available to you in the very
near future. The Bristol-Myers Company has already applied
for FDA permission to market an electrical regeneration bone
fracture healing device for implantation in humans. Dr. Bassett of Columbia University has already obtained FDA permission for limited marketing of his externally applied bone
fracture healing electromagnetic pulse regenerator for human use.*

Well-known examples of regeneration are the ability of salamanders to grow a new tail or leg after amputation and of some lizards and snakes to regrow lost tails. What is less well known is that humans have a limited capacity for regeneration. Children under ten years of age who lose the tip of a finger (above the first joint) often regrow a new one; adults cannot do this. Children who lose a permanent tooth while they still have some baby teeth will sometimes grow a second permanent tooth in place of the first one they lost (as happened, in fact, to one of this book's authors). Many children who have their tonsils removed may partially or entirely grow new tonsils. A child whose spleen is removed may grow several mini-spleens to replace it. These regenerative capabilities are mostly lost by adulthood. Adults can regenerate parts of some organs; for example, skin and liver.

Growth of limbs and other parts of the body develop according to the instructions of a DNA developmental program. An embryo begins as a single cell and grows by cell division. The cells divide synchronously, following the DNA blueprint. Up to the embryonic stage in which eight cells exist in a ball (after three cell-doubling divisions), each cell, if separated and allowed to continue dividing, can develop into an entire and normal animal—as happens in the case of identical twins. After this stage, the cells have been changed (differentiated) so that they are more specialized, destined to become a particular tissue type (nerve, muscle, skin, etc.) and can no longer become a whole organism. The developmental program involves a series of differentiations so that cells are eventually highly specialized for a particular function.

The discovery of control mechanisms for this process of differentiation is considered an extremely important area of research. Since each body cell begins with the same DNA as every other cell, they all have the potential to become any type of tissue, but normally this does not happen because of controls stemming from the genetic (DNA) apparatus. Once a cell has become differentiated into, say, a liver cell, it does not normally turn into another type of cell. Some cells, such as muscle cells, do not normally undergo further division, but others, such as skin, divide to form other cells continuously. These latter normally remain differentiated as skin cells.

When some tissues are injured, cells may become de-differentiated, a reversal of differentiation. The de-differentiated cells form a mass of cells called a blastema, which, as healing proceeds, becomes once again differentiated into the type of cells which originally formed it. In order for regeneration of a limb or organ to take place, some of the specialized cells making up the stump must de-differentiate, to return to an earlier stage of the DNA developmental program.

The electrochemical events controlling this process and that of healing are now becoming understood. Bone, for example, shows a piezoelectric property; that is, when bone is bent, an electric potential is created, with a negative charge on the concave side and a positive charge on the convex side. New bone is laid down on the concave, electrically negative side, while old bone is removed from the convex, electrically positive side. In 1972, Dr. Becker and his associates reported the first successful stimulation of organized limb regeneration in mammals. The forelegs of rats were amputated between shoulder and elbow and an electrical stimulation device was implanted at the stump. Most of the animals regrew at least part of the limb, while a few animals regenerated all tissues more or less properly from the stump down to the elbow. Using a similar technique in human patients with pseudoarthrosis (a persistent nonhealing condition of fractures), Dr. Becker achieved an 80-percent success rate in stimulating fracture healing. Dr. Stephen Smith in 1974 reported success in using small direct electric currents (with an implanted electrode in the stump) to stimulate entire limb regeneration in adult frogs, which do not normally regenerate.

Dr. Bassett and his co-workers have successfully used low-average-power high-peak-power pulsed electromagnetic fields to accelerate the healing of fractured bones. They used coils energized by a battery powered semiconductor pulse generator attached externally over the area of the bone break. Bassett also used low-voltage electrical pulses produced externally by magnetic induction to treat adults and children with pseudoarthrosis (non-healing of fractures), with a high (80 percent) success rate.

The Wall Street Journal of 26 March 1979 reports that Bristol-Myers Zimmer Division has applied for FDA approval to market a device that stimulates healing of broken bones with direct electrical currents. Small electrodes are implanted in the broken bone, a procedure which can be performed under local anesthesia.

FIRM HOPES TO MARKET
BONE-GROWTH DEVICE*

By a WALL STREET JOURNAL Staff Reporter

NEW YORK—Bristol-Myers Co. said it applied for federal approval to market a device that uses an electric current to stimulate regrowth of broken bones.

The device is a product of research that in recent years shows that broken bones tend to regrow and heal faster when they are stimulated continuously by direct electrical current. The method appears particularly useful in so-called nonunion fractures in which the bone is broken completely apart. Frequently, nonunion fractures require surgery to install a bone graft.

Stimulation with direct current to induce the nonunion fracture to heal by regrowth avoids the need for bone-graft surgery. The procedure involves only implanting small electrodes to the broken bone, which can be done under local anesthesia.

Bristol-Myers said its Zimmer direct-current bone growth stimulator was developed in conjunction with orthopedists at the University of Pennsylvania medical school. The application to market the device was made to the U.S. Food and Drug Administration by the company's Zimmer USA subsidiary, a maker of surgical and hospital equipment.

Dr. Becker has studied potential (electrical voltage) differences between regenerating salamander limbs and those of nonregenerating frogs. After amputation, the distal (distant from the body) end of the limbs of both salamanders and frogs become highly positive, but the salamander stump tip soon becomes negative. Regeneration in the salamander proceeds most rapidly during the period of greatest negativity, which peaks at about two weeks. Becker found that the presence of nerves is required for this electronegativity, which causes de-differentiation. Interestingly, tumors are also de-differentiated, losing their specialized tissue properties. They behave rather like de-differentiated cells in a wound which never re-differentiate. Vitamin A can cause some epithelial cells (skin, lung, and intestinal lining are examples) which have become precancerous (de-differentiated) to revert to their differentiated normal state. Some tumors have been regressed by the use of electrical fields which stimulate regeneration.

Recently, Dr. Clarence Cone has found that cells can be stimulated to divide by persistent electrical depolarization of the cell membrane (by causing sodium ions to flow into the cell). Even normally nondividing cells, such as neurons, divide when their membranes are depolarized for long enough. Experiments to learn more about how to control cell division, regeneration, differentiation, and tumor growth by this means are under way.

Part of the aging process suggested by Hayflick's work on cell division, discussed in Part II, Chapter 10, is that irreversible differentiation may eventually block cell division and repair, thereby leading to senescence. It will be very interesting to find out whether the regeneration techniques of Bassett, Becker, Cone, and others can affect the limited number of cell divisions found by Hayflick.

Dr. Bassett is currently experimenting with the use of electrical stimulation to regress cancer and to retard aging. At Columbia Presbyterian Hospital in New York City, he has an effective electrical stimulation clinic for patients with hard-to-heal broken bones. Perhaps the broken-hip problem which permanently ends the active life of so many elderly people will succumb to electrotherapy combined with dihydroxy vitamin D. Electrobiology, Inc., a firm partly owned by Dr. Bassett, is currently selling electrical stimulation devices approved by FDA for use in fractures resistant to healing by other therapies. These devices are said to be spreading widely in use in the United States.

13
Aging Theories Revisited

I don't mean to deny that the evidence is in some ways very strongly in favor of your theory. I only wish to point out that there are other theories possible.

    —Sherlock Holmes, *Adventure of the Norwood Builder*

The aim of science is to seek the simplest explanation of complex facts. We are apt to fall into the error of thinking that the facts are simple because simplicity is the goal of our quest. The guiding motto in the life of every natural philosopher should be, seek simplicity and distrust it.

                      —Alfred North Whitehead

Here is a summary of several different ways we age. A chart displays damage-causing agents, the parts of our body they attack, and the resulting deterioration of our body functions.

Aging theories describe different aspects of the aging process, much as in the tale of the blind men and the elephant (Part II, Chapter 1). While each theory can explain some aspects of aging, it can't explain them all. The proliferation of aging theories and the rapid expansion of the data base for the development of theories make many older classifications of these theories piecemeal and overlapping. For example, the free radical theory, the cross-linking theory, the decline of neurotransmitters, and the biological clock theory all involve free radicals, since free radicals can cause cross-linking and can damage DNA and, therefore, affect aging clocks, and

ATTACKING AGENT	TARGET	TYPE OF INTERACTION	RESULT
free radicals	very large information-carrying molecules: DNA and RNA and their associated polypeptides	mutation	improper expression, repression, or derepression of carried information resulting in abnormal cell function, possibly even cancer or cell death
aldehydes	"	"	"
singlet oxygen	"	"	"
excited triplet oxygen	"	"	"
hydrogen peroxide	"	"	"
organic peroxides	"	"	"
nucleic acid analogs	"	"	"
alkylating agents	"	"	"
viruses	"	"	"
polynuclear aromatic hydrocarbons	"	"	"
aldehydes	very large structural molecules, such as collagen (connective tissue) and elastin (skin, blood vessels)	cross-linking (improper chemical connections)	loss of elasticity, increase of ratio of insoluble to soluble protein fraction, increase in hardness, greater tendency to tear

free radicals organic peroxides oxidants	very large structural molecules, such as collagen (connective tissue) and elastin (skin, blood vessels)	cross-linking (improper chemical connections)	loss of elasticity, increase of ratio of insoluble to soluble protein fraction, increase in hardness, greater tendency to tear
free radicals	lipids (fats)	formation of organic peroxides, hydrogen peroxide, and free radicals	possible consequences include blood clots, peroxidized lipids (carcinogens and mutagens), inhibition of macrophages (white blood cells which attack and eat bacteria, viruses, and cancer cells), damage to cell membranes and membrane-bound enzymes, lipofuscin formation
free radicals hydrogen peroxide oxidants	readily autoxidized compounds; example, L-Dopa	autoxidation, with resultant formation of 6-OH-dopamine, hydrogen peroxide, and free radicals	destruction of dopaminergic neurons in brain, possibly resulting in loss of fine motor control, loss of motivation, decline in function of the immune system.

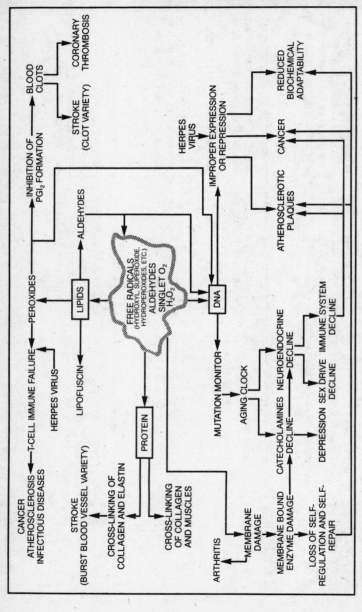

A unified view of aging

may be largely responsible for the damage to neuronal tracts involved in faltering neurotransmitter production and release.

In the two schematic illustrations on pp. 153–55, we summarize several different theories of aging that are somewhat understood and are areas of focus in current gerontological research. The first is a chart that lists attacking agents (the damage-causing entities), subcellular targets for attack by these agents, and the results in terms of aging. (See the individual chapters for details of how these different mechanisms contribute to your aging.) The second is a diagram that represents our own overall view of the interaction of aging processes; that is, who does what to whom. Note that there are many positive feedback loops (circles of cause and effect) which can amplify a modest amount of initial damage into a disaster. Damage begets more damage (as in the howl of a public address system feeding back into the microphone). These positive feedback loops of damage mechanisms may help explain why dying, as opposed to aging, takes such a small part of one's total life span.

PART III
IMPROVING THE QUALITY OF LIFE—IN SICKNESS AND IN HEALTH

I
Some Immediate Benefits of Life Extension Measures

There does not seem to be anything in the nature of the reproduction of tissue which demands its death.... One cause of senility after another will be found and removed, each resulting in only a minor extension of active life. One cannot help wondering what will happen if the causes are all known and found curable. There would be no natural term of life.

—Sir George Thomson, 1937 Nobel Prize winner

Here are a few examples of results you might notice in a short time by taking life extension nutrients. You don't have to wait until you're old to benefit from life extension.

The final proof of the efficacy of an experimental life extension program is, of course, to see how long a follower of that program actually lives. But this may be a very long wait. Consequently, we look at shorter-term changes that may indicate what we can reasonably expect in the long run. With a well-designed life extension regimen, a number of benefits can be expected in a short time.

Take ARTHRITIS, for example. This is usually an autoimmune disease—when part of your immune system attacks part of you (joint membranes and lubricant fluids) instead of undesirables like bacteria, viruses, and cancer cells, you can get arthritis. Such immune system errors in arthritis may in part be due to age-related thymic involution and in part to damage to T-cells caused by free radicals that have been found in arthritic joints. We know that antioxidants (which prevent free radical proliferation) and the proper immune system stimulants can help prevent arthritic attacks. A selection of effective nutrients might include any (preferably all) of the antioxidant vitamins E, A, C, B-1, B-2, B-3, B-5, B-6, calcium pantothenate, PABA, inositol, and selenium, zinc, and cysteine (a sulfur-containing amino acid; do not get cystine, which is the oxidized form of cysteine). (The vitamin niacin, B-3, is not itself an antioxidant but it is used in NADPH, one of your body's natural antioxidants; B-2 is also itself not an antioxidant but is required for the natural antioxidant-recycling enzyme glutathione reductase.) Effective immune stimulant nutrients include C, E, A, selenium, B-1, cysteine, zinc, and arginine or ornithine (amino acids). (See Case Histories in Appendix L.)

Now consider SMOKER'S COUGH. It would be most beneficial, from a life extension standpoint, to stop smoking. But to many people the short-term pleasures and addictive nature of smoking make it unattractive to stop. With proper nutrient supplementation you can get a substantial degree of protection from the damaging effects of smoking (though not 100-percent protection, as yet). The nutrients C, B-1 (a sulfur-containing vitamin), and cysteine (a sulfur-containing amino acid) have been able to protect rats from doses of the chemical acetaldehyde (found in cigarette smoke and also in smog) that killed 90 percent of the control rats (those that did not receive the nutrient supplements). British investigators have found that the acetaldehyde in cigarette smoke actually combines with and destroys cysteine. Cigarette smoke also contains free radicals, which have been detected by electron paramagnetic resonance (epr) spectrometry, so the smoke delivers a double molecular-level injury by simultaneously destroying cysteine and introducing pathological free radicals into the tissues. Vitamins A, C, and E and selenium strongly inhibit carcinogenesis, the process whereby normal cells become cancer cells. The symptoms of smokers' cough can be noticeably alleviated in twenty-four hours with these nutrients. Hydergine® (Sandoz) may be the most powerful antioxidant yet tested. One to three 1-milligram tablets sublingual (held under the tongue) will provide very noticeable smoke protection for your mouth and throat.

Let's think about the effects of aging on OUR APPEARANCE. Under natural conditions, the skin shows age in a variety of unattractive ways, including wrinkling and loss of resiliency, both due to the damage mechanism called cross-linking. (For information on the cross-linking mechanism, see Part II, Chapter 6.) Cross-linking is the process in which proteins are linked together by bonds which prevent them from functioning properly. (This is also what makes your car's windshield-wiper blades, tires, and rubber hoses become brittle and cracked.) Nutrients can be effectively used to inhibit the progression of this mechanism of aging. The tanning of leather is an example of cross-linking; soft supple skin becomes hard, stiff, inelastic shoe leather. Scientists studying the biology of aging have done considerable work in the understanding of cross-linking and the discovery of compounds which can prevent or reverse it. Effective preventive anti-cross-linkers include cysteine, zinc, selenium, vitamins E, C, B-1, and A, and the antioxidant food additives BHT and BHA. Some scientists hope to be able to develop an anti-cross-linking agent that can be put on the skin like a cosmetic but which would actually *unwrinkle* the skin! As mentioned in Part II, Chapter 6, this might be done with proteolytic enzymes—enzymes which dissolve protein, especially those selective for breaking cross-links. Raw pineapple contains bromelain and raw papaya contains papain, both proteolytic enzymes. See Part IV, Chapter 3, "Spices and Other Food Preservatives," for a simple experiment you can do with proteolytic enzymes.

The appearance and condition of SKIN can also be improved quickly with the sodium salt of 2-pyrrolidone-5-carboxylic acid, Na-PCA, the natural humectant (moisturizer) in your skin. As people age, the quantity of Na-PCA decreases, causing the skin to become dry. Old folks typically have about half the Na-PCA in their skin as youngsters. Excessive washing dries your skin because it carries away your Na-PCA. Na-PCA is an ingredient in some premium quality skin-care cosmetics. People used to believe that the oil in skin was what kept it soft and flexible. However, pieces of hardened skin immersed in oils do not regain flexibility. Immersion in water, however, does increase flexibility. The ability of samples of skin to hold moisture is directly related to their content of Na-PCA. A small amount of Na-PCA placed in a bowl and left in the Sahara desert will become a puddle within a few hours because of the water pulled right out of the dry desert air!

How would you like to promptly improve your MENTAL ORGANIZATION, your MEMORY, and your LEARNING ABILITY with a simple nutrient available at many health food and drug stores? Choline has, to a certain extent, done this in human studies. MIT students taking 3 grams of choline a day could learn longer lists of words and could remember better. These results are usually noticeable within a few days. Choline bitartrate, the most common type of choline sold in health food stores, can cause diarrhea. If you use choline bitartrate, you may have to start at a low dose and work it up slowly to avoid diarrhea. Choline chloride (also called choline hydrochloride) does not have this side effect. One friend of ours was a man of few words before he began using choline. After taking 4 to 5 grams a day of choline for a few days, he told us that his speaking vocabulary had increased markedly and that he had become a smooth and eloquent speaker. As he put it, "I couldn't shut myself up!" (See Case Histories in Appendix L.) Choline is also of significant value to many aged patients with memory difficulties. For more about this, see Part II, Chapter 9, and Part III, Chapters 2 and 3. Choline may have a slight drawback for some people because action by bacteria in the intestinal tract can change it into an unpleasant fishy-smelling substance called trimethylamine. This has not happened to most people we know who are using choline. However, it has been reported (in Wurtman and Wurtman's *Nutrition and the Brain*, Raven Press, 1979) that most patients ingesting choline chloride did have this problem. One difference between these patients and people we know who use choline is that the latter group is also taking other nutrients along with the choline. If a fishy smell is a problem for you, try altering your gut bacteria with yogurt, extra dietary fiber, and vitamin supplements.

Even faster MENTAL IMPROVEMENT can be obtained with the hormone vasopressin, released by the brain's pituitary gland and also available in a nasal spray (Diapid®, a prescription drug made by Sandoz). In one study, men in their 50s and 60s taking 16 I.U. of Diapid® nasal spray per day had significant improvements in memory and learning and decreased reaction time (the men were faster!). In several cases of accident-induced amnesia, people recovered their memory in only hours to days after using Diapid®. A nurse we met had suffered amnesia as a result of an automobile accident which covered a period of months, both before and after the accident. Within *seconds* after using the vasopressin nasal spray, she told us that she could feel her mind clearing as if a fog had lifted.

GENERAL STAMINA can be greatly increased in a short period of time. For example, calcium pantothenate, the anti-stress and life extension vitamin, has been shown to increase total muscular output (stamina rather than peak output) in frog leg muscles suspended in a pantothenate solution. Rats taking pantothenate supplements increase their total muscular work output very significantly under conditions of extreme stress (swimming in cold water). Pantothenate plays the same chemical role in human metabolism as in these other animals. It is required for metabolizing fats and carbohydrates to energy and water and carbon dioxide. Thus, people with low energy may have a deficiency of pantothenate. (See Part III, Chapter 9.) CAUTION: Low energy may also be a symptom of diabetes mellitus (sugar-insulin diabetes) or anemia, so be sure to have your doctor give you a complete physical exam if you suffer from chronic fatigue.

You might also increase ENERGY and MOTIVATION to exercise with the nutrient L-Dopa (an amino acid prescription drug). This nutrient may help you put on muscles while eliminating fat. One of its effects is stimulating the release of growth hormone from the pituitary gland in your brain. This hormone is necessary to increase muscle mass, as well as for healing and proper function of the immune system. With L-Dopa, you can get all charged up by exercising and go on and on. Old rats given L-Dopa were able to swim as long and as well as young rats not given L-Dopa. Before receiving the L-Dopa, though, these old rats swam less efficiently and for a much shorter time than the young rats. See Part III, Chapters 8 and 9 on exercise and athletics for further information.

Pantothenate (vitamin B-5) is also essential in the manufacture of fats and oils which are an important part of your skin. Antioxidant nutrients, particularly A, C, E, B-1, B-5, B-6, PABA, zinc, and selenium, protect these fats and oils from free radical autoxidation which causes them to polymerize (join together), like hardening oil paint or epoxy resin, and become less elastic. Vitamin A increases the number of receptors for epidermal growth factor (EGF), a natural hormone which makes your skin grow and heal, thereby increasing your skin's response to a given amount of EGF. Added EGF can slow an aging clock in skin cells in tissue culture, tripling their life span from about 50 to about 150 generations. The use of proper doses of these nutrients can in many cases make your skin feel and look younger within two weeks while, at the same time, slowing further aging.

By intervening in any of these areas, we are taking active steps against our own aging. We can see benefits in the short term, as well as in the more distant future. Aging is made up of a collection of different aging systems. These examples are some of those in which we understand much of the chemistry of the aging events. By understanding mechanisms of action, we can take intelligent steps to intervene. These intelligent steps include the acquisition of more knowledge and our often-cited admonitions to have clinical laboratory tests along with your physician's consultations.

2
Revitalizing Your Brain Power

The mind so strongly depends on temperament and the
disposition of bodily organs, that if it is possible to find
some means which will make men generally more wise
and more clever than they have been till now, I believe
that it is in medicine one should seek it. . . . It is true that
the medicine now practiced contains few things having so
remarkable a usefulness. But, without having any intention
of scorning it, I am confident that there is no one, even
among those whose profession it is, who does not admit
that everything already known about it is almost nothing
in comparison with what remains to be learned, and that
people could be spared an infinity of diseases, both bodily
and mental, and perhaps even the weakening of old age, if
the causes of those troubles and all the remedies with
which nature has provided us were sufficiently well
known.

—René Descartes, *Discourse on Method* (1637)

Are there nutrients and prescription drugs which can im-
prove memory and learning abilities in normal healthy peo-
ple? Yes, there certainly are. We even have a fair
understanding of how some of these biochemicals work in the
brain. Imagine what would be possible for you if you were
more intelligent. Well, this is no dream. Whether you are
young or old, you can improve your mental function right
now by following the suggestions given in this chapter.

In natural aging, your mental functions decline along
with other bodily processes. In fact, many people are more

concerned about senility than about any other infirmity of age. It is particularly sad to see once alert and active parents, relatives, or friends become confused, forgetful, and apathetic. Advancing senility is truly a type of living death in which a once intelligent and alert person gradually turns into a shuffling zombie. Fortunately it is possible with present knowledge to avoid substantially or to delay the natural mental and emotional ravages of aging and even to partially reverse some of the aging damage that may already have occurred in the brain.

CAUTION: Before you assume that any declining mental functions are really due to your age, be sure to consult with your doctor. Increasing forgetfullness, being "too tired" to learn something new, and other symptoms may in fact be due to other conditions such as anemia and diabetes mellitus. If you practice "self-diagnosis," you might be wrong and neglect an important medical disorder. Diagnosis is definitely for professionals.

There are over a dozen chemicals that have been demonstrated to improve animal and/or human intelligence (learning and data processing in particular types of tasks). These include RNA (ribonucleic acid), Isoprinosine® (Newport Pharmaceuticals International, Inc.), vasopressin (Diapid® nasal spray, made by Sandoz), Hydergine® (Sandoz), PRL-8-53, L-prolyl L-leucyl glycine amide (three amino acids strung together to form a tripeptide), Deaner® (Riker), lecithin, choline, amphetamines and related compounds, magnesium pemoline (Cylert® by Abbott), diphenylhydantoin, Ritalin® (Ciba), vitamin B-12, ACTH 4-10, Nootropyl® (UCB), caffeine, Metrazol®, and strychnine (the last two are *extremely* dangerous). There are others, but these compounds are the most interesting to us. Many of them have been used successfully to reverse some manifestations of brain aging in humans. This is due to the fact that some mechanisms of brain aging involve reduction in the quantity and availability of—or receptor sensitivity to—certain brain chemicals. Supplements of these natural brain chemicals or their analogs (similar molecules) or their precursors (molecules that the brain can convert into chemicals it needs) can sometimes be used to replace the missing compounds, resulting in improved mental function. Even in young persons, supplies of neurochemicals are limited—they are costly for the body to make—and mental performance can sometimes be substantially improved by taking such supplements.

For each neurochemical there is an optimal amount which differs for every individual. Above or below this amount, mental function will not improve markedly or will even decrease. Drug effects may be subtle at first, requiring a period of learning for full realization of its benefits.

The schematic diagram in Part II, Chapter 9, "Decline of the Brain's Chemical Messengers," shows how neurotransmitters carry messages between neurons in the brain. An incoming electric impulse stimulates the transmitter neuron to release the message-carrying neurotransmitter chemical from the packets (vesicles) in which it is stored. The neurotransmitter molecules are released into the gap (synapse) between the nerve endings and then bind to the receptors on the nearby receiver neuron. This second neuron is then stimulated by the neurotransmitter in its receptors to fire an electric impulse, which begins the process over again. In other cases, the receiver neuron releases a hormone signal instead of sending out another electric signal. The left-over neurotransmitter in the synapse is either destroyed by an enzyme or recycled back into the transmitter vesicles. Because of recent advances in our understanding of these events, it is now possible to modify some aging changes in the brain's neurochemistry.

Although much remains to be learned in the neurochemistry of memory, a modest amount is understood about how memories are stored and retrieved in the brain. Specific chemicals that are involved have been isolated, and their loss in aging may be compensated for by replacing them with supplemental drugs and nutrients. RNA synthesis is required for memory, and RNA may be a memory-storage molecule; the brain may encode RNA molecules with memory "messages." As people age, they produce less RNA and, consequently, have less RNA available for use in storing memories. In addition to its memory-storage ability, RNA is also an antioxidant that experiments have shown is capable of increasing the life span of rats by about 20 percent. RNA is one nonprescription chemical available in health food stores that we can use to help keep our minds functioning at a level younger than our years.

CAUTION: RNA, however, should not be used by individuals with gout. If gout runs in your family, it is very important to have your doctor test you before taking RNA. When nucleic acids are metabolized, uric acid is formed which, in excessive concentration, can precipitate in joints and kidneys, leading to disability and severe pain. Permanent damage can be done to the joints and kidneys by these crystals. Moreover, the oxidation of RNA to uric acid by the enzyme xanthine oxidase also releases hydrogen peroxide and free radicals. Before using RNA, have an inexpensive clinical laboratory blood test for uric acid. If your serum uric acid and kidneys are normal, you should be able to use oral RNA. (Severe allergic reactions sometimes occur with RNA injections.)

Even if RNA is contraindicated for you, you can take vitamin B-12, which stimulates RNA synthesis in brain neurons. Its administration in rats increased their rate of learning. A dose of 1,000 micrograms (1 milligram) is a reasonable daily dose for an adult human. We know of no evidence that B-12 poses a hazard to people with gout, but suggest that such people watch their urate level while using B-12 to see that it doesn't rise.

Another chemical system involved in memory consolidation (transfer of short-term memories into long-term storage) is the cholinergic system. Acetylcholine is a neurotransmitter in the brain which is thought to be centrally involved in memory. Experiments in humans in which the anticholinergic drug scopolamine was administered to healthy young persons resulted in a pattern of memory deficit that was very like that of senile old age. The nutrients choline and lecithin (which contains phosphatidyl choline) and the drug Deaner® can supply the brain with the choline it needs to manufacture acetylcholine. Plenty of vitamin B-5 (calcium pantothenate or pantothenic acid) is required for this conversion. See Part III, Chapter 3, "Depression, Helplessness, and Aging," for further details. In a very recent mouse study, 13-month-old mice on a choline-enriched diet performed as well as 3-month-old mice on a learning retention task, whereas 13-month-old mice on a choline-deficient diet performed as poorly as senescent (23 months and older) mice. A choline-deficient diet in younger animals may result in learning retention more typical of that of older animals because the older animals cannot produce as much acetylcholine in their brains. Choline has been experimentally demonstrated in humans to improve memory and serial-type learning (a series of words, for example). A single oral dose of 10 grams of choline produced these results. In a study mentioned earlier involving MIT students, 3 grams per day was effective in improving memory and serial learning. The old wives' tale that fish is brain food really has a degree of truth, since fish contains relatively large quantities of both choline and RNA.

As noted in the preceding chapter, choline bitartrate, the most common type of choline sold at health food stores, can cause diarrhea. If you do use it, you may be able to avoid diarrhea by beginning at a low dose and increasing the amount gradually. Choline chloride (also called choline hydrochloride) does not have this side effect. Lecithin was found to be effective at a dose of 80 grams per day in a separate study. The prescription drug Deaner® (Riker) is very effective in increasing the level of cholinergic activity in the brain. Deaner® has also been found to extend the life span of mice by 49.5 percent in one experimental series and by 27.3 percent in another series. Most importantly, the maximum life span of the mice was increased in both experiments—by 36.3 percent and 26.5 percent respectively.

Another important brain chemical in learning and memory is norepinephrine, NE, another neurotransmitter. In experiments in which NE synthesis was blocked or depleted in the brain, memory was impaired. When NE was injected into a specific area in the brain of rats, their memories were enhanced. As we discussed in Part II, Chapter 9, on the brain's chemical messengers, NE is used by certain neurons in the brain to communicate with one another. The messenger chemical is stored in pouches called vesicles on the surface of the neuron's cellular membrane and released into the gaps between nerves (synapses) when the nerves fire. Many popular stimulant drugs increase the level of NE in these synapses, resulting in greater nerve stimulation. Such drugs include amphetamines, Ritalin® (Ciba), phenylpropanolamine (an amphetaminelike compound in many over-the-counter diet aids), magnesium pemoline, and cocaine. These can temporarily improve learning in focusing and attention tasks, as well as memory. However, these effects may be due to general stimulation rather than altered data processing by the nerves. A serious disadvantage of these drugs is that once the stored supply of NE has been released from the vesicles and the NE in the synapses has been metabolized, the drugs no longer stimulate nerve activity (this process is called "tolerance") until the body produces more NE. Depression is very common during the period when NE supply is low owing to the excessive use of the stimulants mentioned above. In addition to causing unpleasant feelings of depression, NE depletion in the brain severely impairs the performance of your immune system because of the brain's failure to send the thymus gland the proper hormone signals. The same growth hormone signal needed by your thymus is also needed for tissue repair; hence stimulant abuse has very serious health consequences. Hyperkinetic children chronically treated with amphetamines or Ritalin® in modest doses often exhibit significant growth retardation over the years. The typical stimulant abuser takes much larger doses; hence the long-term health consequences are apt to be quite severe.

Phenylalanine, an amino acid the brain uses to make NE, can relieve or prevent depressions caused by NE depletion. Typical human doses are 100 to 1,000 milligrams per day, taken either on an empty stomach at bedtime or immediately upon awakening. **CAUTION:** Overdose symptoms are irritability, insomnia, and, rarely, elevated blood pressure. People with high blood pressure should be very cautious about using phenylalanine. They should start with very low doses (100 milligrams) and check their blood pressure frequently as they very gradually increase the dose. Phenylalanine is also useful in restoring energy and vitality after stressful activities. It can provide a lift so that you hop out of bed in the morning instead of dragging yourself out. It is excellent for writer's block, a malady to which we sometimes fall prey. Stress and overwork deplete NE, resulting in mental fatigue and loss of concentration. Phenylalanine helps your brain to replace the lost NE. When you feel mentally "drained," you may be suffering from a drain on your NE stores which has exceeded your brain's ability to replace. You can literally refill the storage pouches on your nerves by using the nonprescription nutrient amino acid phenylalanine. Plenty of vitamin C and B-6 are required for the conversion of phenylalanine and tyrosine to NE. See Part III, Chapter 3, for more information on the use of phenylalanine in depression. The amino acid tyrosine is chemically one step closer to NE than is phenylalanine and has shown antidepressant effects in human studies. It seems, however, more likely to affect blood pressure, elevating it in some people and lowering it in others. **WARNING:** Neither phenylalanine or tyrosine should be used by people taking powerful MAO (monamine oxidase) inhibitors, drugs which are rarely used now in the treatment of depression; extremely hazardous high blood pressure could result.

Recently a new drug was added to the pharmacopoeia of memory-improving drugs: vasopressin. Vasopressin is a natural pituitary-gland hormone which is best known for its regulation of urine volume. It is approved by the FDA for treating diabetes insipidus, a condition of frequent urination (not related to insulin-sugar diabetes) caused by inadequate quantities of vasopressin. A dose of hundreds of units of vasopressin injected intravenously can increase blood pressure. In doses of 16 units a day, vasopressin was found to significantly improve memory and learning in men in their 50s and 60s without any effect upon blood pressure or urine volume. The vasopressin was administered as a nasal spray (Diapid®, made by Sandoz); the dose of 16 I.U. was equivalent to about one spray in each nostril four times a day. We ourselves take daily doses of Diapid® totaling about 40 to 80 I.U. Vasopressin nasal spray has been used to restore memory in amnesia victims (within hours or days). While visiting a doctor in northern California recently, we had occasion to meet and talk with a young nurse, whom we have mentioned elsewhere. She had been in a serious automobile accident about six months before and had suffered head injuries resulting in amnesia, retaining little or no memory of the events that occurred a few months before and after the accident. Within a few seconds of taking a single spray of vasopressin up each nostril, she said, "I can feel a fog lifting in my mind."

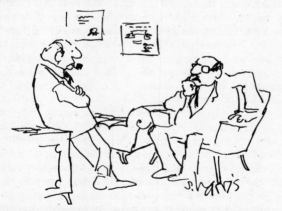

"I can't remember the last time I treated a case of amnesia, and I can't even remember if I ever did treat one."

CAUTION: In patients with angina, use of even small amounts of vasopressin may stimulate angina pains; therefore, its use should be restricted in such cases, even though the clinical literature generally considers these effects to be harmless. Otherwise, there are no contraindications to the use of vasopressin when used at the levels discussed. Caution should be exercised not to "snort" it vigorously, since it can then reach your larynx in a dose large enough to cause laryngeal spasm; this has been reported. Occasionally intestinal cramping or nasal irritation may occur. Diapid® is not approved by FDA for use as a memory- and intelligence-increasing drug, but only for the treatment of diabetes insipidus.

Vasopressin is released by the pituitary gland during trauma (or even in anticipation of severe trauma) and hemorrhage. The dramatic experience that accident victims sometimes report, that "my life flashed before my eyes," may be due to the effects of vasopressin. Vasopressin is also released by the popular drugs LSD, amphetamine, Ritalin®, magnesium pemoline, and cocaine. However, after regular use of cocaine or these other stimulant drugs, vasopressin and NE supplies are depleted, which results in depression. This does not happen with Diapid® because it actually *is* vasopressin, not merely a drug which speeds up its release and destruction. Alcohol and marijuana inhibit vasopressin release, which may explain at least in part why people have memory difficulties when using these drugs. Diapid® will significantly reduce the deleterious effects of alcohol on reaction time and attention. Drinking and driving can still remain lethal, but we would rather encounter a driver on the road who has used both Diapid® and alcohol than one who has had alcohol alone. The orgasm-dulling effects of alcohol are also ameliorated with Diapid®.

One of the effects of aging on the brain that has been most extensively investigated is the accumulation of aging pigment in nerve cells. As we discussed in Part II, Chapter 8, the pigment called lipofuscin is a cellular waste product made up of cross-linked proteins and peroxidized fats. Lipofuscin pigment also collects in skin cells, where it is often called "aging spots" or "liver spots." Although it has not yet been unequivocally proved that lipofuscin causes damage to nerve cells in which it is found, it is generally thought by biological gerontologists that the presence of this material (up to 75 percent or so of the cell volume may be taken up by lipofuscin in old age) leads to seriously disrupted cell function. See the figure showing this effect in Part II, Chapter 8. The body has natural processes by which it removes lipofuscin from cells, involving detergentlike compounds. However, the rate of removal falls farther and farther behind the rate of accumulation. (Even a 3-month-old fetus may have some lipofuscin in some of its nerve cells!) The cholinergic drugs Deaner® and centrophenoxine have been experimentally shown in animals to speed up lipofuscin removal from nerve and skin cells. You can see the brown age spots fade away in the skin over a period of several months to a couple of years. (Freckles, birthmarks, and normal skin pigment are melanin rather than lipofuscin and do not fade away.) The removal of age spots can be achieved in humans through the use of at least 300 milligrams of Deaner® per day plus plenty of nutrient antioxidants, such as vitamins A, B-1, B-5, B-6, C, and E, the minerals zinc and selenium, and so on.

The peroxidation (uncontrolled oxidation) of fatty acids in the brain is probably a causative factor in the development of sensory and cognitive deficits in old age. If so, much of this damage is preventable using antioxidants. In experiments with rats, polyunsaturated fatty acids derived from precursors of linolenic and linoleic acids (found in safflower oil, for example) were found to be important functional components of photoreceptor cell membranes in the eye. The position and number of unsaturated bonds appeared to control the electrical response of the photoreceptor cell membrane. Similar results have been found for the "hair cells" of the cochlea—in the human ear. The sound-sensing nerves in the ear require these highly unsaturated (and highly subject to peroxidation) fatty acids. Zinc deficiency seems to play a role in the loss of taste and odor perception, and zinc helps protect lipids from peroxidation as a part of the antioxidant-enzyme superoxide dismutase.

A drug which can improve brain function is Hydergine®, the prescription drug also produced by Sandoz that has appeared frequently in earlier chapters. As we have mentioned before, this drug has few side effects (it should not be used by persons sensitive to it and in acute or chronic psychosis) and has been used for many years by patients in the United States and Europe. According to a Sandoz representative, Hydergine® is the world's fifth most popular prescription drug. Hydergine® is used for several disparate disorders, but its versatility is less well known in the United States due to FDA restrictions on advertising claims. Hydergine® affects both the noradrenergic (NE) and the dopaminergic nervous systems in the brain. The dopaminergic system is involved in emotions, motivation, brain-stem autonomic activities (the monitoring of breathing, for example), ambitious and aggressive drives, hunger and eating, sexual drive, territoriality, motor activity, and stimulation of release of hormones such as growth hormone. Hydergine® seems to modulate nerve-cell control mechanisms so that the cellular response to the other neural stimuli is neither too great nor too little. Hydergine® "normalizes" the cellular control mechanism involving cyclic AMP, the "second messenger" that responds to nerve signals by carrying the message from the nerve cell's outer membrane to the cell's internal machinery. Although caffeine affects neurons by a similar mechanism, also involving cyclic AMP, Hydergine® acts more selectively than caffeine and hence does not cause the letdowns and jitters that occur after drinking too much coffee.

Hydergine® can do a number of things to help prevent or correct aging in the brain. It increases protein synthesis in the brain (required for memory), stabilizes brain EEG energies even under conditions of low oxygen supply (such as shock, atherosclerosis, drowning, heart attack, emphysema, or stroke), slows by a factor of about four the rate of formation of the age pigment lipofuscin in the brain, improves memory and learning, and stimulates the growth of neurites (nerve cell connections required for forming new memories that are gradually lost during aging). Both the brain's own natural hormone nerve growth factor (NGF) and Hydergine® seem to work by the same biochemical pathway to cause neurite growth. The greatest levels of NGF and highest numbers of neurites in the human brain are found in 2-year-olds. Without a supplement of an NGF-like substance such as Hydergine®, to boost neurite growth, it's downhill all the way after the age of 2. Hydergine® may help you regain that effortless learning ability you had as a child. With Hydergine® therapy it may take at least six months to two years for the regeneration of neurites to achieve optimal improvement in mental function.

Hydergine® can also be of value in hypoglycemia because it helps stabilize the brain's response to energy supply— the brain is normally the part of the body most sensitive to low blood sugar. People who are unable to obtain adequate oxygen because of heavy smoking (the carbon monoxide destroys the oxygen-carrying hemoglobin in the blood and the oxidants can cause emphysema by cross-linking lung tissue), air pollution, or lung diseases can help maintain normal brain energy output with Hydergine®.

In an Italian clinical trial studying the effects of Hydergine® on patients with cerebral arteriosclerosis, the symptoms reported to be significantly improved included headache, dizziness, tinnitus (ringing in the ears), and visual and memory disorders. No side effects were observed at the dose of Hydergine® used (two times daily 300 micrograms of Hydergine® injected intramuscularly for 10 days followed by three times daily 1 milligram Hydergine® orally for the following 10 days).

In France, an indication for the use of Hydergine® is "re-animation," meaning that it can be used to bring very recently dead persons back to life in conjunction with other methods. The basis for this is that, in conditions where oxygen is not adequately supplied to the brain, normally irreversible free radical brain damage begins to occur after about five minutes. However, if Hydergine® can be injected into the carotid artery within a few minutes after death, the brain will not begin to suffer irreversible damage for about thirty minutes. Closed-chest cardiopulmonary resuscitation (CPR) circulates both Hydergine® and more oxygen to the brain. (See Part III, Chapter 20, "First Aid.") Since Hydergine® is a powerful stabilizer of brain metabolism as measured by EEG energy output, French doctors administer it to preoperative patients so that if a crisis such as cardiac arrest occurs while they are on the operating table, the doctors will have more time to handle the situation before they have to worry about brain damage.

The FDA-approved dose of Hydergine® in the United States is 3 milligrams a day; in Europe, the typical dose is 9 milligrams a day. Dramatic effects will probably not be achieved below the typical European dose. Each of us usually takes 20 milligrams per day (10 after breakfast and 10 after lunch for Durk; 7 after breakfast, 9 after lunch, and 3 to 5 after dinner for Sandy). We use Hydergine® in the sublingual form, which means that the tablet is held in the mouth to dissolve, rather than swallowed as in the oral form. If you use the oral form of Hydergine®, you should know that 20 percent will be eliminated in the feces, another 40 percent will be destroyed in the liver, leaving only 40 percent left for the rest of the body, including the brain. The sublingual form gets much more Hydergine® into the brain. However, alcoholics probably should use both oral and sublingual forms because the Hydergine® that gets into the liver provides some protection against the toxic effects of acetaldehyde (a product of alcohol metabolism in the liver). As with all drugs, including nutrients, it is usually best to start at a low dose (perhaps a 1-milligram sublingual tablet a day to start) and increase the daily dose gradually. Although Hydergine® has no toxic effects, annoying nausea or headache may occasionally occur if too much is taken too soon. The use of caffeine in conjunction with Hydergine® is safe, but it does lead to strong potentiation of caffeine's effects. If you develop headache, insomnia, or a "wired" overstimulated feeling, simply discontinue coffee, tea, and cola drinks, at least for a few days.

In a recent study, 12 milligrams a day of Hydergine® (sublingual form) for two weeks resulted in improved performance in normal human volunteers on a variety of tasks requiring alertness and cognitive abilities. As mentioned earlier, although some improvement with Hydergine® is nearly immediate, the full benefits that result, we believe, from increased neurite growth may take from a few months to two years to manifest themselves. We personally know three cases of improvement in sensory function, two involving hearing loss and another involving a man who had had no sense of smell from as early as he could remember to his mid-30s. In one case a man of 32 who had had an inner-ear infection at the age of 12 had suffered severe hearing losses (up to about 90 decibels at mid to high frequencies) in both ears. After taking sublingual Hydergine® for a few months at doses of 12 to 20 milligrams and occasionally more per day, he started hearing high-pitched sounds he hadn't been able to hear for about twenty years. In fact, he had to move to a different neighborhood because the old one now sounded too noisy. The other case of hearing loss was a woman of 36 who had had 6,600-rad X-ray radiation treatment for a salivary-gland tumor. The radiation had severely damaged her inner ear and auditory nerve, although her doctors had not warned her of this side effect of the radiation. Shortly after completing the 6,600-rad X-ray radiation treatment, she experienced tinnitus (ringing) in first one ear and then the other. Eventually her right ear became profoundly deaf to high frequencies, even at levels over 90 decibels, and there was a major loss in her left ear as well. Although her hearing is still below normal, she can hear higher frequencies now after several months of taking 12 to 20 milligrams a day of sublingual Hydergine®. As for the man who was born without a sense of smell, he began taking Hydergine® to improve his mental function and retard brain aging, not thinking that it might have any influence on his missing sense of smell. Before starting Hydergine® therapy he couldn't even smell ammonia, although he felt the burning irritation it caused in his nasal passages. After using 12 milligrams a day of sublingual Hydergine® for a few months, he could smell a banana after peeling it and could not only smell acetone and rubbing alcohol but even discriminate between them—a particularly impressive distinction because these two aromas are quite similar.

Be sure to ask for the Sandoz Hydergine®, because generics are not considered pharmaceutically equivalent (see Part V, Chapter 11, "Caveat Emptor"). Have your doctor specify "no substitutes" in writing on your prescription. Without a written order for "Sandoz Hydergine®—no substitutes," you may be given a generic in California and some other states, even if the prescription says "Hydergine." All the research in the scientific literature and all our own research was done with Sandoz Hydergine®. Although most generics are equivalent to the brand name drugs, there are significant chemical differences between Hydergine® and its generic look-alikes.

Psychopharmacology, the science of drugs which affect psychological functions, offers other interesting materials. The amino acid tryptophan is a safe, nonaddictive sleeping aid which works because it is made into serotonin in the brain. Serotonin is the neurotransmitter which initiates sleep. Tryptophan is found in milk and bananas and can sometimes be purchased in pill form. Two grams of tryptophan just before bed is very helpful in getting to sleep. For best results, take it on an empty stomach. Although milk contains tryptophan, the pure amino acid is more effective. Amino acids have to compete with one another to get into the brain, depending on their electrical charge. Since milk contains a number of amino acids, tryptophan has to compete to get into the brain. With the pure amino acid, you get more of the tryptophan into the brain where you want it. If you take too much tryptophan, you can get headaches, sinus congestion, or constipation. (See Part III, Chapter 4, for more information on sleep problems.)

ACTH 4-10, a seven-amino-acid polypeptide (small protein) section of the pituitary gland's ACTH (adrenocorticotropic hormone) and the tripeptide L-prolyl L-leucyl glycine amide provide learning enhancements in animals and humans. These drugs are very expensive at present and are therefore not really practical for experimentation. However, polypeptide synthesizers are dropping in price rapidly, despite inflation. A polypeptide synthesizer (a small Japanese tabletop model made by Peninsula Laboratories) is now available for less than $2,500 (see Appendix I). Clearly, ACTH 4-10 and other peptides will be much more available in the near future, though this availability may be confined to the gray and black markets because it would be very difficult for their manufacturers to obtain permission from the FDA to market these neurochemicals. This is most unfortunate since it is much more difficult for consumers to ascertain the quality of products offered in the gray and black markets than in the open marketplace, where large pharmaceutical firms with long-standing track records for quality supply such products. Of course, large-scale manufacture—if and when permitted—would be performed with genetically engineered microbes using equipment much like that found in a brewery or antibiotic factory.

All the above-mentioned drugs represent just the beginning of mind-enhancing technology. Research is currently underway on all types of mood control, creativity, and anti-aging neurochemical compounds. One experimental drug, PRL-8-53, has improved recall in human subjects by as much as 150 percent. The typical healthy adult human can immediately learn a string of about eight digits. With PRL-8-53, one might be able to learn around twenty digits at a glance. When this becomes available on the black market, we expect it to completely replace far less effective amphetamine and Ritalin® use by students cramming for college tests. The opportunity to choose what you want to be is expanding rapidly. The first step you need to take in order to profit from all these advances is to decide what you want to be—and one thing's for sure: you don't want to be senile.

3
Depression, Helplessness, and Aging

The drive to resist compulsion is more important to wild animals than sex, food, or water. He [J. L. Kavanau] found that captive white-footed mice spent inordinate time and energy just resisting experimental manipulation. If the experimenters turned the lights up, the mouse spent his time setting them down. If the experimenters turned the lights down, the mouse turned them up. . . .

A drive for competence or to resist compulsion is . . . a drive to avoid helplessness.

—Martin E. P. Seligman, *Helplessness*

When supplies of certain chemicals made by our brains become depleted, depression can result. When this happens, not only are we emotionally depressed, but our immune systems are also depressed, resulting in a decreased ability to fight off infectious diseases and even cancer. As we age, our brain's ability to produce and respond to many brain chemicals falls off, making depression more likely. Read on to find out what you can do about your own depressions.

We have three reasons for including a separate chapter on depression in this book about life extension: (1) you would not want to live a long time if you were depressed, (2) depression is much more common in old age, and (3) depression has a major deleterious effect on general health and on the probability of surviving stresses.

When events are outside our control, we are helpless. The state of being helpless or believing that one is helpless (even if it is not really true) can cause depression, illness, and sudden death in experimental animals and in people.

Dr. J. M. Weiss believes that the negative physiological consequences of helplessness are caused by depletion of norepinephrine (NE) in the brain. After plunging rats into very cold water for six minutes, he tested their ability to escape shock in a shuttle box which had a low barrier that the animal would have to leap over to reach a shock-free area. These rats displayed helplessness (inability to escape shock by jumping over the low barrier). When measured the NE in the brains of these rats was found to be depleted. Rats that were put into warm water for six minutes did not suffer from NE depletion or from helplessness in the shuttle box (they successfully escaped the shock by jumping the barrier). In later experiments, an NE depletor, alpha-methyl-para-tyrosine, administered to rats also caused failure to escape shock in the shuttle box. If NE depletion is significantly involved in the biochemical events of learned helplessness, then phenylalanine or tyrosine, essential nutrient amino acids used by the brain to make NE, should be very effective in relieving human depressions from a variety of causes.

CAUTION: It is important to keep in mind that serious depression often requires professional help. The points raised in this chapter are not intended as a substitute for those patients in need of help from a psychiatrist or a clinical psychologist. The ideas in this chapter are *not* intended as a guide for any psychotic condition, including manic-depressive psychosis (for which lithium therapy is often most appropriate); professional help is necessary in such conditions.

Helplessness develops when animals or people believe that their success or failure is independent of their efforts. In such a circumstance, there is no incentive to act. Voodoo, in anecdotal reports, may kill its victims in this way—they believe they cannot help dying, so they die. The children of rich parents can suffer from helplessness, even though they have many material advantages, because this wealth has no correspondence to their own efforts to succeed.

Death from helplessness has been widely observed in animals and people. In one study, wild rats forced to swim until exhaustion lasted for 60 hours before they drowned. Rats that were first held firmly in the investigator' hand until they

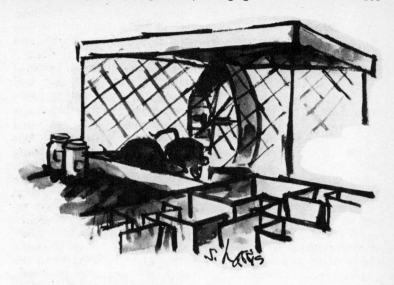

"Treadmills! Mazes! There must be more to life than this."

stopped struggling, and were then put in the water, swam frantically for about 30 minutes, then drowned. Some even died in the hand, before being put in the water. The handled rats behaved as if they were helpless. If the rats were handled but allowed to wriggle out of the experimenter's hand so that they "thought" they "escaped," helplessness did not occur even though the amount of handling was identical. It is a common observation that elderly people in reasonably good health often die very soon after they are placed in a nursing home. People may die of terminal illness just after reaching a meaningful milestone, such as the birth of a child or the celebration of a holiday.

During the year following a major crisis, such as the loss of a loved one, the chances of a serious accident or illness—including cardiovascular disease or cancer—leading to death are markedly increased.

Although it is difficult to ascertain cause and effect, it is noteworthy that in depressed persons the immune system is depressed in its responses to disease and cancer. The useful technique of training cancer victims to focus mentally on their white cells attacking their cancer may be based on the beneficial effects of the improved mental state on the immune system, although advocates of this therapy may not know of this mechanism. They sometimes attribute the beneficial results to some sort of mystic powers. It is also possible that a more positive attitude, engendered by this technique, may simply have led to improved appetites and better nutrition. Among 51 women whose pap-smear cancer checkups had revealed the presence of "suspicious-looking" cervical cells, 18 had suffered a significant personal loss in the previous six months. Of these 18 patients, 11 developed cancer, while only 8 of the other 33 patients, who had not experienced helplessness, developed cancer. Depression does not cause diseases such as cancer, but depression can reduce the effectiveness of your body's protective response to these conditions.

Here is how you might be able to better handle depression. Chemicals in the brain called neurotransmitters transmit the signals from one nerve cell to another. MAO (monamine oxidase) is an enzyme in the brain which degrades the monamine neurotransmitters dopamine, norepinephrine (NE), and serotonin. This enzyme increases in activity with age, thus resulting in lowered levels of these signal-transmitting brain chemicals. Increasing the available supply of monamines by inhibiting MAO has proved of significant benefit in many depressed persons. Procaine—or the procaine compound Gerovital (GH3) developed by Dr. Ana Aslan of Romania—is a mild reversible MAO inhibitor. When using most MAO inhibitors, it is necessary to avoid excessive dietary intake of monamine precursors such as the amino acids tyrosine and phenylalanine to avoid too high levels of the monamines, which can lead to higher blood pressure. Procaine—or GH3—does not seem to require this precaution. Tricyclic antidepressants (such as imipramine) inhibit the reuptake of norepinephrine at synaptic terminals (see diagram in Part II, Chapter 9, "Decline of the Brain's Chemical Messengers"), so that there is an increased concentration of NE at the receptor.

We have had experience with several antidepressive nutrients and drugs. Phenylalanine, an amino acid found in relatively large amounts in meat, milk, cheese, and some other high protein foods, is a very effective and quick remedy for a wide variety of depressions, including the depressive phase of manic-depressive illness and endogenous, schizophrenic, and post-amphetamine depression. When doses of 100 to 500 milligrams of pure phenylalanine per day were taken on an empty stomach for two weeks, most depressed people were entirely relieved of their depressions. Faster results can be obtained by taking 1 to 1½ grams all at once, provided it is ascertained that there is no hypertension (high blood pressure). A day or two at this dosage may alleviate the depression. Phenylalanine was twice as effective as the current prescription "drug of choice" for depression, imipramine, in clinical tests. Of course, phenylalanine or any other drug cannot change reality—if a loved one was lost, the loss remains just as real—but phenylalanine can reduce the time to regain the ability to enjoy life once again. L-phenylalanine is the natural precursor for the neurotransmitters dopamine and norepinephrine; the increase in the supply of these chemicals is why phenylalanine is antidepressive.

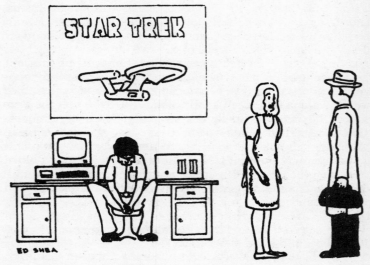

"He's been that way since being relieved of his starship command for losing to the Klingons." © Creative Computing

Phenylalanine has no toxic side effects to metabolically normal people in normal effective antidepressant dosages. It can cause headaches, insomnia, and/or irritability in excess dosage. Reducing the dosage will eliminate these effects. In large enough dosages (depending on the individual), it can increase blood pressure and, therefore, people with high blood pressure should start at a low dose, say 100 milligrams a day, measuring blood pressure at intervals and increasing the dose gradually. D-phenylalanine has recently been discovered to be an effective treatment in some cases for severe pain, because it inhibits the enzymes that break down your brain's natural morphinelike pain killers, the enkephalins. In order to maximize the amount entering the brain relative to that in the remainder of the body, phenylalanine should either be taken on an empty stomach just as you go to sleep or immediately when you wake up in the morning, a half hour or more before breakfast. Using it later in the day is more likely to lead to insomnia.

There are two varieties of phenylalanine you should know about. D-phenylalanine and L-phenylalanine are mirror images of each other, like a right- and left-handed glove. The D form, as mentioned above, is effective, in many cases, against severe pain. The L form is effective against depression. For use against depression, then, the L-phenylalanine or DL-phenylalanine (a mixture of the two kinds) is usually best. Vitamins C and B-6 are both required for converting nutrient precursors such as phenylalanine and tyrosine to norepinephrine and dopamine. The relations between these compounds are shown in a figure in Part II, Chapter 9. Note that the amino acid tyrosine is actually one step closer to being a neurotransmitter than phenylalanine. If you do not achieve satisfactory results with C, B-6, and phenylalanine, you might try comparable doses of C, B-6, and tyrosine. The high blood pressure precautions also apply to tyrosine; start at 100 milligrams and increase dosage slowly, while monitoring blood pressure, and do not use with prescription MAO inhibitors. Tyrosine sometimes causes decreases rather than increases in blood pressure. Tyrosine has also exhibited potent antidepressive effects in human experiments.

A deficiency of acetylcholine, another neurotransmitter, can also lead to depression. Deaner®, a prescription drug, increases acetylcholine levels in the brain. It is both an active analog and a precursor of acetylcholine and is effective in many old people as an antidepressive—it reduces apathy and increases motivation, as well as improving memory and learning in old subjects and hyperkinetic children. Choline and lecithin (which contains phosphatidyl choline), are both acetylcholine precursors that have been shown to improve memory and learning in normal human subjects and can be expected to have antidepressive effects in many people as well. Three grams a day of choline or 80 grams a day of lecithin are reasonable doses for many persons. Your brain's conversion of choline or lecithin into acetylcholine requires ample vitamin B-5 (pantothenic acid or calcium pantothenate). Inadequate B-5 may be why some people, especially institutionalized older people, do not have a good mental response to choline or lecithin. Our experiments with choline have always involved supplemental B-5 and have been quite promising. The acetyl group that must be added to choline to convert it to acetylcholine is transferred by an enzyme called acetylcoenzyme-A. Half this molecule is vitamin B-5, and the remainder can be manufactured by your body. The universal energy molecule ATP is also required for the conversion, and ATP production in the Krebs cycle (see Part II, Chapter 4) requires plenty of B-5. (For example, rats given extra B-5 can swim far longer in cold water than rats receiving normal levels of B-5.) We suggest starting with about 100 milligrams per day of B-5, gradually increasing the dose to 1 gram per day. Since vitamin B-5 increases choline conversion to acetylcholine in the gut, and the acetylcholine makes the gut muscles contract, too much too soon may result in a laxative action or a stomachache. (In fact, large doses of B-5 are an excellent laxative; most laxatives are either irritants, lubricants, or water-balance-modifying diarrhea inducers, whereas B-5 is a specific peristaltic stimulant; see Part III, Chapter 2, "Revitalizing Your Brain Power.") **WARNING:** Acetylcholine precursors should not be used in the depressive phase of manic-depressive psychosis since they can deepen *this* type of depression.

Hydergine® (Sandoz), which is discussed in detail in "Revitalizing Your Brain Power," gives a lift like coffee but without the letdown or jitters you get with coffee. It can be very effective in many cases of old age apathy, lack of self-care, confusion, and related symptoms, if used for an adequate length of time (it may take from several weeks to six months for noticeable effects and up to two years or so for full therapeutic effects to develop). Hydergine® stabilizes brain metabolism, even under conditions of great stress (such as low oxygen, low blood sugar, or alcohol intoxication). It improves human memory and learning, slows lipofuscin (age pigment,

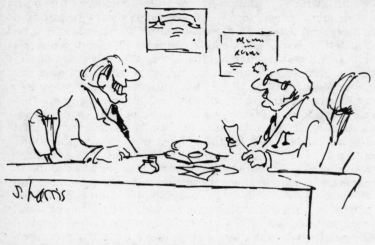

"I'm always like this, and my family was wondering
if you could prescribe a mild depressant."

a waste product) accumulation in the nerve cells, and even
stimulates nerve regeneration in the brain, since one of its
biochemical actions simulates the natural hormone nerve-
growth factor. Be sure to ask your doctor to specify Sandoz
Hydergine®, because generics of this particular drug are not
pharmaceutically equivalent (see Part V, Chapter 11). Excessive stimulation, headache, irritability, and insomnia can occur in a few people who use Hydergine® with caffeine
(coffee, colas) or theophylline (tea). Although this is not dangerous, it can be uncomfortable. Reducing or eliminating
these stimulants will solve the problem.

4
Sleep and Aging

Science consists in grouping facts so that general laws or conclusions may be drawn from them.

—Charles Darwin

Sleep is a complex state controlled by a number of different brain chemicals. In aged individuals, these brain chemicals may not be made in as great a quantity as in youth. Brain cells may become less sensitive to the chemicals. As a result, sleep difficulties become more common with age. But with our growing understanding of the various control systems underlying sleep, we may be able to do a lot to improve our ability to sleep soundly, using nutrients and certain prescription drugs. For nearly everyone, young or old, proper sleep patterns are essential to good health.

One of the most common disorders in old age is the development of faulty sleep patterns. Uncontrolled flights of thought may keep an older individual awake for hours after going to bed. Or a person may fall asleep easily but wake again in the night and have difficulty getting back to sleep. The consequences of disrupted sleep patterns like these are more serious than just weariness and irritability.

CAUTION: Keep in mind that sleeplessness can sometimes be an indication of an underlying medical disorder that may require your physician's intervention. Before you try any of our suggestions, check with your doctor to make sure that these are not the symptoms of a serious illness. Do not attempt self-diagnosis.

There are patterns of chemical changes that occur in the brain and body during sleep. One especially important biochemical rhythm is the release of growth hormone (GH) shortly after sleep begins. Adequate GH is necessary for proper function of the thymus and its "troops," the T-cell immune system that defends the body against bacteria, atherosclerotic plaques, viruses and cancer, and autoimmune self-attacks such as in rheumatoid arthritis. If sleep is delayed or interrupted, GH release can be eliminated, reduced, or aborted. And without a healthy T-cell system, aged persons are susceptible to disease and cancer. (In fact, the old wives' tale that kids' growth can be stunted by not sleeping well is true. Children have to have adequate levels of growth hormone in order to grow properly.) The reduction in nighttime GH in the aged cannot be *entirely* accounted for by age changes in sleep patterns. The lower levels of dopaminergic signals in the aged brain play an important part too.

The cholinergic nervous system in the brain is what controls body movement and sensory sensitivity during sleep. Too much or too little can cause excessive motor activity, such as sleepwalking or endless tossing and turning. In aged persons, there is a sharp decline in activity of the cholinergic system which leads to faulty sleep, particularly involving restlessness and frequent awakening not caused by urinary urgency.

Another sleep disturbance often encountered in older people is increased need to urinate during the night, leading to frequent awakenings. This may be due to insufficient production and/or release of the pituitary hormone vasopressin, which controls urine volume. Vasopressin (Diapid® nasal spray) can help, but it has a short life in the body and may wear off before morning. In men, an enlarged prostate gland is the most likely cause of this nighttime urinary urgency. Bromocriptine (Parlodel®, Sandoz), 1¼ to 2½ milligrams before bedtime, or GABA (gamma aminobutyric acid), an amino acid neurotransmitter, in doses of 20 to 40 milligrams per day (in tablets held under the tongue) may help decrease this problem by suppressing the release of the hormone prolactin by the pituitary gland. Excess prolactin can be a contributing cause of prostate enlargement. Any possible case of prostate enlargement should be promptly checked with a urologist, since prostate cancer becomes much more common with advancing age. There is growing evidence that prolactin is an

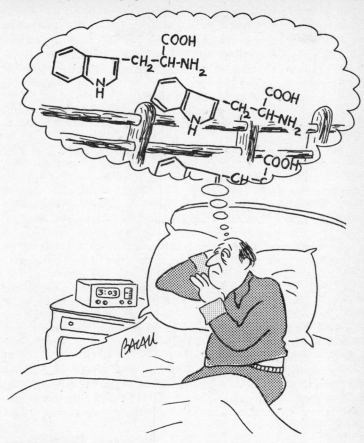

© 1981 Aaron Bacall

immunosuppressive hormone. If this is so, bromocriptine will have a double-barreled effect in prostate enlargement by both reducing the excessive tissue growth stimulation and by helping to restore immune competency so that your T-cells can more readily destroy any abnormal or precancerous cells present. A third possible cause of urinary urgency is kidney damage, which is all too common in advancing age. The most common cause of kidney damage is high blood pressure, though there are many other possibilities. Kidneys do not have the extensive regenerative ability of the liver or spleen; hence any hint of kidney problems calls for a prompt visit to your physician so that the damage can be stopped before you become a dialysis patient dependent on an artificial kidney.

Serotonin is a neurotransmitter which has important inhibitory functions in the brain, to prevent excess nervous stimulation at night so that sleep can occur. It is also a growth hormone releaser. Old people do not make as much serotonin as younger people. This is an important part of aging problems in sleep patterns.

What can be done about these sleep problems? One way is to increase the supply of serotonin in the brain by taking the essential amino acid tryptophan (found in milk and bananas, for example). That hot cup of milk (nonfat is just as good) before bedtime really can help you sleep. Tryptophan is a basic building block that the body can convert to serotonin. Increasing serotonin levels usually improves ease of falling asleep and may reduce the problem of waking up in the night. Tryptophan is much more effective used as the pure material taken on an empty stomach because amino acids in food compete for transport into the brain. Two grams of tryptophan taken at, not before, bedtime is a typical adult dose. Both vitamins B-6 (100 milligrams) and C (1 gram) are required for the conversion of tryptophan to serotonin. Excess serotonin can cause vascular headaches, nasal congestion, or, more rarely, constipation.

Another approach to the problem involves the use of dopaminergic stimulants which increase GH output to help make up for the old-age deficit in GH. In fact, GH levels can be returned to young adult levels. Drugs which increase GH output include:

• L-Dopa, an amino acid and prescription drug that has been shown to extend the life spans of mice. Side effects at low dose levels (say $\frac{1}{4}$ to $\frac{1}{2}$ gram per night) may include nighttime or early morning nausea at first, but this goes away within a week or two. Overdose may cause irritability and insomnia, but tolerance to these effects develops rapidly.

• Arginine and ornithine, two amino acids found in relatively large concentrations in chicken meat. Both can increase levels of growth hormone in doses of a few grams per day. The pure amino acids are much more effective than eating foods which contain them. These amino acids are available at some health food and drug stores and should be taken at bedtime on an empty stomach for maximum benefit.

Acetylcholine precursors (chemicals that are converted in the body to acetylcholine) will increase brain acetylcholine levels for proper control of motion and sensory activation during sleep. Effective precursors include lecithin, choline, and the prescription drug Deaner® (Riker). These substances are also effective in many cases of hyperkinesis, involving excessive movement and poor mental focus in children. (For further information, see Part II, Chapter 9, and Part III, Chapters 2 and 3.)

Another neurotransmitter system has been discovered which affects sleep. Valium®, Librium®, and Dalmane® (all made by Hoffmann-La Roche) are compounds which are chemically known as benzodiazepines. These compounds—especially Dalmane®—are effective sedatives which are safer than barbiturates. Dalmane® in particular does not suppress dreaming REM (rapid eye movement) sleep, unlike barbiturates. Without REM sleep, one's mind tends to become unglued during the day, with fragmentary dream images thrusting themselves into your consciousness, thereby interfering with mental focus and concentration. The portions of the brain that these compounds act on have been named the benzodiazepine receptors. It has just been discovered that niacinamide (also known as nicotinamide, a form of vitamin B-3), is a natural activator for this benzodiazepine receptor. This may explain why people who take megadoses of niacinamide (or niacin, which can be converted to niacinamide in the body) find that it makes them drowsy. You may use this effect to your advantage to improve the quality of your sleep by taking a large dose of niacin or niacinamide at bedtime. (Niacin causes more temporary flushing and itching than niacinamide.) Try a dose of between 100 milligrams and 2 grams, always starting out conservatively and increasing your dose slowly. Inositol, another nutrient which you can get at most health food and many drug stores, also works on the benzodiazepine receptors to promote sound sleep. One to 10 grams at bedtime is a reasonable dose, and it works best with niacinamide. These are not sedatives like the barbiturates, and large doses of these nutrients will not kill you by respiratory failure, unlike most sleeping pills. Barbiturates, moreover, are highly addictive, and mixing barbiturates and alcohol is *very* likely to be fatal. Sudden barbiturate withdrawal will cause insomnia, terrible nightmares, and sometimes even death by convulsions. The nutrients niacinamide or niacin and inositol do not have these hazards, even when used with alcohol.

If you feel you cannot get to sleep without a sleeping pill (assuming you cannot find tryptophan), you might want to try taking ½ the normal nightly sleeping pill dose in conjunction with swallowing one to three 1-milligram tablets of Hydergine®, for which you would need a prescription from your doctor. The total effect has been reported to be a reduction in the requirement of sleeping pill dose along with full sleep-promoting potency, and less sleeping pill hangover in the morning. Do not expect your doctor to have heard of this use for Hydergine®, since this is not an FDA-approved use for this drug; hence Sandoz is forbidden to tell physicians about it. The practice is safe, however, and is widely used in France, where it was derived from the practice of using both Hydergine® and barbiturates together in preparing patients for surgery. And because many sleep aids (including barbiturates) alter sleep patterns (barbiturates reduce dream time), it is better not to use them at all or to slowly reduce the dose you do use. **WARNING:** If you have used barbiturates for years, do not suddenly discontinue their use, or death by convulsions can occur. Consult a physician for withdrawal from chronic barbiturate use.

There are reports of a few individuals who require almost no sleep, in a few cases as little as fifteen minutes a night. The life styles of some of these people have been studied, especially to determine whether they are sleeping during the day, in short catnaps, or in some way entering the physiological states of sleep without appearing to do so. So far, EEG measurements indicate that there really are a few people who are able to live seemingly normal lives while sleeping as little as fifteen minutes a night. We have no explanation for this as yet, but they probably have an alternative mechanism of growth hormone release. We would like to see studies of the pituitary temporal release patterns and biochemical releasing mechanisms of growth hormone and vasopressin (the release of which triggers REM sleep) in these people. Since we spend a third of our lives unconscious while asleep, finding ways to get along without sleep or even cutting it down is a way to extend subjective life span. Although living without sleep would not increase the number of years we live, it would seem to us that we lived many years longer because we would be able to spend the extra time enjoying life rather than being unconscious. We have been able to cut our sleep time down by about an hour by using Deaner® (Riker). Some people find that BHT (an antioxidant food preservative) allows them to reduce sleep time. Phenylalanine (an amino acid found in foods such as meats and cheese and sold in some health food stores) can significantly reduce the requirement for sleep, but watch out for the development of insomnia if you use too much phenylalanine.

Finally, here's a little experiment you can try with a very safe sleep-affecting drug, vitamin B-12. This vitamin can cause spectacular intensification of colors in dreams or sometimes even produce colors in dreams of people who never before had colored dreams! It works about half the time in the small group of people we know who've tried it. (Sometimes the colors are so vivid they can wake you up!) A dose of 1,000 micrograms or so is effective. Take it *just* as you get into bed to sleep. If you take the B-12 half an hour before bed, the dream-enhancing effect·rarely works. Tolerance to this vitamin effect on dreams develops rapidly. So if you use large doses of B-12 every day, it is rather unlikely that this effect will occur.

5
Life Extenders Do It Longer: Sex and Aging

In spring a young squirrel's fancy turns because the days
are getting longer, and exposure to longer light periods
sets off a chain reaction involving the brain and pituitary
gland, resulting in release of hormones that affect sex
hormone levels and in turn cause the sex glands to enlarge
and produce their sex hormones.

—Joseph Meites

*In terms of our sex drive and capacity, it seems all downhill
by middle age. But reduced levels of hormones and certain
other chemicals made in the brain can be brought back up to
more youthful levels. Depressed sex drives can be increased.
And sexual orgasms can be prolonged and intensified with a
natural nonsteroid hormone.*

Sex drive and capacities decline with age. In males, testosterone (the male steroid sex hormone) begins to fall off
after the late teens. In females, estrogens (female sex hormones) begin to decline in the 30s and continue to fall until
menopause results. After menopause, the reproductive apparatus, including the vagina, shrinks markedly and loses
normal function unless estrogen-containing hormone supplements are used.

There are several ways to help maintain sexual capacities
or to possibly increase a depressed sex drive:

· Take antioxidant nutrient supplements, such as vitamins
A, E and C, zinc and selenium. Certain cell tracts in the hor-
mone-responsive areas of the sexual apparatus are particular-

ly sensitive to oxidative damage. As we discussed in Part II, Chapter 10, on aging clocks, we think these areas may act as mutation-damage monitors that eventually cause the sex drive to be shut down by biological clocks in both the brain and the testicles or ovaries. Shutting down would prevent defective (mutated) sperm or ova from developing into defective offspring and using valuable scarce parental and kin resources.

• When used properly, steroid sex hormone supplements are effective stimulants of sex drive. In addition to increasing the sex drive in both males and females, testosterone increases aggressiveness. (**CAUTION:** Females may experience side effects such as reversible facial hair growth and irreversible lowering of voice pitch if testosterone is used to excess.) Systemic (all through the body) effects of sex hormone supplements can be minimized by using them in certain chemical forms topically, that is, directly on the penis or vagina. Certain forms of the sex hormones, such as testosterone cypionate and estradiol dipropionate, have relatively little systemic circulation when applied topically in small amounts because the molecule is too large and nonpolar to move very far very fast. Too much systemic testosterone or estrogen-progestin can reduce levels of the brain hormone LHRH, a natural built-in aphrodisiac, and cause *decreased,* instead of increased, sex drive; systemic hormones may also facilitate the growth of certain cancers.

• The neurotransmitters (chemicals used by the brain's nerve cells to communicate with each other) associated with primitive drives such as sex include norepinephrine (NE), dopamine, and acetylcholine. Increasing the levels of these brain chemicals may increase sexual interest and activity. The amino acid L-Dopa (a prescription drug) increases brain levels of both dopamine and NE. Velvet beans (an animal feed used in the southeast) are a food source of L-Dopa. Another dopaminergic stimulant is the prescription drug bromocriptine (Parlodel®, Sandoz). Bromocriptine seems to be able to reset the biological aging clock involved in the regulation of sexual cycling in women and other female mammals. It has reinstated menstruation in some postmenopausal women and experimental animals, as well as seeming to increase their sex drive. The most common side effect of L-Dopa, bromocriptine, and other dopaminergic stimulants is nausea. This is not a toxic reaction. It is caused by an unusually high level of dopaminergic stimulation in the automatic control circuits of the brain stem. Reducing the dose usually relieves this problem, and gradual dose increases result in tolerance to the nausea-producing effect.

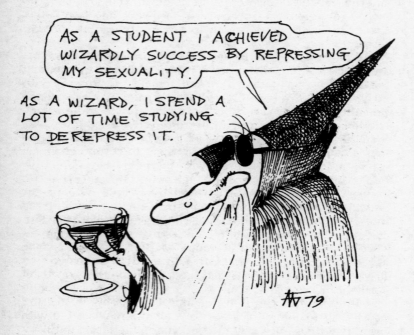

The prescription drug Deaner® and the nutrients choline and lecithin increase brain levels of acetylcholine, which also may stimulate sexual activity. Such sexual stimulation is rarely seen in people in their teens or 20s but is a fairly common reaction to these substances after the age of 40. Acetylcholine is also a chemical transmitter that causes your mucous membranes to release moisture, an important part of the physiological preparations for sexual activity. (See Part II, Chapters 9 and 10, Part III, Chapters 2 and 3, and Appendix L for further information on how to maintain proper levels of brain neurotransmitters.)

There has been much confusing discussion in lay publications concerning the use of hormonal-replacement therapy in postmenopausal women. Many people believe that it is very risky to do this. What are the facts? First, estrogen replacement is necessary in order to prevent vulva-vaginal shrinkage and loss of normal sexual function after menopause. Without adequate estrogenic stimulation, the vagina becomes dry, easily irritated, and often chronically infected. One of the problems in the hormonal replacement therapy commonly used is that only estrogens (the female sex hormones) are given, whereas ovaries of normal premenopausal women also manufacture progestins and about 1 to 2 milligrams per day of testosterone in addition to the estrogens. When estrogens are taken after menopause, progestins and androgens (male sex hormones, such as testosterone) are also needed to avoid excess estrogenic stimulation. In fact, in many cases of breast cancer, androgens are given as therapy; breast cancer and other cancers of sexually responsive female tissues are sometimes stimulated by estrogens.

Ideally, a hormonal-replacement mix of testosterone, progestins, and estrogens might be used as a salve topically in the vagina. This would provide maximum concentration where the hormones are most needed and minimum systemic concentration (such as in breasts, or particularly the ovaries and uterus, which cannot be examined externally). Lipophilic testosterone esters (preferably testosterone cypionate) combined with lipophilic estradiol esters (preferably estradiol dipropionate) in an absorption base do a good job of maintaining the vaginal mucosa while combatting estrogenic overstimulation of the breasts and ovaries. Testosterone cypionate is used for once-a-month depot injections for androgen replacement in males. The hormone slowly diffuses into the general systemic circulation over a period of a month or more. Estradiol dipropionate is so immobile that it is rarely used for depot injections; after a year, half of the hormone may still be at the injection site. The use of a topically applied, relatively low mobility testosterone ester ensures that there will be relatively little systemic effects (such as virilization) while, at the same time, there will be a relatively high hormone concentration in the target tissues. The use of topically applied estradiol ester that is much less mobile than the testosterone ester results in very little systemic dosage of estrogen, with those relatively very small systemic effects being counteracted by the relatively higher levels of the more mobile testosterone ester. This particular combination of esters results in a markedly higher estrogen-to-androgen ratio in the target tissues of the vagina to which it is topically applied than elsewhere in the body. This topical combination provides adequate hormone stimulation to maintain a healthy, moist, well-lubricated vaginal mucosa which is not easily irritated by sexual intercourse and is more resistant to chronic infections.

Without such treatment, many—probably most—post-menopausal women will experience pain, burning, and soreness during intercourse, particularly if it is prolonged or frequent. (A small percentage of premenopausal women also suffer from this problem.) In our limited experience, the following topical formulation works well: ½ to 1 percent testosterone cypionate plus 0.1 percent estradiol dipropionate in any standard lipophilic (compatible with materials soluble in oils and fats) absorption base. This is a prescription drug. It will have to be specially compounded by your pharmacist since we know of no commercial equivalent. Use the *minimum* amount required; your gynecologist can tell you when your vaginal mucosa is in good condition. About $\frac{1}{16}$ teaspoon per day of this salve rubbed into the vagina with a finger has been effective in our experience. This gives a systemic daily androgen dosage of less than 1 milligram and a systemic daily estradiol ester dosage of far less than 50 micrograms. These systemic doses are small compared to the normal endogenous (produced within your body) sex steroid production. Fractional measuring spoons are available in the culinary equipment department of most department stores. For the reasons mentioned above, a topical cream, if available, is preferable to the sex steroid pills for this purpose. However, a topical cream may not provide enough systemic stimulation to prevent postmenopausal vasomotor instability (hot flashes).

CAUTION: Women, especially those using any form of estrogens, should have a pap smear test at least once a year to detect the presence of possible abnormal cervical cells. Estrogens must not be used in the presence of an abnormal pap smear.

The amount of estrogen needed to prevent hot flashes is individual. We know of one case where the above topical hormone formulation and dosage was adequate to eliminate postmenopausal hot flashes (vasomotor instability) with no additional systemic hormones. In this case, the woman was also using 2.5 milligrams a day of Parlodel® and large doses of Hydergine®, both of which may have contributed to the effectiveness of this approach. Since only about half of the hormones in the salve are absorbed, the daily locally absorbed dose was about 1 milligram of testosterone cypionate and about 100 micrograms (0.1 milligrams) of estradiol dipropionate. The systemically circulated doses of these hormones are considerably lower, particularly for the estrogen. Let us compare these doses to those found in a traditional estrogen replacement oral tablet, Estrace® (Mead-Johnson). The active ingredient is estradiol. The recommended daily dose is 1 to 2 milligrams of estradiol per day for 21 days, then off the hormone for 7 days, then back on for 21 days, etc. There is a commercial vaginal suppository for the topical application of hormones, Test-Estrin Vaginal Insert® (Marlyn Pharmaceutical), which contains 5 milligrams of testosterone and 500 micrograms (0.5 milligrams) of estradiol. The absorbed dose is about half of that applied. The estradiol and testosterone are relatively mobile and rapidly enter the general systemic circulation; however, this topical product exposes the rest of the body to 4 to 8 times less estrogen than the conventional pills. Moreover, adequate testosterone is supplied by this product to help prevent excessive estrogenic stimulation. Our suggested topical vaginal treatment with testosterone cypionate and estradiol dipropionate exposes the rest of the body to $\frac{1}{10}$ or less of the hormone dose of the commercial vaginal suppository, and to only a few percent of the hormone dose of the conventional tablets. (See Part III, Chapter 7, for further comments on topical sex hormone delivery systems.) While cyclic (21 days on and 7 days off) use of the topical treatment is most conservative, it may not really be necessary due to the presence of the testosterone, the very low total estrogen dose, and the extremely low systemic estrogen dose. Follow your gynecologist's recommendations and have regular pap smears.

The amount of estrogen needed is individual. Birth control pills, such as Ortho-Novum $\frac{1}{50}$ #21, probably have a hormone balance better than the usual simple estrogen replacement pill. The right dose can be found by starting at the lowest possible dose (say $\frac{1}{4}$ the lowest potency tablet), increasing it slowly until hot flashes disappear (Hydergine® and Parlodel® may help with this symptom of vasomotor instability) and having a gynecologist examine the vagina until it takes on a youthful appearance. If you can get a testosterone cypionate–estradiol dipropionate topical cream to take care of the vaginal mucosa, your systemic oral hormone dose can usually be much lower than would otherwise be necessary.

The dangers of birth control pill use have been grossly exaggerated. Note in the figure below that the mortality associated with birth control pills is lower than the mortality associated with the use of no birth control at all ages except for smokers over the age of 40. Up to the age of 30, risks are low and about equal for the major birth control methods— pill, IUD, diaphragm, condom, or first trimester abortion. Risks are well below those for no fertility control. After 30, risks for nonsmoking pill users and those using traditional methods without abortion backup increase moderately but remain well below health risks to women who use no fertility control at all.

We do recommend that pill users also take nutritional antioxidant supplements, since both B-6 and C levels are known to be reduced in pill users. The increase observed in cardiovascular problems in users of birth control pills who are older and who smoke is to be expected; aging, smoking, and the pill each cause a lowering of B-6 and C serum levels. The combination of these three risk factors can lead to a hazardous B-6 and C deficiency. B-6 and C deficiency leads to such cardiovascular problems, and such pre-existing problems can be corrected (at least partially) in experimental animals with B-6 and C supplements.

Many people in middle age or later suffer from a depressed sex drive due to an excess of the hormone prolactin. Many cases of male impotency (20 to 25 percent) stem from this cause. Most people suffering from this problem have no signs of breast enlargement or lactation; only a clinical test measuring prolactin levels can tell for sure. Two common symptoms of excess prolactin in males are prostate problems and tender, painful, varicose, or atrophied testes. Bromocriptine (Parlodel®, Sandoz) in doses of 1.25 to 2.5 milligrams per day, or GABA (the amino acid gamma amino butyric acid, an inhibitory neurotransmitter), in doses of 20 to 40 milligrams per day held under the tongue, is sometimes effective. The prescription drug and amino acid L-Dopa, at ¼ to ½ gram per day (just before bed), is useful, but see Part II, Chapter 9, for information on the increased antioxidant requirement when using L-Dopa.

· The amino acids phenylalanine and tyrosine (found especially in meats and cheeses) are precursors of (chemically converted to) NE (norepinephrine, the brain's version of adrenalin) and dopamine in the brain. When people are depressed, they almost always lose interest in sex. Phenylalanine

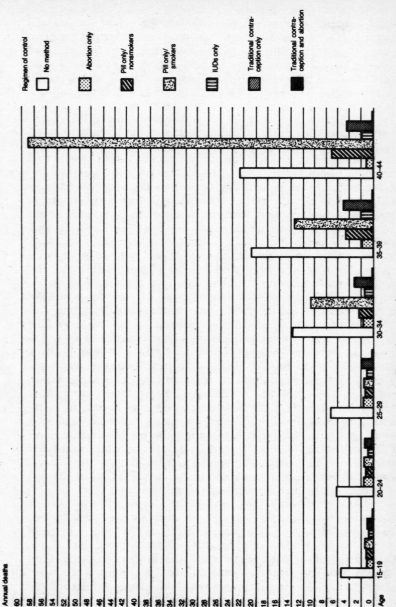

Annual number of deaths associated with control of fertility and no control per 100,000 nonsterile women, by regimen of control and age of woman

is one of the most effective (and possibly the safest) known antidepressant. In doses of 100 to 500 milligrams a day for two weeks, most types of depression (postamphetamine, schizophrenic, endogenous, etc.) are completely relieved. And, of course, sexual interest may be revived. Supplements of vitamins B-6 and C are required for best results. **CAUTION:** People with elevated blood pressure should read the precautions in Part III, Chapter 3, before using these materials.

   • For sexual performance, stamina can be increased by taking certain nutrients, including calcium pantothenate (vitamin B-5). See Part III, Chapter 9, on athletic performance.

   • Vasopressin, or antidiuretic hormone (ADH), has several known functions, including regulation of electrolytes, and urine volume and in very high intravenous doses, blood pressure. In low dosages (16 I.U. per day), it has been shown to stimulate memory and learning abilities in humans without having any effect on blood pressure electrolytes, or urine volume. Since neither of us have high blood pressure, abnormally low daily urine volume, or angina pectoris, we have been experimenting with higher doses, though still well within the range of customary medical use. We have both been using vasopressin daily in doses ranging up to 80 I.U. per day and have noted its remarkable effects on memory and learning. Another effect we noticed that was not reported in the scientific literature is an intensification and prolongation of orgasms! Since vasopressin is destroyed in the brain within an hour or two, you'll need to take it fairly promptly before sex to get these effects. Fortunately, vasopressin begins to work within minutes. Vasopressin is available as a prescription nasal spray (Diapid®, Sandoz). Side effects include occasional nasal irritation (the spray is acidic because vasopressin is more stable in acidic solution, and acids help open the blood-brain barrier) and gastrointestinal tract cramping (uncomfortable, but not dangerous); in people suffering from angina pectoris, vasopressin can precipitate angina attacks. **CAUTION:** In the last condition, the use of vasopressin should be restricted.

   • Release of histamines from body stores is a requirement for achieving orgasm. Often, men and women who cannot reach orgasm respond to supplements of the vitamin niacin which causes release of these histamines. Histamine release during sexual excitation is what causes the sex flush described by Masters and Johnson (blushing in face, neck, shoulders, chest, etc.). The histamine released by niacin results in this same flushing effect, whether there is sexual excitation or not. We often take niacin about fifteen minutes or a half hour before engaging in sex to enhance the natural sex flush that occurs when histamines are released in preparation for orgasm. The niacin-caused histamine release also causes the mucous membranes of mouth and sexual organs to secrete mucus, which enhances the natural mucus formation in response to sexual activity. Since vitamin B-6 is required to turn the amino acid histidine into histamine, supplements of B-6 and eating foods high in histidine (meats and cheeses, for example) may also be beneficial. See the Case Histories in Appendix L.

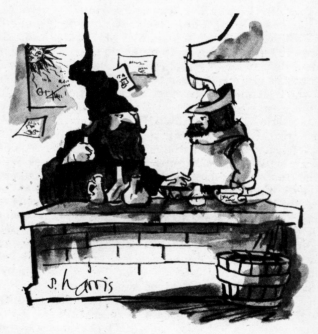

"Gold and silver from base metals is OK, but what I'm trying to transmute is angelica root, mugwort and tincture of marigold into an effective aphrodisiac."

• Some sexual problems can be traced to genital herpes virus infections. These infections are extremely common; in fact, genital herpes is now the number one venereal disease in the United States. The infections can be very unpleasant, interfering with sexual pleasure by burning and itching, dulling sensation, and causing soreness. But herpes virus infections can be more serious than just ruining your fun. They can kill you. Herpes viruses have been associated with some forms of human cancer—in particular, cervical cancer, nasopharyngeal cancer, Burkitt's lymphoma, and perhaps others. It is a good idea not to allow genital herpes infections to persist.

BHT (butylated hydroxytoluene) is an antioxidant used as a preservative in foods, rubber, plastics, fuels, and drugs. In recent experiments, BHT killed all tested small-nucleic-acid-core-diameter lipid (fatty) coated viruses, including herpes viruses. In animal feeding experiments (including rhesus monkeys), BHT has a low toxicity. We know several people who have used BHT at our suggestion to control genital herpes virus infections—$1/4$ to 1 gram of BHT taken immediately before bed eliminated symptoms within a week. Then a maintenance dose of $1/4$ to 1 gram per day taken just before bed prevents the reappearance of the infection. We told a friend of ours who is a clinical-research-oriented physician about BHT's usefulness in cases of chronic herpes (both type I and/or II) infections. He has applied this BHT treatment to over one hundred human cases of chronic herpes (type I and/or II) with complete success and without detectable adverse side effects. He typically uses 2 grams per day for two weeks, repeating the treatment if the symptoms recur. Herpes viruses alter the DNA in persons infected by splicing copies of herpes DNA into their own DNA. The spliced herpes virus DNA instructs the victim's cells to manufacture more herpes virus particles. BHT destroys herpes viruses particles, probably by stripping off the protective lipid coat that conceals them from the immune system and nucleases (enzymes that break down nucleic acids) and that is required for them to be able to penetrate cell membranes. BHT cannot do anything about the herpes virus DNA that has been inserted into the infected person's DNA, so once you have herpes, you have it for life, but regular use of $1/4$ to 1 gram of BHT per day can promptly destroy any free virus particles and prevent both overt signs of infection and communication of the disease. **CAUTION:** Don't take BHT with large amounts of alcohol or barbiturates—it intensifies their effects (but those doses of BHT mixed with either alcohol or barbiturates do not cause respiratory collapse, as a combination of alcohol and barbiturates can). See our list of suppliers in Appendix I for a source of BHT.

CAUTION: You should not assume that a decline in sexual functions or interest is necessarily due to the aging process. Diabetes mellitus is often undiagnosed and is a common cause of impotence in males. Infections and anemia are among the other causes. Therefore, see your doctor before you embark upon our suggestions. With the help of your physician and improved nutrition, life extenders really can do it longer. And to us, that makes living a long time a lot more attractive!

6
Looking as Young as You Feel

One fact about the future of which we can be certain is
that it will be utterly fantastic.

—Arthur C. Clarke, science-fiction author

*You don't just want to feel younger, you want to look younger
too. So do we. In this chapter, we tell you how you can slow
down the wrinkling of your skin using nutrients you can get
at your local health food or drug store. We tell you about your
most important natural skin moisturizer and how it can be
used to regain the youthful, plump, moist appearance your
skin used to have. And we tell you how oral doses of a natural
carotenoid plant pigment can give you a beautiful tan without solar ultraviolet-light-induced skin damage.*

Skin is the largest and most visible of all the organs. As aging progresses, the skin shows the results of aging damage by
becoming wrinkled and losing its elasticity. Except for UV (ultraviolet light) damage, the aging condition of the skin probably reflects that of the rest of the body. Even here, resistance
to UV damage (in the absence of topical UV absorbers) correlates fairly well with resistance to aging damage mechanisms.
We might, therefore, see in this accessible system how well
(or not so well) we are dealing with our own aging processes.

The various aging mechanisms damage skin in the same
manner as other body systems. Skin is also subject to the damage produced by the ultraviolet light in sunlight. This type of

damage does not occur in other parts of the body except the eye. As explained in Part II, Chapter 6, ultraviolet light causes uncontrolled cross-linking (undesirable bonds) between protein molecules in skin which can be recognized in the form of wrinkles. (Chemically caused cross-links also occur in arteries, leading to the so-called hardening of the arteries in which these vessels lose their elasticity and become brittle, hard, and stiff.) Ultraviolet light causes the lipids in skin to undergo several types of free radical damage, including peroxidation and cross-linking addition reactions. The skin is the third most fatty organ in the body, after the spinal cord and brain, and consequently is particularly susceptible to free radical attack. Studies have shown that people with a greater exposure to cross-linkers such as alcohol (converted to acetaldehyde in the liver), tobacco smoke (contains aldehydes), and sunlight (contains ultraviolet) are more wrinkled. The greater the exposure, the greater the wrinkling. People who smoke and drink heavily (without protecting themselves with the proper nutrients) usually look old beyond their years. In fact, they have prematurely aged themselves. If you prefer to do these things, perhaps you should try to protect yourself.

As we have seen, the rate of the undesired random damage of cross-linking may be slowed by taking antioxidants such as E, C, cysteine, and B-1. These compounds interfere with the chemical reactions that cause the cross-linking. In order to bring a higher concentration of these materials into the skin, "miracle" ointments containing some of these compounds are commonly sold. This can be an effective stratagem; however, it is important to know that the shelf life of these ointments is limited because some of the active ingredients—particularly lipids and vitamin E—become inactive or even harmful in the presence of air, light, heat, and moisture.

The skin may be protected from ultraviolet-light damage rather easily. One way is to stay out of the sun. Another way is to use topical sunscreens containing esters of PABA (p-aminobenzoic acid), a vitamin. These PABA esters dissolve into the skin's oils and don't wash out as easily while swimming, from perspiration, etc., as does plain PABA, which is water soluble. The PABA and its esters absorb the energy from the ultraviolet light, thus shielding the skin and its sensitive molecules (such as DNA) from attack. Large oral doses of PABA are fairly effective, too, though not as thorough as a topical sun block.

Skin appearance can be markedly improved by using Na-PCA, the sodium salt of 2-pyrrolidone-5-carboxylic acid, the principal natural humectant (moisturizer) in your skin. The ability of skin to hold moisture is directly related to its Na-PCA content. The ability of Na-PCA to pull water out of the air is amazing. If you put out a small amount of dry Na-PCA in the Sahara Desert, in a few hours it will become a puddle because of the water removed from the very dry air there! Older people have about 50 percent less Na-PCA in their skin than young people, thus contributing to a dry, hard skin condition. Bathing and swimming can lead to dry skin because your natural Na-PCA is leached out. Na-PCA can be found in some premium quality skin-care cosmetics. Look at the labels to see if it is listed as an ingredient.

Here's a simple experiment you can do that will demonstrate the fact that it is water, and not oil, that keeps skin soft and supple. Cut some small pieces of hardened leather from an old shoe, and soak one piece overnight in baby oil, another piece in water, and a third in a 15 percent solution of Na-PCA in water (see Appendix I for a supplier of Na-PCA). Next day, remove the pieces of leather from the liquids, dry them off with a paper towel, and compare them for flexibility and softness. The pieces soaked in the Na-PCA and water and the water alone will both be soft, whereas the oil-soaked piece will be much less soft. Now hang the pieces up to dry. The piece soaked in plain water will rapidly dry out and harden, whereas the piece soaked in the Na-PCA solution will remain moist, soft, and supple.

Many people taking our personal experimental nutrient mix or ones like it (although generally at a dose level $\frac{1}{2}$ to $\frac{1}{10}$ or less of our dose level) notice a distinct improvement in the appearance of their skin over a period of about two weeks. This may occur as a result of improved growth and injury repair, more effective immune system surveillance of the skin cells, protection against cross-linkers such as ultraviolet light and aldehydes, and of course factors of which we are unaware. For example, vitamin B-5, pantothenate, is required for your skin to synthesize protective fats and oils that are essential to skin function. Vitamin A increases the number of skin cell receptors for epidermal growth factor (EGF), the natural skin growth and repair hormone. Skin appearance is a sort of "proof of the pudding" for anti-aging treatments. Skin is as subject to most, if not all, the aging mechanisms as other organ systems. Hypothetically, you should *look younger* if your body is really becoming younger. It is interesting to note that your nerves are derived from the same fetal cells as your skin cells and these two types of cells have much in common biochemically, both with respect to damage and repair mechanisms. Both skin and nerve cells can accumulate age pigment (lipofuscin) and become cross-linked, and both are stimulated to grow by structurally very similar hormones, called epidermal growth factor (EGF) in skin, and nerve growth factor (NGF), in the brain. With the exception of ultraviolet light damage, your skin is, in a sense, a window to your brain. You can remove those ugly brown age spots (lipofuscin age pigment) from your skin with the prescription drug Deaner®. As mentioned in Part II, Chapter 8, a friend of ours, a man in his 60s taking 300 milligrams a day of Deaner®, found that after a few months the age spots on his skin started fading away and eventually disappeared. Furthermore, Deaner® not only removes lipofuscin from skin but also from nerve cells in which it is found. There is a lot more to looking younger than cosmetic cover-ups. See Part III, Chapter 1, "Some Immediate Benefits of Life Extension Measures"; Part II, Chapter 8, "Accumulated Wastes"; and Part II, Chapter 6, "Cross-linked Molecules and Aging" for further information. Be sure to read the material in this last chapter on the "sun tan" carotenoid Orobronze®, now available in Canada. You can now have a beautiful golden tan from the inside out (it will not wash off) without exposing your skin to the harsh cross-linking, carcinogenic, prematurely aging ultraviolet rays of the sun or a tanning booth. You no longer have to look worse later in order to look better now.

7
Male Pattern Baldness and What You Can Do About It

... Just as the pigment of the hair is destroyed by phagocytes, so also the atrophy of other organs of the body, in old age, is very frequently due to the action of devouring cells which I have called macrophages.

—Elie Metchnikoff, *The Prolongation of Life* (1908)

Male pattern baldness is an example of an aging clock. When the time comes, the hair from the affected areas falls out, even if it has been transplanted into a normally nonbalding area of the head. We have learned something about the molecular events that cause balding. Using this knowledge, we can reset the balding aging clock to prevent and even partially reverse it by using the right nutrients and techniques. You don't have to go bald any more. You might be able to grow back some of the lost hair. Durk has a lot more hair now at age 37 in his male pattern baldness areas than he did ten years ago. You too might turn back the aging clock in your scalp.

This chapter deals only with male pattern baldness, the most common cause of male hair loss, and not with other types of baldness. **CAUTION:** Before proceeding with the approach presented here, have your physician give you a complete physical; hair loss can also be due to serious medical disorders such as diabetes mellitus (sugar-insulin diabetes).

Knowledge of how hair follicles produce hair and what causes them to stop is increasing rapidly. We know that hair follicles have a growing and resting cycle. In male pattern balding, the hair follicles in particular areas of the scalp begin to spend more of their time in the resting phase. Meanwhile, hairs continue to fall out. Eventually, there are no macroscopic normal hairs left in that area. However, the atrophied follicles are not necessarily dead and might be induced to begin growing hair again by using the proper growth stimulants.

Male pattern balding is an example of a biological clock. As we mentioned in Part II, Chapter 10, on aging clocks, if you remove some hairs (along with their follicles) from the balding area and transplant them to a nonbalding area of the scalp, the transplanted hairs fall out right on schedule, along with the other balding area hairs. If you transplant hairs from a nonbalding area into the balding area, the transplanted hairs continue to grow, while the hairs all around them are falling out. We do not yet know everything about how this aging clock works, but we do know how to slow and possibly reverse the clock.

It is well accepted that dihydrotestosterone, a hormone formed by metabolism of the male hormone testosterone or from cholesterol, causes these follicles to go into their resting phase. When the time comes to go bald, the hair follicles in the male pattern baldness areas markedly increase their production of testosterone 5-alpha reductase. This enzyme converts testosterone to dihydrotestosterone, which in turn makes the hair stop growing. Female hormones topically applied to the scalp in the balding area can prevent further fallout (by inhibiting dihydrotestosterone formation and blocking its receptors) but usually causes little or no regrowth of hair. In order to avoid other effects of estrogens, such as increased breast growth, you should use topically applied, slowly diffusing forms, such as estradiol cypionate or dipropionate. This can penetrate the scalp to give a high concentration at the follicles, but relatively little estrogen gets into general circulation.

The follicle aging clock of male pattern baldness can also be partially blocked with large doses of testosterone compounds applied directly to the scalp. This both inhibits the formation of dihydrotestosterone (the balding clock compound) and blocks its access to the receptor sites in the DNA of the follicles. A testosterone salve can greatly slow or even halt the progress of male pattern baldness, but hair regrowth averages only about 10 percent after one year. We recommend that testosterone be applied as the cypionate to reduce systemic effects.

One of us (Durk) has used topical estrogens and androgens to help control his own case of male pattern baldness. He found that the use of the estrogens alone tends to lead to scalp fragility and tenderness, whereas the androgens alone lead to scalp acne. To avoid these side effects, Durk uses a 1 to 15 mixture of estradiol dipropionate to testosterone cypionate in either reagent grade DMSO (preferred) or a 50-50 mixture of acetone and ethyl alcohol as a solvent—a combination that yields somewhat better results than either alone. Each drop of solvent contains 2 micrograms of estradiol dipropionate and 30 micrograms of testosterone cypionate. Each treatment uses about 30 to 60 drops; 10 to 20 on top of the head, and 10 to 20 more at each front side corner, the areas where his hair was receding. The solution is rubbed into the scalp and allowed to dry. About one treatment per week of about 120 micrograms of estrogen and 1.8 milligrams of androgen has halted the progress of Durk's balding. These doses of sex hormones are far too low to have any systemic effect, but they seem to have worked for Durk when applied directly to the scalp.

At this point a brief technical note on the drug delivery system is in order. Ideally, the androgens and estrogens should be delivered only to the hair follicles in the balding area, without appreciable whole body dosage. The proper solvent-hormone system can come close enough to this goal. Early experiments reported in the literature used hormones such as testosterone propionate, which diffuse quite rapidly. When applied to the scalp in an absorption base, the hormone rapidly moves out into the remainder of the body, resulting in both an insufficient amount in the scalp and an undesirable excess in the body as a whole. The cypionate and dipropionate esters should be used because they have a much lower mobility in the body; they are sometimes used as depot injections or implanted pellets which slowly leak hormones over a period of weeks or months. Indeed, the dipropionate esters are so immobile that they are usually unsuitable for depot injections. These esters dissolve well in fats but are very insoluble in water.

The solvent used to deposit these hormone esters in the scalp must be low in toxicity, high in fat solvent power, able to rapidly penetrate the skin, and miscible (mutually soluble) with water. DMSO meets these requirements very well. The testosterone cypionate and estrodial dipropionate dissolve slowly in dry DMSO but precipitate out of solution when a small amount of water is added. This is exactly what happens when the solution is applied to your scalp. The DMSO carries the hormone esters through the dry waxy oily dead outer layer of skin. When it reaches the upper layer of living cells, however, their high water content causes the prompt precipitation of the hormone esters right where you want them. The DMSO soon spreads throughout your body, but most of the very hydrophobic hormone esters are left behind in the scalp where they belong.

Both the quantity and frequency of application of this treatment must be individualized. If you use too little too infrequently, your hair loss will be unaffected. If you use too much too often, you will have acne on your scalp. Here is how you adjust your dose. Comb your hair regularly and save all hair fallout, using a separate envelope each day. You will soon discover by estimation (or preferably by actual hair-root count) your typical daily hair loss rate. In Durk's experience, the proper topical dose of hormone solutions will cause a reduction in hair fallout rate of at least a factor of four (and usually more like a factor of ten to twenty) within two days, with a noticeable effect within twelve hours, and the treatment will remain effective for about a week. When the hair loss rate rises, another application is used.

Do not confuse the approach described above with the early testosterone propionate experiments which, while interesting, were of marginal effectiveness and had unacceptable systemic side effects. Nevertheless, do not forget that Durk's approach is also experimental and has only been tried on a handful of people.

This topical treatment is not commercially available. If you wish to use it, you will either have to be a scientist or have a prescription from your doctor, and your pharmacist will have to special-order the chemicals and mix up a batch for you. Keep it in a cool dark place. Since obtaining the materials could be quite time-consuming, we suggest that you go to an unhappily balding pharmacist for this particular service.

Inositol, a B vitamin, is a natural sugar known as muscle sugar and is a cell membrane stabilizer and antioxidant which has a protective effect on hair follicles, perhaps by protecting them from membrane damage caused by oxidized cholesterol in the scalp, or from destruction by clock-triggered lysosomes (proteolytic enzymes). Lysosomal membranes are principally comprised of phosphatidyl inositol.

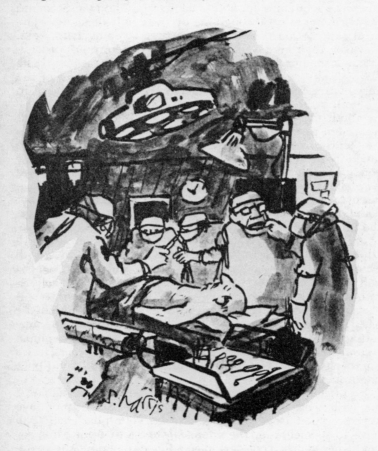

"A heart transplant isn't worth much if he doesn't look good—let's give him a hair transplant, too."

In some species of experimental animals, inositol deficiency causes hair loss and premature graying. In our small sample of human subjects, several grams of inositol alone per day generally noticeably reduced but did not entirely abolish hair loss. In a small percentage of cases, perhaps around 10 percent, there are reports of graying hair darkening back toward its original color.

PABA (p-aminobenzoic acid, para aminobenzoic acid) is also a B vitamin which is an antioxidant and membrane stabilizer. In some experimental animals, PABA retards hair loss and retards or even reverses premature graying. Our own human experiments typically involve doses of 1 to 3 grams per day and suggest a hair response like that obtained with inositol: a reduction in hair loss, no noticeable hair regrowth (at least when PABA is used alone), and a darkening of graying hair toward its original color in perhaps 10 percent of the cases.

Hair is about 8 percent cysteine in composition, so if you want your hair to grow faster, you should take a cysteine supplement. If you can't find it in a health food or drug store as the pure amino acid, you can get some cysteine in eggs or egg powder, about ¼ gram per egg. **CAUTION:** High doses of cysteine can lead to increased cystine (the oxidized form of cysteine) unless high doses of vitamin C are taken to prevent possible formation of cystine bladder or kidney stones. We recommend at least three times as much vitamin C as cysteine. One gram of cysteine plus 3 grams of vitamin C per day is a reasonable dose. Durk's hair used to grow very slowly before he embarked on our experimental life extension program. By using a hair dye marker, he was recently able to measure his hair growth rate—¾ inch in six weeks in most areas, and ⅜ inch at the edge of the male pattern baldness areas.

The vitamin biotin, a growth factor and participant in fatty acid synthesis, seems to have prophylactic value in slowing hair loss. A biotin deficiency leads to hair falling out. People who like to eat foods or drinks containing raw egg should take biotin supplements because uncooked egg white contains avidin, an anti-biotin factor. Take your biotin supplement at least six hours before or after you eat any raw egg white. In one series of tests of biotin in balding men, biotin was used instead of estrogen in a penetrating cream applied to the scalp. The

biotin cream (which also contained niacin, vitamin B-3, a histamine releaser) was applied daily at bedtime. The biotin content was 0.25 to 1.0 percent. Histamine release, such as is
triggered by niacin, is essential for cell growth and reproduction. Histamine release causes a normally healing wound to
become red and itchy. In addition, a shampoo which contained various conditioners to reduce hair breakage and cystine, cysteine, and methionine (amino acids in hair) was used
three times a week. There were no side effects with the biotin. Within six to eight weeks, 89 percent of the nearly 1,200
men in the study (ranging in age from 15 to 69) showed
marked reduction in hair fallout, from losses of 100 to 350
hairs per day to a daily average loss of less than 50 hairs. Regrowth of hair also occurred in the biotin study. Although in-
complete at the time the paper was published, preliminary
data indicated that regrowth (150 to 200 $\frac{3}{4}$-inch or longer
hairs per square inch in bald areas) occurred in about 50 to
75 percent of the subjects. Younger men in the study had better results.

Pulling hairs just short of breaking them or plucking hairs
can stimulate new growth, though its effects are not very impressive.

Such powerful skin irritants as cayenne pepper or, even
more powerful and effective, dinitrochlorobenzene or dini-
trochlorophenol, often cause hair regrowth when rubbed into
the scalp. This is probably at least partly due to histamine release, which stimulates cell division. Experiment on yourself
with pepper, if you wish, but do not self-administer the other
two compounds, which can be very dangerous if misused.

A hair growth stimulating compound that is apparently
often effective has been reported by reputable scientists to
cause an average of 60 percent hair regrowth in just six
months of daily use in many people. This material is approved
by the FDA as a shampoo surfactant and direct food additive
(as an emulsifier, an agent which can cause water and fat
phases to mix). This chemical is called polysorbate 80 (Tween-
80®, Atlas ICI) and its close relative polysorbate 60 (Tween-
60®, Atlas-ICI) and is commonly found in mayonnaise, salad
dressings, and a few liquid detergents. Unfortunately, despite
its very low toxicity and its reported frequent partial effectiveness against balding, the companies offering this chemical
cannot sell it for this purpose. If they did, the FDA could take
them to court because they did not file a new drug applica-

tion, requiring tens of millions of dollars and many years to get approval for use against balding. The FDA has not approved polysorbate 80 or polysorbate 60 for use on balding heads, and hence few people have been able to take advantage of this safe and sometimes effective treatment for baldness.

Polysorbate 80 (which Durk prefers) and polysorbate 60 work in at least two or three different ways. They remove dihydrotestosterone and cholesterol from the scalp. They release histamine (a growth factor). They also probably affect the control of genetic activities in the hair follicle cells since they are able to reverse some of the early tissue disorganization which occurs at the start of some chemically induced cancers. Theoretically, part of the molecule (called a polyoxyethylene chain) should interact with the nucleo-proteins which regulate genetic activity.

If you have access to polysorbate 80 or 60, use it in this manner: Coat the scalp in the bald or balding areas with a thin film of material five or ten minutes before shampooing. A medicine dropper can be used to place several drops in the right areas. Rub the drops into your scalp with the fingertips, preferably vigorously enough for the scalp to be reddened a bit and feel warm. That reddening and warmth is due to histamine release. Then wash it out. Since it is a surfactant, it is a fine principal ingredient for a shampoo. If any gets in your eyes, it will be mildly irritating like most shampoos. It washes out easily with water and will do no harm. You can expect to see new hairs growing within two or three months of daily use if it is going to work for you. At first, the hairs are very thin and short, best seen under bright side lighting and against a black background. Average regrowth reported in the scientific literature was over 60 percent for hundreds of men in their 50s and 60s using polysorbate every day for a year. Beware, though, of organizations selling this material at highly inflated prices (such as $25 per ounce) and claiming it is an exclusive offering. Wholesale cost in 45-gallon drums is about $1 per pound.

This approach is reported as being more effective at promoting hair regrowth than the topical hormone treatments alone, and it has no significant side effects. (For the first week or two there will be an increase in hair loss due to loosening of hairs in resting phase atrophic follicles.) Durk has found it to be a safe and effective treatment for his own personal case of male pattern baldness, best when used in conjunction with the topical hormones and nutritional supplements. In our own observations, the polysorbates appear to be useful but less effective than suggested in the reference literature. This may be because few of our bald acquaintances have really used them daily for an extended period. We personally know of one bald-as-a-billiard fellow who regularly used the polysorbate 80 which we supplied who now has a very nice head of curly (albeit somewhat thin) hair. This was achieved without topical hormones or special nutritional supplements. Male pattern baldness is an aging clock which can sometimes be reset. Durk now has more hair than he did ten years ago when he was 27!

Dandruff is caused by lipid (fat) autoxidation damage to scalp cells, resulting in their proliferation and then falling off. Rancid, musty hair and scalp odors are also caused by autoxidation of lipids in the scalp and on the hair. It can be effectively controlled by shampoos containing antioxidants, such as selenium sulfide (found in Selsun Blue® shampoo) and zinc pyrithione (the latter is a zinc-sulfur compound found in Head and Shoulders® shampoo). Before taking supplementary antioxidants, one of us (Durk) had a lot of dandruff and some hair odor, which he kept under control but could not entirely eliminate with Head and Shoulders® shampoo. Now he does not have to use antidandruff shampoos. But if he goes off his antioxidant supplements, the dandruff and hair odor begin to return in about two weeks. A friend of ours has reported that selenium sulfide shampoo reduced his hair loss.

Durk isn't going bald anymore. But we are both still quite interested in male pattern balding as a convenient readily accessible aging clock. One needs neither laboratory instruments nor decades to observe the impact of experimental manipulations on this aging clock. One can affect it with topical treatments having negligible systemic effect. And if one inadvertently makes this clock tick faster rather than slower, the results are not likely to be fatal (which they could be with the hypothalamic-pituitary clocks) or even permanent. Of course, only some of the things that affect this aging clock will affect aging clocks in general. Topical low-diffusability sex hormones applied with the proper solvent definitely do affect this aging clock but should not be expected to affect aging clocks in general. Both antioxidants and polysorbates 80 and 60 may have more general aging clock effects, since both classes of compounds can cause renormalization of some very early precancerous tissue developmental alterations, and since some aging clocks, such as those in the testosterone-producing Leydig cells in the testes and in the dopaminergic hypothalamic-pituitary nerve tracts, involve lipofuscin-accumulation-induced shutdown which could be a type of "mutation monitor" measuring free radical damage.

Finally, we are currently experimenting with compounds such as minoxidil (Upjohn's Loniten®), diazoxide (Schering's Hyperstat®), and clonidine (Boehringer Ingelheim's Catapres®), all three of which are approved by the FDA for the control of severe high blood pressure. These promote tissue repair where repair does not normally occur; we think they may affect genetic expression. The first two drugs have hirsutism (excess hair growth) as side effects, and the third caused an improvement in memory and learning in some patients with Korsakoff's psychosis (alcoholic brain damage). Of the three drugs, only minoxidil is being tested by its manufacturer for possible eventual FDA approval as a hair restorer. The future undoubtedly holds many more compounds which selectively stimulate tissue regeneration.

8
Exercise: More Is Not Necessarily Better

Americans are in the habit of never walking if they can ride.

—Louis Philippe, Duc d'Orleans (1798)

How much exercise should you do each day? If you're like us, you would rather spend as little time on exercise as is required to maintain a reasonable level of cardiovascular conditioning. Well, we have good news for you. The most effective type of exercise can provide good cardiovascular conditioning in only 30 minutes a week.

Exercise has often been associated with tedious workouts, done as a sort of duty, rather than for pleasure. Recently, there have been attempts to involve people in what are believed to be healthful and enjoyable exercise routines, such as jogging. Some people do enjoy spending an hour or two running each day. However, many others either do not have the time available or else simply prefer to pursue other interests in their leisure hours.

There are four general benefits of regular exercise of the proper type:

1. Muscles, including heart muscle, can be kept in condition, that is, at an efficient level of work output and capable of heavy peak work demands.

2. Regular exercise uses up calories that might otherwise be stored as fat.

222

3. Psychologically, a person who keeps his or her body fit has a sense of well-being and may be able to perform better under physically and emotionally demanding conditions of stress.

4. The proper type of exercise causes the release of growth hormone from the brain's pituitary gland. Growth hormone has an important stimulant effect on the immune system, builds muscles, and burns fats. Recently, however, evidence obtained from the BLSA (the Baltimore Longitudinal Study of Aging, an ongoing study of over 800 healthy persons given a battery of biomedical and sociobehavioral tests at intervals) indicates that in healthy men and women the release of growth hormone in response to exercise ceases after about the age of 30. The physically active adult BLSA men had no greater muscle mass than their age-matched peers who were sedentary, illustrating their loss of exercise-stimulated growth hormone release. In addition, no muscle mass differences attributable to physical activity have been found between older women who are active and those who are sedentary. There are ways for older people to increase pituitary release of growth hormone. We discuss some of these in the next chapter, "Athletics." We and other scientists are continuing our researches in this area and we hope to include additional material in our next book about this important problem.

What is the best type of exercise? That depends first on what type of effects you are looking for. The exercise which is designed for effective cardiovascular system conditioning is not the same as the exercise you should do for athletic prowess. We describe here a system of exercise which is specifically aimed at cardiovascular conditioning, fat loss, and muscle building. It is not designed to make you into an athlete. It should be exercise you enjoy enough to do regularly. Next, the exercise which causes the most rapid cardiovascular conditioning effects, as well as the greatest release of growth hormone in younger people, is *peak effort* expended over a short period of time rather than a less-than-peak effort over a longer time period. Regularly running full tilt up a hill for several minutes conditions the cardiovascular system and, in younger people, causes the release of growth hormone. Jogging for a few miles, unless there is peak effort, releases little or none, and is not very efficient for cardiovascular conditioning. Cardiovascular conditioning can be achieved much more effectively with peak effort exercise.

If you enjoy jogging (it does release the brain's natural morphinelike compounds, the endorphins and enkephalins, giving many joggers a euphoric high), do it—but remember, there is little evidence of health benefits from jogging. The New York Academy of Science held a symposium on the physiology of marathon runners—but the papers delivered at the meeting reported that no health benefits were found. However, recent evidence suggests that marathon running may increase serum content of HDL (high density lipoproteins), which provides protection against heart attacks. In order to make sure that runners do not have high HDL to begin with (rather than increasing the level by running), we need to see studies which examine before *and* after HDL levels. Such studies are necessary because we do know that marathon runners constitute a low-risk group for other factors: they tend to be lean nonsmokers, highly educated, health and nutrition oriented, and generally without such disorders as hypertension. A sample of runners is unlikely to contain many chain-smoking, alcoholic, obese, sedentary, junk-food junkies, which might mean that the observed results were caused by a selection bias. Another recent study found an increase in fibrinolytic (blood clot dissolving) activity in healthy adult humans who participated in a ten-week vigorous physical conditioning program.

Dr. Lawrence E. Morehouse, in the excellent book *Total Fitness in 30 Minutes a Week,* reports his findings that about ten minutes of *peak* effort every other day gave the most benefits in terms of cardiovascular conditioning. Ten minutes every other day will earn you 80 percent of the cardiovascular conditioning benefits of exercising for hours every day! You need not spend a lot of time doing exercises. And you can choose any type that appeals to you, provided *peak* effort is required. You will find that this type of exercise raises the heart rate considerably. This is how you know when you are exerting the desirable peak output. The book contains a chart which tells you how high a heart rate you should work for, given your age and physical condition and how rapidly you can safely approach this heart rate target. If this sounds too good to be true, we should mention that Dr. Morehouse was formerly the director of NASA's manned space flight physiology research program and was the founding director of the Human Performance Laboratory of the University of California at Los Angeles. Dr. Morehouse's statements are not wild opinion; they are facts firmly based on careful instrumental measurements of human exercise performance. Dr. Morehouse has written a fine book on this subject for laymen which is available in paperback. **WARNING:** Do not attempt a peak-output exercise program without this professional guidance. (If you have active heart disease, discuss this program with your physician before you start.) We hope that you will buy this book, written by Dr. Morehouse and Leonard Gross. It will be the best investment in exercise that you have ever made!

9
Athletics: Improving Your Performance with Nutrients

I want to be the best-built man in the world, I said frankly.

— Arnold Schwarzenegger, *Arnold: The Education of a Bodybuilder*

There are two different types of athletic performance: 1) stamina, and 2) peak output. Stamina depends on the ability of your muscles to put out energy for a prolonged period of time. Peak output, on the other hand, is your muscles' ability to put out a maximum amount of energy over a short time. It is now possible to take old rats—the age equivalent of about 80 years for a human—and rejuvenate some of their athletic performance and coordination back to roughly their young adult level. We have applied these techniques to a few humans—and to a significant extent they work. There is still a lot to learn about the processes underlying muscular activities. But, using current knowledge, we have greatly increased our stamina and the size of our muscles with only a few minutes of exercise a week AND the right nutrients.

The biochemistry underlying athletic performance is, like that of aging, becoming increasingly understood. With current knowledge, it is possible to greatly improve athletic output while decreasing the effort required to achieve that output. For example, you can improve stamina (total muscular output) using the proper nutrients. These techniques apply to young as well as older individuals. It is also a good idea to seek advice from a doctor in the relatively new field of sports medicine. Some useful methods are described below.

226

• The citric acid cycle (also called the Krebs cycle) is the chemical pathway of aerobic (oxygen is required) energy production in animals. Oxygen, the electron donor (the fuel), various enzymes, and various food acids are required. See the figure showing the citric acid cycle in Part II, Chapter 4, "Molecules of Life and Life Extension." The energy generated by the oxidation of food to carbon dioxide and water in the citric acid cycle is stored in high-energy phosphate bonds of the ATP molecule (adenosine triphosphate). Energy in the form of ATP is also produced *without* oxygen via glycolysis. Glycolysis is the primary energy pathway used in short interval high-output athletic events, such as sprints. However, it is not an efficient means of ATP production—only a net gain of 2 molecules of ATP is obtained from each molecule of glucose metabolized to pyruvic acid, compared to 38 molecules of ATP per molecule of glucose converted to carbon dioxide and water via the citric acid cycle. Moreover, anaerobic (without oxygen) glycolysis produces toxic lactic acid, which causes that burning sensation in fatigued muscles and the mental confusion which accompanies maximum-output athletics.

Stamina can be increased by increasing the availability of molecules and enzymes used in the citric acid energy cycle: the vitamin pantothenic acid (an essential part of the enzyme acetyl-CoA), malic acid, citric acid, fumaric acid, succinic acid, etc. Nicotinamide or nicotinic acid is also required. In an experiment with calcium pantothenate (a stable form of vitamin B-5, pantothenic acid, a required factor in the citric acid cycle), three groups of rats were provided with a diet that was deficient, adequate, or high in calcium pantothenate. The animals were then put in a tank of water at 18 degrees C (64 degrees F) and allowed to swim to exhaustion. Swimming times for the three groups markedly increased with the amount of calcium pantothenate in their diets as follows:

deficient   16 +or—   3 minutes
adequate   29 +or—   4 minutes
high   62 +or— 12 minutes

Experiments on human volunteers subjected to cold water stress agree with these results. Addition of calcium pantothenate also doubled total work output (but not peak output) of isolated perfused frog muscle preparations in separate experiments.

In order to increase stamina with citric acid cycle food acids, doses of a few grams to several grams are required. The compounds are water soluble and, therefore, are excreted rapidly from the body. In our personal experiments, we have taken them every three or four hours for the duration of the athletic performance.

• Hydergine® (Sandoz) is a prescription drug which is effective in slowing down some of the aging processes in the brain (see Part II, Chapter 9, and Part III, Chapters 2 and 3, for more information). For athletic performance, Hydergine®'s ability to stabilize the brain's energy metabolism is relevant. In one series of experiments, blood was withdrawn from anesthetized cats, reducing cerebral blood flow to a critical level; EEG (brain wave) energy values were reduced by 50 percent within 15 minutes. However, in cats which had been pretreated with Hydergine®, EEG energy was maintained at a normal level for 45 minutes despite the withdrawn blood. Admittedly, in athletics you aren't likely to lose much blood, but after long fatiguing effort the oxygen available to your brain will be diminished due to muscular demand. Hydergine® can maintain normal brain energy levels during these stresses, probably resulting in better judgement and superior neuromuscular control. In our experiments, it seems excellent for mountain climbing or any other athletics at high altitudes (where there is low oxygen availability).

• Acetylcholine is a neuromuscular messenger (enables nerves to communicate with muscle cells) and a neurotransmitter (it carries messages between nerves). This chemical is required for muscular control and proper muscle tone. Both lecithin, which contains phosphatidyl choline, and choline can be used by the body to make acetylcholine. Vitamin B-5 (pantothenate) is required for this conversion. Deaner® (Riker), a prescription drug, increases acetylcholine levels in the brain, where the regulation of movement takes place.

• Vasopressin is a hormone secreted by the posterior pituitary gland of the brain. Also called antidiuretic hormone, vasopressin has several known functions, including the retention of fluids in the body (antidiuretic effect) and pressor effects (blood pressure increases at hundreds of times the antidiuretic dose), as well as causing contraction of smooth muscle such as intestine and uterine walls and blood vessel walls. In addition, vasopressin has beneficial effects on memory and learning in humans. It increases performance in tests requiring attention, fast reactions, precise visual discrimination, coordination, concentration, and focus. Therefore, we expect it to be of value to athletes. The effective memory-improving dose is 16 I.U. per day, well below the maximum frequently used antidiuretic dose and far below the pressor (blood pressure increasing) dose. It may be obtained as a convenient nasal spray called Diapid®, a prescription drug made by Sandoz. Possible overdose side effects include brief headaches, pallor, and intestinal cramps, and it sometimes stimulates angina pains in patients with angina pectoris. **CAUTION:** People with angina should avoid the use of vasopressin.

• Growth hormone (GH) is released by the pituitary gland in the brain in response to exercise, fasting, hypoglycemia, sleep, trauma, dopaminergic stimulants, and other factors. It has many functions, including maintaining the immune system, stimulating muscle growth, and burning fat. Exercise in which there is briefly sustained muscular *peak* output releases growth hormone; exercise at less than peak effort, even when prolonged, releases little or no GH. Recent evidence (from the Baltimore Longitudinal Study of Aging) indicates that growth hormone release in response to exercise ceases by the age of 30 or so, however, although GH release in response to other factors continues. Jogging usually involves less than peak output and, therefore, usually results in no release of GH. As noted in Chapter 8, some recent research has found higher HDL levels in runners. HDL (high density lipoprotein) is a fraction of fat-protein compounds in the blood that provides a reduction of risk of heart attacks. However, the studies have not compared the HDL levels before subjects began running to HDL levels after becoming runners. It is possible that runners may have a high HDL to begin with; we do know that runners tend to be highly educated, well nourished, health-oriented, lean nonsmokers, who are generally free of disorders such as hypertension. Since lazy obese people rarely choose to become marathon runners, some of these apparently pro-running results may be caused by subject selection bias.

There are several nutrients and prescription drugs which cause GH release. These include the amino acids arginine and ornithine and the prescription drugs L-Dopa (another amino acid), bromocriptine (Parlodel®, by Sandoz), and vasopressin (Diapid®, Sandoz nasal spray). In one study, ½ gram per day of L-Dopa increased the growth hormone output of men in their 60s (who were not suffering from Parkinson's disease)

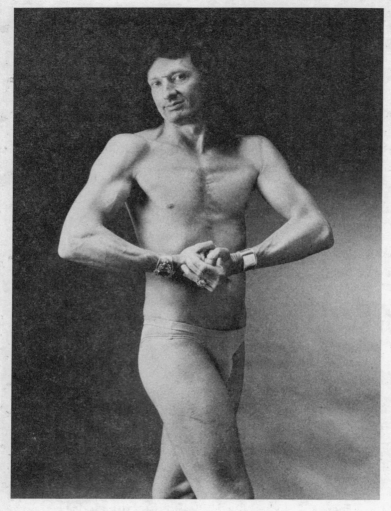

I am not an amateur body builder. Even with our nutritional GH release techniques, the 30 seconds that I exercise before going to bed doesn't put me into the body builder class. I am a 6'4", 177 lb., 37-year-old sedentary scientist, yet I now have a better ratio of muscle to fat than I had in my teens. I eat a high calorie diet like a teenager.

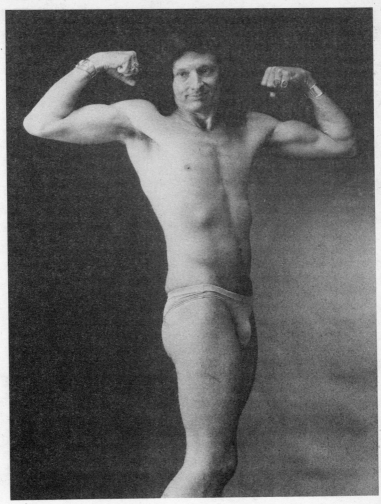

Literally, 85 percent of my time is spent in a swivel chair, an easy chair, or on my water bed, the last being where most of my athletic activities take place. My 30 seconds of exercise is merely lifting a pair of 34 pound dumbbells over my head less than a dozen times. (There are undoubtedly far better exercise routines, but I have not yet studied this area.) I had been doing these exercises for about two months when these photos were taken. It took me a total of about 30 minutes of exercise to build these muscles.

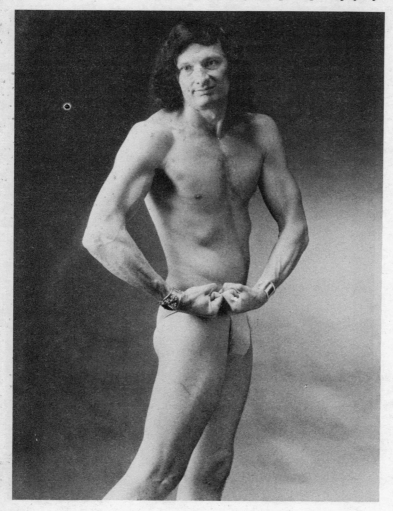

Sandy has been taking much larger quantities of GH releasing nutrients than I, with a more accelerated muscular development; I will be increasing my doses to a comparable level. As Dr. James Watson (Nobel laureate, codiscoverer of the structure and function of DNA) said, "Never confuse hard work with hard thinking." I am dedicated to hard thinking, not hard workouts. I wonder what a person with Arnold Schwarzenegger's dedication could do with these techniques! (Standard body builder diffuse lighting was employed for these photos, but no posing oil or sweat was used to enhance muscular definition.)

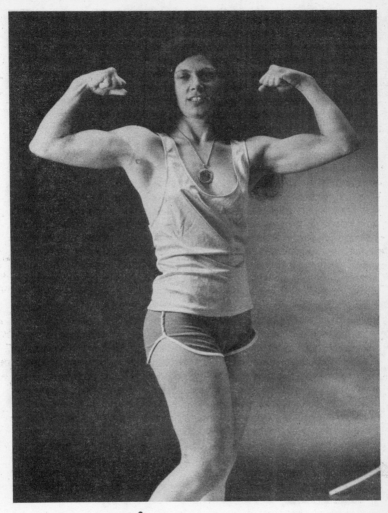

I work out (using a Bullworker®, a well-designed, easy-to-use exercise aid) less than 3 minutes a week. The several grams of growth hormone releasers I take daily are an important part of what has enabled me to build up my muscles and reduce body fat while being an almost entirely sedentary research scientist.

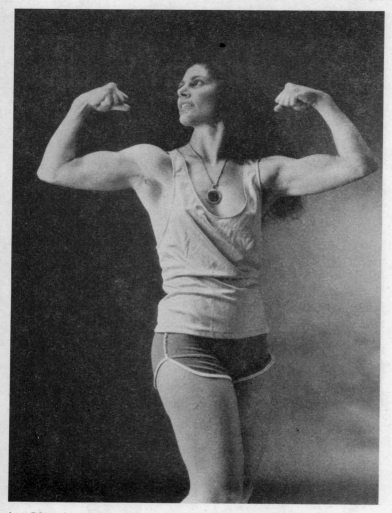

I am 5'3" and weigh 114 pounds, less than I weighed at the age of 22, yet I am far less physically active now and I eat as much. I am much more muscular now than I was then.

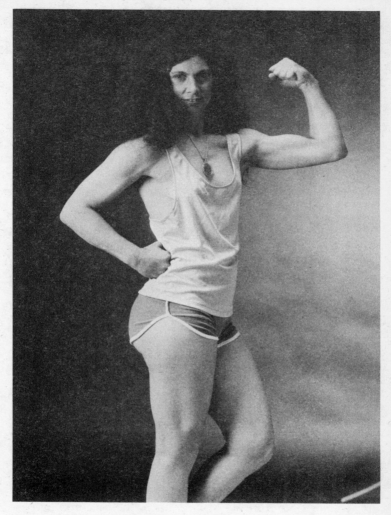

Although women in my family tend toward short, chunky bodies, accumulating fat on the hips and thighs after young adulthood, I have happily been able to avoid this genetically determined fate.

back up to near young adult levels. This may be a partial solution to the problem of cessation of exercise-stimulated growth hormone release in persons over the age of about 30. We and others are doing much research in this area.

GROWTH HORMONE CAUTION: Inappropriate use of GH releasers may have adverse consequences. They should not be used by persons who have not completed their long-bone growth (that is, who have not grown to their full height) unless they have been advised to do so by their physician. After full height is attained, GH will not cause further height increases. Excess GH will cause the skin to grow so rapidly that it becomes noticeably coarser and thicker; this effect is reversible when excess GH is withdrawn. Very excessive GH over an extended period of time can cause irreversible enlargement of joint diameter (which may be unsightly but is usually not dangerous) and lowering of voice pitch due to larynx growth. The maintenance of extremely high levels of growth hormone (above normal teenage to young adult levels) for extended periods of time requires further safety research. In some GH releaser experiments on animals either previously or subsequently given cancer, the GH releasers usually caused an improvement. At Cornell University Medical Center, however, hypophysectomy (surgical removal of the hypothalamus) in women with advanced metastatic breast cancer has sometimes produced dramatic improvements. Since this procedure affects many other hormones besides GH, including LHRH, LH, FSH, TRF, TSH, thyroid, prolactin, estrogens, progestins, endorphins, beta lipotropin, etc., it is not yet clear what is going on here.

In recent research, it was found that L-Dopa given to old rats could restore their swimming abilities to that of young adult rats. The old rats, before getting L-Dopa, swam in a more vertical position and used the energy they did have in a very inefficient manner, sinking under the water after a relatively short time. The old rats, after getting L-Dopa, swam in a more horizontal position (like the young rats) and were indistinguishable from the young rats in their swimming performances. L-Dopa is used in the brain to make dopamine and norepinephrine. Dopamine is a major neurotransmitter involved in motor (muscular movement) control. Parkinsonism patients, who have lost their fine motor control and developed tremors, are often benefited by L-Dopa or other dopaminergic stimulants. (In many cases, a combination of bromocriptine [Parlodel®, Sandoz] plus a somewhat reduced dosage of L-Dopa provides better control of Parkinsonism with fewer side effects.) L-Dopa, like other catechols, is a good antioxidant and has been used for radiation protection. **CAUTION:** Long use at high dose levels, especially without adequate intake of other antioxidants, can lead to undesirable autoxidation side effects.

• Proteolytic enzymes—enzymes that dissolve proteins—increase the turnover rate for proteins by stimulating protein manufacture and repair. Examples of common proteolytic enzymes are bromelain (in raw pineapple) and papain (in raw papaya). Cooked or canned pineapple and papaya do not contain these enzymes, which are destroyed by heating. These enzymes can slowly dissolve away damaged protein tissues, speeding up healing and repair. They have been used to reduce inflammation and edema and to treat many athletic injuries. If you eat raw pineapple or papaya for these enzymes, watch out for the development of sore and tender corners of your lips (they are tenderized in the same way that proteolytic enzymes tenderize meat). When this occurs, stop eating these fruits. Promptly washing your mouth after eating raw pineapple or papaya is a good idea, if you eat them frequently. **CAUTION:** Do not eat raw pineapple or papaya if you have an ulcer. Athletes frequently take tablets of Ananase® (Rorer), a prescription form of bromelain, for athletic injuries.

It has been observed that women athletes sometimes stop menstruating. Recently, Harvard researchers suggested a possible reason. They noted that girls at the start of menstruation need to have a body fat content of about 17 percent or menstruation will not begin. When nonathletic women lose 10 to 15 percent of their body weight, including about a third of their body fat, they usually stop menstruating. The researchers suggest that this may be an adaptation to prevent skinny women from becoming pregnant, because until recently an adequate body store of fat was necessary to survive food shortages, which were frequent. See also Part III, Chapter 13, "Controlling Your Weight."

• Athletic injuries are common. DMSO (dimethyl sulfoxide) is very helpful in reducing damage in many injuries. In crushing injuries, including bruises, blood leaks into the damaged tissues. When the red blood cells hemolyze (break down), they release copper and iron, which stimulate the production in these injured tissues of free radicals (see Part II, Chapter

7, "Our Subversive Free Radicals"). DMSO is an especially effective scavenger of a particular type of free radical, the hydroxyl radical. When DMSO (a clear liquid) is placed on the skin over the injury, it actually moves through the skin and into the deeper tissues, where it inhibits destruction by free radicals, allowing healing to proceed more rapidly. DMSO has been used successfully in some cases of spinal cord injury where, if a solution in physiological saline is injected soon enough (within a few hours after the injury), it has helped prevent the development of paralysis. DMSO is available as a prescription drug and is also sold in some health food stores. Be careful that you buy a high-purity grade of DMSO; see Part III, Chapter 20, "First Aid."

Biochemistry has a great deal more to offer the athlete, whether amateur or professional. It is actually possible to remodel your body, adding muscles and eliminating fat, with far less effort than with conventional means. The aging effects that eventually end all athletic careers can be delayed for at least several years, and perhaps for decades. A whole book could be written on this subject—in fact, we are writing one. Look for it in two or three years.

10
Smoking: Making It Safer with Nutrients

The true and lawful goal of the sciences is none other than this: that human life be endowed with new discoveries and powers.

—Francis Bacon, *Novum Organum* (1620)

We have good news for you, whether you are a hard-core smoker or simply live or work with smokers—which can be equivalent to smoking several cigarettes per day. You can reduce the health risks of tobacco by using the proper nutrients, available at health food stores. Or you can use any of a number of simple techniques to smoke less without reducing your pleasure—and without getting fat! You can even eliminate most of the bad odors of cigarette smoke that cling to your home's rugs, draperies, and walls, while at the same time making it a cleaner and healthier place to live—whether you give up smoking or not. Through scientific research, we now know why people smoke, what real psychological and behavioral benefits smoking provides, what the major molecular mechanisms are which make smoking hazardous, and, finally, how to reduce the hazards of smoking without reducing those benefits of smoking pleasure.

If you are a smoker, you are probably used to reading and hearing preachy messages from friends and strangers about how you should quit smoking. From the point of view of optimal health, it is, of course, sound advice. But most committed smokers, who have quit smoking repeatedly, will

239

doubtless be happy to know that there is another solution to their dilemma. There are a number of ways to make it safer for you to smoke—not as safe as not smoking, but considerably safer than it is now. Many of these ways of reducing smoking risks involve the use of nutrient supplements that you can purchase in any health food store.

Let's consider why people continue to smoke. They don't quit because smoking gives them certain benefits. Many campaigners for the elimination of cigarette smoking have not realized that people would lose these benefits, as well as the health risks. Tobacco has significant effects on behavior and psychological state. Recent research has shown that cigarette smokers (and others who use tobacco) find that tobacco use makes it easier to cope with overstimulation like city noise and overcrowding. That's because the nicotine in cigarette smoke is a stimulus barrier, a substance that makes it easier for a person to function in an overstimulating environment. Human brain-wave activity can be measured by putting electroencephalograph electrodes on a person's head. When a subject is subjected to a sudden unexpected stimulus (like a loud noise), you find out how much the brain responds to these stimuli. The brain of a person who has used nicotine responds less to these distracting stimuli than the brain of someone who doesn't smoke. In this way, the nicotine makes it possible for some people to cope with the overstimulation found in most cities by reducing their brain's reactions to the extraneous stimulation. In one laboratory experiment, for example, rats given nicotine showed less response to painful heat stimuli than rats that did not receive nicotine. When people quit smoking all of a sudden (cold turkey), they suffer from withdrawal symptoms which include an increase in their brain's response to outside stimuli. The rebound effect of no longer using the stimulus barrier of nicotine results in an unpleasant reversal of the nicotine effects, so that the outside stimuli cause a greater response by the brain than if the person had never used the stimulus barrier (nicotine) at all. This makes it difficult for would-be nonsmokers to concentrate. No wonder that quitting smoking is so hard for many people.

Tobacco, and its major psychoactive alkaloid nicotine, is used widely throughout the world. One fascinating aspect of tobacco use, of which few smokers in this country are aware, is that it is used to produce a "trip" (psychedelic experience) in some countries. In Surinam and French Guiana, for example, tobacco is used in combination with the alkaline ash of the bark of sterculia trees, to intensify and accelerate the action of the nicotine. The tobacco is prepared by placing tobacco leaves in a small tin, sprinkling ash under and between the leaves, adding water, and pressing the mix to produce a dark-brown liquid. This is taken as a liquid snuff by inhaling it into the nostrils. It is used during the course of daily activities rather than as part of a special ritual. The drug experience of a user unaccustomed to tobacco was reported as follows: . . . "immediately after inhalation there is an overwhelming feeling of ecstasy, accompanied by a not-unpleasant sweet taste at the back of the mouth. The light-headedness lasts only a few minutes and then gives way to feelings of disorientation, a strong urge to vomit and finally a cold sweat. All effects subside after 20–30 minutes." Needless to say, this type of tobacco use is far different from that of most tobacco users in this country. This form of usage does not involve the smoking of tobacco and hence avoids many of the health hazards associated with smoking.

In order to reduce the risks of tobacco smoking without giving up its benefits, we must first understand how the harm is caused. Only then can we do something sensible to counteract it. We know of several important ways that smoking tobacco diminishes health. The most serious risks are those of increased rates of cancer and cardiovascular disease. The "tars" of tobacco smoke contain a class of chemicals that are believed by many scientists to cause between 40 and 80 percent of all internal human cancers—the polynuclear aromatic hydrocarbons. These substances can cause mutations in the DNA blueprint material of your cells. Such mutations can result in cancer and can also lead to the formation of atherosclerotic plaques. In their role as mutagens, these polynuclear aromatic hydrocarbons first bind to the DNA molecule and then chemically damage it. There are several nutrients able to interfere with this process and, thereby, reduce the risks of getting cancer and atherosclerosis from cigarette smoking. These include vitamins A, E, and C, and the minerals selenium and zinc. Selenium has recently been found to be a powerful inhibitor of cancer formation. In animal experiments, selenium has been used to suppress the formation of cancers caused by exposure to toxic chemicals. People who live in cities where the drinking water is high in selenium have lower cancer rates than people in cities where the drinking water contains low levels of selenium. The National Cancer Institute is now recommending that people take about 200 micrograms of selenium every day as a prophylactic against cancer. They are trying to get the Food and Drug Administration to recommend this in their Recommended Daily Allowances. Such a recommendation would require that the FDA abandon its dogmatic position that all nutrients normally needed or desirable are provided by well-balanced meals, so the delay is likely to be extended. If people took this much selenium every day, cancer rates might eventually decrease by about 70 percent, based on several human and domestic animal epidemology studies both here and abroad, and also based on several animal and tissue culture experiments as well, as reported by Dr. Johan Bjorksten and Dr. Ray Shamberger. We currently prefer to take our selenium in the form of sodium selenite, the form subject to most research to date. Although selenocystine and selenomethionine increase blood levels of selenium more rapidly, these seleno amino acids are less effective than sodium selenite in elevating serum glutathione peroxidase levels. Mammals and birds do not seem to be capable of distinguishing between seleno and sulfur amino acids. Sodium selenite was also superior in inhibiting Ehrlich ascites tumor cell growth in mice. (One type of selenium containing yeast has recently shown good glutathione peroxidase elevation, however. See the chapter notes.)

Another hazardous chemical contained in cigarette smoke is acetaldehyde (and closely related formaldehyde), which is also found in smog and in the bloodstream of alcohol drinkers (the acetaldehyde is made from alcohol principally by the liver). This toxic chemical is known as a cross-linker because it makes undesirable chemical bonds via free radical reactions between molecules in the body, such as proteins and nucleic acids. (See Part II, Chapter 6, "Cross-linked Molecules and Aging.") Although a certain amount of controlled cross-linking is necessary, there are also uncontrolled cross-links in the wrong places. When undesired links form between such molecules, they no longer function normally. Examples of cross-linked proteins are wrinkled, inelastic skin and inelastic, hardened arteries. Emphysema is caused to a substantial extent by cross-linking of lung tissues. The emphysema and lung fibrosis found in victims of the current U.S. paraquat treatment of cannabis program is caused by the fact that paraquat is a powerful free radical initiator which results in extensive lung cross-linking. The use of paraquat on cannabis (grass or hash) greatly increases its health hazard. Since free radicals are often mutagens and carcinogens, smoking paraquat-contaminated cannabis may also cause lung cancer. Vitamin B-3 has reduced paraquat toxicity in experiments on rats.) The hardening of rubber windshield wipers is also a cross-linking process. Fortunately, a very effective nutrient combination against undesirable cross-linking is vitamin B-1, vitamin C, and the amino acid cysteine (found in eggs and sold as the pure material in some health food stores). When Dr. Herbert Sprince gave large doses of acetaldehyde to rats, 90 percent of them died, but when he gave another group of rats the same dose of acetaldehyde after fortifying them with B-1, C, and cysteine, none of the rats died.

Nicotine, although not as much of a health problem as the polynuclear aromatic hydrocarbons or aldehydes, has risks of its own. Nicotine causes blood vessels to constrict (become smaller in diameter), thus increasing blood pressure. Also, nicotine causes an increase in blood fats, such as cholesterol. But these effects can be largely countered with nicotinic acid. You can see from the name that nicotinic acid is closely related to nicotine. The drawings below, showing the structures of nicotine and nicotinic acid (vitamin B-3, which is also called niacin), reveal the similarity. Unlike nicotine, however, the vitamin niacin causes dilation (widening) of the blood vessels and a reduction in blood fats like cholesterol. In one human study, a dose of 3 grams of niacin per day reduced the cholesterol level in the bloodstream by 26 percent after only two weeks. Other studies have found that these desirable results continue as long as people take the niacin.

N = nitrogen
O = oxygen
C = carbon
H = hydrogen

CH₃

cut here and
add oxygen

A nicotine molecule,
the stimulus barrier
psychochemical in tobacco.

A nicotinic acid molecule,
also called niacin,
a form of vitamin B-3

As mentioned previously the vitamin niacin has, for some people, annoying—but harmless and transitory—side effects of flushing and itching (due to the dilation of blood vessels and also the release of histamine). To minimize the effects, start with niacin at a low dose (perhaps 100 milligrams), taken on a full stomach. Work your way up to one gram after each meal. Usually, you'll find the side effects diminish, often disappearing completely when you use the niacin regularly. Since niacin is acidic, it is wise to neutralize it with an antacid if you use large doses of more than a gram per day; (see below for more about this).

Cigarette smoke also contains heavy metals, particularly lead, radioactive polonium, and arsenic. These heavy metals all poison certain enzyme reactions in your body, particularly those with sulfhydryl groups, which are often protective antioxidants. Vitamin C provides considerable protection against these heavy metals by helping to keep them in solution so that they can be eliminated from the body in the urine. Vitamin C can also block the formation of cancer-causing nitrosamines, made from nitrates and nitrites in cigarette smoke and amines such as nicotine and other amines found in your daily food. Vitamin C can even help prevent that scourge of all smokers, the smoker's cough. (It works for sore throat too.) Add a teaspoon of vitamin C crystals (available at many health food stores) to a glass of cold water or fruit juice and sip this drink while smoking. (The vitamin C is acidic, so you may want to add ½ teaspoon of baking soda to neutralize it. Don't use baking soda if you are on a low-sodium diet or have essential hypertension; in the latter case, try powdered limestone or calcium carbonate instead.) Don't save what you don't drink, because vitamin C is destroyed by autoxidation in water within only a few hours. Smoker's cough can also be prevented or ameliorated with Hydergine®. Simply hold one or two 1-milligram sublingual tablets under your tongue while smoking. Hydergine®, a powerful antioxidant, can provide protection from the major damaging agents in smoker's cough, free radicals.

Cigarette smoke also contains carbon monoxide and nitrogen oxides. These dangerous gases can be found in smog in small quantities, but they are a major problem in cigarette smoke. Carbon monoxide destroys the ability of your blood to carry oxygen. Nitrogen oxides damage your throat, lungs, DNA (cell blueprints), and abnormally oxidize your body's fats

BASIC VITAMINS AND MINERALS FOR SMOKERS

(dose per day)

Selenium, trace element	250 micrograms
Vitamin A	10,000 to 20,000 international units
Vitamin E	1,000 to 2,000 international units
Zinc (gluconate or other chelated form)	50 milligrams
Vitamin B-1	½ to 1 gram
Vitamin B-2	100 to 200 milligrams
Vitamin C	3 to 10 grams
Cysteine (not cystine)	1 to 3 grams (at least three times as much vitamin C as cysteine)
Vitamin B-3 (niacin, not niacinamide)	300 milligrams to 3 grams (100 milligrams to 1 gram taken 3 times a day on a full stomach), starting at 100 milligrams
Vitamin B-5 (pantothenate)	250 to 1000 milligrams
Vitamin B-6	250 to 500 milligrams
Choline	1 to 3 grams
PABA (a B vitamin)	500 milligrams to 1 gram
Beta Carotene	20,000 to 60,000 international units

via a free radical mechanism, turning them into cancer-causing substances. Fortunately, the antioxidant vitamins, which block abnormal, uncontrolled oxidation reactions (including vitamins A, C, E, B-1, calcium pantothenate or pantothenic acid, B-6, and PABA), provide very effective protection from nitrogen oxides.

Some additional advice for smokers on their vitamin/mineral formulation:

CAUTION: Do not start out taking these high doses. Do not start to take this formula on an empty stomach, either. Start at about ⅛ of these amounts per day and slowly increase your doses. Be sure to divide the total daily dose into three parts and take it with meals to slow its absorption and to minimize the gastric effects of acidic vitamins such as C and niacin. This allows your body time to adjust to all these extra nutrients. If you take too much initially, annoying (but not hazardous) side effects may occur, such as upset stomach, diarrhea, and brief skin flushing and itching. It is a good idea to consult your doctor before you start to take these substances. If you skipped over the Disclaimers in "The Engraved Invitation" at the beginning of this book, we suggest you read them now.

CAUTION: Persons with diabetes mellitus (sugar insulin diabetes) should use large doses of vitamins C, B-1, and the amino acid cysteine with caution and *only* under the supervision of their physician. This nutrient combination is capable of inactivating insulin by reducing some disulfide bonds, including one or more of the three disulfide bonds that determine insulin's tertiary structure (three dimensional shape). We have clinical laboratory serum glucose determinations (use the hexokinase method only) on about two dozen nondiabetic adults using these nutrients, and all serum glucose levels have been normal, and all urine samples have been sugar free. However, we have *not* seen test results showing its effects on diabetics.

Vitamins B-1, B-2, B-3 (niacin), B-5 (also known as pantothenate), B-6, PABA, and C, and the amino acid cysteine, should be taken in three or four divided portions (which add up to the daily dose). This is because these vitamins are rapidly eliminated via the urine and must be replaced several times a day to maintain high levels in the bloodstream. You can demonstrate this for yourself by taking a 50-milligram vitamin B-2 tablet, which will color the urine a bright yellow a half hour or so after taking it. In about three or four hours, the urine will have become pale again, indicating how quickly the B-2 (and other water-soluble vitamins) is eliminated. The other supplements (choline, selenium, vitamins E and A, and the chelated zinc) do not have to be taken in divided doses throughout the day, but may be if desired. Otherwise once a day is adequate for these.

It is important that at least three times as much vitamin C be used as cysteine. In people who do not take adequate quantities of water-soluble antioxidant nutrients such as vitamin C, it is possible for cysteine to be converted to cystine (the oxidized form of cysteine). Cystine can form damaging stones in the kidneys or urinary bladder, but cysteine can't.

Some people experience dizziness or headache when first using niacin. This is caused by the widening of blood vessels in the brain, particularly when they have been chronically narrowed by nicotine. The dizziness and headache usually disappear with regular niacin use. When niacin is not taken on a full stomach, flushing and itching are more likely to occur. These symptoms may be alarming but are not harmful. **CAUTION:** The acidity of niacin should be neutralized when large doses are used and particularly if it is taken on an empty stomach.

Vitamin C in the form of crystals or powder is preferred. Sodium ascorbate (nonacidic vitamin C) is best unless you are on a low-sodium diet. Vitamin C, which can provide partial protection against most of the hazards of smoking, is markedly lowered in concentration in the serum of smokers.

Vitamin B-5 (pantothenic acid or calcium pantothenate) is an antioxidant which will provide noticeable and rapid improvement in the appearance of your skin. The cross-linking pollutants in cigarette smoke cause premature skin wrinkling.

Vitamin B-6 levels of smokers are known to be lower than those of nonsmokers. Since vitamin B-6 can help prevent undesirable oxidation reactions in the body (like the ones that turn fats in your body into cancer- and atherosclerosis-causing substances), vitamin B-6 supplementation is especially important for anyone who smokes.

Vitamin A, an antioxidant and a specific regulator of epithelial tissue growth, such as skin and cells lining the lung, throat, and gastrointestinal tract, is markedly reduced in the serum of smokers. See Part III, Chapter 19, "Cancer," for details.

The B vitamin PABA provides protection against ozone damage to the lungs. Ozone is found in smog, cigarette smoke, and the smoke of almost anything that burns. PABA should not be used at the same time as you are taking a sulfa drug because the PABA can prevent the sulfa drug from being effective. (Sulfa drugs work by resembling PABA and fooling bacteria into substituting them for real PABA, thereby giving the bacteria a vitamin deficiency because the sulfa drugs don't do the jobs done by PABA.)

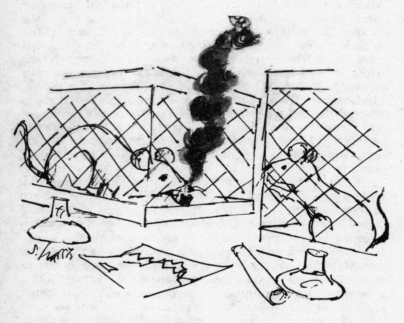

"I can't complain. Last week they had me on martinis."

Vitamin B-2 is required for the protective enzyme glutathione reductase. The added cysteine makes more glutathione, which in its reduced form is an antioxidant. Glutathione reductase reduces oxidized glutathione, thereby recycling it for reuse.

CAUTION: Keep in mind that vitamins B-3 (niacin) and C (most widely available as ascorbic acid) are acids, so if you take megadoses, it is advisable to take an antacid, such as baking soda (bicarbonate of soda), to avoid irritating the stomach or, under rare conditions, even causing an ulcer. You can test the pH (acidity or alkalinity) of your urine (to be sure it is properly neutralized or somewhat basic) with pH paper or litmus papers available at any drugstore. The pH of normal urine is 4.8 to 8.0. Neutral pH is 7.0; lower pH numbers indicate an acid, while higher pH numbers are basic (alkaline). When your urine makes pink litmus paper dipped in it turn pale blue, the urine is basic.

Psychologist Stanley Schacter found that people who had an acidic urine smoked more than people with an alkaline urine. In his investigation of this phenomenon, he gave one group of smokers 4 grams of antacid baking soda per day (we suggest 1 gram between meals and a gram before bedtime), which reduced their craving for smoking. In the fifth week of the study, this baking soda group of smokers were using only 0.14 cigarettes per person each day, whereas 7.8 cigarettes per person were smoked per day by another group taking vitamin C (which increased acidity) and by a third control group receiving a nonactive placebo. Scientists know the reason for these findings. The nicotine is eliminated through the urine. When the urine is acid, more of the nicotine is eliminated than when the urine is alkaline. Since one of the main reasons smokers smoke is for the stimulus-barrier effect of the nicotine, they smoked more often when the urine was acid, to keep their blood and brain levels of nicotine up. In the group taking the baking soda, the nicotine was not eliminated as fast, so the smokers did not need to smoke as often. If you have essential hypertension or are on a low-sodium diet, use powdered limestone (calcium carbonate), dolomite, or some other low-sodium antacid recommended by your physician instead of baking soda, which is sodium bicarbonate.

One of the most serious problems confronting smokers who are able to quit smoking is that of weight gain. It is not a very good bargain to quit smoking in exchange for becoming obese. It is well known that obese persons have higher rates of cancer and cardiovascular diseases, as well as many other dangerous conditions, than people of normal weight. In fact, the risks are much higher (much more than additive) for people who are both fat and smokers. One of the major reasons for these problems of the obese is the abnormal, uncontrolled oxidation of fats in their bodies. Fats in the body can be converted into poisonous oxidized fats by oxygen in the tissues and by other free radical oxidation initiators or oxidizers like acetaldehyde, nitrogen oxides, and ozone (found in almost any kind of smoke and smog). These oxidized fats have several negative effects on health: they are carcinogens (cancer-causing agents) and they can damage DNA (the cell's blueprints), leading to abnormal cell function. Damage to DNA is believed to be a major factor in aging, as well as the usual cause of cancer.

The oxidized fats inhibit certain white blood cells (macrophages) which normally attack and eat bacteria, viruses, cancer cells, and other undesirables in the body. But in fat people, who are full of oxidized fats, white blood cells are deterred from attacking these enemies. The result is that fat people get sick more often than people of normal weight. Many antioxidant nutrients provide protection against these abnormal, uncontrolled oxidations (that's why these nutrients are called antioxidants), including vitamins A, C, E, B-1, B-5, B-6, and PABA, the amino acid cysteine, and the minerals zinc and selenium. Even with protection, though, it is better not to be obese.

One possible reason for the obesity problem that plagues people who quit smoking is that eating may replace nicotine as a stimulus barrier. There are ways of circumventing this problem. Nicotine is a cholinergic substance, meaning that it stimulates that part of the brain where nerve cells communicate with one another using the brain chemical acetylcholine. People who smoke may require a high level of cholinergic stimulation. It may be possible to substitute choline, a vitamin and cholinergic substance, for the nicotine. Choline is used by the brain to make acetylcholine (see Part II, Chapter 9, for more about this and other nutrients and your brain). Acetylcholine is used by the brain's system that controls how much outside stimulation gets into the brain. Without enough acetylcholine, outside stimuli come pouring in. Choline may be able to provide the same type of stimulus barrier effect as nicotine without the risks associated with the use of nicotine (which are especially large in smoked tobacco). Regular use of choline has several benefits, including stabilization of membranes (like those in your joints and lungs) and increase of human intelligence and memory (in MIT students taking 3 grams per day and involving the learning of lists of words). Furthermore, choline has been found to increase the life span of experimental animals.

Another way to avoid obesity is to take the appetite-reducing amino acid phenylalanine, discussed in several previous chapters, including the chapter on weight control, but worth repeating here. This amino acid is found in such foods as meats, cheeses, and milk. In fact, you probably get about 2.8 grams a day in your diet (about $\frac{1}{10}$ ounce). The best way to use phenylalanine is as the pure amino acid, available at a few health food stores. Take between 100 and 500 milligrams in the evening on an empty stomach just before bed. Once you have reduced your weight, it may be a good idea to also reduce your intake of phenylalanine, or even eliminate it altogether, if you can maintain your weight without it. (It is better to use the pure amino acid rather than foods containing the phenylalanine because the phenylalanine has to compete with other amino acids to get into the brain. Foods contain a lot of these other amino acids, so only a little phenylalanine can get into the brain this way. And only the material that reaches the brain can help reduce appetite.) Phenylalanine should be distinguished from phenylpropanolamine, an appetite depressant used in many over-the-counter diet pills. The brain uses phenylalanine to make norepinephrine (NE), a chemical needed for communication between certain nerve cells that are involved in appetite regulation. Phenylpropanolamine cannot be used by the brain to make more NE, but it does cause the brain to use its supplies of NE, eventually depleting them. When the supply of NE runs low, after a couple of weeks or so of using phenylpropanolamine, you suffer a letdown and will probably go on a rebound eating binge. This does not happen with phenylalanine, since it is the natural nutrient used in your brain to make more NE. **CAUTION:** It is important to stress, as we have earlier, that in large doses (more than the amounts mentioned here) phenylalanine can increase blood pressure. People with high blood pressure should begin at a very low dose (perhaps 100 milligrams) and have frequent blood pressure readings to make sure it isn't rising. If you become irritable or aggressive, or have headaches or insomnia, you should reduce your dose of phenylalanine, or perhaps take it midway between breakfast and lunch. Continuous use of high doses of phenylalanine on an empty stomach, to increase its availability to the brain, has not been tested for chronic toxicities. Such use must be considered experimental. In the brains of newborns who have extremely high circulating levels of phenylalanine, due to a serious genetic defect (phenylketonuria, an absence of an enzyme in the brain), this amino acid and its breakdown products lead to destruction of brain tissue and mental retardation.

SELF-DEFENSE FOR NONSMOKERS

Some of you reading this book are nonsmokers wondering how you can protect yourself, your family, and your loved ones from cigarette smoke produced by smoking relatives, coworkers, friends, and strangers. In a study of middle-aged subjects, Drs. James R. White and Herman F. Froeb found recently that nonsmokers who inhaled tobacco smoke in their workplace had a significant reduction in the small-airways function of their lungs compared to nonsmokers not so exposed. This reduction in lung capacity was similar to that seen in light smokers and smokers who did not inhale but was not as severe as that seen in heavy smokers. The same nutrients that provide protection to smokers will also help protect nonsmokers. Particularly effective are vitamins C, E, B-1, A, and PABA, the amino acid cysteine, and the minerals zinc and selenium. Remember that sidestream smoke (the smoke that enters the air directly from the burning tobacco) contains far more of the carcinogenic tars and smoke particles than inhaled smoke, which has been filtered through a mat of tobacco. A recent EPA study conducted by Drs. Repace and Lowrey has quantified the effects of this sidestream smoke on innocent bystanders. A typical nonsmoker who either lives or works with a smoker is involuntarily exposed to particulates and carcinogens, equivalent to smoking 4 to 20 cigarettes per day! Simply being in the same room with a smoker forces you to become a smoker. A recent study conducted in Japan compared the incidence of lung cancer in nonsmoking women who lived with nonsmoking husbands to that of "nonsmoking" women who lived with husbands who smoked. The "nonsmoking" women whose husbands smoked had about twice the incidence of lung cancer of the nonsmoking women with nonsmoking husbands. Involuntary exposure to tobacco smoke in public places is, in our opinion, a far more serious public health hazard than smog, automotive or industrial pollution, or low level radiation. Although this problem may be politically intractable due to the tobacco state Congressmen's pursuit of what they perceive to be their own states' best interests, it is readily subject to a technological fix on an individual home and business basis.

The proper type of room air purifier can provide complete protection from the hazards of tobacco-smoke-laden air and from the sticky film of carcinogenic tar that tends to coat everything in a smoker's room, and almost complete protection from the unpleasant odor of stale smoke. There are two basic types of air cleaners that are suitable for this purpose:

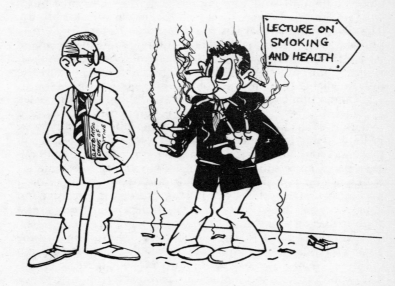

the HEPA filter type and the electronic precipitator type. The HEPA (high efficiency particle absolute) filter was originally developed to remove tiny radioactive plutonium particles from the air of nuclear weapons factories. They are so effective that they remove not only all smoke and tars from the air but also all pollen and bacteria, as well as most viruses. The HEPA filter air cleaner requires little maintenance: every six to twelve months you replace a prefilter (cost about $2), and every few years you replace the HEPA filter (cost about $60).

The electronic precipitator type has a prefilter like the HEPA unit. The small-particle filter is an electronic collector cell that pulls tiny particles from the air the same way that static electricity on a comb or record attracts dust. As the collector cell must be washed with warm water containing dishwashing detergent every few months, the electronic precipitator is a bit less convenient than the HEPA unit, though both are equally effective if properly maintained. Power consumption and sometimes noise tend to be lower in the electronic type.

Activated charcoal filters are available as an option on both the HEPA and the electronic precipator units. Activated charcoal is a universal odor grabber; whether your problem is stale smoke, fried onions, or a wet dog, it will suck it right up. The activated charcoal has to be replaced one to four times per year, so get a unit which holds granular activated charcoal in a refillable basket or frame. When the odors come back, simply dump out the old charcoal granules and pour in the new (available from any air conditioning contractor).

In addition to giving you a safer and more pleasant place in which to live or work, these air cleaners (the HEPA filter and the electronic precipitator) can pay for themselves by greatly reducing the need to repaint, clean draperies, furniture, and rugs, and even dust and vacuum clean! Do not confuse these air cleaners with "negative-ion air fresheners," which are far less effective for this purpose. (See Appendix I for sources of air cleaners.) Furthermore, the negative-ion generators produce a free radical, superoxide, from atmospheric oxygen and water.

You don't have to have a doctor's prescription to purchase an air cleaner—but if you do get a doctor's prescription for an air cleaner you can deduct it from your taxes as a medical expense. Common medical indications for an air cleaner prescription are airborne allergies, asthma, and emphysema.

A very simple way to reduce smoking risks is to use those cigarettes which are highest in nicotine compared to tars. The lowest-tar cigarettes are not always safer than higher-tar ones. Research has shown that smokers tend to smoke on the basis of nicotine content. If a cigarette is low in nicotine, a smoker will smoke more of them to get a satisfactory level of nicotine. With high-nicotine cigarettes, smokers tend to smoke fewer of them. You may be able to reduce your cigarette consumption by smoking cigarettes that have the highest ratio of nicotine to tars (nicotine content divided by tar content). Some comparisons for several popular brands are:

BRAND	NICOTINE*	TAR*	NICOTINE/ TAR RATIO
	(milligrams)		
Triumph Filter	0.4	3	.13
Kool Super Lights	0.7	7	.10
Carlton Soft Pack	0.1	1	.10
Viceroy Rich Lights	0.8	9	.089
Virginia Slims Lights	0.8	9	.089
Tareyton Lights	0.4	5	.080
Salem Lights	0.8	10	.080
True	0.4	5	.080
Winston Lights 100s	1.0	13	.077
Merit Kings	0.6	8	.075
Marlboro Lights	0.8	12	.067
Merit 100s	0.7	11	.064
Benson & Hedges Lights (menthol)	0.7	11	.064

*These tar and nicotine values are as shown on cigarette packages of these brands (as taken from latest FTC report or determined using FTC method) in April 1980.

We would like to see cigarettes fortified with nicotine to greatly increase the nicotine-to-tar ratio and, thereby, reduce the number of cigarettes smoked. This would reduce the health risks associated with smoking. Under current rules of the FDA and the Treasury Department's Bureau of Alcohol and Tobacco Tax, adding nicotine to cigarettes is not allowed, and tobacco companies, even if they were permitted to do this, would not be allowed to claim any health benefits for the nicotine-fortified cigarettes, even though these cigarettes would be healthier to use than those with a lower nicotine-to-tar ratio. The added nicotine would cost less than $1/100$ of a cent per pack, and you would be smoking less and enjoying it more than ever before.

You can avoid most of the health risks of smoking while still getting the stimulus-barrier benefits of nicotine by using snuff or chewing tobacco. Although these forms of tobacco are much safer than cigarettes, they are not completely safe and certainly are rather messy to use. Few houses and offices have spittoons nowadays. We have long thought that a nicotine-containing chewing gum would be an excellent way for smokers to stop smoking without giving up nicotine. Such a product may soon be available in the United States. A nicotine chewing gum called Nicorette is now being sold in Canada (prescription only) and in Switzerland (over the counter). The Dow Chemical Company, which is selling the gum in Canada under license to the Danish company A/B Leo, is not sure what approach it will take when it applies for FDA permission to market the gum in the United States. The FDA does not approve recreational drugs—even when they replace older, more hazardous recreational drugs such as cigarettes.

Each stick of Nicorette gum contains either 2 or 4 milligrams of nicotine. A pack of fifteen sticks is intended to replace a pack of twenty cigarettes. The gum has done well in clinical trials with 3,000 volunteers. Minor side effects of use can include a taste some people don't like, throat irritation, excessive salivation, and hiccups. The side effects will not include lung cancer or emphysema. Although Nicorette is not yet available in the United States, it will be possible for many people to get it in Canada. And we don't think there will be a heavy penalty for amateur nicotine smuggling!

Using some of these simple methods, it is possible for smokers to suffer less from their smoking while getting all the benefits. The stimulus-barrier effects of nicotine can be obtained by using nonsmoked forms of tobacco, such as snuff, nicotine chewing gum, and chewing tobacco, or possibly by substituting choline for nicotine. The cancer-causing polynuclear aromatic hydrocarbons and acetaldehyde can also be avoided by using nonsmoked tobacco. Or you can use high-nicotine-to-low-tar cigarettes. Or you can use nutrients which protect you from the hazards of smoking. Yet another way is to make your urine alkaline to help keep the nicotine in your brain. Whatever you decide to do, you have the opportunity to choose your own habits at your own desired risk level.

Besides the nutrients, there are two prescription drugs, mentioned earlier, that are helpful to a smoker, but your doctor may not be aware of this use for these drugs because of the FDA's rules preventing drug companies from telling doctors about new (FDA unapproved) uses for their products. The first is the remarkable drug Hydergine® (Sandoz), which has appeared often in previous chapters. It can not only help prevent damage to health when you smoke, it can even undo some of the damage that has already been done. Hydergine® is a very safe drug. The only contraindications for its use (that is, medical conditions that make it undesirable to use Hydergine®) are sensitivity to the drug (we do not know anyone who experienced this) and acute or chronic psychosis. The dose recommended in this country (as set by FDA) is 3 milligrams a day. In Europe, the dose typically used is 9 milligrams a day.

What does Hydergine® do? We originally came to study Hydergine® as part of our research into aging processes because of its potential for life extending effects. Hydergine®, which has been shown to be a very powerful antioxidant, slows aging in the brain caused by several different aging mechanisms. Hydergine® can maintain the normal brain energies of an animal (as measured by EEG) for forty-five minutes, even when the animal's oxygen supply has been reduced to a dangerously low level (without Hydergine®, we would see brain damage within fifteen minutes). Hydergine® is routinely used in many European countries for emergencies such as stroke, heart attack, drowning, electrocution, etc., and can often be useful in the revival of apparently dead patients if given soon enough. What can Hydergine® do for smokers? It protects the brain and the heart from the oxygen-depleting effects of the carbon monoxide in cigarette smoke, from the blood-vessel-constricting effects of nicotine, and from the abnormal oxidizing effects of the aldehydes and nitrogen oxides in cigarette smoke. Sublingual Hydergine® promptly combats smoker's cough, too. For further information on Hydergine® and its remarkable effects on the brain, see Part III, Chapter 2, "Revitalizing Your Brain Power."

The second prescription drug of interest to smokers, called diphenylhydantoin, has been used successfully to allow smokers to quit without withdrawal symptoms. Mentioned earlier, this drug has been used safely in humans for decades; in experimental animals it was found to improve their learning ability under certain conditions, and even to increase their life span. Diphenylhydantoin has been used for many years by epileptics to control their epileptic seizures. Many epileptics use diphenylhydantoin every day of their lives, often starting in childhood. Diphenylhydantoin is also a stimulus barrier (like nicotine) which has been used successfully in smoking-withdrawal trials with human subjects. It works very well. The reason this treatment is not being widely used is because the drug is approved only as a treatment for epilepsy, not for smoking. In fact, since smoking is not considered a disease, the FDA may *never* approve any treatment, no matter how safe, specifically for the purpose of stopping smoking. (Considering how many people are killed by smoking each year, this FDA policy is difficult to understand.) If all else has failed and you would like to try to cut down on your smoking with the help of diphenylhydantoin, you can chew a 50-milligram children's tablet when you crave a smoke. It is wise to begin using only two tablets a day and work up to as many as six a day, if necessary, starting out slowly to get used to the drug's sedative effects. If you use over 100 milligrams a day and want to stop taking it, you should taper off the drug slowly. Otherwise you may experience some withdrawal symptoms. Smokers report that it is much easier to withdraw from diphenylhydantoin than from cigarettes. Once you have stopped smoking, slowly reduce and finally discontinue the diphenylhydantoin. Prolonged use has some undesirable effects, such as occasional overgrowth of the gums (particularly in people with poor dental hygiene), and it may produce sedation during the day when you do not want such an effect.

CAUTION: If you consider using the vitamin and other drug suggestions in this chapter, you should remember that chronic smokers may have stomach or duodenal ulcers. These can be aggravated if acidic vitamins are taken on an empty stomach. Therefore, consult with your doctor first, before taking our suggestions.

IMPORTANT LAST MINUTE ADDITION: A recent study indicates that beta carotene provides substantial protection to smokers against lung cancer. See Appendix K (References and Chapter Notes) for this chapter.

11
You Can Protect Yourself from Pollution

Every man takes the limits of his own field of vision for the limits of the world.

—Arthur Schopenhauer

Political processes have been slow, inefficient, and ineffective in dealing with pollution. So why don't you deal with it yourself—at least, with the effects of pollution on your own body? Nutrients you can buy at any health food store provide remarkably effective protection.

Preventing people from polluting the environment you live in is very difficult. Such mass action depends on unreliable political processes. Don't rely on laws; they may not happen. And even when laws have been enacted, they have often controlled the wrong things, and at far too great a cost. For example, a nonsmoker living or working with a smoker may double his or her chances of contracting lung cancer, yet EPA regulations ignore this ubiquitous and lethal form of pollution while wasting billions of our tax dollars controlling pollutants of far less consequence.

You can protect yourself and your loved ones against the most pervasive forms of pollution, without waiting for others to take action. Here are some ways:

• Chlorine (an oxidant) and some chlorinated organic compounds in your water supply can promote cancer and contribute to heart disease. The chlorinated organics are broken down in the body by the mixed-function oxidase enzymes, which are found in all cells but are particularly active in the liver. Upon breakdown, the chlorinated organics are converted to free radicals, which do damage that can lead to cancer and cardiovascular disease. Singlet oxygen, a highly reactive form of oxygen which does similar damage to free radicals (and can even produce free radicals), can be easily made in the lab by reacting salt, water, hydrogen peroxide, and sodium hypochlorite. Chlorinated drinking water contains significant quantities of hypochlorite. Therefore, it can be expected that drinking chlorinated water will increase the levels of dangerous singlet oxygen in your body, since hydrogen peroxide and salt are found there. It is simple and inexpensive to remove these water pollutants in your home by installing a water filter combining coarse filtration (to remove particulates) and activated charcoal, which removes organics and chlorine from the water as it flows through. A suitable water filtration unit (such as the one we use) can be purchased inexpensively from Sears for about $20. The filter cartridge (replaceable for $5.00) lasts about 6 months, some time after which you can begin to taste chlorine again. That's the time to replace the filter cartridge. We think the filtered water tastes delicious—as good as expensive bottled water—and it is ideal for cooking as well. Note that this type of filter does not remove minerals, which have health benefits (there is a positive correlation between heart attacks and soft water, which is low in minerals). Water distillation units not only remove the desirable minerals, but they have the additional disadvantage that organics and chlorine will distill over with the steam in all but extremely expensive research laboratory units. We are *not* suggesting that chlorination of public water supplies be halted. The potential hazards of water-borne diseases like typhoid fever are far greater than the carcinogenic hazards of the chlorination products. But after the chlorine has disinfected the water, you can remove it and its byproducts from the water that you use for drinking and cooking. The EPA has proposed that all municipal water systems treat their water with activated charcoal after chlorination. This approach is needlessly expensive, since only a tiny fraction of the water will ever be used internally by humans..

• Ozone is a strong oxidizing agent found in all polluted city air and also over green countryside. Pine trees in particular produce ozone and free radicals by releasing hydrocarbons which interact with air and ultraviolet light. The Blue

Ridge Mountains of Virginia and the Great Smoky Mountains were covered with this photochemical smog long before the white man arrived in America. Los Angeles, too, already had heavy smog by the time the white man arrived. (In fact, the Indians living here called it "the valley of ten thousand smokes.") Vitamins E and PABA have both been demonstrated to protect rats against ozone damage. Dietary supplementation of 100 milligrams of dl-alpha-tocopheryl acetate per kilogram of diet extended lethal time for survival of 50 percent of the animals exposed continuously to one part per million of ozone from 8.2 to 18.5 days. Another nutrient group effective in providing protection against carcinogenic effects of air pollutants in experimental animals are the precursors to vitamin A, the retinoids, vitamin A itself, and the carotenoids, such as beta carotene (which give carrots their yellow color). Singlet oxygen is created during some reactions of ozone. Both alpha tocopherol and beta carotene (more effective than alpha tocopherol) can quench (terminate chain reactions of) singlet oxygen. Because of its particular molecular structural relationship to beta carotene, we think that the red carotenoid canthaxanthin should be even more effective at quenching singlet oxygen.

• Nitrates and nitrites, used in many meats to prevent growth of ultratoxin-producing botulism organisms and carcinogen-producing *Aspergillis flavus* mold, can combine with amines found in the meats to form carcinogenic nitrosamines. However, vitamin C, in adequate doses, can block nitrosamine formation. In fact, some meat packers add sodium ascorbate, a form of vitamin C, to the meat, along with the nitrites. However, there is an FDA-set legal limit on how much C can be added, preventing the packers from providing better protection from nitrosamines. The food industry has filed a request for the FDA to permit higher ascorbate additions to meat.

• Most urban lead pollution is found in particles in the air and dust. (Small children may suffer from the *much* greater hazard of eating lead paint chips, and a few very old urban areas such as parts of New York, Boston, and London are still served by dangerous lead water pipes.) Air particles also contain carcinogenic tars from smoke in the air, which are a far greater health hazard. These particles can be easily removed from the air you breathe at home by installing an electrostatic precipitator. This device has a fan which sucks air through the unit, where air particles are electrically charged by a fine wire electric grid. The charged particles are then attracted to an oppositely charged metal plate, where they become stuck fast. The cleaned air is blown out the other end. Many electrostatic precipitators also contain a charcoal filter to remove odors. The electrostatic collector cell will need washing every few months or so—which can be simply done in the sink or shower. Electrostatic precipitators are available from Sears, Montgomery Ward, and other large appliance stores. If you

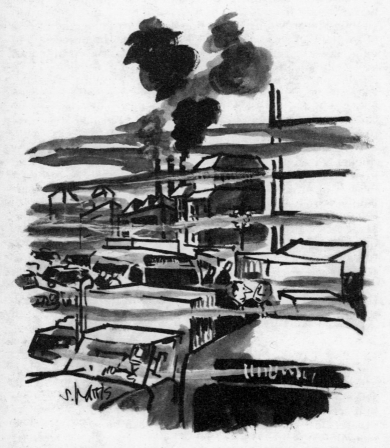

"The only other solution is that we may evolve into a species immune to all this junk."

smoke, you don't have to subject the other members of your family to potentially lethal smoke too, simply by being in the same room. You can get an electrostatic precipitator. Another excellent type of air cleaner is the HEPA filter unit, originally developed to remove plutonium particles from the air in nuclear weapons plants. Although more expensive, it requires less maintenance (see Part III, Chapter 10, for further information). If a doctor prescribes such a unit for medical reasons, it is tax deductible.

The combination of EDTA (a prescription-drug chelating agent) and vitamin C is quite effective in removing lead accumulations in bone and in the brain. EDTA alone does not remove much of the lead in the brain, where it probably does most of the damage. Lead also appears to be an immune system suppressant and definitely inhibits the actions of free radical–scavenging compounds which contain sulfhydryl (SH) groups. Lead from leaded gasoline is not a significant hazard except in chronic direct contact with leaded gasoline. (Some careless auto mechanics and possibly guards in some old, poorly ventilated automotive tunnels may have this problem).

The oceans naturally contain as much mercury in solution as about 10 million times man's present annual rate of production of mercury and its compounds. Thus, sea animals, both fish and mammals, have evolved biological means of handling mercury. The most common method is to inactivate the mercury by forming very much less toxic mercury selenide. Sea animals get the selenium they need for these reactions directly from the sea. (Selenium has many other useful properties; e.g., it is a powerful antioxidant which works synergistically with vitamin E and other antioxidants.) Selenium supplements can help protect you against mercury. Although there have been tragic incidents of local mercury pollution, such as Minamata Bay in Japan, the average mercury content of tuna and other fish has *not* increased in the past few thousand years, as shown by analysis of fish from Roman and Egyptian tombs.

• Sunlight is not often thought of as a pollutant. However, ultraviolet light can damage DNA in skin and contributes to skin aging and is the number one cause of human skin cancer. Several substances are effective in preventing ultraviolet damage. PABA, a vitamin, is used widely in tanning lotions and sunblocks to protect skin by absorbing UV energy and scavenging singlet oxygen and free radicals. Although you can make PABA in your body, you do not have a large enough concentration in the skin to provide optimal UV protection. PABA is effective both orally and topically. Topical PABA esters are even more effective since they resist being washed off the skin by sweat or while swimming. Orally administered BHT, a powerful antioxidant food additive, was very protective in experiments with hairless mice in preventing skin cancer. Oral Vitamin A is another effective protectant against UV induced skin cancer. Oral carotenoids are also useful, including beta carotene and canthaxanthin. Our experimental antioxidant formula roughly triples the amount of ultraviolet light required to cause our skin to burn. See Appendix L, "Some Case Histories."

• The polynuclear aromatic hydrocarbons (PAH) are pollutants formed from burning organics (such as wood, coal, oil, gasoline, candles, tobacco, cannabis, etc.). These compounds are carcinogenic—the PAH free radical reactions attack cellular DNA, resulting in altered, broken, and deformed chromosomes. Antioxidants tend to provide protection against the epoxides and free radicals produced by PAH. This includes vitamins E, C, B-1, and calcium pantothenate, cysteine, zinc, and selenium. Even more effective are the synthetic antioxidants BHT and BHA.

• Radiation is a worry to some people. Microwave radiation, below the level that causes heating, does no damage because the microwave photons each carry 100,000 times too little energy to break chemical bonds and create free radicals. The photons of ordinary light are vastly more energetic and dangerous. If you are concerned about microwaves, you can buy an inexpensive device to detect them at most stores which sell microwave ovens. Microwaves do not create free radicals, mutations, or cancer. Radioactive heavy metals, such as radon, thorium, radium, and polonium, are dangerous. These metals are generated from coal-burning power plants and are released to the atmosphere on very small respirable particles of fly ash. Most fly ash this fine is not caught by any known practical stack-gas cleaning apparatus. If you breathe in these particles, the metals concentrate in the bones and remain there for life (unless removed by chelation). Coal-burning power plants, even if they could meet the very strict and exceedingly expensive—and probably impractical—1985 EPA standards, actually release more radiation of a hazardous kind per unit of energy than do nuclear power plants. Another source of radiation is potassium-40 and carbon-14, both naturally occurring radioactive forms. Radiation causes cellular damage by creating free radicals. Free radical scavengers are, therefore, effective protectants, especially BHT, BHA, vitamin E, and cysteine. In self experiments, we have found that our experimental antioxidant mixture roughly triples the X-ray dosage required to cause our skin to redden and burn.

• Aldehydes are a harmful class of chemical pollutant formed during the burning of fuels; for example, they are found in automobile exhaust, cigarette smoke, and smog and are also formed by the liver from alcohol. Aldehydes autoxidize to produce free radicals and are cross-linkers, mutagens, and carcinogens, and evidence supports the idea that they make a significant contribution to aging processes. The damaging effects of aldehydes can be largely blocked by taking adequate quantities of supplemental antioxidants. In rat experiments, a combination of vitamins C and B-1, and the amino acid cysteine enabled rats to survive a dose of acetaldehyde large enough to kill 90 percent of another group of rats not receiving the C, B-1, cysteine supplements.

Emphysema victims suffer from hypoventilation, an inability to breathe in through their damaged lungs enough air for adequate oxygen supplies. Their brains, in particular, suffer from the reduced oxygen supply. One serious consequence of the low oxygen in the brain is an increase in production of free radicals, atoms or molecules with an unpaired electron which can cause severe damage to many cellular components (especially to the lipid membrane-dependent enzymes and also to the DNA genetic material, where damage may result in cancer-causing mutations). Oxygen in normal quantities helps to control these free radicals. But emphysema victims cannot breathe in enough air to get this much oxygen. Hydergine® has been shown to provide high levels of protection against free radical damage in the brain, as under conditions of reduced levels of oxygen supply, such as occur in emphysema or impaired cerebral circulation.

Most cancers and cases of emphysema in the United States, however, are caused by smoking and drinking, *not* air or water pollution. In fact, about 35 percent of all cancer deaths are due to high-tar cigarettes coupled with excess alcohol consumption, and about 45 percent are caused by improper nutrition (a combination of excess caloric intake, excess fat intake—polyunsaturated fat being particularly hazardous—low fiber diet, deficiency of retinoids and antioxidants, and obesity). Smoking greatly amplifies the hazards of air pollution. Smoking inhibits the motions of cilia (tiny hair-like projections) which carry mucus and pollutants out of the lungs. Essentially all coal miners suffering from black lung disease (caused by half a pound or so of coal dust in their lungs) are smokers. Many of these smoking coal miners who have contracted black lung disease are now collecting billions of dollars of your tax money. But is it a wise public policy to subsidize people who choose to cause injury to themselves? Nonsmoking miners breathe in just as much coal dust, but they have not destroyed the ability of their lungs to remove this trash. Smoking also seriously damages the ability of the immune system to locate and destroy cancer cells in the lungs. As P. B. Medawar, the Nobel Prize–winning tumor biologist, has pointed out, everyone probably gets cancer thousands and possibly even millions of times in his life, but these cancers are almost always detected and destroyed by your immune system long before they become noticeable. World War II shipyard asbestos workers who did not smoke may have a slightly elevated incidence of lung cancer, but those who smoked have an extremely high incidence of parenchymal cancer, an otherwise rare and very deadly type of lung cancer. Uranium miners who do not smoke may or may not have a very slightly elevated risk of lung cancer, but those who do smoke have an extremely high risk of lung cancer. Most human cancers are the result of an individual's voluntary choice of life style, not of an involuntary consumption of chemical pollutants in the general environment. (The most important exception to this is lung cancer induced by the involuntary breathing of other people's tobacco smoke.) Both the EPA and OSHA (Occupational Safety and Health Administration) regulate according to the congressionally legislated doctrine that protection must be designed and enforced for the most susceptible individuals in our society, even if this susceptibility is self-chosen, as is smoking. As a result of this, nonsmokers are forced to pay billions of their tax dollars per year for costs whose benefits are reaped largely by smokers. In our opinion, it is time to terminate these immense hidden subsidies to smokers. Either let the smokers pay these greatly increased pollution control and safety costs, or let them protect themselves with the proper nutrients, or let them suffer the consequences of their own voluntary actions. (See Part III, Chapter 10, "Smoking: Making It Safer with Nutrients.")

12
Alcohol: Making It Safer with Nutrients

I understand that the effects of whiskey are many and varied. In my own experience, however, the effects of the absence of whiskey, rather than its presence, have been most startling.

—W. C. Fields, *W. C. Fields by Himself* (1974)

This chapter is not a preachy temperance tract that treats social drinkers as if they were skid row bums. Alcohol, the world's most popular recreational and social drug, can be used with a great deal of safety if you know how. This chapter is about you, your enjoyment of alcohol, and your good health. We tell you how you can continue to enjoy alcohol and yet greatly improve your health with simple nutrients and, optionally, certain prescription drugs. This chapter will tell you how to get the benefits of alcohol while avoiding much of alcohol's health hazards. We explain how alcohol acts in the brain and body and how simple nutrients provide considerable protection against undesirable alcohol effects. We even explain recent findings about the underlying causes of alcoholism—how it is inherited like gout and diabetes and is not, therefore, some sort of moral weakness—and how simple nutrients offer substantial protection against the age-accelerating effects of too much alcohol and may even offer hope of a cure for alcoholism. In fact, the techniques we tell you about will prove beneficial to both social drinkers and alcoholics.

This chapter isn't merely a theoretical treatise. It is filled with practical information that you can use right now! How to prevent hangovers—without drinking less; how to cure a hangover—without drinking more; how to greatly reduce your chances of alcohol-induced cardiovascular disease and cancer by adding a few simple vitamins, minerals, and other nutrients to your diet; how to slow alcohol-caused premature skin wrinkling. You can enjoy your alcohol without embalming yourself.

If you are an alcoholic, we have some amazing new scientific discoveries to tell you about—information that may lift a big load of guilt from your shoulders. We explain how we now know that alcoholism is due to an inherited metabolic defect and how the right nutrients may change an individual's biochemistry from that of an alcoholic (inherited) to that closely resembling an ordinary social drinker.

Alcohol has been a favorite recreational drug of a large portion of the human race since prehistoric times. Mesopotamian pottery depicting scenes of fermentation have been found that date back to 4200 B.C. A small wooden model of a brewery dating circa 2000 B.C. is on display at the Metropolitan Museum of Art in New York City. The Brooklyn Museum of Natural History has an ancient Egyptian stone bas-relief of a priest holding a special flask for distilling wine into brandy. And the people who make and use alcohol have always seen special qualities in alcohol. For example, the word "whiskey" comes from the Gaelic *uisge beatha* or *usquebaugh,* meaning the "water of life." Many American Indian tribes had their favorite fermented drinks which provided them with B vitamins as well as alcohol. According to government records of 1810, some 6.5 million gallons of distilled spirits were produced in Pennsylvania alone that year. In fact, alcohol drinking was even more popular in America during the early 1800s than it is now. This prompted the English naval officer Frederic Marryat to write in *A Diary in America,* "They say that the English cannot settle anything without a dinner. I am sure the Americans can fix nothing without a drink. If you meet you drink, if you part you drink, if you make an acquisition you drink. They quarrel in the drink, and they make up with a drink." George Washington is even credited with the first distilling of rye whiskey in America. If you enjoy alcohol, you are in plenty of good company!

People have different reasons for drinking alcohol, the

most popular recreational drug in the world. Sometimes people use it to forget something. Alcohol is good for that since it impairs memory (more on that later). Yet other people use alcohol to disinhibit their higher brain centers to allow boisterous or playful activities. Some people use alcohol as a stimulus barrier. A stimulus barrier is a drug or meditation technique which helps a person filter out unwanted stimulation from the environment. For example, a person who works or lives in a noisy area might use a stimulus barrier like alcohol or nicotine to help handle the stimuli. You can measure the effect of a stimulus barrier by measuring the EEG (electrical brain wave output) of a person's brain while you spring unexpected stimuli (like bright lights or loud noises). The stimulus barrier will cause a person's brain to show less response to these suprise stimuli. Common stimulus barriers, beside alcohol and nicotine, include most tranquilizers and sedatives. One of the problems of using stimulus barriers is that withdrawal results in the opposite of the stimulus-barrier effect, an increase in sensitivity to outside stimuli. For a person withdrawing from alcohol, excessive stimuli come pouring in!

All healthy mammals, including people, make a small amount of alcohol in their bodies as part of normal metabolism. The average person makes about one ounce of alcohol every day by normal metabolism. In order to metabolize this internally created alcohol, man and the other mammals have special enzymes, particularly in their livers. These enzymes handle both the internally made alcohol and also alcohol drunk in beverages. In the first step, the enzyme called alcohol dehydrogenase converts alcohol to acetaldehyde, a chemical which can damage the body in several ways. It can create abnormal chemical bonds in important large molecules like proteins (resulting in skin wrinkling and artery hardening and loss of elasticity), and damage DNA (resulting in abnormal cell function, birth defects, and even cancer). This abnormal chemical bonding process is called cross-linking and is the same process that causes your car's rubber windshield wipers to harden and become brittle and that converts (tans) soft, moist cattle skin into hard, dry, stiff leather. It is also the same process used to embalm cadavers, which employs close chemical relatives of acetaldehyde such as formaldehyde and glutaraldehyde. When cross-linking takes place in the lungs, we call the result emphysema. Another way acetaldehyde causes damage is when it is nonenzymatically oxidized in the body, creating dangerous and reactive chemical fragments called free radicals. These free radicals can cause cancer, birth defects, cross-linking, atherosclerosis, and are implicated as major causative factors in aging.

Our bodies don't just leave this dangerous acetaldehyde hanging around, though. We have another enzyme (called aldehyde dehydrogenase) which enzymatically oxidizes the toxic acetaldehyde into essentially harmless acetate (a form of acetic acid, common vinegar). Unfortunately, long-term heavy use of alcohol leads to free radical liver damage which impairs the performance of this enzyme system. This results in less acetaldehyde being harmlessly destroyed enzymatically and more acetaldehyde self-oxidizing to free radicals which do further damage, and so forth, in a destructive chain reaction.

Normal people who do not drink excess alcohol have no trouble converting all the internally created alcohol into acetate via the alcohol-handling enzyme system. When we drink alcohol, though, we can overload the enzyme system. If we drink alcohol fast enough, acetaldehyde may be made by the enzyme alcohol dehydrogenase faster than can be eliminated by the aldehyde oxidizing enzyme. *That's* when the trouble begins. Alcohol itself is much less harmful than acetaldehyde. Acetaldehyde and its free radical autoxidation products cause nearly all the damage to brain and body that we blame on alcohol—the increased risk drinkers have of developing cancer or cardiovascular disease, premature skin wrinkling, atherosclerosis, liver damage, brain damage, cataracts, decreased resistance to disease (due to suppression of our body's police force, the immune system), alcohol addiction itself, and even hangover!

Scientists recently discovered that alcoholics have a metabolic defect that results in their having twice as much of the harmful acetaldehyde in their bloodstream after a drink as normal people. Even some nondrinking relatives of alcoholics make more acetaldehyde from alcohol than normal people; they have inherited this tendency. The tragedy of alcoholism has emerged not as a lack of morality or willpower but as an inherited condition which makes alcoholics either create too much acetaldehyde too rapidly from the alcohol they drink or destroy the acetaldehyde slower. In one study, adopted boys whose natural parents were alcoholics tended to become alcoholics themselves. The boys whose natural parents were not alcoholics tended not to become alcoholics even when their adoptive parents were alcoholics. Heredity, rather than environment or weak will, causes alcoholism.

Alcohol itself provides a degree of protection against the unpleasant effects of the acetaldehyde by scavenging some of the dangerous reactive free radicals created when the acetaldehyde is abnormally oxidized in the body. This abnormal oxidation occurs when the acetaldehyde produced from the alcohol piles up and overwhelms the supply of the acetaldehyde-destroying enzyme called acetaldehyde dehydrogenase. The vicious cycle of alcoholism is now revealed: Acetaldehyde is made from alcohol mostly in the liver by our enzymes; the acetaldehyde and its free radicals make the drinker feel lousy so he drinks more alcohol, which not only makes him feel better but actually helps protect him against acetaldehyde poison and dangerous free radicals—*until* the liver makes *more* acetaldehyde out of the additional alcohol, so the drinker drinks more alcohol. And on and on. Before we understood this metabolic pathway in alcoholics, alcoholism seemed a nearly hopeless problem, with complete abstinence the only solution.

Alcohol addiction is not due to weak will or moral depravity; it is a genetic metabolic defect, just as Durk and most males in Durk's father's family have a genetic metabolic defect resulting in gout. For centuries it was thought that gout was the result of "immoderate living," "weak will," or "moral depravity." Sound familiar? We now know that gout can be caused by at least 85 different inheritable metabolic defects. A proclivity to alcohol addiction is genetic, not moral. If you have a high ratio of the enzyme alcohol dehydrogenase (which turns alcohol into nasty acetaldehyde) to the enzyme acetaldehyde dehydrogenase (which turns nasty acetaldehyde into harmless acetate), you will find it hard to stop drinking if you ever start.

It is interesting to note that there are racial differences in the average levels of these two enzymes. (Note that we are speaking of group averages, not individuals. There are far greater differences between individuals within a race than there are differences between racial averages.) For example, the incidence of alcoholism is higher than average among the Irish and among American Indians (and several other groups as well). These groups have a higher average ratio of acetaldehyde-producing to acetaldehyde-destroying enzymes. An

American Indian may *start* drinking because his home, land, culture, and livelihood were stolen from him at cavalry gunpoint, but such genocidal treatment is not the cause of the alcohol *addiction*. Personal or job problems can lead one to start drinking but cannot make one an alcoholic. (Remember that only 5 to 10 percent of regular drinkers ever become alcoholics; this is genetic, not environmental.)

New knowledge brings new solutions. A scientist named Dr. Herbert Sprince has found a combination of nutrients which provide remarkable protection against acetaldehyde and its free radicals. He gave a group of rats a dose of acetaldehyde large enough to kill 90 percent of them. He gave another group of rats the same dose of acetaldehyde, but he also gave this group vitamins B-1 and C and the amino acid cysteine (found in eggs and sold in some health food stores). None of the rats receiving the supplemental nutrients died! For many years, interns have given themselves B-1 shots for hangovers. You may remember the old wives remedy for hangover: a raw egg stirred into a large glass of orange juice. This is really a good idea. The egg contains about 250 milligrams of cysteine, and the orange juice contains about 250 milligrams of vitamin C. Larger doses of the nutrients provide even more protection. A reasonable dose for a hangover might be a gram each of vitamin B-1 and cysteine and 5 grams of vitamin C. Regular heavy drinkers should consider using these nutrients on a regular basis. They offer alcohol drinkers considerable protection against the major source of drinking damage—acetaldehyde and its free radicals made in the body from alcohol. We suspect, too, that it might be possible for these nutrients to enable alcoholics to control or even cure their alcohol problem by blocking the effects of the excessive amounts of acetaldehyde that they have in their blood after drinking alcohol. Behavioral therapy might be required to teach alcoholics to reach for the nutrient bottle, not the booze bottle, when feeling hung over. Further research on this possibility would be very desirable.

Hydergine® (Sandoz), a prescription drug, is currently the fifth best-selling prescription drug in the free world outside the United States. In France, where alcoholic drinks such as wine are consumed in large quantities, Hydergine® is the number one prescription drug. There is a remarkably low rate of alcohol-associated complications (such as cirrhosis of the liver) in France compared to Italy and similarly large difference in Hydergine® usage. We have investigated Hydergine® because of its potential life extending properties and have been interested in the significant degree of protection Hydergine® offers against alcohol damage in both the brain and the liver in experimental animals. Its clinical properties strongly suggested to us that it should be an extremely potent antioxidant—that is, a powerful free radical scavenger. We arranged for Sandoz to supply a sample of pure Hydergine® (without tablet fillers or binder) to Dr. Harry Demopoulos, a free radical pathology expert, for testing. His laboratory biochemical tests showed that Hydergine® is a powerful antioxidant, probably the most potent antioxidant yet tested.

In chronic alcoholics, a serious condition may develop in which there is severe loss of recent memory and confusion. This is called Korsakoff's psychosis (alcoholism-induced brain damage). The ability of Hydergine® to protect the brains of experimental animals from alcohol damage suggests that regular Hydergine® use by alcoholics may prevent some of the damage causing this condition. Very recently, another prescription drug, clonidine (Catapres®), improved the mental function of Korsakoff's psychosis patients. Memory improved and some patients became more alert and had improved learning ability. Catapres® is FDA approved to control high blood pressure but not to treat Korsakoff's psychosis. However, your physician can prescribe it for any condition he wishes. You will probably want to provide a copy of the scientific paper because the FDA has made it a crime for the manufacturer of an approved drug to tell physicians about new scientifically sound but non-FDA approved uses. See Appendix B for information on these papers.

Most of the damage to the brain resulting from strokes and insufficient brain circulation is caused by the dangerous free radicals mentioned earlier. These free radicals, you see, are not just formed when acetaldehyde is nonenzymatically self-oxidized. They are necessary in certain normal metabolic reactions. And although we have enzymes to keep the free radicals under control, the controls are not perfect, so some of the free radicals escape and do damage. Free radicals are also formed when fats in the body are nonenzymatically self-oxidized and then broken down. In recent years scientists have found that antioxidant nutrients (including vitamins A, B-1, B-5, B-6, C, and E, the amino acid cysteine, and the minerals zinc and selenium) are an important part of our natural control system for free radicals. Without the control enzymes and antioxidants, we would quickly die. These nutrients and

Hydergine® are useful in protecting both the brain and the liver from the damaging free radicals.

The nutrients choline and lecithin and the prescription drug Deaner® (Riker) are used by our brains to make the important chemical acetylcholine. Acetylcholine is used by certain nerve cells in the brain to communicate with each other, and it is required for memory, appetite, and sexual behavior. It is also important in controlling how responsive we are to both external and internal stimuli. For example, acetylcholine is what turns down our responsiveness to our environment so that we can sleep. Many hyperkinetic children respond to choline, lecithin, or Deaner® with improved mental focus. These materials may be of value to drinkers who use alcohol as a stimulus barrier by helping to control response to stimuli in our environments. Three grams of choline per day is a reasonable adult dose. Since vitamin B-5 is required to convert choline to the neurotransmitter acetylcholine, at least a few hundred milligrams to a gram of B-5 should also be taken per day. Choline, vitamin B-5, and Deaner® are also free radical scavengers.

One of the reasons that alcohol remains a problem is that its manufacturers are not allowed to add nutrients to it that would help protect drinkers against its hazards. Half a century or so ago, an alcoholic vitamin tonic called Hadacol was quite popular in the United States, especially in the South. Hadacol contained enough nutrient additives to be a genuinely safer form of alcohol than simple distilled liquor. What happened to Hadacol? The FDA killed it. They called this action "protecting the consumer." Recently, a major distiller, who realized that vitamin B-1 could help prevent cirrhosis of the liver and brain damage, proposed adding vitamin B-1 to his alcohol products, but he discovered that if he did so the Treasury Department's Bureau of Alcohol Tax, which controls alcohol, would either consider it illegally adulterated alcohol or a drug that should be controlled by the FDA. The FDA, however, wouldn't touch it; (it doesn't handle recreational drugs). The FDA approves only drugs which prevent, ameliorate, or cure diseases. It won't approve a recreational drug no matter how safe it is or how much of an improvement it is over another recreational drug. So long as our distiller did not add nutrients to his booze, he could continue to market his products without complications. It is no wonder that nothing was ever done.

An ideal solution to the alcohol problem would be to develop new recreational drugs which provide the desired alcohol high without the damaging side effects. There is, in fact, such a drug. It was invented by Alexander Shulgin, synthesized, and tested in humans (test subjects couldn't distinguish between the drug and a few martinis). However, this drug is not FDA approved, and it is not likely to be approved in the foreseeable future.

Dr. Harry Demopoulos and others discovered that free radicals can be partially controlled by oxygen in our blood. When there is either too much or too little oxygen, these free radicals get out of hand and do a lot of damage. When the brain does not get enough oxygen, as when arteries are atherosclerotic and narrowed, the free radicals run wild and cause brain damage. Tobacco smoking makes this problem worse because nicotine narrows the brain's blood vessels even further and the carbon monoxide destroys oxygen-carrying hemoglobin in red blood cells. (See Part III, Chapter 10, "Smoking: Making It Safer with Nutrients," for ways to nutritionally prevent this problem.) Alcohol drinkers can have a lot of these free radicals in their brains as a result of the abnormal nonenzymatic self-oxidation of acetaldehyde made from the alcohol they drink. But Hydergine® (Sandoz) can provide a great deal of protection against these free radicals. Experiments have been done in cats in which their brains did not receive adequate oxygen to function normally. Irreversible brain damage occurred in fifteen minutes. But in cats whose brains were equally deprived of oxygen but who also received Hydergine® (in a dose properly scaled down from the usual amounts a person uses in this country), there was no brain damage for forty-five minutes. Because of this protective property, Hydergine® is administered in many countries in Europe just before an operation so that if anything goes wrong, doctors will have more time to correct the situation before brain damage occurs.

Experiments in rats have shown that Hydergine® helps protect the liver, as well as the brain, from alcohol damage too. Hydergine® is used in an oral (swallowed) and a sublingual (dissolved in the mouth) form. The sublingual form delivers a higher percentage of the dose to the brain (it passes directly through the mucous membranes of the mouth into the blood vessels going to the brain), while 40 percent of the oral form is taken up by the liver. So, an alcohol drinker would get protection to both liver and brain, particularly if both forms were used.

Hydergine® does even more. The acetaldehyde-created free radicals are particularly apt to do damage to delicate fibers which connect nerve cells in the brain and enable these cells to communicate with each other. These delicate fibers, called neurites, are absolutely essential to learn, see, feel emotions, or do any other brain activity. One reason you can't teach old dogs new tricks is that their ability to grow neurites is badly impaired. People have a natural hormone, nerve growth factor, which stimulates the growth of these neurites. But we have less and less of this hormone as we grow older—in fact, we have the most neurites we're going to have at the age of about 2! It was recently found that Hydergine® acts like the nerve growth factor which stimulates the growth of neurites. So it is actually possible to recover from some alcohol damage which has already taken place in the brain! Some Korsakoff's psychosis patients may also be able to recover some brain function by using Hydergine®.

In a short-term study, Hydergine® at a dose of 12 milligrams per day for two weeks improved the memory and intelligence of normal persons. It even improved the ability to do abstract thinking (finding and logically relating patterns in sets of line drawings). Hydergine® benefits have been tested in senile older persons and in normal young and middle-aged persons and provided startling benefits to both. The recommended dose in this country is 3 milligrams per day. In Europe, 9 milligrams per day is typically used, and there is a move to go to 12 milligrams per day. We both use about 20 milligrams of Hydergine® per day. We would be surprised to see any vivid benefits at the low dose (3 milligrams per day) recommended in this country. (Start out by taking 1 milligram per day and slowly increase the dose to avoid possible upset stomach, diarrhea or headache.) Hydergine® is particularly likely to produce these annoying but harmless side effects, and insomnia as well, if it is used with large doses of the stimulants caffeine (in coffee or cola soft drinks) or theophylline (in tea).

Another prescription drug which can benefit alcohol users is Diapid® (Sandoz). This is a synthetic version of a natural hormone, vasopressin. Diapid® has been tested in men in their 50s and 60s with amazing results: their memories and intelligence improved (in tasks requiring focus and concentration), their sensory discrimination and alertness improved, and it caused faster sensory-motor reactions. Since the use of alcohol often results in a poorer memory (alcohol inhibits the brain's release of vasopressin), in reduced alertness and sensory discrimination, and in slowed reactions, Diapid® can be of value if you have to perform a task while under the influence of alcohol. While it would be much better not to drink and then drive, we would far prefer that drinking drivers also use Diapid®. Diapid® does not interfere with the relaxing, euphoric, and social disinhibiting effects of alcohol. If you drink for fun, you will probably like it. But if you drink to forget, don't use Diapid®—it will help you remember!

Withdrawal from alcohol addiction is extremely hazardous. Even in the finest hospitals, with the best of care, about 5 percent of advanced alcoholics die in withdrawal. This is far worse than heroin withdrawal! Diphenylhydantoin is a drug which has been used safely for many years by epileptics to control their seizures. It can also be used to help control the convulsions which can be experienced during alcohol withdrawal. Diphenylhydantoin has also been used to help cigarette smokers withdraw from smoking without withdrawal symptoms (see Part III, Chapter 10, "Smoking: Making It Safer with Nutrients"). Alcohol withdrawal in advanced alcoholism *must* be handled by a physician experienced in this field.

Another nutrient which can help counteract the foggy mental effects of alcohol is vitamin B-12. This vitamin has, in animal experiments, improved learning ability. It increases the brain's manufacture of RNA, which is necessary for memory and learning.

Drinking alcohol during pregnancy can lead to one of alcohol's most tragic consequences: the fetal alcohol syndrome (FAS). FAS refers to a collection of birth defects which occur together, including impaired brain development, growth deficiencies, and abnormal facial appearance. The blood level of alcohol in the unborn child is the same as that in the drinking mother. In studies where alcohol was included in the diet of newborn rats (fed through a tube into their stomachs), brain weight was 19 percent below that of normal littermates. Their body growths were comparable. We do not know to what extent the nutrients and drugs we've discussed here can reduce the risks of FAS. These experiments have not yet been done, though free radical pathology theory suggests that antioxidant nutrients may be quite useful. Until this information becomes available, however, we can only very strongly suggest that you keep away from alcohol if you are pregnant! This is the sort of high-priority research which we believe the

FDA should pursue, instead of wasting our tax money and their personnel on attempts to make high-potency vitamins into prescription drugs and to prevent people from making and selling thymosin.

Among alcoholics, there is a high incidence of depression. Vitamins C and B-6, destroyed by the acetaldehyde produced in the liver from the alcohol, are absolutely necessary in order for the brain to make special chemicals called neurotransmitters which allow brain cells to send messages to each other. Decreased vitamin C and B-6 serum levels in heavy alcohol users means that the brain may not make large enough quantities of the neurotransmitter called norepinephrine (NE). Too little NE causes depression. This depression can usually be remedied by taking supplemental phenylalanine (an amino acid the brain uses to make NE) and vitamins B-6 and C (so that the phenylalanine can be converted into the NE). In one study, 100 to 500 milligrams of phenylalanine per day for two weeks eliminated depression in most people with a depression from a number of causes, including amphetamine abuse, schizophrenic, endogenous, and other types. (See Part III, Chapter 3, "Depression, Helplessness, and Aging.") In addition, the acetaldehyde can chemically react with certain neurotransmitters in the brain to form addictive, consciousness-impairing substances known as isoquinoline alkaloids, which are related to morphinelike compounds.

It is a well-known fact that smokers tend to have very low vitamin C serum levels (about half that of nonsmokers), which is thought to be a predisposing factor for lung cancer and cardiovascular disease. Most people realize that smokers have a greatly increased risk of cancer. However, few know that users of alcohol are also at a greatly increased risk of cancer.

For several years it has been known that the cancer-inducing effects of both smoking and alcohol together are far worse than additive. A person who is both a heavy drinker and heavy smoker is *much* more likely to get cancer than one who is either a heavy drinker alone or a heavy smoker alone. Part of this effect is undoubtedly due to the fact that both drinking and smoking destroy antioxidant, free radical–scavenging nutrients such as vitamins A, B-1, B-5, B-6, C, and E, and cysteine. The cancers that are most strongly promoted by this combination of smoking and drinking—cancers of the lungs, mouth, larynx, esophagus, liver, and urinary bladder—are principally caused by polynuclear aromatic hydrocarbons

(PAH, found in tobacco combustion tar), which are metabolically activated to PAH epoxides, the actual active carcinogens. People who both drink and smoke can form PAH epoxides by another abnormal route: Excess ingestion of alcohol leads to the formation of more acetaldehyde than the body can enzymatically destroy. This acetaldehyde autoxidizes via a free radical route to peracetic acid, an organic peroxide which is so efficient at converting unsaturated compounds (such as PAH) to epoxides that it is used industrially to make epoxy resins. This peracetic acid can rapidly and efficiently convert the tobacco tar PAH to its carcinogenic PAH epoxide, thereby causing a multiplicative risk when tobacco smoking is mixed with heavy alcohol use. If you both smoke and drink, the use of antioxidant free radical–scavenging nutrients may save your life. The requirement for some of these supplemental nutrients is made even greater by acetaldehyde damage impairing the liver's ability to metabolically process and activate some of these nutrients.

Additional problems are caused by the high caloric content of alcohol, about 20 calories per teaspoon. A pint of 86-proof liquor supplies half the normal daily adult caloric requirement, but these alcoholic calories are utterly empty of nutrients. The heavy drinker who eats less food worsens an already severe vitamin deficiency; if food intake is *not* reduced, many of the extra alcohol calories are converted to fat, resulting in high serum triglyceride and cholesterol levels and obesity. These fats are subject to further free radical autoxidation. Three grams of niacin (vitamin B-3) per day (one gram with each meal) can lower these serum lipids in many people by about 25 percent within two weeks.

When acetaldehyde autoxidizes in one's body in the presence of unsaturated fats and oils, there ensues a literal chain reaction of destruction involving acetaldehyde, acyl radicals, peracetic acid, hydrogen peroxide, superoxide radicals (which are destroyed by the enzyme SOD, superoxide dismutase), hydroxyl radicals, alkyl radicals, peroxyl radicals, epoxides, organic peroxides and hydroperoxides, hypochlorite, chlorohydrins, singlet oxygen, and others. This results in DNA-damaging mutations, cross-linking, suppression of formation of the natural hormone PGI_2 (which prevents abnormal blood clots), and damage to the brain, liver, heart, and other muscles, damage to your immune system, frequently resulting in cancer, birth defects, and cardiovascular disease.

Fortunately for us, the same promiscuous high-energy chemical reactivity that makes these free radicals so dangerous also makes them susceptible to reactions with certain free radical–controlling molecules called free radical scavengers. Vitamins A and B-1, the B-2-dependent enzyme glutathione reductase, the B-3-dependent biochemical NADPH, B-5, B-6, C, E, and the cysteine-dependent biochemical glutathione are all free radical scavengers, as is the zinc-dependent enzyme SOD, and the selenium- and cysteine-dependent enzyme glutathione peroxidase. The dangerously reactive organic peroxides formed by the free radical autoxidation of fats and oils are destroyed by some of these compounds too, particularly by glutathione peroxidase. Your biochemistry is quite complex and involves many protective mechanisms, which is why there are so many different nutrients in our suggested protective nutrient formula.

A GOOD NUTRIENT FORMULA
FOR PEOPLE WHO ENJOY ALCOHOL

total dose per day,
to be divided into three doses and taken *with meals*

Vitamin A	10,000 to 20,000 I.U. (international units)
Vitamin B-1	1 gram
Vitamin B-2	100 to 200 milligrams
Vitamin B-3 (niacin)	600 milligrams to 3 grams
Vitamin B-5	2 grams
Vitamin B-6	500 milligrams
Vitamin B-12	500 micrograms
Vitamin C	3 to 10 grams (at least three times as much C as cysteine)
Vitamin E	1000 to 2000 I.U. (international units)
Choline	3 grams
Cysteine (not cystine)	2 grams
Zinc (chelated)	50 milligrams
Selenium	250 micrograms

Do not start out taking these high doses. Do not start to take this formula on an empty stomach, either. Start at about one eighth of these amounts per day and slowly increase your doses. Be sure to divide the total daily dose into three parts and take it with meals to slow its absorption and to minimize the gastric effects of acidic vitamins such as C and niacin. This allows your body time to adjust to all these extra nutrients. If you take too much initially, annoying (but not hazardous) side effects may occur, such as upset stomach, diarrhea, and brief skin flushing and itching. It is a good idea to consult your doctor before you start to take these substances. If you are diabetic, be sure to see the caution on B-1, C, and cysteine use in Part III, Chapter 10, and also see your physician. If you skipped over the Disclaimers in "The Engraved Invitation" at the beginning of this book, we suggest you read them now.

OPTIONAL PRESCRIPTION DRUGS
FOR ALCOHOL DRINKERS

Hydergine®*	9 to 12 milligrams per day
Diapid® (Sandoz)	16 I.U. (international units per day)

*Note: specify Sandoz Hydergine®—no substitutions—generics are not biologically equivalent. (The official FDA dosage recommendation for Hydergine® is 3 milligrams per day.)

A well-known hazard of alcohol use is the many interactions which occur between alcohol and other drugs. Some of the most common of these interacting drugs follow:

1. Barbiturates: The result of interaction is enhanced effect of both alcohol and barbiturates during alcohol intoxication. Chronic alcohol use reduces the barbiturate effect when there is no alcohol present and increases the effect when there is. At high enough dosages of these two drugs in combination, respiratory collapse can occur, resulting in death. In fact, several thousand people every year die in just this way. Worse yet, when a person dies of barbiturate/alcohol-induced respiratory collapse, their insurance company often is reluctant to pay off, alleging that these deaths are suicide. In fact, this is often the case, since this form of suicide is one of the easiest and least unpleasant.

2. Antihistamines: In combination with alcohol there is enhanced depression of the central nervous system (reduced responsiveness, reaction, etc.)

3. Tranquilizers (such as Valium® and Librium®): With alcohol, there is enhancement of effects of the tranquilizer. Recently, Valium® and Librium® were discovered to act in the brain by fitting into brain receptors called the benzodiazepine receptor (like keys into locks). Valium® and Librium® cause tranquilization only because they fit into these special receptors. But we also have natural brain chemicals which fit into these receptors and induce calm and tranquility. The form of vitamin B-3 called niacinamide seems to be one such compound. The B vitamin inositol and the amino acid gamma aminobutyric acid (GABA) enhance niacinamide binding to the benzodiazepine receptors. Alcohol promptly increases the effectiveness of both GABA and Valium®-like compounds at their active sites in the brain, increasing their anti-anxiety effects in the short run. In the long run, however, heavy alcohol use decreases the number of these anti-anxiety receptor sites and damages them, reducing their sensitivity. This is why addiction to alcohol plus Valium® or Librium® often develops more rapidly than addiction to alcohol alone. Moreover, this alcohol-induced anti-anxiety nerve receptor damage is likely to play an important part in the chronic anxiety found in most alcoholics. Users of Valium® and Librium® may find that nutrients are able to substitute satisfactorily, in whole or in part, for these tranquilizers. If you use these drugs, we suggest you try a combination of niacin or niacinamide, inositol, and GABA in place of part or all of the prescription tranquilizers. Using the nutrients, you can avoid the Valium® and Librium® side effects, which unfortunately include inducing higher levels of the enzyme alcohol dehydrogenase, which results in a greater liver production of toxic acetaldehyde after drinking alcohol. A reasonable dose might be 1 gram of niacin or niacinamide, 3 grams of inositol orally, and 500 milligrams of GABA sublingually. *Note*: Many people flush and itch after they take niacin because this vitamin causes the release of histamines. (The release of histamines also causes blushing and the Masters and Johnson sexual flush and is required for orgasm.) Usually this effect lasts only a short time (twenty minutes or so) and is not harmful. To avoid this, you can use niacinamide, which causes less of the flushing and itching than niacin but does not reduce blood lipids

(fats) as niacin does. The flushing is greatly reduced if you take the niacin on a full stomach, starting at a very low dose (100 milligrams after meals) and increasing it slowly. If you use the niacin regularly, you will quickly develop tolerance to the flushing effect—the flushing lessens or disappears and doesn't reappear at its original strength as long as you take the vitamin regularly.

4. Oral anticoagulants: There is an enhanced effect during alcohol intoxication, reduced effects with chronic alcohol use.

5. Phenothiazines (Thorazine®, Mellaril®, Compazine®): These have an additive effect with alcohol.

There are many other alcohol-drug interactions. For a longer list, see *Drug Interactions* published by Medical Economics, Oradell, NJ 07649 ($3.95). This is a good investment, particularly if you are unwilling to remind your physician that you drink every time a drug is prescribed for you. Of course, the most prudent approach is to both remind your physician every time *and* to purchase and use the book, too.

13
Controlling Your Weight

Appetite comes with eating.

—Rabelais

All human history attests
That happiness for man—the hungry sinner—
Since Eve ate apples, much depends on dinner.

—Lord Byron

Excess weight is not only unattractive but unhealthy as well. The fat person has much higher risks of cardiovascular disease and cancer than the person of normal weight. Our brains contain a weight control center, which is responsible for setting and maintaining body weight. It is by altering the brain's weight control center that we can ultimately control our own weight. If you are fat and want to be slim, you will find a variety of effective techniques in this chapter. Once you understand a little about the biochemistry that controls your weight, you can accomplish a lot with very little effort. Sandy lost over 20 pounds by using the right nutritional supplements, together with about two minutes of exercise a week—no dieting and no "diet pills"! The calories burned by the exercise accounted for only one ounce of fat of the 20+ pounds lost. Here's an easy way to lose weight—and, if you wish, you can replace that fat with hard, youthful muscles.

Being overweight is more than just unattractive, it's downright unhealthy. You probably agree. Many people think that overweight is harmful because it forces the heart to work harder, pumping blood to these pounds of extra fat cells. However, this is an old wives' (old doctors'?) tale. The heart of a sedentary obese person works no harder and may even work less than hearts of physically active individuals. It is not extra work that causes overweight people to have much higher rates of cancer and heart disease, and lower life expectancies.

The excess quantities of fats stored in an overweight person's body accumulate peroxides as they are nonenzymatically autoxidized over time. These peroxidized (rancid) fats are potent immune system depressants because they inhibit the activities of the macrophages (white blood cells which patrol the body looking for invaders such as bacteria, viruses, and cancer cells, which they kill and eat). Also, being overweight depresses the levels of some hormones, such as growth hormone, which is important to immune system function. In a fat person, there is an increasing load of these peroxidized fats as times goes on (in the absence of adequate supplements of antioxidants). These peroxidized fats are formed in the body by the unregulated attack of oxidizing chemicals (including oxygen) on fats. Thus, in the obese person the macrophages are increasingly inhibited, rendering the body more and more susceptible to infectious diseases and to cancer. In addition, peroxidized fats are mutagens (damage DNA) and carcinogens (cause cancer). Moreover, peroxidized fats inhibit the enzyme prostacyclin synthetase which manufactures PGI_2, the hormone that prevents abnormal platelet aggregation and blood clots in arteries. These abnormal clots cause heart attacks and about 85 percent of all strokes. Overweight people are carrying around many pounds of fat containing these poisonous peroxidized fats.

Some recent events of human evolution give an insight into the pervasive problem of overweight. During the last Ice Age, people who could store fat within their bodies in times of abundant food were better able to survive the frequent famines of those hard times. Natural selection favored the fat storers. Those peoples who came from northern (harsh, cold) climates, such as the Slavs, developed a short chunky physique that reduces heat loss. The fat acts as insulation and also as energy reserves in case of starvation. People living in the tropics typically have long slender limbs to get rid of body heat and usually store fat only in the buttocks and belly. Apparently, the unfortunate tendency of many people to put on weight has come about as a survival trait inherited from earlier times when food was hard to come by. Even as late as the

Renaissance, female beauty was pictured as very plump by modern standards. Such women were more likely to survive the frequent famines and have surviving offspring than thin women.

Using any of a number of diets, it is possible to lose several pounds a week. However, if a person on such a diet discontinues it, he or she often rapidly gains back at least the weight that was lost. Why is this? Again, we must look at evolutionary mechanisms. If a person loses more than about a pound or two a week, the body's weight and hunger metabolic control system (the hypothalamus in the brain) "thinks" that there's a famine. Thus, when this person goes back to eating a normal diet, the body tries to store as much fat as it can before food again becomes scarce. (Reliably abundant food is a *very* recent phenomenon!) The moral of this is that you should lose weight slowly, no more than a pound or two per week, if you want to remain slim after dieting stops.

A sudden jump in body weight occurs in many people after they enter their twenties. People who might have been slender may balloon by ten to twenty or even more pounds. This change is due to alterations in hormone levels that take place at that time. Although the full details have yet to be uncovered, we do know that growth hormone levels start to fall off and that, by the age of about 30, exercise no longer acts as an effective growth hormone releaser. (In addition to being a thymic immune stimulant, growth hormone causes the body to burn fat and build muscle.) One important hormone involved in weight control, dehydroepiandrosterone, falls more than any other hormone yet known in the 20- to 30-year age period. These hormonal changes are thought to be due to a developmental program clock located in our cellular DNA.

Here are some helpful and effective methods for losing weight:

• Get a precise scale and weigh yourself every day at the same time, preferably just before dinner. This provides biofeedback data for your weight control center in the brain. A precision of ¼ pound or better is desirable. We like the Heath or Dunhill electronic scales, which read to ¹⁄₁₀ pound, and the Sears physician's-type balance.

• Buy a good full-length mirror for your bedroom and take the time to look at yourself nude each day. Particularly focus on those areas where you want to lose weight. More biofeedback. The best time is just before a large meal. Get a plate

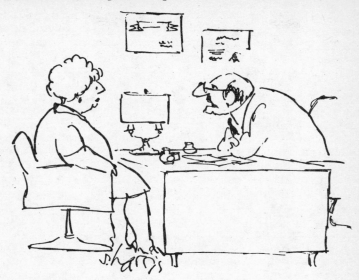

"It's partly glandular and partly 8,500 calories per day."

glass or float glass mirror; otherwise you'll look wavy and distorted, which is not the type of feedback that you want or that your mind will trust.

• Drugs that can reduce appetite exist, though most (phenylpropanolamine, amphetamine, Ritalin®, fenfluramine) are stimulants that are effective for only a few weeks and often have undesirable behavioral side effects. Phenylalanine, an essential nutrient amino acid, can inhibit appetite by increasing the brain's production of the neurotransmitter NE (norepinephrine). Phenylalanine also causes the brain to release the hormone CCK (cholecystokinin), which has been shown to inhibit eating in experimental animals. Amphetamine works by causing the brain to release NE from its stores and by blocking its recycling. But, unlike amphetamine, phenylalanine does not cause a depressive crash when the weight loser stops taking it. That's because phenylalanine causes the brain to increase both its production and its stores of NE, rather than depleting the stores as amphetamine does. Dr. James G. Gibbs, Jr., of Cornell University has used L-phenylalanine successfully in rhesus monkeys to reduce their eating. (The L-phenylalanine seems to be more effective in weight loss than D-phenylalanine. D-phenylalanine is more effective for relief of pain and has a euphoriant quality. For depression, the comparative effects of D- and L-phenylalanine depend on individual response.) The amino acid (prescription drug) L-Dopa and the nutrient amino acids L-arginine and L-ornithine are also able to stimulate weight loss. L-Dopa increases NE. L-Dopa, L-arginine, and L-ornithine trigger the release of growth hormone, which burns fat and helps put on muscle. Vasopressin (Diapid®, Sandoz, nasal spray), a hormone released by the pituitary in the brain, causes the release of both growth hormone and beta lipotropin, another hormone which causes fat to be burned. Thyroid hormones can promote growth hormone release. Bromocriptine (Parlodel®, Sandoz) causes release of growth hormone and, used in conjunction with L-Dopa and/or L-arginine, is even more effective in reducing fat and increasing muscle mass. See Part V, Chapter 7, "Our Current Personal Experimental Life Extension Formula" and Appendix G for our personal dose levels for these substances.

Phenylalanine is found in foods such as meats, cheese, and milk. You probably get about 2.8 grams a day in your diet. A reasonable dose would be between 100 and 1000 milligrams. Start out at 100 milligrams and increase the dose slowly over a period of weeks. It usually takes several hours for the phenylalanine to be converted to NE by the brain, so the first effects are not noticeable until that much time has passed. Vitamins C and B-6 are required for this conversion and should be taken as well. Since the NE is stored in the brain for a few days, there will be a lag of a few days between dose changes and full response to the dose change. Side effects can include irritability, insomnia, or headache; if any of these occur, reduce your dose of phenylalanine. In large doses (larger than the suggested appetite-reducing doses), phenylalanine can increase blood pressure. **CAUTION:** People with high blood pressure should proceed very cautiously, beginning with a very low dose (100 milligrams) and taking frequent blood pressure readings while using the nutrient to make sure their blood pressure isn't rising. It is advisable for such people to consult with their physician before using phenylalanine. Remember that it is phenylalanine in your brain that controls eating, and it is mostly phenylalanine in the rest of your body that affects blood pressure. By taking the phenylalanine on an empty stomach, you maximize the ratio of appetite suppression to blood pressure increase. Used this way, phenylalanine has a far better ratio of hunger suppression to blood pressure elevation than any of the appetite-depressant stimulants, such as amphetamine or phenylpropanolamine.

Phenylalanine should be distinguished from phenylpropanolamine, an appetite depressant used in many over-the-counter diet pills. The phenylpropanolamine causes the brain to use up its stores of NE, without stimulating it to produce more. After your supply of NE runs out (after two weeks or so), you feel let down, and very probably you will go on a rebound eating binge when you stop taking the pills. Amphetamines and other stimulants have a similar but more severe effect. Since phenylalanine does not deplete the supply of NE (in fact, the brain uses it to make more), you don't have the letdown and rebound-eating binge problem. A more serious side effect of phenylpropanolamine, reported in the 12 January 1980 *Lancet* (a respected British medical journal), is "potentially dangerous" increases in blood pressure in 16 of 71 healthy volunteers taking medications containing either 50 milligrams or 85 milligrams of phenylpropanolamine. We have seen over-the-counter diet capsules containing up to 130 milligrams of phenylpropanolamine. Prolonged use of high doses of phenylalanine may not be advisable for all people, since, at abnormally high concentrations, this amino acid and its breakdown products damage the brain of newborn infants, as in the genetic disease phenylketonuria, where an enzyme involved in phenylalanine metabolism is deficient.

Growth hormone causes one to put on muscle and burn fat. Everybody knows that most teenagers can eat like horses without becoming obese, even if they are sedentary. A middle-aged person eating the same food and getting the same exercise will usually become fat. The higher growth hormone levels in teenagers have a great deal to do with this difference. Obese (more than just overweight) people do not have a normal growth-hormone response to L-arginine, L-ornithine, L-Dopa, fasting, hypoglycemia, exercise, or sleep. This may be a big part of their problem. We and others are currently doing research on this and we hope to report useful results in our next book.

The amino acids L-Dopa, ¼ to ½ gram, and/or L-arginine, 5 to 10 grams, and/or L-ornithine, 2.5 to 5 grams, and/or tryptophan, 1 to 2 grams, taken on an empty stomach at bedtime, cause growth hormone release. The L-Dopa, tryptophan, and L-arginine/L-ornithine cause the release of growth hormone by different mechanisms, so they are even more effective when taken together. These techniques can easily make a normal 65-year-old's growth hormone levels resemble those of a young adult or even a teenager. The nutrient stimulated release of growth hormone and beta lipotropin may not be the only mechanisms responsible for the observed muscle building and fat loss. Dopaminergic stimulation of the hypothalamus and pituitary can, to some extent, reset biological aging clocks, and many brain neurohormones undoubtedly still await discovery.

The type of exercise good for losing weight is the kind that causes release of growth hormone. As we explained in Part III, Chapters 8 and 9, on exercise and athletics, this type of exercise is a peak-output type rather than prolonged periods of less-than-peak effort (as in jogging). Exercise alone is not an effective growth hormone releaser for most people over 30 years old. We and others are currently doing research directed toward correcting this deficit.

Scientists are studying the brain's mechanisms for controlling the setting of appetite (and consequently weight) level. The brain's hypothalamus gland is thought to be the location of this control system. By making small lesions in the hypothalamus surgically, or with electrodes, scientists can cause rodents, dogs, cats, or monkeys to either starve themselves to death or eat themselves to death, depending on the location of the lesion. Nobel Prize winner Rosalyn Yalow recently reported finding that genetically obese mice contain only a third of the hormone cholecystokinin (CCK) in their cerebral cortex as their normal sized littermates. James G. Gibbs, Jr., a scientist at New York's Cornell University, believes that CCK may be a "satiety signal" in the brain, telling the animal when to stop eating. Like electrical stimulation, CCK can cause an animal to literally starve itself to death in the midst of plenty. The hormone is released when food enters the intestine (duodenum), where it causes secretion of pancreatic enzymes and bile acids. A CCK nasal spray would be a splendid reducing aid, but don't hold your breath waiting for the FDA to approve it. Dr. Gibbs has recently found that the amino acid L-phenylalanine (but not its mirror image D-phenylalanine) causes the release of CCK, resulting in less eating in rhesus monkeys. Thus, either DL- or L-phenylalanine is an excellent nutrient for weight control.

Here are additional weight control suggestions:

• Do not let yourself go hungry. Nibbling between meals is OK if you eat snacks high in fiber or high in protein, low in carbohydrates (starches and, especially, sugars) and low in fats.

• Do not eat large evening meals; large breakfasts and lunches are OK.

• Eat snacks with high protein and/or high fiber about thirty to forty-five minutes before main meals, to reduce appetite. Meats and cheeses contain tyrosine and phenylalanine, which are converted in the brain to norepinephrine (NE). NE is an appetite-inhibiting neurotransmitter. The conversion takes a little time but can suppress appetite later. If used regularly, high-protein snacks help keep brain levels of NE high and, as a result, appetite down. High fiber moves food through your gastrointestinal tract quickly, resulting in the absorption of fewer calories, as well as mechanically making you feel full.

• Use small plates and utensils to make meals appear bigger.

• Pantothenate (vitamin B-5), a stimulant of intestinal peristaltic contraction, decreases the transit time of food through the digestive tract, thus reducing the calories absorbed. In doses of 1 to 3 grams per day, B-5 can reduce gut residence time from the three days typical of a low-fiber Western diet to the one day found in native peoples eating high-fiber diets. Fiber, although it decreases transit time of food and absorbs bile acids (which carry cholesterol and other fats), also absorbs vitamins and minerals. The relative absorptions of various fiber sources has yet to be determined. The health benefits of any particular type of fiber seem to vary from species to species.

• Dr. Richard J. Wurtman has found that high-carbohydrate meals (starches and sugars) result in an increased passage of the amino acid tryptophan into the brain, where it is converted to serotonin, the neurotransmitter. Experimental animals, as a consequence of this effect, then prefer to eat high protein meals. Therefore, tryptophan may be helpful in weight control by shifting the hunger from high-carbohydrate to high-protein meals. **CAUTION:** High-protein meals increase the requirement for vitamin B-6 (see Part III, Chapter 16).

• When you eat, know what it is that you are eating for. For example, if you have a craving for chocolate, it is far better to eat a chocolate bar than to gorge on chocolate-covered cereal or chocolate chip cookies. Cereal and cookies are a higher-calorie way of getting chocolate, because you have to eat a lot of other stuff to get the chocolate. Many people crave chocolate because it contains the stimulants beta-phenylethylamine and theobromine. Beta-phenylethylamine is an effective mood elevator in some people who are depressed because of broken love affairs. Such people are known to frequently gorge themselves on chocolate after breakups of intense love relationships. From a weight point of view, it would be better to use a beta-phenylethylamine salt directly rather than eat a lot of calories containing a small amount of it. Theobromine is a somewhat milder stimulant than its chemical cousins theophylline (in tea) and caffeine.

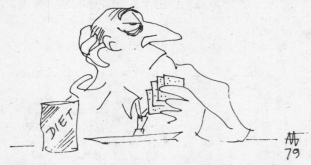

"Who am I fooling? Four RyKrisp and a diet drink doesn't beat a pair of fried eggs with three rashers of bacon."

• When you eat, pay attention to your eating! You feel full and stop eating because your brain releases CCK hormone. What you think and what you perceive controls this release, NOT the number of calories consumed. Eliminate distractions while you're eating. Turn off the TV or radio. Put down that newspaper. Pay close attention to the aroma, taste, mouth feel, and appearance of your food. It's fun! Eat slowly and deliberately. You will be amazed at how little food it takes to fill and satisfy you if you pay very close attention to your eating. If you eat slowly, you give your hypothalamus time to release CCK and make you feel full. If you wolf your food down, you will consume far more calories than are necessary for complete satiation, due to the delay for CCK release.

• You are not doing yourself any good to stuff yourself rather than "waste" food. Because human beings had to struggle for food until very recently (and many still do), we have evolved both genetic and cultural mechanisms to use food efficiently. Wasting food is a definite no-no. But if you want to lose weight or maintain it, you will have to stop eating when you feel comfortably full, not when you have cleared your plate.

• Genetically obese mice release abnormally large amounts of the morphinelike hormones, the endorphins, in response to food. Endorphins are the brain's natural morphine or heroin-like painkillers. The warm euphoric glow you feel after a big meal is a miniature version of what the heroin addict feels after taking a shot. Like heroin, these endorphins are addicting, and it is more probable that people with many obese relatives will have extra trouble with food addiction, because of likely hereditary factors. In fact, Dr. Candace Pert and her co-workers report that they administered an opiate antagonist called naltrexone to young obese mice for five weeks and found that the treated mice gained weight more slowly than the control mice. Beta endorphin levels were lower in the animals' pituitary glands and bloodstream. Dr. Irwin Stone found that vitamin C (30 grams a day to start, tapering off to a maintenance dose of 10 grams a day in divided doses after a few weeks) enabled addicts to quit heroin without withdrawal symptoms. The vitamin C makes this possible by slowing the breakdown of the enkephalins (other natural short-acting heroinlike compounds) in the brain. Vitamin C may also affect the sulfhydryl groups (SH) at the active receptor sites for endorphins. Vitamin C is a good reducing agent and may act this way. It is therefore likely that frequent high doses of vitamin C can reduce the addictive withdrawal symptoms of dieting. D-phenylalanine and D-leucine both retard breakdown of endorphins and enkephalins. The prescription high-blood-pressure medication clonidine hydrochloride (Catapres®) has also been shown to reduce heroin withdrawal symptoms and may be of particular value to people who are both obese and have high blood pressure, a very common combination. Finally, the behavioral treatment of obesity and overeating as a type of addiction is described in Dr. William Rader's *No-Diet Program for Permanent Weight Loss* and in *Behavioral Treatments of Obesity,* edited by John Paul Foreyt (see Appendix K for references and chapter notes).

• Another approach to weight control is to alter the digestion of foods in the gut. The Howard Hughes Medical Foundation has done research in this area. Phaseolamin, a protein found in raw kidney beans, prevents your natural starch-digesting enzyme alpha amylase from working. As a result, if you use phaseolamin, you can't digest starches at all. You could gorge yourself on pasta, spaghetti, bread, and potatoes and not gain an ounce. In fact, if that's all you ate, you could starve to death! This product, phaseolamin, is not yet approved by the FDA for sale to the public in this country. Cooked kidney beans do not contain any phaseolamin, which is destroyed by heating. You should *not* eat uncooked kidney beans because they contain liver and kidney damaging substances. One reason people have been so successful in dominating this planet is that people can eat many more types of foods than other animals because cooking food destroys many harmful substances. The way that phaseolamin is obtained is by extraction from kidney beans, followed by purification. The details are given in the reference in our bibliography.

CAUTION: Overweight individuals are particularly prone to high blood pressure and heart disease. It is highly advisable to consult with your physician before starting on any of the suggestions in this chapter. Sodium restriction is often a part of the management of these disorders and care should be taken to avoid vitamin and drug preparations that contain sodium if your physician has recommended a low-sodium diet.

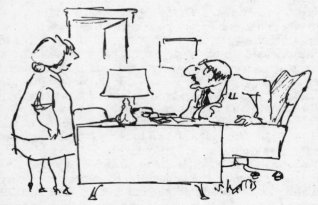

"Let me put it this way:
you're an addict, and your grocer is a pusher."

APPETITE-REDUCING AGENTS

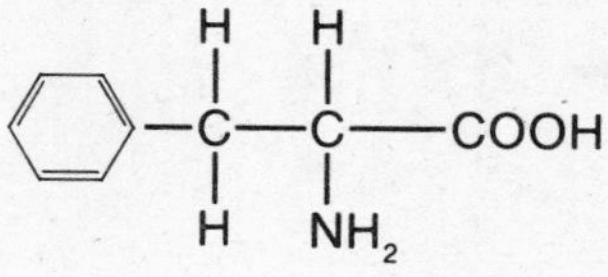

PHENYLALANINE, an amino acid which is converted in your brain to NE (norepinephrine), a neurotransmitter which controls hunger.

Here are some of the phenylalanine look-alikes found in diet pills:

PHENYLPROPANOLAMINE

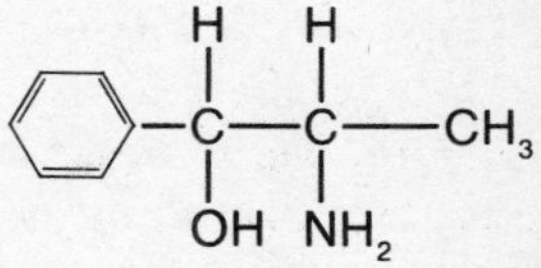

AMPHETAMINE

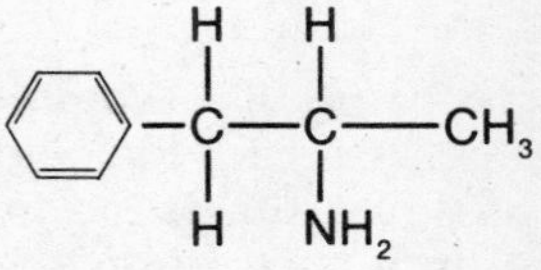

CHLORPHENTERAMINE

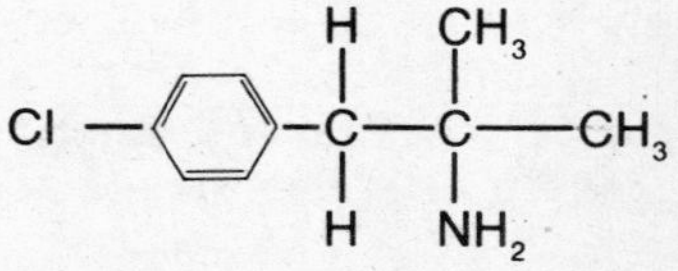

14
Arming Your Immune System against Arthritis

Science is built up of successive solutions given to
questions of ever increasing subtlety approaching nearer
and nearer towards the very essence of phenomena.

—Justus von Liebig (eminent German chemist, 1803–73)

*Arthritis occurs when your immune system makes a mistake
and attacks your body's normal tissues, damaging the cells in
your joint membranes and degrading your joint lubricating
fluids. By improving the immune system with the right nutrients, you can prevent or even regress arthritis. Unlike most
prescription arthritis drugs, these nutrients neither cover up
pain nor depress your immune system's ability to fight dangerous entities such as bacteria, viruses, and cancer cells.*

Arthritis is a common degenerative disease of aging. In
recent years, understanding of the underlying basic chemical
causes of arthritis has greatly increased, along with effective
means of prevention and treatment.

Arthritis can result from several different diseases, including rheumatoid arthritis, bacterial infections, and a serious disorder, systemic lupus erythematosus. All these
conditions involve the production of free radicals by the immune system. Before you engage in dangerous "self-diagnosis," consult with your physician about your arthritis and
about our vitamin and other drug suggestions. Proper diagnosis requires the experience of a professional.

It is now thought that arthritis is caused by free radical damage (see Part II, Chapter 7, "Our Subversive Free Radicals"). The atoms or molecules with an unpaired electron which constitute free radicals are highly reactive, attacking and damaging DNA, lipids (fats), the synovial fluid (joint lubricating fluid), synovial membranes, and other tissue components. Superoxide free radicals can be producing during the autoxidation (in which a molecule spontaneously oxidizes itself) of various natural biochemicals, including hydroquinones, catecholamines (brain neurotransmitters), thiols, reduced flavins (like vitamin B-2), tetrahydropteridines, and hemoproteins. Superoxide radicals can be formed in enzymatic reactions, also.

Both superoxide radicals and hydrogen peroxide are necessary to destroy the lubricating properties of the synovial fluid by depolymerizing it (breaking down its components). In rheumatoid arthritis, an autoimmune T-cell failure (white cells from the thymus) is involved. Certain leukocytes (white blood cells), the polymorphonuclear variety, produce both hydrogen peroxide and superoxide radicals as a lethal weapon to destroy bacteria, which the white cells then eat. In rheumatoid arthritis, an influx of these white cells into the affected joints occurs, with subsequent damage by the superoxide radicals produced by the white cells and hydrogen peroxide (which can be produced by the reaction of superoxide radicals with the hyaluronic acid present in the synovial fluid). Dr. Joe M. McCord's studies suggest that both superoxide and hydrogen peroxide are required to depolymerize the hyaluronic acid (a polysaccharide, or long chain starchlike molecule). Superoxide dismutase (SOD), a group of natural enzymes made in your body to protect you against superoxide radicals, can prevent damage to the synovial fluid and membranes. One form of SOD contains zinc and copper, while another contains manganese. SOD constitutes the fifth most abundant protein in our bodies, after collagen, albumin, globulin, and hemoglobin. The enzyme catalase, which breaks down hydrogen peroxide to harmless products, is also effective in providing protection to the synovial fluid. Superoxide dismutase is found mainly in the fluids inside cells, so that superoxide radicals generated outside of cells can do a lot of damage. Superoxide dismutase injections into arthritic joints have sometimes been dramatically effective. SOD is used extensively in race horse training to alleviate the joint inflammations of these thoroughbreds. Scientists have recently discovered that complexes of copper and aspirin (copper salicylates) have superoxide dismutase properties, rapidly quenching superoxide radicals. That old wives' tale about wearing a copper bracelet for arthritis turns out to be true. Copper can be absorbed from a copper bracelet, provided the bracelet does not have an impermeable finish (such as varnish) on the copper. It is, of course, easier to take a copper gluconate supplement, which also allows better control of the dosage.

Hydroxyl free radicals are the actual agents which attack the bonds holding hyaluronic acid together, according to McCord. This radical is formed when superoxide reacts with hydrogen peroxide. A piece of supporting evidence is that an experimental arthritis treatment, DMSO, is effective in some cases in restoring function and eliminating stiffness and pain—DMSO is a powerful hydroxyl radical scavenger. Inositol (muscle sugar, a B vitamin) is a less potent but very safe hydroxyl radical scavenger that you can buy in any health food store. DMSO is now available as a prescription drug, a 50 percent solution of DMSO in water. The new product, called RIMSO-50®, is manufactured by Tera Pharmaceuticals, Inc. in Buena Park, California, and is distributed by Research Industries Corp., Pharmaceuticals Division, Salt Lake City, Utah. The DMSO solution is FDA approved as a treatment for interstitial cystitis but is not currently approved for any other use. DMSO works best in conjunction with antioxidants like vitamins A, C, E, B-1, B-5, and B-6 and cysteine, zinc, and selenium, since the DMSO is converted to the less hazardous sulfoxide free radical when it destroys a hydroxyl radical, and this sulfoxide radical must in turn be destroyed by other antioxidants in your body.

These findings suggest that an effective way to prevent the development of arthritis (or to use in its therapy) is to take nutrient free radical scavengers, including the antioxidants: vitamins A and E, selenium, vitamins C, B-1, B-5, B-6, and PABA (also a membrane stabilizer), inositol, BHT, and thiodipropionates. Immune system stimulation with agents such as arginine, ornithine, and cysteine (amino acids) and vitamins A, E, and C (see Part II, Chapter 5, "Aging and the Immune System") should also help prevent or treat arthritis caused by an autoimmune mechanism, since autoimmune reactions are caused by inadequate activity of T-suppressor white cells.

Many polyvalent (capable of existing in more than one oxidation state) metal ions, including copper and iron, can stimulate (catalyze) the production of free radicals. As mentioned in Part II, Chapter 6, substances which can remove excess unneeded quantities of these metals, chelating compounds, can help reduce the quantity of free radicals and the damage caused by them. D-Penicillamine, a chelating prescription drug, has been used in successful alleviation of the signs and symptoms of severe active rheumatoid arthritis unresponsive to conventional therapy. (L-Penicillamine, on the other hand, is a very dangerous substance that can be lethal.)

The correct dose of antioxidants for effective arthritis therapy must be determined by experimentation. The effective dose may be quite high. For example, a friend of ours who is a well-known artist in his fifties developed arthritis in his hands. This man's hands became so painful and stiff he could no longer use his fingers to remove the caps from his tubes of paint. He tried vitamin E at increasing dose levels. It was not until he got up to 10,000 I.U. of E and 20,000 I.U. of A per day that he obtained relief from the pain and crippling stiffness. His hands are now flexible and can be used to draw without difficulty. But they remain so only as long as our friend takes 10,000 I.U. of E and 20,000 I.U. of A a day, not less (he's tried).

Dr. John M. Ellis (author of *Vitamin B-6: The Doctor's Report*) now uses 500 milligrams to 2 grams per day of vitamin B-6 in treating patients for arthritis, with considerable success reported.

"Rheumatism" is a common problem that develops with age. People may awaken with hands or arms numb, tingling, and painful to flex and use. Sleeping on such hands or limbs in an ordinary bed contributes to the development of the condition and increases its severity.

Demopoulos at NYU and others have found that, under conditions of low oxygen availability to nerve tissue (as occurs in advanced atherosclerotic narrowing of arteries, strokes, etc.) the tissues are damaged by a greatly increased rate of formation of free radicals there (Part II, Chapter 7). In addition, damaged blood vessels (as in injuries, bruises, strokes, etc.) leak blood into surrounding tissues. Demopoulos and others showed that copper and iron in the leaked blood act to stimulate the production of free radicals. Chelation of the copper and iron with D-Penicillamine was partially effective in reducing the extent of damage in crushed spinal cord injuries in cats.

When people sleep on an arm or a leg in an ordinary bed, they can restrict or cut off the blood flow to the limb. The reduced blood supply means less oxygen is available to quench free radicals forming in these tissues. Free radicals are mutagenic, carcinogenic, cross-linkers, and destabilizers of membranes. Damaged membranes in blood vessels of affected joints may leak blood, releasing copper and iron which further accelerate the production of damaging free radicals. Incapacitation is usually progressive unless prompt corrective steps are taken.

There are several ways to interfere with this progressive destruction of limb function:

• Take antioxidants to scavenge the free radicals. Especially effective in "rheumatism" is vitamin B-6 (as reported by Ellis). Other antioxidants include vitamins A, E, B-5, C, and B-1, cysteine zinc, selenium, inositol, choline, and PABA.

• Take membrane stabilizers that help prevent damage to joint membranes. These include PABA, inositol, and choline. Vitamin C and bioflavonoids form a powerful combination to increase capillary resistance to damage by free radicals (as in injuries, arthritis, and bruises).

• Sleep in a water bed. In a water bed, limbs and other body parts are not subjected to the concentrated crushing weight of a heavy body during sleep. The water provides uniform support, preventing the problem of restricted blood supply to limbs. If you want to consider this option, keep in mind these seven hints for best results:

1. Buy a heavy-gauge lap-seam vinyl bag and liner for durability.

2. Get a top quality heater. Water has a high thermal conductivity (heat or cold will be efficiently transferred to you). As little as a couple of degrees too high or low will lead to discomfort. Too cool water will result in your waking with aches and pains. You'll want a good heater for adequate temperature control.

3. Place a well insulated blanket or mattress pad over the water bag for better thermal isolation—this makes exact temperature control less critical.

4. When the water bag is first filled, it may take a few days to reach the desired temperature. It may take you a week to finally adjust the temperature to the most comfortable level.

5. Adjust the water fill to your taste. More water leads to less rocking.

6. Get a leak repair kit. Durk's water bed has had one minor leak in seven years.

7. Any apartment or building fit for human occupation is adequate to handle the weight of a water bed. A double-bed-size unit weighs about as much as six husky men; if your floor can't handle that, you had better move.

15
A Brief Note on Allergies and Asthma

... it is not worthy of a philosopher to deny phenomena only because they are inexplicable in the present state of knowledge.

—Pierre Simon LaPlace

Nutrients may provide substantial improvements in allergies and asthma.

When we planned this book, we had no intention of including information on allergies and asthma. However, our science editor, Beatrice Rosenfeld, who suffers from asthma, encouraged us to say something about this subject. Our observation of a few dramatic improvements in long-term chronic problems of this sort which occurred in people engaging in self-experimentation with antioxidant nutrients finally changed our minds. Of course, these cases are anecdotal data, not double-blind placebo controlled experiments on a large group of experimental subjects. In themselves, they prove nothing, but they are interesting leads. There are, however, mechanisms that have been demonstrated in the laboratory which suggest that the improvements observed were causally related to the antioxidants. Please keep in mind that these are brief notes, not an attempt at an overview of the field. It is also a good idea to remember that the symptoms that are termed "asthma" can be caused by allergies, a variety of lung diseases, and heart failure. Do not engage in self-diagnosis and unassisted self-treatment; consult with your doctor first about your "asthma."

It is known that asthmatic and other allergic responses are mediated at least in part by the immune system. People with lots of allergies tend, for example, to have higher levels of IgE (immunoglobulin E). IgE has been among the least studied of the immunoglobulins, which are large protein molecules made by B-cells, apparently under T-cell orders. IgE is very powerful and exists in tissue in very low concentrations, making its study more difficult than the other immunoglobulins. High levels of IgE may have evolved as a defense against internal parasitism, a severe health problem before the days of shoes, modern sanitation, and high-technology food production and processing techniques. Nowadays, internal human parasites are a minor health problem in technologically advanced societies, though these parasites are still a major cause of disability and death in the primitive world. Although plenty of IgE was a net benefit to our ancestors, it no longer affords us such a large positive health payoff, while the allergic side effects are unabated. (Yes, natural medicines produced by your own body have side effects too. Nothing is perfectly safe.)

As we age, our T-cell immune system function declines faster than that of our B-cells. (See Part II, Chapter 5, "Aging and the Immune System.") One family of T-cells whose function is impaired by aging is the T-suppressor cell system. The T-suppressor cells do what their name implies; they suppress self-damaging immune system activities. The functional decline of T-suppressor cells with age is involved in many autoimmune diseases such as rheumatoid arthritis and is quite likely to be involved in the frequent tendency of allergies and asthma to worsen with age, both in terms of the severity of their effects and with respect to the range of allergens provoking the response. Anything sufficiently safe that improves T-cell function is a reasonable candidate for testing on allergies and asthma. Indeed, thymosin—a natural T-cell stimulating thymic hormone—has shown good results in preliminary human clinical trials on some patients with life-threatening asthma, as well as on some autoimmune diseases and some cancers. (See subject index for more on thymosin.) As discussed in Part II, Chapter 5, "Aging and the Immune System," Part II, Chapter 7, "Our Subversive Free Radicals," and Part III, Chapter 14, "Arming Your Immune System Against Arthritis," many antioxidants have been shown to improve T-cell immune system function in aging animals. This may be a significant factor in the improvement that we have observed.

Antioxidants are involved in other ways as well; see Durk's case history for the effect of vitamin B-2 on his allergic conjunctivitis. Vitamin B-2 is required for the enzyme glutathione reductase, which recycles oxidized glutathione back to reduced glutathione, one of the body's major antioxidants. Autoimmune, allergic, and asthmatic reactions frequently involve the immune system's inappropriate release of powerful oxidants such as free radicals, singlet oxygen, and hydrogen peroxide in the target tissues, which are thereby damaged. Adequate appropriate antioxidants can reduce this damage.

Leukotrienes are a class of polyunsaturated fats with three double bonds that were first found while studying the responses of leukocytes, a type of white cell. Recent research shows that leukotriene oxidation products are extremely powerful bronchoconstrictors, which have long-lasting effects. Like histamine, they cause inflammation and constriction of the lung's air passages, but they are not blocked by antihistamines. Dr. Bengt Samuelson and his colleagues have made a good case for these substances being an important factor in human asthma. Antioxidants can help prevent the formation of the active form of these compounds and also help destroy them after they have been formed. We suspect that these autoxidation-produced bronchoconstrictors may be involved in breathing difficulty in S.I.D.S. (sudden infant death syndrome, also called crib death).

Histamine is also a major factor in allergies and asthma. It is well known that vitamin C is involved in the destruction of histamine.

Hydergine® (Sandoz) is effective in helping about 60 percent of the asthma sufferers who try it. These effects probably stem from two quite different mechanisms. First, Hydergine® is an extremely potent, yet low toxicity antioxidant. Second, Hydergine® elevates an intracellular messenger hormone called cyclic AMP, as does theophilline (a major caffeinelike stimulant in tea), which has been used in asthma medications for better than half a century. Higher levels of cyclic AMP often reduce the bronchoconstriction.

Details can be found in the case histories of "Mr. Smith," Beatrice Rosenfeld, and Durk. Antioxidants are certainly not a cure-all for allergies and asthma, but they do seem to be worth a try. We suspect that many of the underlying mechanisms involved in allergies and asthma will become correctable over the next decade or so as a result of both basic and directed research on the immune system, much of it funded by pharmaceutical companies. Whether you will be able to get a prescription for these new drugs depends more on FDA regulations than on scientific progress, however. The eight to twelve years and $56 million required on the average for a new drug to receive FDA approval is often an insurmountable hurdle. Thymosin was first used on humans in 1965. It has been a remarkably safe and frequently spectacularly effective immune system stimulant. Thymosin is exceedingly expensive when extracted in the laboratory from calf thymus glands; however, Hoffmann-La Roche has developed methods for its economical large-scale production. Where is thymosin today? It is lost in the FDA's bureaucratic regulatory limbo. Since the patents (which last for seventeen years) are about to expire, we doubt that thymosin will ever become available from your physician and pharmacist—not unless the FDA is made into an advisory agency without the power to prohibit the marketing of prescription drugs.

POSSIBLE ALLERGIC REACTIONS TO TABLET BINDERS AND FILLERS

Fillers and binders comprise the bulk of the contents in many vitamin tablets. We have seen people who exhibited adverse side effects (such as headaches, rashes, hives, itching, and upset stomach) to large doses of vitamin tablets who did *not* have these adverse reactions to the same vitamin doses taken as the pure vitamin powders in gelatin capsules.

Dr. Hunter Harang is an oral surgeon who uses megavitamins in his practice, and who does clinical research on allergies. He has observed many such undesirable reactions (including headache, arthritis, joint pain, chronic fatigue, depression, personality changes, gout attacks, and even chronic earaches and infections in children), and hence he set out to find the source of the problem. He discovered that the allergic reactions are generally to tablet fillers and binders, not to the vitamins themselves. (Of course, even pure vitamins can cause trouble in excessive doses.) Dr. Harang found that 8 to 10 percent of his tested clinical population is allergic to cornstarch and other corn products, and about another 10 percent to soy products. He has also noted frequent allergic reactions to yeast in B vitamin products, and sometimes even to the cod liver oil in vitamin A capsules. These allergies can be sufficiently severe to produce very unpleasant symptoms when megadoses of vitamins using these fillers and binders are taken. Dr. Harang uses vitamins from M Squared Ethical Pharmaceuticals (P.O. Box 174, West Chicago, Illinois, 60185), which in his experience have been relatively free of allergic complications.

16
Cardiovascular Disease, Its Prevention or Amelioration: Atherosclerosis

Death in old men, when not from fever, is caused by the veins which go from the spleen to the valve of the liver, and which thicken so much in the walls that they become closed up and leave no passage for the blood that nourishes it.

The incessant current of the blood through the veins makes these veins thicken and become callous, so that at last they close up and prevent the passage of the blood.

—Leonardo da Vinci

Atherosclerosis, hardening of the arteries, kills hundreds of thousands of Americans each year. We now understand much of the how and why. By using the correct nutrients, we can reduce our chances of developing atherosclerosis. It is even possible to gradually reduce atherosclerosis if we already have it.

Atherosclerosis is a disease in which small tumors (plaques) grow in the lining of arteries, accumulating cholesterol deposits that lead to the narrowing of these arteries. Blood clots develop on these plaques which can break loose and lodge elsewhere, causing a coronary thrombosis or stroke. It was not realized until 1970 that these plaques were a type of tumor, when this was discovered and reported by Dr. Earl Benditt. Thus the failure of the immune system which results in cancer can also lead to formation of these plaques. In humans about 60 percent of the plaques grow from a single cell (a monoclonal tumor), whereas the other 40 percent grow from more than one cell. Herpes viruses have been demonstrated to cause the formation of the latter type of plaque in both chickens and rabbits, and possibly in man. Herpes viruses are believed to have a causative role in human cancers, including nasopharyngeal cancer, Burkitt's lymphoma, cervical carcinoma, and others. Recently, a herpes virus has been found to be closely associated with human liver cancer. There is a vaccine against the atherosclerosis-causing herpes virus in chickens—Marek's disease vaccine. Until this veterinary vaccine was made available by a large pharmaceutical company, these herpes virus infections were responsible for the death of a large number of chickens, placing a burden on the poultry industry and, of course, raising the price of chicken. The loss of chickens was so great that the USDA allowed the sale of infected chickens, provided the tumors present were not too gross.

T-cell immune function can be greatly improved by taking a number of dietary supplements, as described in Part II, Chapter 5, on the immune system. Particularly effective are C, E, A, arginine, ornithine cysteine, selenium, and zinc. All these, except the amino acids arginine and ornithine, are antioxidants, which can prevent the formation of peroxidized (rancid) fats in the body. These peroxidized fats, since they are mutagens and carcinogens, are able to initiate plaque formation. Polyunsaturated fats and cholesterol are particularly likely to be converted into these carcinogenic peroxidized fats because they are very susceptible to oxidation. These peroxidized fats are also immune suppressants which prevent the desirable destruction and removal of plaque tissue. When a cholesterol deposit forms in the lining of your arteries, specialized white blood cells called phagocytes approach the cholesterol and eat it. In so doing, the phagocytes, which produce a variety of oxygen-related free radicals whenever they eat something, cause the cholesterol and other fats to become oxidized.

It is known that, within the bounds of normal diets, the cholesterol content of the diet does not determine serum cholesterol levels. The body can manufacture about 1.5 grams a day of cholesterol. If dietary cholesterol is reduced, the body, via a feedback mechanism, increases its manufacture of cholesterol in about 40 percent of people. Low cholesterol diets alone may, therefore, be ineffective in reducing serum cholesterol. Further, there is little strong evidence that high serum cholesterol levels themselves *cause* heart disease. It is

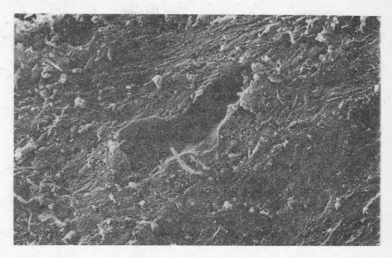

Figure 1. This specimen shows an oblique slice through a normal cat brain capillary about 10 microns in diameter. This scanning electron microscope photograph is enlarged about 1000 X. The cavity in the center of the photo is the inside of the capillary blood vessel. Note that the inner surface is smooth and free of sticky debris.

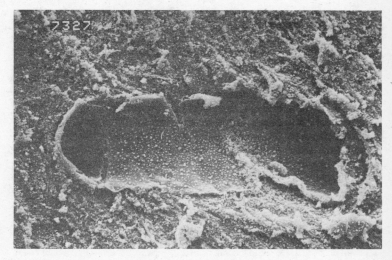

Figure 2. The cavity in the center of the photo is an oblique slice through an abnormal blood vessel containing adherent platelets. The white specks clinging to the inner surface of the blood vessel are the platelets caught in the first stages of the thrombosis (clotting) process. About 600 X magnification.

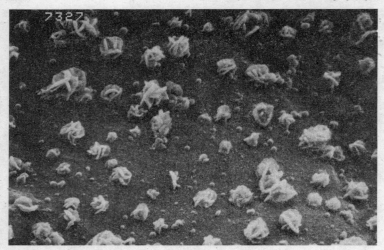

Figure 3. This is about a 10,000 X magnification of the inner surface of the blood vessel in Figure 2. The light ridged octopuslike particles are the adherent platelets.

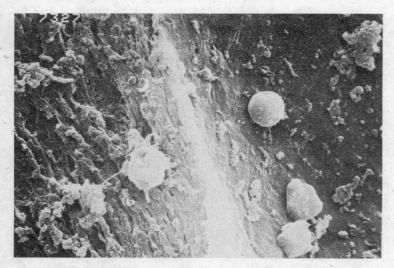

Figure 4. Three misshapen red blood cells (the large light blobs) and aggregated adherent platelets are stuck to the inner surface of the blood vessel in the right half of this electron micrograph. About 2400 X magnification.

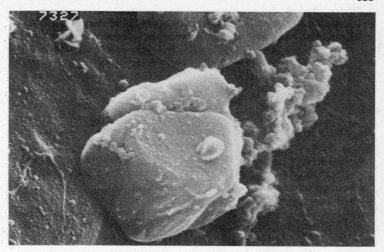

Figure 5. Higher magnification of Figure 4 showing a platelet on a misshapen red blood cell stuck to the blood vessel wall. About 12,000 X magnification.

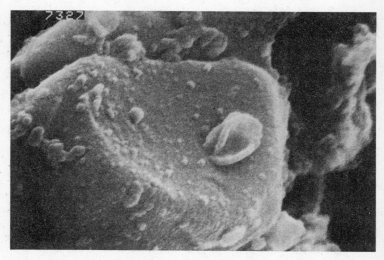

Figure 6. Still higher magnification of Figures 4 and 5. At about 30,000 X the surface of the clotting red blood cell is severely damaged, as is the platelet stuck to it. This red blood cell nearly fills the whole photo. Leakage of iron and copper from such damaged red blood cells powerfully catalyzes free radical autoxidation of fats which suppresses production of the anti-clotting hormone PGI_2, leading to further platelet and red blood cell aggregation and clot growth.

known that oxidized cholesterol is a mutagen and plaque tumor initiator. The oxidized cholesterol and peroxidized polyunsaturated fats also enhance plaque formation by preventing the synthesis of PGI₂ (prostacyclin) in blood vessel walls. This substance prevents platelets in the blood and red blood cells from sticking to the vessel wall. Plaques continue to build up because platelets and red blood cells keep sticking to them, since the oxidized fats have turned off PGI₂ production in the area of the plaque. The iron and copper leaking from the hemolyzed red blood cells in the clot are very powerful catalysts of free radical oxidation, worsening the problem in a deadly feedback loop. The March 1981 issue of *Trends in Pharmacological Sciences* reports that "S. Moncada, another of the co-discoverers of PGI₂, suggested that small doses of a synthetic prostacyclinlike substance might be all that is required as a prophylactic in vascular disease." See the electron photomicrographs above for the first published pictures of the earliest stages of arterial thrombosis (clot) formation.

An important indicator of the risk of heart attack is the ratio of HDL (high density lipoproteins) and LDL (low density lipoproteins) in the blood. Lipoproteins are fat-protein molecules which, among other functions, either carry cholesterol to tissues (principally LDL) or remove cholesterol from tissues (principally HDL). The authors of this book eat diets that include plenty of butter, milk, meat, and so forth, yet our serum cholesterol levels are very low, and the ratio of our high density lipoproteins (HDL) to low density lipoproteins (LDL) shows the highly desirable ratio of high HDL to low LDL. (See Appendix L.) Thus, the amount of fats eaten may not be as important as the way the body metabolizes these fats. We happen to be among the fortunate people who have favorable HDL/LDL ratios, and we can tolerate a high fat intake. But not everyone can. An alert T-cell system can prevent formation of atherosclerotic plaques, and a high HDL/low LDL can help prevent deposition of cholesterol in arteries.

Deficiency of vitamin B-6 can also lead to development of atherosclerosis. It was noticed early in the 1900s that feeding rabbits diets high in protein induced atherosclerosis. But the diets also contained high cholesterol, and when the cholesterol-causes-atherosclerosis theory became popular, the possible protein link to atherosclerosis was forgotten. In the early '60s, investigators discovered a new disease in which young children died of rapidly developing atherosclerosis. These children were excreting large amounts of homocystine in their urine. Dr. Kilmer McCully studied this disease and found out what was causing it. When the amino acid methionine (but *not* cysteine) is broken down in a normal healthy body, it is converted to the hazardous pro-oxidant homocysteine and then, with the help of vitamin B-6 as an enzyme facilitator, to the nontoxic antioxidant cystathione. When there is a deficiency of vitamin B-6, the homocysteine is not converted to cystathione, but instead does free radical damage to arteries. (See Part II, Chapter 7, "Our Subversive Free Radicals.") Homocystine, the oxidized form of homocysteine, is excreted in the urine. Evidence supporting this idea includes the fact that smokers, who have elevated risks for cardiovascular disease, typically have low vitamin B-6 levels in their blood serum. Women who use oral contraceptives, who have higher risks of cardiovascular disease than nonusers, also have lower serum levels of vitamin B-6. People fed a low vitamin B-6 diet for three weeks began excreting homocystine in their urine. Vitamin B-6 (especially in conjunction with vitamin C) has been used successfully to cause atherosclerotic damage to shrink back. Eating a diet with a great deal of methionine in it and with little vitamin B-6 is, therefore, potentially atherogenic (atherosclerosis-causing).

Here at last we seem to have at least part of the solution to the Eskimo-diet–cardiovascular disease puzzle. Eskimos who eat a traditional diet and live a traditional life-style rarely suffer from cardiovascular disease, even in old age. This observation was troublesome, because the traditional Eskimo diet is raw fat and meat, with the fat constituting about 90 percent of the calories in their diet. (Of course, the traditional diet provides very high levels of vitamin A from the livers of fish and marine mammals.)

When Eskimos move into a modern house, cardiovascular disease often moves in soon thereafter, even if the same type of food is eaten. There is a difference in the diet, however; the fat and meat are cooked before eating, and here seems to lie the problem. Cooking fat in the presence of air leads to the production of atherogenic, mutagenic, carcinogenic, immune system depressing, free radical–initiating organic peroxides. Moreover, vitamin A is a temperature-sensitive antioxidant,

and substantial amounts are destroyed in cooking, as is also
the case for the antioxidant vitamins B-1 and C, which are already marginal in the raw diet. Perhaps most important of all,
Dr. McCully has experimentally demonstrated that the ratio
of B-6 to the amino acid methionine in a piece of raw meat
is high enough to prevent homocysteine accumulation in experimental animals, but that the vitamin B-6 destruction
caused by cooking is sufficient so that the cooked meat does
lead to atherogenic, free radical–initiating homocysteine accumulation. Does this mean we should eat all our meat raw?
Definitely not! Raw meat is all too likely to have other hazards, including parasitic worms and possibly even slow viruses
which can cause slow progressive neurological deterioration.
The moral of this story is to take B-6 supplements, avoid oxidized fats, and enjoy your medium rare lean steak.

Another factor in the low incidence of heart attacks among
Eskimos eating a traditional diet has been found. A fatty acid
called eicosapentaenoic acid acts as a competitive inhibitor of
the enzyme cyclo-oxygenase, preventing prostaglandin formation. Thromboxane, the clot-promoting prostaglandin, is
not produced in as large amounts under these conditions. Eskimos living in coastal villages in Greenland eat seafoods rich
in large amounts of the n-3 variety of polyunsaturated fatty
acids structurally related to eicosapentaenoate. As a result,
these Eskimos have a prolonged bleeding time and a low incidence of abnormal blood clots.

Atherosclerosis can be induced by exposure to low oxygen conditions. When there is too little or too much oxygen,
free radicals are generated. These reactive chemical fragments can attack and damage artery walls, leading to atherosclerosis. Carbon monoxide, a gas found in nearly all smoke,
can induce atherosclerosis. The gas reduces oxygen carried in
the blood by reacting with the hemoglobin in red blood cells,
preventing the hemoglobin from carrying oxygen. Antioxidant nutrients, including vitamins A, E, C, B-1, B-5, B-6, the
amino acid cysteine, and the minerals zinc and selenium, can
provide a significant degree of protection against the free
radical damage induced by low oxygen conditions. Hyder-
gine® is an extremely powerful antioxidant prescription drug
that should be useful.

There are effective ways to reduce the size of plaques
after they have formed. Vitamin C, alone and in conjunction
with vitamin B-6, has been used to regress atherosclerotic

plaques in rabbits. (Vitamin C is also sometimes effective in large doses against other types of tumors; see Part III, Chapter 19, on cancer.) Other T-cell stimulants can also be expected to be effective in reducing existing plaques: e.g., arginine, ornithine, vitamins A and E, selenium, cysteine, and zinc.

Excess intake of table sugar (sucrose) can contribute to the development of atherosclerosis. Sucrose stimulates the release of insulin, which is required in order to utilize the sugar for energy. Sucrose, however, is metabolized quickly, while the insulin remains circulating in the bloodstream for hours. This excess insulin is thought to cause cholesterol and other lipids in the blood to be deposited in arterial walls. Diabetics using insulin to control their blood sugar often develop serious cardiovascular complications, such as atherosclerosis. Diabetics who are able to control their blood sugar levels adequately by dietary means do not generally develop these complications. For example, diabetic retinopathy, blindness in diabetics resulting from damage to the blood vessels of the eyes, occurs in diabetics using insulin but not in diabetics who can control blood sugar via diet. It appears, therefore, that the insulin diabetics take so they can utilize glucose in their blood (metabolism of this sugar is the body's main source of energy) is responsible for many of these complications. There is now a home computer program (written in BASIC) available which calculates the proper insulin dose based on a patient's eating schedule, diet, exercise, and urine sugar content (measured with Clinistix®, which may be purchased at many drugstores). This program helps to lessen the chances of using too much or too little insulin. (See Steve Faber's paper in the references to this chapter in Appendix K.)

An association has been discovered between heart disease and drinking soft water. Minerals have been removed from soft water, and certain minerals—especially selenium and zinc, required by the body as parts of the antioxidant enzymes glutathione peroxidase and superoxide dismutase—are necessary to maintain disease-free arteries. It is undesirable, then, to drink soft or distilled water that lacks these minerals unless one takes an appropriate mineral supplement. For those of you who would like to drink water with minerals but without chlorine and free-radical–inducing chlorinated carcinogens that are formed as a chlorination byproduct, a Sears activated charcoal filter ($19.95) is an inexpensive and effective answer. The water tastes great, too!

Since atherosclerotic plaques are a type of tumor, the T-cell immune system is responsible for preventing their growth. Free radicals, including oxygen-related radicals and lipid peroxides, may be responsible for *stimulating* tumor growth because these free radicals stimulate the production of cyclic guanosine monophosphate (cGMP). In high levels, cGMP induces most types of cells to undergo rapid cell division. Antioxidants, which can lower cGMP, help prevent cell division and tumor formation, while simultaneously helping the blood vessels maintain their production of PGI_2 to keep platelets and red blood cells from piling onto the plaques. Thus, immune system stimulation, such as we have discussed in Part II, Chapter 5, and Part III, Chapters 14 and 19, can help prevent atherosclerosis formation and development.

The physical "hardening" of the arteries by free radical–induced cross-linking leads to loss of vascular elasticity, thereby further elevating blood pressure already increased by the arterial narrowing caused by plaques and blood clots. This is the same type of cross-linking damage that makes rubber automobile parts become inelastic and brittle over the years. Antioxidants retard this process, both in rubber and in the blood vessels. See Part II, Chapter 6, for further information.

Some physicians are now using a diagnostic instrument called an ultrasonic doppler blood velocimeter. This device can measure blood velocity in veins and arteries near the surface by simply moving the sensor head along the skin over these blood vessels. Partial occlusions (blockages) are detected by the speedup in blood flow as it passes by them. Unlike diagnostic X-rays, this technique can be used as often as desired to monitor either the progress or the reversal of occlusive vascular disease.

WARNING: If you have a disorder that is caused by atherosclerosis (coronary artery disease leading to a "heart attack," kidney disease, brain damage, or poor circulation to your legs), you must remain under your doctor's care. The vitamins and other drugs that we discuss in this book are *not* a substitute for your doctor's treatment of you. With his or her consultation, the antioxidant nutrients may enhance the overall treament by assisting your body's natural repair mechanisms and by augmenting your body's natural protective mechanisms.

17
Cardiovascular Disease, Its Prevention or Amelioration: Stroke

Happy he who could learn the causes of things and who put beneath his feet all fears.

—Vergil, *Georgics I*

Every year, 400,000 Americans suffer strokes, a dreaded occurrence of aging. Many tens of thousands of these stroke victims die. About 85 percent of strokes are due to blood clots in the brain; the rest are due to internal bleeding (hemorrhage). By taking the right nutrients, you can greatly reduce your chances of having a blood clot or hemorrhage in your brain. You can prevent much of the brain damage, even if a stroke occurs. Most surprising of all, you will learn how you can promote substantial repair and regeneration in your own brain, whether or not you've had a stroke.

A leading cause of disability and death, strokes occur almost entirely in older individuals, resulting from failures of the blood circulation system in the brain. Strokes can be of two types, hemorrhage or clot(s) blocking a blood vessel. More strokes, though, are due to clots (85 percent) than to hemorrhage (15 percent). Often, an individual can have many small strokes long before a fatal attack. These small strokes can cause progressive deterioration in mental and physical functions. What causes them?

In one scenario of stroke occurrence, atherosclerotic plaques form in the lining of arteries leading to or in the brain. Platelets (clot-forming particles in the blood), red blood cells, and cholesterol and other lipids are deposited in the lining of these injured vessels, narrowing them and making it more difficult for oxygen to move through the blood vessel walls. Thus, the brain cells supplied by these narrowed atherosclerotic arteries do not get adequate oxygen, a condition known as hypoxia. Hypoxia and peroxidized fats reduce the production of PGI_2, the arteries' natural clot-prevention hormone. Eventually, a blood clot forms in the narrowed artery (or lodges there, having broken off another plaque upstream), causing further damage by cutting off most of the oxygen, producing a region of severe hypoxic damage. The area of brain cells killed in such a stroke is called the infarct. It may do so little damage to brain function that it is unnoticeable, or it may cause paralysis or death. The earliest stages of arterial clot formation are shown in the photomicrographs in Part III, Chapter 16.

Dr. Harry Demopoulos and others have found that free radical activity is greatly increased under conditions of inadequate oxygen concentration. Most strokes, brain damage during birth, heart attacks, and the organs of aged people have low to poor oxygenation. Rarely do we see *no* blood flow. Free radical–damaging mechanisms operate most rapidly in conditions where there is low to poor oxygenation. Ordinary oxygen (O_2) can interact with free radicals to terminate the chain reaction. Oxygen's presence at a proper level in the tissues (neither too high nor too low) helps control free radical activity. Therefore, free radicals (see Part II, Chapter 7) are a major source of damage under conditions where there is hypoxia (low oxygen) because of insufficient circulation. Hypoxic conditions are far more frequent than anoxic states such as cardiac arrest, when there is *no* blood flow. Free radical damage is most severe when there is partial flow and partial oxygenation, as occurs in most strokes, birth traumas that lead to cerebral palsy, and the low blood-flow conditions seen in most organs of people as they age. Taking antioxidants (such as vitamins C, E, A, B-1, B-5, and B-6 and cysteine, zinc, and selenium) and Hydergine® (Sandoz) would be expected to provide substantial protection against the free radicals and low oxygen condition prevailing in many aged brains. Hydergine® protects the brain from free radical damage under conditions of inadequate oxygen, whether due to blood clots blocking blood vessels or hemorrhage. In one experiment, blood was withdrawn from a cat until its blood pressure fell to about half normal. After about fifteen minutes, the cat's EEG (electroencephalograph, brain wave) readings indicated the start of irreversible brain damage. In another cat from which the same amount of blood was withdrawn but which received Hydergine® (at a blood concentration typical of a human using Hydergine®), there was no brain damage for forty-five minutes, or three times as long as the unprotected cat! It will work similarly in your brain via the same mechanisms. Although the patents on Hydergine® have expired, the Sandoz Corporation still spends about 40 percent of their research budget on this truly remarkable drug. As a result of this and other data (there are over 3,000 research papers on Hydergine® in the scientific literature), we hypothesized that it must be an extraordinary antioxidant and arranged for Sandoz to supply some of the material to Dr. Demopoulos for testing. In experiments that have been reported to Sandoz and other researchers, Demopoulos has found Hydergine® to be an extremely powerful antioxidant and to protect lipids. (For further data on Hydergine®, see the subject index.)

Another way strokes may occur is when a blood vessel bursts or hemorrhages. In addition to the damage mentioned in the last paragraph, the arteries may be hardened due to a process called cross-linking. Just as in the gradual deterioration of rubber parts on your car (an example of cross-linking), the arteries become stiff, hard, and brittle. Cross-linking is an end product of free radical reactions. The vessels lose their flexibility. Under conditions of unusual stress, these hardened blood vessels may burst, resulting in a stroke, just as the radiator hose on an old car may burst while climbing a long steep hill on a hot day. The blood that enters the tissues from broken vessels introduces copper and iron into fatty tissues of the brain. Iron and copper can induce and speed up free radical reactions a million-fold, thereby destroying cells.

There are six basic aging mechanisms involved in strokes that we can do something about. One is mutagenesis, which appears to be the major cause of plaque formation in humans and is mostly due to free radicals. Another is the T-cell immune failure that allows the development of the atherosclerotic plaques (a type of tumor) by failing to destroy them. A third is the free radical–caused cross-linking process. The fourth is abnormal clotting due to organic peroxide (free radical–oxidized fats and oils)-induced deficiency of the natural anti-clotting hormone PGI_2 (prostacyclin) in the artery lining. The fifth is the free radical damage to the brain caused by the stroke. The sixth is neurite destruction, both directly by free radicals and indirectly by lipofuscin accumulation, which is caused by free radicals and stimulated by hypoxia.

We have reviewed these aging mechanisms in their own chapters, so there is no need to go into great detail here. We do know that the T-cell immune system can be made to function at a greatly improved level by taking specific nutrients in adequate doses, including A, E, C, cysteine, zinc, selenium, ornithine and arginine. (See Part II, Chapter 5.) Among other things, the antioxidant nutrients protect cell membranes against spontaneous free radical damage, which is occurring all the time and which distorts cell surfaces. The T-cell immune system requires normal cell surfaces and receptors in order to function. The nutrients may help in this regard. Vitamins C and B-6 have been used to regress (to cause to shrink) atherosclerotic plaques in rabbits. We also know that much cross-linking and mutagenesis can be prevented by taking antioxidant nutrients, including C, E, cysteine, B-1, BHT, and selenium (see Part II, Chapter 6). BHT is also very effective against herpes viruses (see Part III, Chapter 5), and herpes viruses have been implicated in atherosclerosis.

There is even more that can be done. In individuals who have already had strokes, the prescription drug Hydergine® (Sandoz) can improve brain function by stabilizing the brain's energy levels (as measured by EEG output), increasing synthesis of protein (necessary for memory), and stimulating growth of neurites in brain cells (necessary for learning and proper communication between nerve cells). (See Part III, Chapter 2, and Part II, Chapter 9, for further information, dosage, and precautions.) Several months to two years may be required for full effects.

Deaner® (Riker) can even improve memory and learning in some senile individuals. Of course, the worse the impairment, the longer it will take for these drugs and nutrients to make a perceptible change. Sometimes several months to two years are required for full effects. (See Part III, Chapter 2, and Part II, Chapter 9, for further information, dosage, and precautions.

Vasopressin (Diapid® nasal spray, made by Sandoz) can also be very useful in stroke victims whose memory difficulties or outright amnesia are due to inadequate release by the pituitary gland of this memory hormone. If benefits occur, they will be quite prompt, sometimes appearing within seconds, sometimes taking as long as a week or so. (See Part III, Chapter 2, and Part II, Chapter 9, for further information, dosage, and precautions.)

CAUTION: As we have indicated in our other chapters, the nutrients and drugs mentioned here should be reviewed with your doctor. Those substances are *not* intended as a substitute for other treatments, such as low-dose aspirin.

18
Cardiovascular Disease, Its Prevention or Amelioration: Heart Attacks

New associations and fresh ideas are more likely to come out of a varied store of memories and experience than out of a collection that is all of one kind.

—Dr. E. L. Taylor

Over a million people suffer heart attacks each year and, of these, about 350,000 survive. Even the survivors often die within a year or so of another heart attack, sometimes very suddenly. But the understanding of what causes heart attacks has led to ways to reduce their occurrence. One readily available drug can reduce the rate of death from a second or subsequent heart attack by 74 percent. The right nutrients provide protection against abnormal clots. Eventually everybody will be taking advantage of this new knowledge. You can do that right now!

There is a widespread notion, promoted by some nutritionists, that until this century there were few heart attacks, and that this demonstrates a flaw in our modern diet or lifestyles. It is true that heart attacks are far more common today than they were several decades ago and earlier, but perhaps not for the reason that many people believe. Broda Barnes, M.D., offers his own theory: During World War II, the incidence of heart attacks decreased greatly in Europe. People thought this was because of a lack of availability of high cholesterol foods. However, the real reason, according to Dr. Barnes, may have been that tuberculosis had increased in incidence more than heart attacks had decreased. Patients were being killed by TB *before* they could have a heart attack, but autopsies of TB victims revealed that coronary artery damage was double the prewar level. Later, when antibiotics against TB were available, deaths from TB dropped and heart attacks rose. As Dr. Barnes observed, "In the adults having died from tuberculosis, advanced atherosclerosis was the rule.... It would appear that the individual susceptible to any infectious disease is highly vulnerable to atherosclerosis." This is an attractive theory. And since we now know that atherosclerosis occurs at least partly as a result of a T-cell immune system failure, the comparison of susceptibility to infections and atherosclerosis is very appropriate. It is, in fact, the T-cells that fight tuberculosis. Barnes has found that patients with too little output of thyroid hormone are particularly susceptible to heart attacks. Adequate thyroid hormone is required for proper function of the immune system.

Thyroid hormone acts as an immune system stimulant by causing the pituitary to release growth hormone. Thyroid hormone may stimulate the immune system by another route as well. The hypothalamus in the brain measures the amount of thyroid hormone in the blood. When thyroid hormone levels are too low, the hypothalamus sends a hormone message of TRF (thyrotropin releasing factor) to the pituitary in the brain, which, in turn, releases TSH (thyrotropin, or thyroid stimulating hormone) which then causes the thyroid gland to release thyroid hormone. As the level of thyroid hormone rises in the blood, less TRF and TSH are released; thus, if you take thyroid hormone, your blood levels of TRF and TSH fall. This effect may be important because there is some evidence that TRF has immune system suppressant effects.

Barnes recommends a simple measurement of underarm temperature to spot low thyroid hormone output. In the morning, before rising or talking or doing anything else, place a thermometer in the armpit for a few minutes. Normal armpit temperature should be between 97.8 and 98.2 degrees Fahrenheit. If the temperature is lower than this, low thyroid hormone output should be suspected. The clinical tests run for thyroid function, T3 and T4, may give results that disagree with other symptoms, such as cold extremities. This is because the quantity of thyroid hormone is measured rather than its biological effectiveness. Reduced numbers of thyroid hormone receptors or insensitivity of receptors are not detected by these tests, which may indicate normal levels of thyroid hormone when the actual biological hormone effect is abnormally low.

Another belief in wide circulation is the theory that reducing dietary cholesterol can reduce serum cholesterol and lead to a healthier cardiovascular system. This theory has been examined in several large clinical studies. In the Framingham study, 437 men and 475 women were observed for periods up to ten years. There was no correlation found between dietary intake of cholesterol and serum levels of cholesterol. This result has been repeated in other studies. But there were additional findings. There was no clear relation between serum cholesterol and deaths due to heart disease and, therefore, no proof that simply reducing serum cholesterol is capable of reducing the heart disease death rate. However, a low calorie diet should be of great value for overweight persons. High blood cholesterol levels, together with elevations in uric acid (hydrogen peroxide and free radicals are released during its production), blood sugar, triglycerides, and unfavorable patterns of blood lipoproteins offer a more complete picture of your risk of atherosclerosis. Low cholesterol diets alone have not been demonstrated to provide protection from heart attacks because many other nutrients are involved in protecting the vessels against atherosclerosis and the associated stickiness of platelets, which is caused by free radical damage. Nutrients of importance include vitamins A, B-1, C, E, and B-6 and zinc, selenium, and other antioxidants.

A recently developed indicator of risk for heart disease, mentioned in Part III, Chapter 16, is the ratio between two fractions of lipoproteins (lipid-protein molecules which are important constituents of cellular membranes) in the bloodstream. The ratio of the HDL (high density lipoproteins) to LDL (low density lipoproteins) can indicate high or low risk of heart disease. A high HDL to LDL ratio is considered protective, while a low ratio (high LDL to HDL) indicates high risk. Both fractions carry cholesterol, but LDL seems to deposit the cholesterol in arterial walls, while the HDL removes the cholesterol from the arterial walls. In addition, LDL carries considerably more polynuclear aromatic hydrocarbons (produced whenever fuels are burned) and other carcinogens. Thus, high LDL levels might also contribute to a higher cancer risk. Clinicians are looking for factors which affect HDL, the fraction which seems to provide protection against the development of heart disease. Factors which are associated with lower HDL levels (increasing the risk of heart disease) include cigarette smoking, obesity, diabetes, elevated LDL, and elevated triglycerides. Factors which are associated with increased levels of HDL include being female and physical activity. Measurements of total cholesterol do not give any indication of the amounts of HDL and LDL. There are not many testing laboratories able to perform differential lipoprotein measurements at present. However, it would be well worth looking for a lab that does.

A visible indicator of heart attack risk recently discovered is the earlobe crease. (See photo. Arrow points to tell-tale crease.) Other creases on the ear have no known correlation. The crease, as shown in the photo, either on one or both earlobes, was noticed by several doctors as being much more prevalent among heart attack patients than among non-heart attack control patients of the same age or even older. In coronary heart disease patients in one study, 47 percent had the earlobe crease. At the Mayo Clinic, Dr. Sternlieb found that in his study of 121 coronary artery disease patients, the earlobe crease plus symptoms of heart attack (such as chest pains) meant a heart attack 90 percent of the time. But in people with heart attack symptoms and *no* earlobe crease, the chances were about 90 percent that the people did *not* have coronary artery disease. Other reports suggest the possibility that the correlation between the diagonal earlobe crease and heart disease may differ among races. Rhoads et al. found a very low frequency of earlobe crease among male Japanese Americans in Hawaii. Petrakis and Koo reported an age-related increase in the frequency of the crease among white, black, and Latin-American groups, but not among Chinese.

What is the reason for the appearance of the earlobe crease? We think it may be a result of cross-linking processes, such as occur in the formation of facial wrinkles. Cross-linking of the rich bed of blood vessels in the thin-skinned earlobe could cause such a crease and also reflect similar damage to other blood vessels, including the coronary arteries. Cross-linking of blood vessel walls reduces flexibility, thereby contributing to high blood pressure, and alters arterial oxygen diffusion properties—that is, decreases the ability of oxygen to migrate through the artery wall to reach the tissues. The most common environmental cross-linking agents are aldehydes, such as acetaldehyde (formed in the liver from alcohol) and malonaldehyde (formed in the breakdown of peroxidized fats in the body). The process of forming the cross-links involves

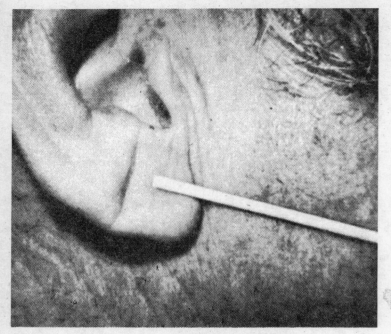

The ear-lobe sign—a deep crease in the lobule portion of the auricle.

free radical reactions and can be inhibited by the use of the right antioxidants. Aldehydes are also mutagens and carcinogens and, therefore, able to stimulate plaque formation. A very effective antioxidant combination against aldehyde damage is vitamin C, B-1, and the amino acid cysteine (see Part III, Chapters 10 and 12).

Dr. David Bresler of the Center for Integral Medicine had another hypothesis about the earlobe crease when we discussed it with him a few months ago. He told us that the vagus nerve which controls the heart also has an ending in the earlobe. Thus, the crease may reflect damage to this nerve. We do know that one very common type of fatal heart attack is caused by abnormal rhythms in the heart stimulated by the vagus nerve. In one experiment, such heart attacks in dogs could be prevented by severing this nerve. Some new drug therapies for people at risk for heart attack work by stabilizing or inhibiting the vagus, for example the drug Anturane® (more on this below).

Several nutrients provide substantial protection against heart attacks. Vitamins E and C can prevent abnormal clot formation. In double blind studies in humans, 1 gram of vitamin C daily reduced incidence of deep vein thrombosis (blood clots) by half. Lower doses of C that have been used in similar clinical trials failed to provide significant protection. Thus C doses must be high enough to provide this protection. Another study in 60 geriatric patients, utilizing 1 to 3 grams of vitamin C per day, provided protection against thrombotic (abnormal clots) episodes for up to $2\frac{1}{2}$ years. Vitamin E slows the formation time for abnormal clots when injected interperitoneally into rats. Vitamin E also prolongs clotting time of recalcified human plasma, although it does not prevent normal clotting at a wound. Antioxidants such as E and C, and especially antioxidants which contain reduced sulfur (such as cysteine), are anti-cross-linkers and may help prevent the type of damage which causes the formation of the earlobe crease. In human subjects, 3 grams of niacin (nicotinic acid) per day reduced serum cholesterol by 26 percent after a year. More importantly, niacin especially reduces the quantity of VLDL, the very low density lipoproteins. Niacin also acts as a vasodilator—skin reddening caused by niacin is due to widening of blood vessels in the skin and release of histamine stores there. In the 4th edition of the medical textbook *The Pharmacological Basis of Therapeutics,* the authors, L. S. Goodman and A. Gilman, state on page 768 that "this agent [nicotinic acid] has its greatest usefulness in the treatment of patients with elevated very-low-density lipoproteins and a lesser or limited usefulness in the treatment of those with elevated low-density lipoproteins."

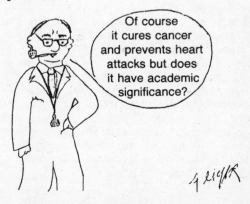

It is not too late to improve your cardiovascular system using these nutrients, even if you have already had a heart attack. **CAUTION:** Vitamin E use can cause a transitory initial rise in blood pressure, so people with heart disease or hypertension should start vitamin E at a low dose (perhaps 100 I.U. per day) and under a doctor's supervision (see particularly Dr. Wilfred E. Shute's book, *Vitamin E for Ailing and Healthy Hearts*). This is a specific example of why your doctor must be consulted if you plan to take any suggestions that appear in this book.

A Ciba-Geigy drug approved for the treatment of gout, Anturane® (sulfinpyrazone), has been discovered in a human clinical study to reduce the chance of death from a *second* or subsequent heart attack by 74 percent. This is important, since many patients survive their first heart attack but die from a second or subsequent heart attack within five years. This is a case of a drug approved for one use (gout) which has another use (preventing heart attacks) for which the FDA has not approved it. We would be unable to report this new use if we owned any Ciba-Geigy stock or worked for the company. And yet, why should people be disqualified from free speech because they are connected with the company that developed the drug? If a statement is scientifically correct, it is correct regardless of who says it. If you have had a heart attack, especially within the past six months, ask your physician for Anturane®.

A class of drugs known as beta blockers is now being used to reduce blood pressure and to prevent abnormal heart rhythms which can result in sudden death. These drugs block certain adrenaline receptors so that the "fight or flight" syndrome is suppressed. Until recently, there was only one drug of this type approved in the United States, propranolol. There are over a dozen beta blockers available in Europe, where they have been used effectively for many years. A new beta blocker, Sandoz's Viskane®, has just been approved for human clinical trials in the United States. This same class of drugs is now being used successfully in the treatment of phobias such as fear of flying, stage fright, etc. (See Sandy's experiences in Appendix L.) Beta blockers have undoubtedly played an important role in the age-corrected reduction in the United States heart attack rate which has taken place over the past ten years. In one study, propranolol reduced heart attack deaths by about 25 percent.

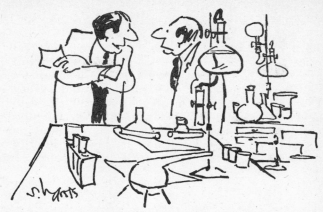

"Just for kicks, let's come up with something that has a good side effect."

Biofeedback can be used to help control hypertension. In a recent study, doctors found that 43 percent of high blood pressure patients could reduce their blood pressure by at least 10 mm Hg (systolic and/or diastolic) by simply measuring their own blood pressure twice a day for a month. This should provide a powerful motivation to such patients to buy and use a blood pressure gauge every day.

Home blood pressure measuring devices range from the traditional mechanical units to high technology units containing a microcomputer. Sears, Montgomery Ward, and some mail order firms, such as J S & A Sales, sell these units and a companion device, the pulse rate counter. These inexpensive pulse rate measuring devices can also be used for the biofeedback control of blood pressure. It took about fifteen minutes for each of us to learn to will our pulse rate lower by fifteen to twenty beats per minute, with an accompanying reduction of blood pressure.

Aspirin has been effective in reducing the risk of abnormal blood clots in males in some studies, as in one reported in the *New England Journal of Medicine* of 13 July 1978. A Canadian study found that aspirin reduced the incidence of big strokes (but not small ones) and of death by 48 percent in males. There was no reduction with aspirin in females. A recent American Heart Association study on aspirin was disappointing, however.

Ballistocardiography is a research technique for measuring the elasticity of the cardiovascular system by detecting the "jiggling" of the tissues in response to cardiovascular pulses, as the heart beats (much like the jiggling of Jell-O®). It can be very helpful in following the effects of therapies on atherosclerotic blood vessels. We hope this technique will be used much more widely in prevention-oriented medical clinics. The patient simply lies on an instrumented table for a few moments, and a computer does the rest. This technique was born and died in the early 1950s—a time when a computer cost as much as a hospital. But now a far more powerful computer can be purchased for the cost of one week's hospital fees for a single room.

19
Cancer, Its Prevention or Amelioration

There is but one safe way to avoid mistakes; to do nothing, or, at least, to avoid doing something new. . . . The unknown lends an insecure foothold and venturing out into it one can hope for no more than that the possible failure will be an honorable one.

—Albert Szent-Gyorgyi, Nobel Prize winner for the discovery of vitamin C

When the control system (in or around the DNA blueprint material) that governs a cell's reproduction is damaged, one of the most deadly and feared diseases can result: cancer. It is the job of the immune system to detect these cancerous cells and kill and eat them. We can greatly improve the effectiveness of our immune system surveillance by taking the right nutrients. The correct nutrients can both reduce our chances of getting cancer and improve our chances of recovery if we already have cancer.

Cancer is a word that still strikes fear in the modern heart. Despite the many billions of dollars that have been spent on cancer research, many hundreds of thousands of people die of this dreaded disease each year. Yet we are on the brink of new breakthroughs in understanding the process by which cancer cells emerge from normal cells (transformation) and escape detection by the body's immune system to become tumors. Nobel Prize–winning tumor biologist P. B. Medawar has said that probably every person develops cancer thousands, perhaps millions, of times in his or her life. Only rarely do tumors result, and that is when the T-cell immune system fails to do its job of protection.

Prevention of cancer is now an advanced area of research. Many available nutrients may be taken in safe doses which have prevented the development of many types of cancer in experimental animals. These nutrients include: vitamins E, A, C, and B-1; cysteine, an amino acid; arginine and ornithine, amino acids; the minerals selenium and zinc; and BHT and BHA, common antioxidant food preservatives.

How do these substances inhibit the development of cancer? First, by stimulating the immune system (see Part II, Chapter 5). Only cancer cells that escape detection by the immune system have the opportunity to become tumors. Only rarely do tumors escape detection by the immune system, which usually destroys the abnormal cells before they proliferate enough to be noticeable as a tumor.

Another way these nutrients help prevent cancer is by deactivating free radicals, a type of very reactive chemical entity that is produced in normal metabolism, by exposure to ultraviolet light and X-ray irradiation, in the breakdown of peroxidized fats (rancid fats) in the body, and by ozone, nitrogen oxides, and some other pollutants. Free radicals damage important parts of human cells, especially the genetic blueprint material (DNA and RNA) which controls the metabolism of the whole cell. When a part of the DNA's growth control apparatus for the cells is damaged, cancer can result. Many anti-cancer drugs have the property of terminating chain reactions of free radicals. If cancer runs in your family, it is particularly important to take nutrients that can help protect you from developing cancer.

Selenium is a powerful antioxidant and inhibitor of cancer initiation and development. In a 1965 study, higher selenium levels in soil and crops correlated with lower human cancer death rates in the United States and Canada. Higher levels of selenium in human blood correlated with lower human cancer death rates in several cities. Independent reports by Dr. Bjorksten and Dr. Shamberger on a number of human and farm animal epidemiological studies and laboratory animal and tissue culture experiments suggest that the incidence of cancer can be reduced by about 70 percent with adequate selenium supplements. The National Cancer Institute is attempting to get the FDA to set a Recommended Dietary

Allowance for selenium at around 200 micrograms a day. Selenium in its sodium selenite form is the least expensive. In recent tissue culture experiments, sodium selenite has directly killed certain types of cancer cells at levels which did no noticeable harm to normal mammalian cells. We currently prefer to take our selenium in the form of sodium selenite, the form subject to most research to date. Although seleno-cystine and selenomethionine increase blood levels of selenium more rapidly, these seleno amino acids are less effective than sodium selenite in elevating serum glutathione peroxidase levels. Mammals and birds do not seem to be capable of distinguishing between seleno and sulfur amino acids. Sodium selenite was also superior in inhibiting Ehrlich ascites tumor cell growth in mice. (One type of selenium containing yeast has recently shown good glutathione peroxidase elevation, however. See the chapter notes.)

BHT and BHA, antioxidant food preservatives, inhibited the development of cancer under conditions in which there was contact of a carcinogen with the target tissue, such as cancer of the stomach in mice fed the carcinogens benzo(a)pyrene (BP) or dimethylbenzanthracene (DMBA), tarry products of partial combustion. The BHT and BHA also suppressed the development of cancer when the carcinogen acted at a site far from the point of administration, such as inhibition of mammary tumor in rats given oral DMBA. In studies in which the antioxidant BHA or BHT was added at a concentration of 5 milligrams per gram of food along with the carcinogen BP at a concentration of 1 milligram per gram of food, the BHA or BHT inhibited BP's carcinogenic effects. Normally, a single 0.1 milligram dose of BP will cause cancer in most of these rodents. In the United States, people get a couple of milligrams per day of these antioxidants in their foods. (At least, they were getting that much back in 1974. Since then, the misinformed public clamor against adding any synthetic chemicals to foods has resulted in the removal of BHA and BHT from many products in which they were formerly contained.)

Several viruses have been implicated in some animal and human cancers, including herpes viruses (thought to be a factor in such human cancers as Burkitt's lymphoma, nasopharyngeal cancer, and cervical carcinoma) and hepatitis B virus (implicated as a cause of liver cancer). These viruses may turn out to be just "passengers" and not be causal, but it may be important to note for other viral diseases that BHT is toxic to all small nucleic-acid-core-diameter, lipid-coated viruses, of which herpes is one. Others include some influenza viruses, measles viruses, rabies virus, mumps virus, and most "C" type viruses (most animal-tumor-causing viruses known are "C" types), as well as others. Other small-core-diameter, lipid-coated viruses have not yet been tested with BHT, but the method of inactivation postulated by Dr. George Rouser at the City of Hope Hospital should work equally well.

Some lipid-containing viruses, such as herpes, are also implicated in some slow virus degenerative diseases, such as multiple sclerosis, kuru, Creutzfeldt-Jakob disease, muscular dystrophy, diabetes, and others. It may be, at least in the early formative stages of such slow virus diseases which involve lipid-coated viruses, that BHT might be of therapeutic value. In our experiments, 250 milligrams of BHT per day has been effective in all people so far tested for both type 1 herpes (oral) and type 2 (genital) infections. This therapy has since been used by a research-oriented physician on over one hundred cases of chronic herpes of both types. He normally administers about 1 gram of BHT each night for two weeks, with the treatment repeated if the symptoms return. The results have been complete suppression of symptoms and infectivity as long as at least 250 milligrams of BHT is taken each night. No adverse side effects have been observed in these patients. See Appendix L, "Some Case Histories" for further data.

The mixed-function oxidase enzyme system of the liver is also capable of modulating the formation of cancer-causing chemicals. Many carcinogenic compounds are acted upon by the liver before getting into the general system. This is termed "metabolizing the carcinogen," and the process can convert the chemical into an active substance, or the metabolic activity can inactivate and detoxify the chemical. Inducers of increased activity of this system include the carcinogens themselves, phenothiazines (a widely used class of antipsychotic drugs), alfalfa, Brussels sprouts, cabbage, turnips, broccoli, cauliflower, spinach, dill, and celery. Many of these vegetables also contain substances called indoles which inactivate chemical toxins and carcinogens.

It is far easier to prevent than to treat cancer. However, there are treatments available which have been used with some success in cancer patients. Vitamin C, for example, was given in a dosage of 10 grams per day to terminal cancer patients in a study in a Scottish hospital by Linus Pauling and

Ewan Cameron. The 1,000 control patients (who received only painkillers and no supplemental vitamin C) lived an average of 50 days after the study began. The 100 experimental patients (given the painkillers and supplemental 10 grams of C per day) lived an average of over 200 days, over four times as long. Of the original 100 vitamin-C-treated terminal cancer patients, thirteen are still alive today and free of cancer. The Mayo Clinic recently also tested C in terminal cancer patients. Unfortunately, this experiment was not an actual replication of the Pauling-Cameron experiment. Very few of the Pauling and Cameron patients had received immune-system-destroying chemotherapy, whereas the Mayo Clinic patients had generally undergone such treatments. Vitamin C is itself poisonous to certain cancer cells at levels tolerated by normal cells; probably its major actions, though, are to activate the T-cell immune system and to increase your body's production of interferon, an anti-virus and anti-cancer chemical. We hope someone will attempt to repeat this very interesting experiment with cancer patients who have not had their immune systems compromised with chemotherapy. Pauling is currently preparing to do another study of the same type with 20 grams of vitamin C per day given to another group of terminal cancer patients. See Appendix A for the address of the Linus Pauling Institute of Science and Medicine.

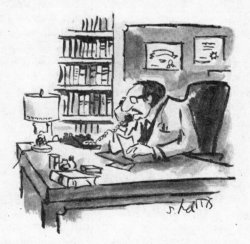

"Take some interferon, and call me in the morning."

Vitamin C is very effective in inhibiting malignant transformation of mouse fibroblasts (connective tissue cells) in cell culture caused by the addition of methylcholanthrene, a combustion tar PAH mutagen and carcinogen. Levels of ascorbic acid as low as 1 microgram (one millionth of a gram) per milliliter can inhibit this transformation. This amounts to only about 1 milligram of ascorbic acid in one quart of culture medium! Vitamin C can also prevent the formation of carcinogenic nitrosamines in your gut from amines (from protein) and nitrites (most of which are produced in the gut by bacteria, rather than eaten as an anti-microbial food additive).

An interesting treatment, although of very limited availability (because of FDA failure to approve it), is the thymus hormone thymosin. The thymus gland behind your breastbone is the heart of your immune system, producing T-cells and generally controlling your body's self-defense forces. As mentioned in Part II, Chapter 5, on the immune system, thymosin, discovered by Dr. Allan Goldstein of George Washington University in 1965, has been used to successfully treat a wide range of diseases due to immune system failure, including cancer. Thymosin is effective in about 50 percent of the restricted types of cancer cases in which it has been used. There is a simple blood test administered in advance which is a predictor of whether thymosin treatment will be of value. In this test, the patient's white cells are challenged in a test tube with sheep red blood cells. If the immune system is able to respond better with added thymosin—the white blood cells being better able to recognize and attack the alien red blood cells—the patient's immune system is 95 percent likely to improve its function with thymosin therapy. Unfortunately, this unusually safe and promising therapy is still considered experimental by the FDA, and there seems little likelihood that the FDA will be willing to approve it the near future. Indeed, it is unlikely that anyone will attempt to get FDA approval, since the patents on thymosin are about to expire, thereby eliminating any possibility of recovering the immense cost of seeking FDA approval to market it. Thymosin is being manufactured and used in Israel, as is interferon.

In terminal cases of cancer, when all else has failed, institutions that offer advanced life support systems during intense chemotherapy, such as the Janker Clinic in Germany, might be considered. There they administer chemotherapy and radiation treatments, pushing them to their limits by carefully monitoring the patient's condition. They often follow drugs and radiation with immune stimulation therapy. While it is usual practice in treating cancer patients to stop drugs or radiation when white blood cell counts fall too low, the Janker Clinic does not do this. Instead, they use antibiotics to control possible infections, while keeping treatments going at the highest dose level the patient can tolerate. These treatments are not pleasant, but the Janker Clinic has had a good survival rate in some types of cancers including advanced testicular cancer, pancreatic cancer, lung cancer, stomach cancer, and others.

Radiation and chemotherapy work by being—hopefully—slightly more toxic to the tumor than to the patient. The philosophy at this clinic is to provide life support systems to keep the patient alive during therapy that would normally be fatal. Chemotherapy usually severely suppresses the immune system; hence it usually must be applied vigorously enough to kill all the cancer cells, not just 99 percent of them. Surgery and thymus-sparing radiation therapy are valuable even when they miss some cancer cells, since they reduce the mass of often immune-suppressing tumor tissue which your immune system must destroy. For more information about the Janker Clinic, contact Hans Hoefer-Janker, M.D., Hospital Director, or Wolfgang Scheef, M.D., Medical Director, The Janker Clinic, Baumschulallee 12–14, 5300 Bonn, Federal German Republic (telephone: 02221/637747).

It is widely believed that perhaps 40 to 80 percent of human cancers (excluding the very common ultraviolet-light-induced skin cancers) are caused by carcinogens like those in cigarette smoke, which are called polycyclic or polynuclear aromatic hydrocarbons (PAH). These materials are produced when almost anything burns, including tobacco, gasoline, paper, wood, coal, fat, oil, etc. One strategy for avoiding cancer is, of course, to keep away from these carcinogens. Stop smoking. Avoid cooking smoke. Don't eat charcoal-broiled meats. And so on. Another strategy is to prevent these carcinogens from causing cancer by taking nutrients which interfere with the cancer-causing process. These PAH (polycyclic aromatic hydrocarbons) are not carcinogens in themselves. They are converted in the body to the carcinogenic form by an enzyme system—the mixed-function oxidase system mentioned earlier—which detoxifies poisons and other compounds. The synthetic antioxidants BHT and BHA modify the PAH metabolism, so that less of these compounds is converted to a cancer-causing (carcinogenic) form. Indoles found in foods such as cabbage and cauliflower can also modify PAH metabolism and prevent carcinogenic activation of PAH. BHT, vitamins C and E, and selenium inhibit chromosome breakage by the PAH carcinogen 7,12-di-methyl-benz-a-anthracene.

It has recently been discovered that some people who have unusually low serum cholesterol levels exhibit a higher incidence of cancer. Although the cause of this has not been demonstrated, we believe that we can suggest some plausible, testable mechanisms.

The most commonly used method of lowering serum cholesterol is to substitute polyunsaturated fats for saturated fats in the diet. This tends to block cholesterol synthesis. Polyunsaturated fats are much more subject to free radical autoxidation that creates carcinogenic and immune-suppressant organic peroxides. Both animals in experiments and humans in long-term cardiovascular studies have exhibited an elevated incidence of cancer when saturated fats were replaced with polyunsaturated fats.

Dr. Harry Demopoulos and others have shown that cholesterol—in its unoxidized form—is one of the body's major antioxidants. Cholesterol is the only major antioxidant we know of that an animal can make without dietary trace elements such as zinc, selenium, manganese, copper, and iron. Most biochemicals produced in the body are made under closed-loop feedback control; that means that they are produced in greater quantities when more is needed. (Your home's furnace and thermostat are an example of a closed-loop feedback control system.) In our opinion, the high serum cholesterol observed in smokers, drinkers, the obese, and atherosclerosis patients is due to a high level of free radical damage stimulating the body to produce more of the protective antioxidant cholesterol. (This concept is supported by the fact that most low-toxicity antioxidants tested, whether nutrients or artificial food additives, will lower serum cholesterol in both experimental animals and humans.) The body's use of cholesterol as an antioxidant does have disadvantages (side effects), however. Oxidized cholesterol, such as cholesterol epoxides and cholesterol hydroperoxides, are immune suppressants, blood clot initiators, mutagens, and mild carcinogens. These oxidation products certainly are a less immediate hazard than the original uncontrolled free radicals, but in the long run (as you grow old), they can lead to cardiovascular disease and cancer. We would very much like to see a clinical laboratory test developed to measure the serum ratio of reduced cholesterol to oxidized cholesterol. We suspect that this would be a useful predictor of cardiovascular disease (and probably cancer), as the ratio of HDL to LDL is.

If cholesterol is low because free radicals are being effectively scavenged by other protective molecules, our hypothesis predicts a low incidence of free radical pathology, such as cardiovascular disease and cancer. If cholesterol is low because its synthesis has been blocked or because of a genetic defect, we predict an elevated incidence of free radical pathology. Indeed, children with cystic fibrosis have a genetic defect which drastically impairs cholesterol biosynthesis, and some of their tissues are badly cross-linked, presumably by inadequately controlled free radicals. In addition, they suffer from chronic respiratory infections and exhibit abnormally low serum levels of vitamins A and E—reasonably consequences of inadequately controlled free radicals. Our extremely low cholesterol levels are due to our high intake of other antioxidants.

Two closely related drugs have a dramatic effect on cancer incidence in rodents. Hydergine®, an extremely potent antioxidant, reduces the incidence of spontaneous breast cancer (in a breast cancer prone strain) by about 60 pecent at a serum level corresponding to typical human use in Europe (9 milligrams per day). Bromocriptine (Parlodel®) has a related chemical structure and is likely to be an antioxidant. It increases the production of the immune system stimulant growth hormone in normal persons, and it suppresses the production of prolactin, a breast growth stimulating hormone which evidence suggests is an immune system suppressant as well. A PAH combustion tar (found in tobacco and other smoke) component called DMBA is normally quite effective in producing breast cancer in most experimental animals. In recent experiments, bromocriptine completely prevented the development of breast cancer in animals exposed to DMBA at levels which would normally cause this cancer every time.

Feces of normal people contain mutagenic (mutation causing) substances (as assayed by the Ames test) which may be causative agents for colon cancer. Because scientists believe that these substances may be N-nitroso compounds, Bruce and his associates fed ascorbic acid and alpha tocopherol to human volunteers. They found that the vitamin combination was able to reduce the level of mutagens in the feces to 25 percent of the level in the control (no vitamin supplements given) subjects. The reason for providing both vitamins is that one (ascorbic acid) is soluble in the water phase, while the other (alpha-tocopherol) is soluble in the fat phase of intestinal contents.

Other treatments which seem to have had some beneficial effects include BCG and levamisole immunotherapy. These substances increase the effectiveness of the patient's own immune system in attacking his or her cancer. BCG (Bacillus Calmette-Guerin) is a cow tuberculosis bacterium which is used in some provinces in Canada and elsewhere as a vaccine to immunize people to human tuberculosis. In one Canadian study, hundreds of thousands of Canadian schoolchildren given a single BCG superficial skin immunization had half the leukemia rate of similar schoolchildren not receiving BCG. Two inoculations reduced leukemia by about 70 percent, and three inoculations provided 80 to 90 percent protection. Given in a series of inoculations, BCG has, in some people, caused a degree of recovery from cancer. In other people there is no improvement; rarely, it causes the cancer to accelerate. Most serious side effects occurred from deep injections, rather than the usual superficial skin inoculations. BCG should be used only in people with functioning T-cell immune systems (see section on clinical tests). Levamisole is a veterinary drug approved and used for the treatment of parasites and worms. Curiously, its immune system stimulating effects have been helpful to some human cancer patients. Both these treatments are of limited availability in the United States because neither is approved for cancer therapy by the FDA.

It is well known that people who smoke have a much higher incidence of cancer. Ninety percent of lung cancers and about 50 percent of cancers of the urinary bladder occur in smokers. It is less widely realized that people who drink alcohol—particularly in large quantities—also have a much higher cancer incidence. As noted earlier, people who both drink and smoke have far more cancers than either smokers only or drinkers only. The cancer risks for each group are multiplied together, not merely added! Ninety percent of cancers of the mouth, larynx, esophagus, and liver are in smokers who also drink. Acetaldehyde, a pollutant found in smog, in cigarette smoke, and made from alcohol in the human liver, is a carcinogen and mutagen. It autoxidizes, producing free radicals and peracetic acid; the latter can activate

PAH (carcinogenic tars) to their active carcinogenic DNA-damaging epoxide form. It also destroys an important antioxidant, cysteine, and adds onto cellular molecules by free radical addition reactions. The combination of vitamin C, vitamin B-1, and the amino acid cysteine provided significant protection to rats given huge doses of acetaldehyde, sufficient to kill 90 percent of the unprotected rats.

WARNING: *If you have cancer or know someone who does, it is essential that a course of treatment include surgery, even if the tumor cannot be completely removed, radiation (for sensitive types of cancer), as well as therapy with immune stimulants, such as we discussed in this chapter. Do not just take vitamin C and other immune system–stimulating nutrients. Surgery, radiation, and these nutrients may be much more effective. A big tumor can overwhelm your immune system, particularly if it grew large before being detected by your immune patrols. If the tumor mass is substantially reduced by surgery and/or radiation, your immune system will have a much greater chance of destroying what is left. Do not say no to your surgeon if he can only remove two thirds of the tumor. Vitamin C supplements will not interfere with surgery (in fact, they can markedly speed recovery) or radiation treatment. Vitamins are also not a substitute for follow-up visits to your doctor if you have cancer. Together with your doctor's ongoing treatments, the nutrients, such as ascorbic acid and selenium, may enhance your response.*

WARNING: While nutritional supplements can often be used to improve the performance of one's immune system and, hence, help the surgeon and radiologist to fight cancer, there is one kind of cancer which should be treated with nutritional *restraint.* Pigmented malignant melanoma produces its black melanin pigment by the autoxidation of aromatic amino acids such as tyrosine, phenylalanine, and L-Dopa. Experiments have shown that melanomas may obtain over 60 percent of their metabolic energy from this autoxidation process. In both experimental animals and in the relatively small number of humans tested to date, marked slowing of tumor growth was obtained with diets low in tyrosine and phenylalanine. (These are essential amino acids and cannot be entirely eliminated.) If you do not have access to a nutritionally-oriented oncologist, the type of diet used on children with PKU should be discussed with your physician. PKU, phenylketonuria, is an inherited disorder in which there is an inability to properly metabolize phenylalanine. Infants with

PKU will be brain damaged unless they are given a diet quite low in phenylalanine and tyrosine. This is not a particularly rare problem and physicians will generally have PKU diets, even though they may not yet be aware of the usefulness of diets low in aromatic amino acids for the treatmet of pigmented malignant melanomas.

The thymus gland is very sensitive to radiation; a dose of radiation of 20 rems does significant detectable damage to it. Unless you have a rare thymic cancer, it is imperative that your thymus be protected during radiation therapy. Very few radiologists understand the central importance of the thymus in the immune system and the necessary part that the immune system must play if cancer is to be cured. *You* are going to have to make sure that your thymus is not inadvertently knocked out by radiotherapy. Get a written estimate of the expected thymic radiation dose from the radiologist *before* treatment starts. Ask for a lead shield for your thymus well in advance—just one dose of radiation can be a disaster. *Insist* that a radiation-measuring film badge (for the 0-to-50-rem range) be placed over your thymus during each treatment and that you be informed of the measured thymic dose *before* your next treatment. If the radiologist your surgeon recommends is reluctant to protect your thymus gland from radiation damage or claims that it is unnecessary, PROMPTLY HIRE ANOTHER RADIOLOGIST, SINCE IT IS YOUR LIFE AND YOUR MONEY!

GROWTH HORMONE CAUTION: Inappropriate use of GH releasers may have adverse consequences. They should not be used by persons who have not completed their long-bone growth (that is, who have not grown to their full height) unless they have been advised to do so by their physician. After full height is attained, GH will not cause further height increases. Excess GH will cause the skin to grow so rapidly that it becomes noticeably coarser and thicker; this effect is reversible when excess GH is withdrawn. Very excessive GH over an extended period of time can cause irreversible enlargement of joint diameter (which may be unsightly but is usually not dangerous) and lowering of voice pitch due to larynx growth. The maintenance of extremely high levels of growth hormone (above normal teenage to young adult levels) for extended periods of time requires further safety research. In some GH releaser experiments on animals either previously or subsequently given cancer, the GH releasers usually caused an improvement. At Cornell University Medical Center, however, hypophysectomy (surgical removal of the hypothalamus) in women with advanced metastatic breast cancer has sometimes produced dramatic improvements. Since this procedure affects many other hormones besides GH, including LHRH, LH, PSH, TRF, TSH, thyroid, prolactin, estrogens, progestins, endorphins, beta lipotropin, etc, etc, it is not yet clear what is going on here.

FOR IMMEDIATE RELEASE

BCG VACCINE AVAILABLE-
POSSIBLE PROPHYLACTIC AGAINST LEUKEMIA

Studies performed by Dr. S. R. Rosenthal, et al, at Cook County Hospital in Chicago show that infants vaccinated with BCG as a prophylaxis against tuberculosis showed significantly lower incidence of leukemia and other childhood cancers than non-vaccinated infants. A study done in Quebec also suggested that BCG might have a prophylactic effect against childhood cancers.

U.S. produced and FDA licensed BCG vaccine is now available in virtually unlimited quantity from Research Foundation, 70 West Hubbard St., Chicago, Ill., 60610, according to a Foundation spokesman.

This announcement was made to put to rest rumors that American BCG was not available or in extremely short supply. Distribution was interrupted by a move of the production laboratory to improved and larger facilities. Unpredictable construction delays caused an unanticipated long-term suspension of production. However, the Bureau of Biologics of the FDA has now licensed both the new establishment and the BCG produced therein.

The Tice strain, also known as the Chicago BCG, is the only FDA licensed BCG vaccine produced in this country.

*   *   *

1976 press release on BCG

20
First Aid: Don't Let Accidents Kill You

You don't have to let your body die
You can come back again if you try
           if you try
           if you try

     —Paul Kantner, Jefferson Airplane,
      "Alexander the Medium"

As aging comes under our control, accidents will become relatively greater threats to our survival. Don't go to a lot of trouble to develop a life extension program and then get killed by choking on your own dinner. In many cases, you can save yourself and other accident victims by using simple first aid techniques and/or the right nutrients and, in some cases, prescription drugs. It is even possible in some cases to restore both life and normal mental function to apparently dead persons. If your heart stops or fibrillates, you may even be able to apply cardiac resuscitation to yourself long enough to get to a hospital or for the paramedics to get to you. Thanks to science, you can perform your own "miracles"!

Although it is important to be prepared for at least the most life-threatening types of accidents, this chapter is not an attempt to provide a comprehensive course in first aid or cardiopulmonary resuscitation. For this, take a Red Cross or paramedic course. But the methods described here can be used in many different situations where bleeding, wounds,

344

burns, and shock play a part. Remember, first aid means just that. It is aid administered before medical care arrives. Do not try to treat a serious problem with just first aid. If in doubt, call for medical assistance. Your taxes and insurance premiums pay for it in most cases.

Vitamin C is very effective in treating shock, a common accompaniment to wounds and serious injuries of all types, even emotional shocks. In shock, blood pressure falls, sometimes catastrophically. That's why the skin becomes pale and clammy. If the victim is conscious, drinking salt water (about 3 teaspoons of salt per quart) can help to maintain blood pressure and is useful in replacing fluids lost in bleeding or from burns. In a series of experiments, weights were dropped onto the legs of anesthetized guinea pigs. When vitamin C was injected shortly after the trauma in concentrations of 100 milligrams of sodium ascorbate per kilogram of body weight, the treated animals would always survive, even when all untreated animals died. (The untreated animals received normal levels of dietary C.) The vitamin C may be administered orally, of course, though it will take a longer time to take effect.

Wound healing promoters include ornithine, L-Dopa, and arginine (amino acids), zinc, and vitamin C. The healing properties of vitamin C have been known for several decades, yet it is rare that surgical patients are given vitamin C before and after operations. You can provide this for yourself. Hospitals do not routinely include C in their intravenous fluids. Ask for it—such IV solutions are commercially made. When scheduled for surgery, state in advance that you want vitamin C in the postoperative intravenous drip solution. Most hospital pharmacies do not stock this solution, so they will have to order it in advance. (See Appendix I, "A Few Suppliers.") People can tolerate large quantities of vitamin C, arginine, and ornithine. At levels of several grams a day, C (as ascorbic acid) requires neutralization, since it is an acid. Since arginine and ornithine are usually sold as the free base, they may provide adequate neutralization if they are taken along with the C. Otherwise, use ordinary antacids, such as calcium carbonate or Maalox® (for people without essential hypertension, baking soda works very well and is preferred). Arginine, ornithine, and L-Dopa stimulate wound healing by causing the pituitary gland to release growth hormone. Arginine and ornithine can also be converted into growth stimulant polyamines.

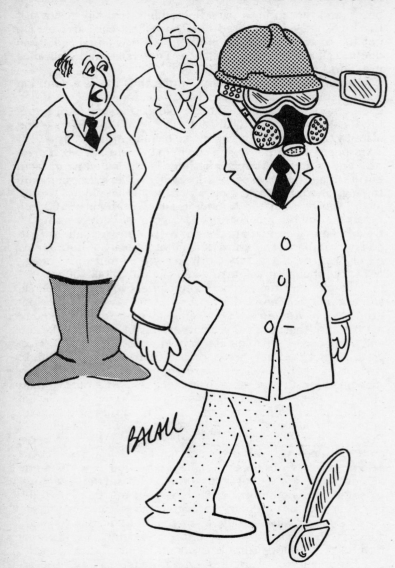

"That's our safety director. He takes safety *very* seriously."

© 1981 Aaron Bacall

Injured tissues release histamines, which can be toxic to other tissues in the excess quantities released during injuries. Antihistamines can be helpful in blocking these histamine effects. Vitamin C is also effective in detoxification of histamine in stress situations.

A good first aid for minor burns is to plunge the burned area into cold water; then add ice. Then coat vitamin E on the burn to hasten healing and reduce scarring. Do not buy bottles of vitamin E oil; unless they contain very potent antioxidants, such as BHT and BHA, the oil is apt to rapidly become badly autoxidized. Instead, use a pin to punch a hole in a fresh, soft gelatin capsule of vitamin E, and squeeze out the entire contents at one time. Use the smallest capsules per unit of vitamin E potency to avoid potentially peroxidized filler oils. Do not buy vitamin E in safflower or other polyunsaturated oils. In serious burns, one of the biggest problems is loss of water and salts from the damaged area. Vitamin B-3 (niacin, nicotinic acid) is a nutrient that can significantly reduce this fluid loss.

A fast and effective treatment for bruises, crushing injuries, pulled or wrenched muscles, and similar injuries is dimethyl sulfoxide (DMSO). DMSO is a powerful scavenger of hydroxyl free radicals, which are responsible for much of the damage which occurs following a crushing injury and which have also been implicated in arthritis. When the damaged blood vessels in the injured area leak blood into the surrounding tissues, the copper and iron contained in the blood stimulate the production of free radicals. Antioxidants such as vitamins A, C, E, B-1, B-5, and B-6 and cysteine, zinc, and selenium can help control these free radicals. But these materials are distributed throughout the body rather than concentrated in the injured area. The DMSO (often as a 50 to 90 percent solution in water) can be applied (externally) to the injury where it can do the most good. The DMSO actually penetrates the skin, acting as a powerful inhibitor of free radical activity. Some of it even spreads into the rest of the body—you may be able to taste the garlic-oyster DMSO taste in your mouth in a couple of minutes. (Extremely pure DMSO has only a slight odor and flavor.) If DMSO is applied quickly enough to an injury (before symptoms appear), it is possible to abolish entirely any bruising (the colors you see in a bruise are due to free radicals chemically attacking certain tissue constituents). DMSO reduces the free radical damage and thereby allows faster healing. DMSO in physiological saline, given by injection, has been used to reduce the paraplegia resulting from crushing spinal cord injuries in experimental animals (cats). This might work as well for people, if administered within an hour or two after injury. The Brain Edema Center of San Francisco General Hospital has recently approved the use of an intravenously administered solution of DMSO as its primary drug treatment, in an experimental brain trauma program. Dr. Harry Demopoulos of New York University is currently attempting to have New York City paramedics experimentally equipped with DMSO for prompt use on brain and spinal cord trauma victims. Note that DMSO does *not* itself cause regeneration of injured tissues, either in spinal cord or elsewhere. (See Part II, Chapter 9, "Decline of the Brain's Chemical Messengers," and Part III, Chapter 2, "Revitalizing Your Brain Power," for possible nervous system regeneration with Hydergine® by Sandoz.) A DMSO solution (50 percent by weight in water) is now available with a prescription. The product, called RIMSO-50, is manufactured by Tera Pharmaceuticals, Inc. in Buena Park, California and distributed by Research Industries Corp., Pharmaceuticals Division, Salt Lake City, Utah. The RIMSO-50 (DMSO) solution is FDA approved for the treatment of interstitial cystitis but has not been FDA approved for any other condition. DMSO works best in conjunction with other antioxidants such as A, C, E, B-1, B-5, B-6, cysteine, zinc, and selenium, since it turns into a free radical (usually a sulfoxide radical) in the process of destroying more dangerous radicals. These DMSO radicals must in turn be destroyed by other free radical scavengers. The rabbit cataracts caused by immense doses of DMSO were probably due to an absence of adequate antioxidant scavengers for the DMSO sulfoxide radicals, which oxidized the sulfur-amino acids in the rabbits' eye lenses and corneas to sulfoxides.

Recently, DMSO, supposedly "for solvent use only," has appeared in many health food stores and hobby shops, typically priced at about $1.00 an ounce. We have mixed feelings about this. We condemn the FDA's track record on DMSO as a travesty of science. We believe that DMSO has plenty of legitimate medical uses and that it should be available for topical use as an OTC (over-the-counter; that is, nonprescription) drug.

But since the material is supposedly sold as a solvent,

there are no accompanying instructions cautioning occasional external use only (when used without a physician's advice) on limited areas of the body, nor are there suggestions of a potentially increased need for nutrient antioxidants.

Worse, this DMSO is often really impure industrial-solvent-grade material; the DMSO will carry these impurities through your skin. *Never* put industrial-solvent-grade DMSO on your skin! If the DMSO has even the slightest tinge of either color or haze, do not use it. Unfortunately, clear DMSO may still be industrial-solvent-grade and may still contain hazardous impurities, some of which (nitrogen oxides and benzene) can be carcinogenic. The following three grades of DMSO are scientifically (but not legally) suitable for human use: ACS reagent grade, spectrophotometric grade, and pesticide quality grade.

The FDA's policies have done little to prevent harmful misuse of DMSO; however, these same policies have made the proper and reasonable use of DMSO far more difficult. The FDA is directly responsible for the presence of solvent-grade DMSO (in a market that would otherwise use high purity material) because it has placed restrictions on the sale of DMSO. These restrictions are relatively easily enforced in the scientific supply house market with its small-scale sales of high-purity DMSO from a rather limited number of vendors. These restrictions are simply impossible to enforce in the high-volume industrial-solvent market. So what do people have to use? Just try to buy a bottle of reagent-grade DMSO from a chemical supply house! Usually, people get an industrial solvent from a hobby shop. We find this to be very disconcerting. Paradoxically, you would be safer if the FDA made no attempt to limit DMSO availability but rather acted in an advisory capacity by performing and publishing peer-reviewed research on potential hazards and, in particular, their underlying fundamental biochemical mechanisms. Take your tax money away from the FDA legal and regulatory bureaucrats, and give it to their scientists instead. Medical safety is better served by test tubes, microscopes, and publishers than by lawbooks, guns, and bureaucrats.

It is wise when traveling to remote areas where medical treatment cannot be obtained to take along some strong painkillers (Talwin® is a good nonnarcotic prescription pain reliever which is effective for many, but not all, people) and antibiotics.

If you are going on such an expedition, ask your doctor for prescriptions for 100 each 250 milligrams tetracycline, 100 each 250,000 unit penicillin, and (if you are willing to pay a high price for a very good antibiotic) some erythromycin. Store them dry and in the refrigerator. If you haven't used these antibiotics before, have your doctor check you for sensitivity with a skin test (some people have fatal allergic reactions to penicillin, for example). Do *not* use antibiotics for random minor illnesses, and do *not* try to treat such illnesses yourself if you can reach a doctor. Many infections are resistant to most antibiotics; hence a clinical laboratory antibiotic sensitivity test (or, at least, a doctor's clinical experience) is required in choosing your antibiotic treatment. *Self treatment with antibiotics is strictly for major emergencies when no physician is available.*

Hydergine® (Sandoz) in doses of 3 to 12 milligrams per day is very effective in preventing brain damage from hypoxia (insufficient oxygen) in emergencies such as drowning, smoke or carbon monoxide poisoning, heart attack or stroke, or severe brain concussion. If you use Hydergine® regularly, you will be much less likely to suffer severe brain damage from these injuries. If you don't regularly use tablets of Hydergine®, it is available in an injectable form for use by physicians in emergencies (3 to 12 milligrams can be injected intravenously or, better yet, directly into the carotid artery in the neck, which leads directly to the brain). It would be very desirable for physicians and paramedics to carry injectible Hydergine® for protecting the brain from hypoxic damage during heart attack, stroke, and accidents, including brain and spine concussion. The basis for this recommendation is available in the references we have provided, particularly the experiment in which EEG energies were measured during severe blood loss. The tragedy of hypoxic brain damage may often be easily and safely preventable. Perhaps someday the FDA will even approve Hydergine® for "reanimation," as the French drug approval authorities have.

People who appear to the uninitiated eye to be dead are often capable of being resuscitated if proper mechanical action is taken quickly to re-establish heart and lung action. Two cases in the United States of such resuscitation illustrate the possibility of recovery from apparent and extended death without obvious brain damage. In one case, a child was hit on the head by a lightning bolt during school recess. A registered nurse at the school detected no pulse or respiration. When the ambulance arrived, one of the medics applied cardiopulmonary resuscitation (CPR) "just for the hell of it." The child revived, even though clinically dead for twenty-six minutes. Although initially exhibiting considerable mental confusion, within about two months, the child was perfectly normal. An IQ test administered at that time showed no significant change from a test given about three months before the accident. A second case involved a period of death of about forty-five minutes. A child fell through the ice into a frozen river and was carried under the ice by the current. Rescue personnel recovered the body forty-five minutes later. In addition to CPR, bicarbonate and corticosteroids (membrane-stabilizing antioxidants) were repeatedly administered to assist in re-establishing brain circulation. (Loss of circulation in the brain rapidly leads to damage-caused swelling, which restricts circulation even further, leading to further hypoxic damage and more swelling.) The child recovered and after an initial period of confusion of a few weeks became fully normal. In this case, the cold temperature helped prevent damage in the brain by inhibiting free radical reactions (see Part II, Chapter 7, on free radicals). See the chapter notes on "First Aid" in Appendix K for references on the prompt use of injectable antioxidants in cases of severe spinal cord and brain trauma. In some cases, they can make the difference between lifelong paralysis and complete recovery.

Over 50,000 people a year are killed in automobile accidents and many tens of thousands more in home accidents. Many of these accidents involve fatal bleeding. Paramedics cannot now carry blood to aid these accident victims because blood, even serum (all cellular particles, including red and white blood cells, are removed from serum), requires constant refrigeration. In addition, both blood and serum may carry infectious hepatitis virus, and whole blood must be immunologically matched to the recipient, using tests, or the white cells and antibodies in the new blood may attack the already weakened accident victim. New synthetic bloods, made from fluorocarbons, have been used with great success in Japan for emergency replacement of lost natural blood, even when up to 80 percent of the person's blood was replaced by the synthetic. These fluorocarbons carry much more oxygen (dissolved in the liquid) than natural blood, so much so that animals such as rats and dogs have continued to live while submerged in tanks of these fluorocarbons for hours. They just "breathed" the liquid fluorocarbon in and out. Patients receiving the fluorocarbon blood also avoid the risk of hepatitis that can be contracted from natural blood transfusions. Moreover, fluorocarbon emulsion replacement blood is immunologically inert, so that the potentially lethal delay for blood typing can be eliminated. It might be possible to treat emergency cases of carbon monoxide poisoning by replacing part of the victim's blood with fluorocarbons (carbon monoxide doesn't have any effect on the oxygen-carrying ability of the synthetic blood). These synthetic bloods are not yet approved by the FDA for use in the United States.

Closed-chest cardiopulmonary resuscitation, CPR, can keep a person's brain and body alive for several *hours* after the heart has stopped beating and/or he has stopped breathing, provided it is started soon enough. People have been revived without brain damage after more than six hours of prompt, manually applied CPR, during which they had no natural heartbeat or respiration. No equipment is required. Anyone who lives with someone having a serious heart condition should learn this simple technique. Your local Red Cross or paramedic group will be glad to teach you how to do it. You can bring a loved one back from the dead with your breath and your bare hands—if you know how.

Researchers have recently examined CPR to determine its major mechanism of action. Prior to this work, the most accepted assumption was that pressure applied to the chest actually squeezed the heart to cause it to pump blood. Evidence now suggests that the major CPR mechanism is higher pressure within the thorax (chest), which forces blood from inside the chest to the rest of the body. J. Michael Criley of UCLA has found that a patient whose heart stops can keep his blood circulating by simply coughing strongly (about once every two seconds), which greatly increases the intrathoracic pressure. Each cough delivers over twice as much blood to the brain as a simple CPR chest compression. After the heart stops, you have only about fifteen seconds to act before you black out; thus, self-applied coughing CPR must be begun promptly in order to maintain consciousness and the ability to continue coughing. One of Dr. Criley's patients, a doctor, was able to keep himself alive after his heart went into fibrillation by coughing all the way to the hospital!

CPR
IN BASIC LIFE SUPPORT

Place victim flat on his back on a hard surface.
If unconscious, open airway.

Neck lift, head tilt **or** Chin lift, head tilt

1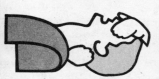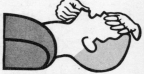

2 **If not breathing, begin artificial breathing.**

4 quick full breaths.
If airway is blocked,
try back blows, abdominal or
chest thrusts and finger probe
until airway is open.

3 **Check carotid pulse.**

4  **If pulse absent, begin artificial circulation.** Depress sternum 1½" to 2".

One Rescuer	Two Rescuers
15 compressions	5 compressions
rate 80 per min.	rate 60 per min.
2 quick breaths	1 breath

CONTINUE UNINTERRUPTED UNTIL
ADVANCED LIFE SUPPORT IS AVAILABLE

AMERICAN HEART ASSOCIATION
7320 GREENVILLE AVENUE, DALLAS, TEXAS 75231

77-006-A Rev
77-100-M
6-78-75M
© 1977 American Heart
Association

It has recently been found that, after a crushing injury to the spinal cord of pentobarbital-anesthetized adult cats, the natural opiates (endorphins) released by the brain cause a drop in blood pressure. This drop in blood pressure results in a reduced quantity of oxygen available to the tissues. In the injured area of the spinal cord, this hypoxia (deficiency of oxygen) stimulates free radical activity that, we believe, leads to the severe neurological damage resulting in partial paralysis of the limbs. Cats which were given injections of the opiate antagonist naloxone (which blocks endorphin receptors), however, developed much less neurological damage and recovered more quickly. The naloxone prevented the endorphin-mediated drop in blood pressure. These results suggest that naloxone would be a useful addition to a paramedic's emergency medical kit, especially in cases of neurological injury and sharp drops in blood pressure resulting from shock. Dr.- Harry Demopoulos of New York University and his co-workers have done experiments with naloxone and spinal cord injuries in cats. He tells us that naloxone is an antioxidant and therefore a free radical scavenger. He says naloxone should be administered within one to two hours after injury for best results.

Accidental choking, particularly on food, is a rather frequent cause of death. The chart that follows shows how to rapidly dislodge an object caught in a person's throat.

Accidental poisonings are a common cause of death, particularly among children. Every home medicine cabinet should contain a bottle of activated charcoal, a nearly universal antidote. This material, available in drugstores, can be used even when the identity of the poison is unknown, since activated charcoal is quite general in its absorption powers. Even the enterotoxins of food poisoning are soaked up by this material, so be sure to take some along when traveling to lands where sanitation is primitive. Barbiturate overdoses, too, can be counteracted by activated charcoal, provided the victim is still conscious enough to safely swallow it. First, *call the paramedics*, then if the victim is conscious, give him or her two tablespoons of activated charcoal stirred into a glass of water.

Activated charcoal is for use in acute poisonings, not for everyday use to absorb environmental toxins, because it will absorb the vitamins in your gut too.

First Aid for the Choking Victim
The Heimlich Maneuver*

with the VICTIM STANDING or SITTING

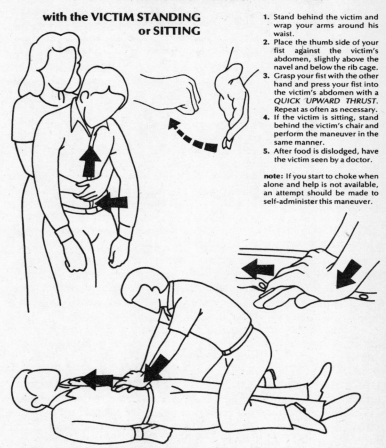

1. Stand behind the victim and wrap your arms around his waist.
2. Place the thumb side of your fist against the victim's abdomen, slightly above the navel and below the rib cage.
3. Grasp your fist with the other hand and press your fist into the victim's abdomen with a *QUICK UPWARD THRUST.* Repeat as often as necessary.
4. If the victim is sitting, stand behind the victim's chair and perform the maneuver in the same manner.
5. After food is dislodged, have the victim seen by a doctor.

note: If you start to choke when alone and help is not available, an attempt should be made to self-administer this maneuver.

when the VICTIM HAS COLLAPSED and CANNOT BE LIFTED

1. Lay the victim on his back.
2. Face the victim and kneel astride his hips.
3. With one hand on top of the other, place the heel of your bottom hand on the abdomen slightly above the navel and below the rib cage.
4. Press into the victim's abdomen with a

QUICK UPWARD THRUST. Repeat as often as necessary.
5. Should the victim vomit, quickly place him on his side and wipe out his mouth to prevent aspiration (drawing of vomit into the throat).
6. After the food is dislodged, have the victim seen by a doctor.

This is an adaptation of a poster prepared by the New York City Department of Health for display in restaurants.
*Patent pending

21
Getting Your Child's Immune System Off to a Good Start

When health is absent, wisdom cannot reveal itself, art cannot become manifest, strength cannot fight, wealth becomes useless, and intelligence cannot be applied.

—Herophilus, physician to Alexander the Great

CAUTION: This is the *only* chapter in this book which provides health advice for children.

Your child's immune system has evolved so that exposure to bacteria and viruses are necessary for learning and self-programming. That's why vaccinations for common diseases are so important. For example, polio in early infancy is usually no worse than a bad cold. Adult or childhood polio is much more serious, with paralysis a likely complication, but polio vaccination prepares your child to resist the disease as an adult. Don't just educate your child's mind. Educate his or her immune system, too!

Modern medicine has practically eliminated certain diseases which were once great killers, including smallpox, polio, and plague. However, in doing so, the pattern of development of immune responses to these diseases in children has been altered from that of even a few score years ago. It is important to understand how immune responses develop and to ascertain that your child will not be unnecessarily susceptible to infectious diseases by failing to develop immunity.

For example, consider polio. Before modern sanitation practices were used widely, polio virus-containing sewage filled the streets and rivers and most children got mild cases of polio while still very young. The symptoms were usually like those of a bad cold. Development of paralysis was rare under those conditions, and afterward the child had a lifelong immunity to polio. Nowadays, however, children rarely are exposed to polio. In the absence of vaccination, their immune system's B-cells (which make antibodies) do not make polio antibodies. Later, an older child or adult who does not have immunity to polio can develop a serious case, including possible paralysis and death. Though polio is uncommon, the more children that fail to acquire immunity by vaccination, the more cases of polio with serious consequences may develop. It is very prudent indeed to see that your children are vaccinated against polio.

Your child can develop immunity by simple vaccination to several other diseases that can be serious in non-immune older children or adults: diphtheria, pertussis (whooping cough), tetanus, measles, rubella, and mumps. In order for the immune system to develop the optimal amount of immunity, the vaccinations should be provided on a particular time schedule. Below is the schedule recommended by the U.S. Department of Health and Human Services (HHS), formerly the U.S. Department of Health, Education, and Welfare (HEW). HHS offers a useful booklet about childhood vaccinations *(Parents' Guide to Childhood Immunization)*, which is available free of charge.

Although smallpox is apparently nonexistent throughout the world today (except in some research laboratory freezers), vaccination against it still may be a wise practice. Smallpox vaccinations (which have a small risk of harmful effects) stimulate the immune system in a general way and can, therefore, improve immunity to other diseases as well. In a few cases, smallpox vaccinations have even resulted in tumor regressions in adults due to this immune system activation.

You might want to consider a BCG vaccination for immunity to tuberculosis. This type of vaccination is used widely in Canada and some other countries but is not generally available in the United States except in cases of exposure to TB and in experimental cancer immunotherapy, where BCG has sometimes been effective in stimulating the patient's immune response against the cancer. In Canada, where nearly all schoolchildren in certain provinces receive BCG vaccinations, very interesting benefits have appeared. The rate of leukemia was halved among about 400,000 Canadian children receiving one BCG vaccination for tuberculosis immunity. Whether this was fortuitous and just a matter of clustering and timing of random events will be determined by the passage of time and additional research, but the sample size reported here is quite large. This result had not been anticipated but seems to demonstrate a powerful immune-system stimulating effect of BCG. Two or three BCG superficial skin inoculations at least a few months apart seem to provide even more protection against leukemia. The side effects that sometimes occur when BCG is used in cancer therapy do not generally occur in these vaccinations, which involve smaller quantities and superficial skin inoculations rather than large, deep injections. If you do decide to have your child BCG vaccinated, choose an area of skin where a scar would not be objectionable, since unsightly local scarring can occur on the first inoculation and is almost certain if subsequent inoculations are given.

Be sure to ask your doctor for his or her recommendations concerning additional vaccinations. Your immune system and that of your child requires adequate stimulation to function well, and the routine immunizations rate a medical "best buy" recommendation. **WARNING:** Remember that your child's immune system requires plenty of vitamin C and other nutrients, too. Ask your physician to recommend a high potency children's vitamin supplement. Immunization of sick or vitamin-deficient infants can result in SIDS—sudden infant death syndrome. See chapter notes for further data.

Notes:

Measles, rubella and mumps vaccines can be given in a combined form, at about 15 months of age, with a single injection.

Children should receive a sixth tetanus-diphtheria injection (booster) at age 14-16 years.

Your doctor may recommend schedules that differ somewhat from those that appear here. Generally, though, the first schedule, below, shows the immunizations that children one through five will get on their first visit to the doctor and on each visit thereafter. The second schedule is recommended for children six years of age and older.

IF YOUR CHILD IS TWO MONTHS OLD . . .

Age	Diphtheria Pertussis Tetanus	Polio	Measles	Rubella	Mumps
2 mos.	*	*			
4 mos.	*	*			
6 mos.	*	* (optional)			
15 mos.			*	*	*
18 mos.	*	*			
4–6 yrs.	*	*			

IF YOUR CHILD IS ONE THROUGH FIVE YEARS OF AGE . . .

First Visit	Diphtheria, Pertussis, Tetanus (DPT) Polio
1 mo. after first visit	Measles, Rubella, Mumps*
2 mos. after first visit	Diphtheria, Pertussis, Tetanus (DPT) Polio
4 mos. after first visit	Diphtheria, Pertussis, Tetanus (DPT) Polio (optional)
10-16 mos. after first visit	Diphtheria, Pertussis, Tetanus (DPT) Polio
Age 14-16 years	Tetanus-Diphtheria (Td)— repeat every 10 years

*Not routinely given before 15 months of age.

IF YOUR CHILD IS SIX YEARS OF AGE OR OLDER . . .

First Visit	Tetanus-Diphtheria (Td) Polio
1 mo. after first visit	Measles, Rubella, Mumps
2 mos. after first visit	Tetanus-Diphtheria (Td) Polio
8-14 mos. after first visit	Tetanus-Diphtheria (Td) Polio
Age 14–16 years	Tetanus-Diphtheria (Td)— repeat every 10 years

Immunization Schedules

WARNING: Immunization of a sick or vitamin deficient infant can result in sudden infant death. These immunizations are recommended only for healthy, well-nourished infants and children. Immunizations and natural infections markedly increase the consumption of the antioxidant nutrients, particularly vitamin C. See Kalokerinos, *Every Second Child*, Thomas Nelson (Australia) Limited, 1974; also published in paperback by Keats Publishing, Inc., New Canaan, Connecticut, 1981 (popular media)

PART IV
NUTRITION AND LIFE EXTENSION

1
Who's Afraid of Cholesterol? or, Fats, Facts, and Fantasy

Every creative act involves . . . a new innocence of perception, liberated from the cataract of accepted belief.

—Arthur Koestler, *The Sleepwalkers*

Recent evidence about the role of cholesterol in heart disease has helped to clear up controversy that has raged for years. In several recent studies in humans, the amount of dietary cholesterol has not determined serum cholesterol in most people. This is because many individuals make 1 1/2 grams or so a day of cholesterol when they don't eat any cholesterol in their diet. When people eat cholesterol, the body tends to make less cholesterol via a feedback mechanism. Reducing dietary cholesterol alone may be of little value in reducing serum cholesterol for many people. Substituting polyunsaturated fats for saturated fats, a strategy for lowering serum cholesterol previously recommended by the American Heart Association for many years and still recommended by many doctors, is a potentially dangerous practice. While this can lower serum cholesterol slightly, the heart attack risk is not necessarily lowered, and risk of cancer may increase because these polyunsaturates turn rancid (peroxidize) more easily and increase the body's requirements for antioxidant nutrients. A newly developed way to measure atherosclerotic risk of heart disease is the ratio of two types of fatty proteins in the blood, HDL to LDL. Understanding how cholesterol is used in the body will help you understand the confusing claims made about dietary and serum cholesterol.

363

Even more controversial than the effects of artificial sweeteners, the role of dietary cholesterol in the origins and development of heart disease has long been debated. At one time, it was widely belived that serum cholesterol could be reduced by simply cutting out dietary cholesterol. In several recent studies, however, the serum cholesterol level was shown to be poorly correlated with dietary intake of cholesterol. For example, in a 1978 study, Dr. Slater and Dr. Alfin-Slater found that in their subjects the serum (blood with the cells and large particles removed) cholesterol level did not reflect cholesterol consumption within the range of intake from 200 to 900 milligrams a day, which comprises the amounts in most diets. This result is due to the fact that many people manufacture about 1 1/2 grams of cholesterol per day if the food they eat contains no dietary cholesterol at all. Thus, reducing dietary intake of cholesterol may stimulate the body, via feedback mechanisms, to produce a greater supply of cholesterol. Low-cholesterol diets may, therefore, be of limited value in these individuals in reducing serum cholesterol. However, the reduction in total calories that may occur in a low-cholesterol diet can be of value for weight control.

Furthermore, there is little evidence of a direct causative relation between serum cholesterol and heart disease. Although many heart-disease patients do have elevated serum-cholesterol levels, there are others who do not. Some persons with high serum-cholesterol levels do not show any signs of heart disease.

As we discussed in Part III, Chapters 16, 17, and 18, on heart disease, certain fatty protein fractions in the blood have recently been found to be associated with high heart-disease risk. The low-density lipoproteins (LDL) are correlated with increased risk of heart disease because this fraction deposits cholesterol in blood vessels. In addition, the LDL may play a significant role in the genesis of many types of cancer, as these lipoproteins carry in the bloodstream the carcinogenic polynuclear aromatic hydrocarbons (PAH), the tarry combustion products found in auto exhausts, smog, wood, coal, and especially cigarette smoke. These PAH structurally resemble cholesterol, and this is why the LDL carry them.

The high-density lipoproteins (HDL), another blood lipid fraction, are thought to be beneficial in the prevention of heart disease by removing cholesterol from the artery walls. The ratio of these two fractions, HDL to LDL, is a recently

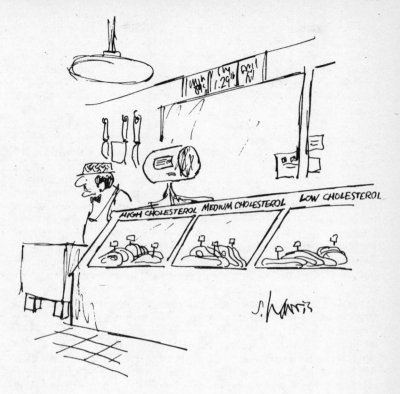

developed measure of heart disease risk, although many medical testing laboratories are not yet equipped to do this test. A high HDL/LDL is considered protective, while a low HDL/LDL is considered an indication of high risk. People with a favorable ratio are fortunate. If the ratio is unfavorable, more attention should be paid to dietary consumption of total fats and calories as well as to intake of antioxidant nutrients.

There are nutrients able to reduce serum lipids significantly, including vitamin C, niacin (vitamin B-3), and lecithin. Niacin can reduce the quantity of very low-density lipoproteins somewhat. A dose of niacin of 3 grams for as little as two weeks reduced serum cholesterol in humans by 26 percent. These results continue as long as the niacin is taken. Five hundred milligrams of vitamin C taken three times a day reduced serum cholesterol in atherosclerotic humans in one study by about 35 to 40 percent by fostering conversion of cholesterol into bile, which is eliminated in the feces. A fair amount of fiber in the diet will then absorb the bile and prevent the reabsorption of the converted cholesterol. Cholesterol removal from the body can be speeded up by sulfation. When Dr. Ralph Mumma fed ascorbic acids to rats, their excretion of cholesterol was doubled. But when he fed them L-ascorbic acid 3-sulfate, a derivative of ascorbic acid, their cholesterol discharge was increased by a factor of 50. We would like to see more research done with this potentially valuable substance.

Cholesterol is subject to peroxidation, resulting in cancer-causing products such as a cholesterol epoxide that has been proved to be a cause of skin cancer. Cholesterol oxidation products are found in high levels in the feces of people with colon and rectal cancer. Thus, a dietary intake of adequate antioxidants is required to prevent excessive formation of these compounds, which are clot promoters, mutagens, carcinogens, and immune-system suppressors. These cholesterol peroxides and epoxides may play a significant role in the formation of atherosclerotic plaques as well, since, as mentioned earlier (in Part III, Chapter 16), these plaques are now known to be a type of tumor. Further, cholesterol oxidation products, like other lipid peroxides, stop the formation of the blood vessels' natural anti-clotting factor, PGI_2 (prostacyclin).

One unfortunate strategy for reducing serum cholesterol which has been widely recommended by the American Heart Association and the American Medical Association is to substitute polyunsaturated fats for saturated fats in the diet. Although this substitution can slightly reduce serum cholesterol, it does not reduce the death rate from heart attacks, and in addition there is an increased incidence of cancer. (In fact, the rising incidence in the first half of this century for most types of cancer may be partially a result of increasing consumption of polyunsaturated fats compared to saturated fats. It is interesting to note that since the start of this century, almost all fat increases in the American diet have been in the amounts consumed of unsaturated vegetable fats, not saturated animal fats.)

Polyunsaturated fats are, as we have previously described, more subject to free-radical oxidative attack than saturated fats and consequently form more of the immune-suppressive, thrombogenic (clot-causing), mutagenic, and carcinogenic peroxidized fats. Again, antioxidant nutrients such as vitamins E, A, C, B-1, B-5, and B-6, the amino acid cysteine, and the minerals selenium and zinc help prevent formation of these carcinogens. The more polyunsaturated fats you eat, the more antioxidants your body requires to remain healthy.

Dr. Harry Demopoulos told us that cholesterol and many other steroidal substances act as antioxidants. These natural antioxidants may be found in such high quantities in some people (its concentration increases with age) because the body is making it in a desperate attempt to stem the tide of abnormal free-radical oxidation. If so, this would explain why, when large doses of other antioxidants are taken (such as A, C, E, B-1, B-5, B-6, and BHT), the cholesterol concentration in the blood decreases. The body would be expected to stop making cholesterol in such large amounts because the other antioxidants are able to provide substantial protection against the undesired abnormal oxidation reactions. Elevated serum cholesterol is an indicator of elevated free radical activity, and it is these free radicals and their oxidation products that cause the cardiovascular damage rather than the nonoxidized cholesterol itself. (See Part III, Chapter 19, for further comments on this subject.)

Our own personal experimental life extension formulas have had a dramatic effect on our cholesterol levels. Sandy's total serum cholesterol is 114 milligrams per deciliter and Durk's total serum cholesterol is 91 milligrams per deciliter. The latter figure is particularly striking since Durk has the genes for hypercholesterolemia (excessively high serum cholesterol). His grandfather, who had this condition, died of a heart attack. His father also has it and has to watch his diet and take anti-cholesterol prescription drugs (but we don't know whether they're doing him any good). At the age of 17, Durk's total serum cholesterol was 185 milligrams per deciliter and his physician told him to either watch his diet carefully or to expect a premature death from cardiovascular disease!

Our extremely low total serum-cholesterol values are not the only serum-lipid effects of the antioxidants and nutrients we take. We also have excellent HDL/LDL ratios. These unusual values were not obtained with the help of a special diet. The two of us together in a week consume: 1 to 2 dozen eggs; about a pound or two of butter; several pounds of beef, poultry, and pork; and 4 to 5 gallons of whole (not low-fat) milk. Such a diet, loaded with dairy products and meat, is enough to make a no-fat or low-fat food faddist cringe, but our ultra-low total serum cholesterol figures indicate that it is possible to eat plenty of tasty meats and dairy products if you take the right nutrients to prevent them from clogging your arteries. *Remember that this approach must still be considered a personal experiment. It cannot be assumed that other people will respond well to a high fat diet as we seem to have so far.* It would be more conservative to have a lower fat diet, but in any case, dietary cholesterol can usually be ignored, polyunsaturated fats should be low and fiber high, and additional nutrient antioxidants should be taken, either in fresh fruit, vitamin and mineral pills, or, best of all, both.

Avoid peroxidized (rancid, autoxidized) fats and oils like the plague! These substances are carcinogenic (cause cancer), atherogenic (cause atherosclerosis), thrombogenic (cause undesirable blood clots), immune suppressive (inhibit your body's security force from destroying cancer cells, atherosclerotic plaques, bacteria, and viruses, and make it more likely to attack you by mistake), cross-linkers (cause hardening of the arteries and loss of tissue elasticity), and are dangerous free radical chain reaction initiators.

Here are some common dietary sources of dangerous peroxidized fats and oils:

• A half-used bottle of polyunsaturated vegetable oil without antioxidant additives is one of the worst offenders. When the oil is fresh, in a full and unopened bottle, the organic peroxide content will be low, but autoxidation starts the moment you open the bottle. Just because the oil doesn't smell rancid doesn't mean that the oil isn't rancid and that it is safe. The peroxide content of vegetable oils has to be about 3 1/2 times as great as for animal fats before a rancid odor is detectable. To avoid peroxides, use a non-polyunsaturated cooking oil which contains potent antioxidants such as BHT, BHA, TBHQ, or propyl gallate, and citric acid. Store the bottle in a cool, dark place, preferably in the refrigerator, although this may cause the oil to solidify. Cooking oils contained in aerosol cans are free from rancidity; we prefer to use them for coating frying pans whenever possible. We also add a teaspoon of BHT to a quart of cooking oil the moment we open it. Note, however, that this addition is ten times the amount of BHT addition permitted by the FDA.

• Leftovers containing fats or oils (including all meats) are likely to become peroxidized (rancid) quite rapidly. Ascorbyl palmitate (fat-soluble vitamin C), a tasteless powder, can be mixed with or used to coat leftovers to help prevent this problem. We often do this and it works well. Sodium ascorbate or ascorbic acid, though less effective, can also be used for this purpose. (See Part IV, Chapter 4.) Prompt refrigeration and tight wrapping to exclude air will help, too. Leftover ground meats are the worst problem.

• Ground meats such as hamburgers, hot dogs, and sausages are particularly subject to peroxidation, for a number of reasons. The grinding process mixes fat and blood, and the red blood cells are broken down and release iron and copper, powerful autoxidation catalysts. Extra fat is often added to ground meats to reduce their cost. The grinding process greatly increases the surface area of the food, promoting autoxidation. We both like hamburgers—but we insist on actually watching the beef being ground from a whole piece of meat from which excess fat has been trimmed. We cook and eat this freshly ground beef within a few hours, and we do not save the leftovers. We also like sausage—but we only buy sausage which contains BHT, BHA, TBHQ, or propyl gallate plus sodium ascorbate, and citric acid.

• Try to minimize the eating of food contaminated with burnt fat. We don't always do so because a char-broiled steak tastes awfully good to us. We don't worry about it too much, though, since we take BHT and other potent anticarcinogens (see Part III, Chapter 19, and Part II, Chapter 7). Your risk can be reduced by carefully trimming off the excess fat before cooking, and keeping the smoke from burning fat away from the meat and out of your lungs. The following lists food preparation methods in terms of carcinogen production from worst to least: meat cooked directly over charcoal, baked or broiled meat, pan-fried meat, microwave-cooked meat, or boiled meat. Carcinogen production is negligible in the last two cooking techniques. Microwave cooking also destroys the least vitamins, whereas boiling causes almost complete loss of water-soluble vitamins. From the standpoint of nutrition, convenience, and safety, microwave cooking is superior.

2
Sugar, Diet, and Longevity

Knowledge once gained casts a faint light beyond its own
immediate boundaries. There is no discovery so limited as
not to illuminate something beyond itself.

— John Tyndall (1820–93)

*From all sides, you hear about the dangers of sugar. You can
hardly eat a doughnut without feeling guilty. Is sugar really
as dangerous as some "nutritionists" claim? Sugar certainly
can be a health hazard when eaten in large quantities, because this can lead to obesity. In addition, to metabolize large
amounts of sugar, the pancreas releases a lot of insulin into
the bloodstream. Excess insulin in the bloodstream is definitely harmful to health. Excess insulin can contribute to
atherosclerosis, hypoglycemia, increased fat synthesis, and
can inhibit the pituitary's release of growth hormone (which
is required for a healthy immune system). You can eat sugar,
but only eat small amounts at any one time and never close
to bedtime.*

We have said little to this point about the influence of
diet on longevity other than the profound effects of antioxidant nutrients and pro-oxidant peroxidized (rancid) fats. Six
sensible rules of eating are:

1. Don't eat too much. Obesity is associated with a markedly shortened life span.

2. Eat the types of foods you like, including some proteins, carbohydrates, fats, and fiber.

370

3. If you like sweets—and you are not overweight or diabetic—eat only small sugar snacks, nibbling throughout the day rather than eating a large sugar snack at one time. Sweets are hard on your teeth, but daily use of a high-potency prescription fluoride mouthwash can almost completely prevent tooth decay, even in sweets nibblers. Moreover, if the high potency prescription sodium fluoride mouthwash also contains calcium phosphate, small dental caries (decay) will actually repair themselves by becoming remineralized.

4. Get your vitamins and minerals in high levels from a bottle, rather than relying on diet. It is difficult to get large amounts of most vitamins in even the best of unsupplemented diets. For example, you are unlikely to be getting as much as 25 I.U. of vitamin E from your diet, even if you are devoted to unprocessed whole-grain foods.

5. Do not eat any significant quantities of polyunsaturated fats which do not contain antioxidant preservatives such as BHT or BHA. If you use even small amounts of oils without such preservatives, it is especially important to take antioxidants as dietary supplements (eg., vitamins E, C, B-1, B-5,B-6, and A, the amino acid cysteine, and the minerals selenium and zinc). Substitute saturated fats for polyunsaturates and, to be extra careful, eat these in moderation.

6. A diet high in fiber and fresh fruits and vegetables (which contain natural antioxidants), relatively low in total fat, and very low in polyunsaturated fat appears to be the safest.

As for our own diet, we eat what we like, which includes meats, lots of whole milk and butter, eggs, plenty of fresh fruits and vegetables, daily high fiber cereal, and even sweets (such as brownies). (We never eat sweet snacks before bed, though, for reasons explained.) We get our high doses of vitamins and minerals from bottles rather than relying on the foods we eat. There is no way that our diets could supply the megadoses of nutrient supplements we take. The rather large amount of total fat (mostly saturated) that we eat must be considered an experiment. The additional antioxidants do not provide complete protection from the free radicals and organic peroxides produced by autoxidizing fats. A more conservative, less experimental diet would involve considerably less fat, though that fat should definitely be mostly saturated.

Much has been written concerning the alleged dangers of sugar. Except for diabetics, however, a single moderate dose of sugar is relatively harmless. Problems can develop when individuals chronically eat large amounts of sugar. When common table sugar (sucrose, a simple sugar) is eaten, insulin is quickly released by the pancreas to metabolize the sucrose. This sugar is quickly used up, but the insulin remains in circulation for hours afterward because it has a much longer half-life (the length of time it takes for the concentration in the blood to drop by half) than the sugar. This insulin can lead to a hypoglycemic rebound because the circulating insulin continues to keep blood sugar down, even though the original sugar meal which caused the insulin to be released has been used up.

Evidence supports the idea that insulin can promote deleterious changes in the cardiovascular system. It is well known that most insulin-using diabetics eventually develop cardiovascular complications such as atherosclerosis. Some scientists now think it is insulin that is primarily responsible for these changes. Insulin can cause lipids to be deposited in arterial walls. It also increases fat storage in adipose (fatty) tissues by stimulating the synthesis of lipids and inhibiting their breakdown.

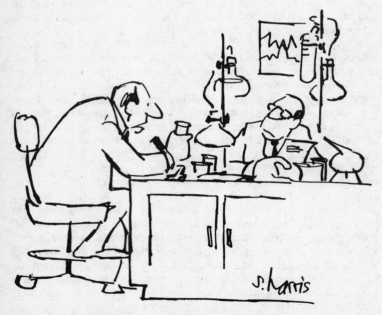

"This sugar substitute is perfect except for one thing. It's salty."

Some sugars that are more complex in structure than sucrose (table sugar) do not cause insulin release and, therefore, do not have the side effects mentioned in the previous paragraph. These noninsulin-requiring sugars include sorbitol, mannitol, inositol (muscle sugar, a B vitamin), and xylitol. Fructose (fruit—but not grape—sugar) releases less insulin over a longer time and consequently causes fewer problems than sucrose (cane or beet sugar) or glucose (grape sugar). There is some evidence, however, that fructose elevates triglycerides more than sucrose does. Honey and brown sugar have the same type of insulin-releasing effect as sucrose and therefore offer no advantages in this respect, although we prefer their taste. Insulin suppresses growth hormone release and may, therefore, impair the immune system's ability to destroy atherosclerotic plaques, bacteria, viruses, and cancer cells. *Since an important amount of growth hormone is released during the first hour and a half of sleep, it is particularly important not to eat table sugar or foods containing large quantities of it within a few hours of bedtime.*

For many cases of adult-onset-type diabetes, the best medicine is control of body weight. If you can keep yourself skinny, you will probably require little or possibly no insulin shots—and you will be in less danger of developing cardiovascular disease and blindness. Part III, Chapter 13, on weight control can help you. You should not try rapid weight reduction by fasting if you are a diabetic, and you should, of course, remain under your doctor's close care. If you are a diabetic, a home computer can help you to adjust your dose of insulin to your exercise and diet. See Steve Faber's article listed in Appendix K.

Cysteine, a sulfur-containing amino acid, can block the effects of insulin by altering its chemical structure (it breaks some S-S cross-link bonds, changing the molecular shape). Cysteine is even more effective when combined with vitamins C and B-1. C, B-1, and cysteine can be quite effective in controlling reactive hypoglycemia. A few grams of this mixture taken orally can reduce a hypoglycemic headache, weakness, nausea, and anxiety by 50 percent in less than twenty minutes. Another way to counteract the effects of insulin is by stimulating the pituitary gland to release growth hormone (See Part II, Chapters 5 and 9, and Part III, Chapters 2, 3, 8, 9, and 14). **CAUTION:** If you have diabetes, however, you should remain under the care of your doctor and *not* experiment by yourself.

What about saccharin and cyclamate? While nothing is completely safe, the risks associated with these artificial sweeteners are less than the risks associated with an amount of sugar required for an equal amount of sweetness. Remember those cancer-scare experiments with artificial sweeteners in rats? If the rats are given 10 percent more calories per day as sugar, their cancer rate increases much more than that caused by the saccharin or cyclamate, even at the immense unrealistic doses used in the scare experiments. While we do not recommend drinking 3,000 cans of artifically sweetened soda pop per day—that is the sort of dose given to the rats— normal use of artificial sweeteners is probably safer than the normal use of sugar. Do we ourselves use artificial sweeteners rather than sugar? No, we use sugar—simply because it tastes better to us than the synthetics, and we are not overweight. If we were overweight, we would substitute the artificial sweeteners to avoid the unneeded calories in sugar wherever possible. We, along with many other scientists, favor an end to FDA restrictions and even bans on saccharin, cyclamate, and Aspartame®. The last is a dipeptide—a string of two amino acids, aspartic acid, and phenylalanine. It is about 160 times sweeter than sugar and lacks the bitter aftertaste many people perceive in saccharin. (The ability to sense this bitter aftertaste is genetically controlled—some people taste this and some don't. If you are an amateur genealogist, check this out on the living members of your family tree, just for fun.)

3
Spices and Other Food Preservatives

You say nothing's right but natural things . . . you fool.
Poison oak is a natural plant—why don't you put some in
    your food?
I don't care if there's chemicals in it, as long as my lettuce
    is crisp!
Preservatives may be preserving you . . . I think that's
    something you missed.

              —Grace Slick, Jefferson Airplane,
              from the song, "Eat Starch, Mom"

Food, like living plants and animals, is subject to aging. We are all familiar with food aging—oils go rancid, bananas become brown, Jell-O® becomes stiff and "weeps," bread becomes hard, leftover beef discolors and develops a stale taste. The aging processes involved in your foods are similar to the aging processes of your own body. Among seekers of improved health, the subject of preservatives is a somewhat controversial topic. But many food preservatives actually retard aging in food by affecting the same processes which take place in our bodies. Food preservatives can help preserve you.

One of the classes of industrial chemicals that has been most subject to attack by self-proclaimed consumer representatives has been food additives, especially preservatives. Many people seem to believe that food preservatives are used to create the impression that bad food is actually good, and that chemicals are used to cover up bad odors and tastes that arise in spoiled, unwholesome food. Actually, modern food preservatives prevent both undesirable and unhealthy chemical degradation and the growth of dangerous microorganisms in foods.

The most interesting class of preservatives, called antioxidants, are chemicals which interfere with, reduce, or prevent undesirable oxidation reactions in foods. These compounds do not kill bacteria or mold. Food containing fats or oils are especially subject to attack by oxidants (such as oxygen, free radicals, and hydrogen peroxide), resulting in the production of mutagenic (mutation-causing) and carcinogenic (cancer-causing) lipid products. Oxygen is eight times more soluble in fats than it is in water, so it is naturally present in fats and oils. Oxygen is a di-radical (it has two unpaired electrons, one on each atom of oxygen) itself and spontaneously oxidizes (autoxidizes, peroxidizes) fats and oils. You have encountered fat and oil oxidation under another name: rancidity. Antioxidant food additives prevent the creation of the rancid (peroxidized) fat poisons in food by chemically blocking the oxidation. It is no trick or illusion that fats and oils that would normally become rancid do not do so for a much longer time when preserved with antioxidants. The food fats and oils containing such antioxidant preservatives as BHT, BHA, propyl gallate, or TBHQ are far safer than unprotected fats and oils.

Since the late 1940s, food producers have been adding one or more of these and other powerful, reasonably nontoxic antioxidants (*much* less toxic than the fat and oil peroxides they prevent from forming). The FDA permits the addition of these antioxidants—singly or in combinations—in food at a maximum concentration of 0.02 percent of the weight of fat or oil contained in the food. In animal or poultry fat, the Animal and Plant Health Inspection Service and U.S. Department of Agriculture regulate the use of BHA, BHT, and propyl gallate, permitting up to 0.01 percent by weight of any single antioxidant, either alone or in combinations totaling up to 0.02 percent. The markedly decreased incidence of stomach cancer in the United States since World War II may be attributable to the addition of such antioxidants as BHT to the food supply and possibly also due to the increased availability of antioxidants in fresh fruits and vegetables made available by our excellent refrigerated distribution system for foods. In countries like Japan, where antioxidants have not been used to any appreciable extent, stomach cancer continues to increase in incidence. In our personal experimental life extension formula, the BHT supplements each of us has taken daily for years amounts to a *thousand* times as much as average Americans get in their diets, and there have been no detectable toxic effects.

Spices have been used for many hundreds or even thousands of years for food preservation. In fact, many spices are antioxidants, preserving food by the same mechanisms as synthetics like BHT and BHA. Examples of effective antioxidant spices are cloves, oregano, sage, rosemary, and vanilla (data from *Autoxidation and Antioxidants*, Vol II, ed. Lundberg, Interscience Publication, New York). So effective are these antioxidant spices that in 1937 and 1938 a patent was granted for a mixture made up of fractions from celery, sage, and cloves. The biblical gifts of frankincense and myrrh are both antioxidants and were used as preservatives thousands of years ago. Extracts of rosemary have been compared in lard with other antioxidants and were found to be more active than BHT and BHA. Because spices and herbs are often antioxidants, they are vulnerable to degradation by exposure to air, light, and heat. We preserve our spices and herbs by storing them in small glass bottles with tight-sealing caps. In these bottles, we place a small piece of cheesecloth wrapped and secured around a teaspoonful of BHT. This system works very well in preserving the potency of the bottles' contents, since the BHT vaporizes and these vapors permeate the contents of the bottle. Herbs that would noticeably lose potency and aroma in a few months are not adversely affected by a year's storage using this technique. Many cereals and convenience foods, in fact, are protected in this manner, with BHT or BHA added to the packaging materials.

When uncured cooked meats are stored for even a short period of time, they often develop an objectionable stale, rancid taste called warmed-over flavor. This warmed-over flavor is caused by exposure of oxygen-sensitive constituents in the meats, particularly the lipids (fats), to air. The peroxidized lipids formed in this manner not only taste bad but are known to be toxic to animals—they are mutagenic (mutation causing) and carcinogenic (cancer causing), immune suppressant, and clot promoting. This problem can be substantially reduced by adding antioxidants such as vitamin E, BHT, sodium ascorbate, vegetable protein, ascorbyl palmitate, or antioxidant spices (as just mentioned), or by smoking the meat (smoke flavoring contains phenolic—that is, BHT-like antioxidants). Commercial U.S. liquid smoke flavors do not contain significant amounts of carcinogenic combustion products. Or food leftovers may be sealed in packaging which excludes oxygen (tightly sealed Zip-Loc® bags with excess air squeezed out, for example). For long-term storage, glass is impermeable to oxygen, unlike plastic.

Almost every organism on earth, including all air-breathing or oxygen-tolerant animals, plants, and microbes, contains antioxidants in its tissues. Some oxidation reactions are necessary for the organism's energy production, but other oxidation reactions are undesirable, causing damage to the organism. Thus, living organisms require protective enzymes and antioxidants to control these oxidation reactions. Once the animal or plant has died, however, it no longer eats or chemically synthesizes the necessary antioxidants and its tissues are rapidly oxidized. Modern food processing can slow this degradation by the addition of antioxidants to our food.

When the two of us shop for foods containing fats or oils, we always try to buy brands which contain antioxidant food preservatives. When we can't find such a brand (usually because the manufacturers have removed antioxidants in response to fears of consumers), we add our own antioxidants, usually BHT and/or ascorbyl palmitate. (For more about this, see Part IV, Chapter 4, "Life Extension Experiments in Your Home.")

Antioxidants play a role of major importance in preventing the random damage of aging that results largely from oxidants. Some antioxidants have been found to extend the life span of experimental animals (see Part II, Chapter 7, on the free radical theory of aging).

The stability of fats and oils, with or without added antioxidants, is generally determined by the Active Oxygen Method (AOM). In this test, the fat or oil is held at 210 degrees F and exposed to a constant flow of oxygen (in air). The peroxides that are formed are measured as the number of hours of exposure it takes to reach the average peroxide value (a quantitative measure of organic peroxide content) at which rancid odors can just be detected by the nose. This peroxide value is about 20 units for animal fats and about 70 units for vegetable oils. Note that the rancidity of vegetable oils is more difficult to smell than that of animal fats, but this does not mean that it is less hazardous. In fact, vegetable oils are more dangerous than animal fats because they become hazardously peroxidized (rancid) long before the odor is perceptible. If you use mayonnaise or salad dressings or other foods containing vegetable oil and you do not plan to add antioxidants to them, you should purchase the smallest size container of such products, keep them refrigerated, and throw them out frequently, even if partly unused. If you don't like going to all this trouble, write the manufacturers and ask them to add antioxidants, or add antioxidants (such as ascorbyl palmitate, which is tasteless) yourself.

Lard is commonly used in cooking and is an animal fat more like human fat than other edible oils and fats. Eastman Chemical Products, a marketer of antioxidants, has done stability tests with lard, with and without added antioxidants. Of course, these tests were done for the purpose of finding antioxidant combinations that extend the life of foods, not the life span of experimental animals or people. The test findings are shown in Charts A and B below.

Chart A

Effectiveness of Antioxidants in Lard

Antioxidant Treatment of Lard Wt %		AOM Stability, as hours to develop peroxide value of 20 meq	Oven Storage Life, as days to develop rancid odor at 145°F (62.8°C)
Untreated (Control)		4	6
Tenox TBHQ	0.005	4	16
	0.010	38	45
	0.020	55	64
Tenox BHA	0.005	27	17
	0.010	36	18
	0.020	42	21
BHT	0.005	12	9
	0.010	18	19
	0.020	33	20
Tenox PG	0.005	12	8
	0.010	20	10
	0.020	42	18
Tenox TBHQ + Tenox BHA	0.010 0.010	59	81
Tenox TBHQ + BHT	0.010 0.010	42	60

PG = propyl gallate
TBHQ = mono-tertiary-butylhydroquinone
Tenox[R] is a registered trademark of Eastman Chemical Products, Inc.

Chart B

Increased Shelf Life of Potato Chips Prepared in Cooking Oil Containing Tenox Antioxidants

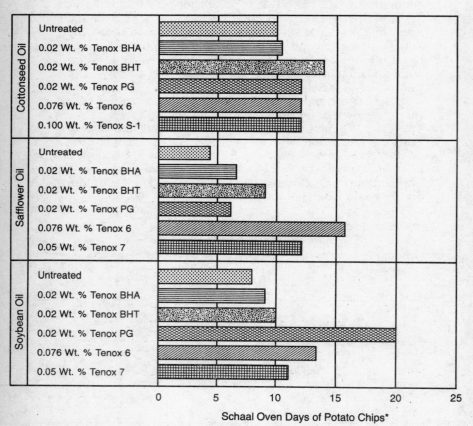

Schaal Oven Days of Potato Chips*

Tenox * BHT and BHA are food-grade BHT and BHA
Tenox® S-1 is 20% propyl gallate (PG), 10% citric acid, and 70% propylene glycol
Tenox® 6 is 10% BHA, 10% BHT, 6% propyl gallate, 6% citric acid, 28% corn oil,
    28% glyceryl mono-oleate, and 12% propylene glycol
Tenox® 7 is 28% BHA, 12% propyl gallate, 6% citric acid, 20% glyceryl mono-
    oleate, and 34% propylene glycol

*The Schaal Oven Test can be briefly described as an accelerated aging test
wherein fats, oils, and food products are subjected to a constant temperature of
145°F (62.8°C) until the first evidence of rancidity can be detected. (Request
Eastman Food Laboratory Standard Procedure No. 20)

Tenox^R is a registered trademark of Eastman Chemical Products, Inc.

Chart C

Oxidation of Soybean Oil, 45 C

Antioxidant[a]	Days to reach 70 meq/kg PV
None	7
0.01% AP	16
0.02% AP	19
0.05% AP	21
0.2% AP	25
0.02% BHA	9
0.02% BHT	10
0.02% TDPA	15
0.01% PG	20
0.02% PG	20
0.02% NDGA	21
0.02% TBHQ	26
0.02% Ascorbic acid	12
0.2% Ascorbic acid	17
0.01% AP + 0.01% PG	27
0.01% AP + 0.01% TDPA	21
0.01% AP + 0.01% BHA	18
0.01% AP + 0.01% BHT	17
0.01% AP + 0.01% NDGA	28
0.01% AP + 0.01% Tocopherol	16
AP at 0.05%, PG, TDPA at 0.01%	42
AP at 0.05%, BHA, TDPA at 0.01%	30
AP at 0.05%, BHA, PG at 0.01%	31
AP at 0.05%, BHT, TDPA at 0.01%	31

[a]AP = ascorbyl palmitate, BHA = butylated hydroxyanisole, BGT = butylated hydroxytoluene, TDPA = thiodipropionic acid PG = propyl gallate, NDGA = nordihydroguaiaretic acid, TBHQ = 2-tertiary butylhydroquinone, PV = peroxide value.

The more polyunsaturated the oil, the more susceptible it is to oxidation. Chart B, reflecting other tests by the same company, shows three vegetable oils treated with antioxidants and the length of time in days it takes for rancidity (detected by the nose) to develop. Note that each oil has its own individual response to the added antioxidants, some oils being much better protected than others.

Some antioxidants, when used together, exhibit a property called positive synergy, which means that the combination is a more powerful antioxidant than the sum of the individual effects of the antioxidants in the mixture. Ascorbyl palmitate (lipid-soluble vitamin C) and thiodipropionic acid, two substances in our personal experimental life extension formula (see Part V, Chapter 7) are powerful antioxidant synergists. Soybean oil kept at 45 degrees C (113 degrees F) takes seven days to reach a particular level of rancidity with no added antioxidant. Chart C shows the results of a third group of tests with various antioxidants in combination.

When you cook with food containing fats and oils, it is wise to include antioxidants if you plan to store any leftovers. For example, you can add vitamin C (a bit sour) or preferably ascorbyl palmitate (better because it is fat soluble and has practically no taste) to the coating mix you use in frying or baking chicken for retaining a fresh taste and wholesomeness longer. Vitamin C added to fruit pies and gelatins with fruits keeps fruits from browning, an oxidative reaction. Weeping of leftover Jell-O® is due to cross-linking and can be prevented with a teaspoon of vitamin C powder. Antioxidants in the gravy in which beef is cooked can help prevent the development of warmed-over flavor (rancidity) in leftovers. The addition of BHT to cooking oils and salad dressings can greatly extend the time it takes for them to develop dangerous and unpleasant rancidity.

Ground hamburger is a particularly rich source of free radicals because it contains a high percentage of fat which, since it is ground, has a large surface area exposed to the air and easily oxidized. In addition, the copper and iron contained in the red blood cells and meat are mixed into the fat by the grinding process, thus exposing the fats to these powerful free radical catalysts. If you enjoy hamburger (as we do occasionally), you should buy fresh lean beef and have your grocer grind it up freshly while you watch. The ground hamburger should be eaten immediately. If stored overnight, it is best to sprinkle the meat with ascorbyl palmitate, knead it to mix it in, and seal it in a Zip-Loc® bag. Usually we do not keep ground meat leftovers.

It is interesting to note that not all cross-linking is undesirable, either in foods or in the human body. The right amount of enzymatically controlled cross-linking provides shape and rigidity to enzymes and structural proteins like collagen. If hair proteins were not cross-linked, hair would dissolve in water! Every time you cook an egg, you are cross-linking proteins. Every time you toast a piece of bread, you are cross-linking carbohydrates. While uncontrolled cross-linking in the body is undesirable, enzymatically controlled cross-linking in the body and the processing of specific foods by cross-linking are highly desirable.

Other preservatives inhibit the growth of dangerous molds and bacteria. Common examples include: propionic acid, calcium propionate, benzoic acid, sodium benzoate, sorbic acid, potassium sorbate, methylparabens, propylparabens,

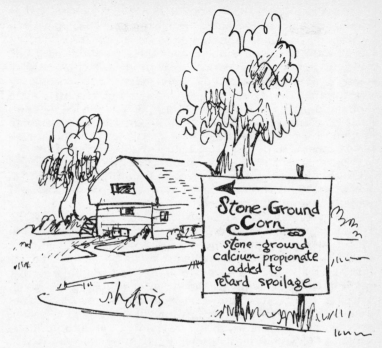

Stone·Ground Corn

stone-ground calcium propionate added to retard spoilage

J. Harris

sodium nitrate, and sodium nitrite. The consequences of foods (other than canned) stored without these additives goes beyond the immediate hazard of food poisoning. Some of the microorganisms that live and grow in food produce carcinogenic toxins which can gradually give you cancer without ever upsetting your digestion. Most important among these is the common mold *Aspergillis flavis,* which produces the powerful carcinogen aflatoxin. Peanuts and corn products are currently the most important aflatoxin sources in the American diet, but other grains and nuts are frequently contaminated by this ubiquitous and dangerous mold. In some parts of the warm humid tropics, aflatoxin-caused cancer is the number-one cause of death. Bacon made without nitrite and nitrate is extremely susceptible to aflatoxin formation as well as to the growth of botulism organisms, which make the most powerful poison known. Only 1,000 molecules of this poison can kill a mouse. Or, to put it another way, one ounce of these toxins would be sufficient to kill everybody on earth. Botulism toxin, not plutonium, is the most poisonous substance known—and it can appear overnight in your own kitchen in improperly stored or unprotected foods.

Because of public concern over these food preservatives, some bacon has been experimentally produced without them. Analysis of this bacon made without nitrite or nitrate additives often showed very dangerous levels of aflatoxin, even though no mold was visible and there was no tattle-tale odor. Rats fed aflatoxin in a daily amount equivalent to a human portion of 4 ounces of the unprotected bacon rapidly developed cancer—70 percent had cancer within two months.

Nitrates and nitrites do react with amines from amino acids (the building blocks of protein) to form carcinogenic nitrosamines. This reaction can be blocked by the presence of enough vitamin C. About two to three times more C is needed in these foods than the maximum now permitted by the FDA. That's right—it's a crime to put too much vitamin C in bacon, even if it reduces the incidence of cancer! Since most of your body's nitrate and nitrite are made by bacteria in your gut, taking all nitrate and nitrite out of food wouldn't do that much good. It certainly would do a lot of long-term harm, however. It is good to know that vitamin C can block carcinogenic nitrosamine formation in your gut as easily as in bacon. Fortunately for all of us, the FDA is not yet able to limit the amount of C we put into our own guts.

Proteolytic enzymes—enzymes that dissolve proteins—increase the turnover rate for proteins in your body by stimulating protein synthesis and repair. As discussed in Part II, Chapter 6, examples of common proteolytic enzymes are bromelain in raw pineapple and papain in raw papaya. Since these enzymes are inactivated by heat, they are not present in canned pineapple or papaya. The enzymes can be used to slowly dissolve away old wrinkled or scarred skin, so that new youthful nonscarred skin can be made to replace it. Several proteolytic enzymes are also immune-system stimulants (see Part II, Chapter 5) that increase your ability to resist diseases, including cancer. You can demonstrate the ability of bromelain or papain to dissolve proteins by adding some raw pineapple or papaya to your next Jell-O® dessert. The dessert won't be able to gell, because the proteins that give it its structure are broken down by the enzymes in the same way that meat tenderizer, which contains proteolytic enzymes, breaks down and tenderizes meat.

4
Life Extension Experiments in Your Home

There is no end to our searchings. . . .
No generous mind stops within itself. Its pursuits are
without limit; its food is wonder, the chase, ambiguity.

—Montaigne (1533–1592)

The ability of words to convey ideas is limited. Even when we think we understand concepts we've read about, a simple demonstration or hands-on experience may convey a surprising amount of additional understanding, clarity, and conviction. In this chapter, we suggest a few simple life extension experiments you can do in your own home.

THE SKIN PINCH TEST

Skin aging is the most readily observable sign of increasing age. Elasticity decreases and wrinkling appears, primarily due to cross-linking damage (inappropriate bond formation between protein molecules, especially between adjacent sulfur atoms—see Part II, Chapter 6, on cross-linking). Examples of agents which promote cross-linking are the ultraviolet rays in sunlight (a major cause of skin aging) and aldehydes (chemicals found in cigarette smoke and smog, created in the liver during alcohol metabolism, and produced by the breakdown of peroxidized fats).

You can test your skin's elasticity by performing the skin pinch test (see photos in Part II, Chapter 6):

1. Place your hand palm down on a hard, flat surface, spreading your fingers wide.

2. Take a fold of skin on the back of the hand (not the loose skin over the knuckles) and pull it up taut, holding it for five seconds. Release the fold and observe how long it takes for the skin to return to its original position. Young skin literally snaps back. Old skin may take a minute or more to return to normal. Compare your skin to that of friends and relatives of younger or older ages. People do not age at the same rate, so you may find these comparisons interesting. You will find it particularly educational to compare the skin elasticity of heavy smokers and drinkers to their more moderate or abstaining chronological (but not physiological) age mates.

COOKING OIL SHELF LIFE TEST

Cooking oils, like fats in the body, form peroxidized compounds when attacked by oxidants, such as oxygen in the air. Eating peroxidized (rancid) fats and oils is a serious health hazard because these materials are powerful mutagens and carcinogens, promote blood clots, and also inhibit certain white blood cells (macrophages) which are involved in defense against disease organisms and cancer cells. Peroxidized fats and oils directly adversely affect the intestinal tract and are also absorbed as the peroxides into the circulation and other tissues.

Even when cooking oils still smell fresh (just before your nose can detect rancidity, the smell given off by peroxidized oils), there can still be a hazardous amount of rancid oil present. Antioxidants added to oils in adequate quantities are able to prevent oxidative attack—it takes much longer to become rancid. In a similar way, taking antioxidant nutrients helps protect the body's fats (which include important cell membranes) against oxidation. FDA-approved addition levels for each of the powerful antioxidants such as BHT is 0.01 percent by weight of the total amount of oil or fat present, or 0.02 percent for a combination of two or more. You can do an experiment that demonstrates the protective ability of antioxidants in your cooking oils:

1. Pour a small amount of cooking oil, say ½ cup, into a glass bottle without a cap to allow oxygen in the air to react chemically with the oil. Add the same amount of oil to a second uncovered glass bottle of the same size.

2. Add ¼ teaspoon of BHT crystals to the cooking oil in one of the bottles and stir. The crystals require several hours to dissolve. (Setting the glass of BHT and oil in a bowl of hot water will speed the dissolution, particularly if the oil is vigorously stirred. If you do this, be sure to heat the untreated control cooking oil the same way, so that the treated and untreated oil will be handled exactly the same except for the BHT.)

3. Label each bottle so you can identify the contents.

4. Have a friend or spouse relabel each bottle to cover your own label, keeping a coded record, so that you won't know which one contains antioxidant and which one doesn't. (This is a standard scientific technique to help prevent the experimenter's biases from influencing his or her judgment of the results.) From your friend's record of the original label and the one that covered it, you can find out later the contents of each bottle.

5. Store at room temperature and smell each sample daily. Record the number of days it takes for the contents in the jars to become rancid. The larger your group of sniffers (called an organoleptic panel in the food industry), the more reliable your results, so have the whole family smell each bottle daily, writing down their findings individually before discussing it. (You don't want one person's opinion to bias the perception of the other family members.) Discard all the oil after the test. Do not eat.

PLASTIC MILK BOTTLE TEST

Plastics, like skin, are subject to cross-linking. You can see how ultraviolet radiation cross-linking makes plastic brittle with this simple test.

1. Place a plastic milk bottle outside on a windowsill in direct sunlight.

2. After several months, check the flexibility of the plastic. Compare it to an identical plastic milk bottle kept in your closet. This test can also be done with outdoor rubber objects such as windshield wiper blades (which probably have some added antioxidant protection) and indoor rubber objects like baby bottle nipples (which often don't contain antioxidants).

THE COOKIE SHELF LIFE TEST

Cookies usually require a large amount of shortening or butter, both of which are subject to peroxidation. With added antioxidants, cookies can last much longer before becoming rancid. You can demonstrate this for yourself by adding the antioxidant BHT (or ascorbyl palmitate) to your next batch of cookies.

1. Add 0.02 percent by weight of BHT and/or 0.05 percent of ascorbyl palmitate to half the butter or shortening you will be using in the cookie batter. Use freshly purchased butter or shortening. Do this *just* before making the cookies so that the mixture when used is fresh and low in peroxides. Do not add antioxidant to the other half of the butter or oil.

2. Store the experimental cookies (with added antioxidant) and the control cookies (no antioxidant) in separate containers placed next to each other.

3. Have a friend label the cookies so you do not know which is which. Then another friend can put another label over the first label, recording the information on paper for your use later. Now no one knows which cookies have been treated (but the information is on paper).

4. Compare the cookies for taste and smell every few days. Which one smells rancid first? Discard old rancid cookies after testing.

EXTENDED COOKED-CHICKEN SHELF-STORAGE LIFE TEST

1. Add 1 teaspoon of ascorbyl palmitate to half the coating mix for 3 pounds of chicken. Ascorbic acid may be used in place of ascorbyl palmitate in the chicken coating, but it is less effective because it is not fat soluble. Whereas the palmitate form is nearly tasteless, ascorbic acid crystals are sour and less effective because they do not dissolve well in fats. Ascorbic acid crystals are especially compatible with foods having sour flavor notes, such as those which contain vinegar, lemon juice, or sour cream.

2. Coat half the chicken with the ascorbyl-palmitate-augmented coating and the other half with plain coating. Cook as usual.

3. Package each half of the chicken identically for refrigeration. Have a friend label each package, so that he or she knows which one is which, but you don't.

4. Store chicken in refrigerator. Check each day for taste and odor. Discard the old rancid chicken after testing. Do not eat left over rancid foods.

We have suggested BHT and ascorbyl palmitate (fat-soluble vitamin C) in these experiments, although these are normally available only to food processors to be used as additives (for supply sources, see Appendix I). We would have preferred to include experiments using antioxidants which are readily available in health food stores—vitamins E and C (ascorbic acid is the easily obtained form). However, these antioxidants are not in any appreciable use as antioxidant food additives (except C for curing meats, such as bacon) because the synthetics (such as BHT, BHA, propyl gallate, TBHQ) are much more effective antioxidants and are less expensive. In order to determine the antioxidant levels of vitamins E and C (ascorbic acid) that are effective as food preservatives, experiments must be done. We are currently involved in investigating these antioxidants, both singly and in combinations. (We hope to publish these results in our next book.)

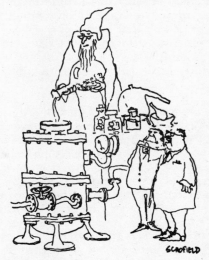

"We're combining technology with tradition."

THE WATER-SOLUBLE VITAMIN LOSS TEST

Your body cannot store megadoses of water-soluble vitamins such as B-1, B-2, B-3, B-5, B-6, C, and H (biotin). If you wish to have high levels of these nutrients in your body, you must take them three or four times a day. Here is a simple demonstration. Take 50 milligrams of the yellow vitamin B-2. Within about half an hour, your urine will be colored bright yellow by the B-2 being eliminated through the kidneys. Within a few hours, you will have lost so much of that B-2 dose that your blood levels will be roughly back to normal and your urine color will have returned to its previous state. If you take vitamin B-2 often enough to keep your urine bright yellow, you are taking it often enough to keep your blood levels markedly elevated. Not all water-soluble vitamins taken in large doses are lost at exactly the same rate, but this little experiment vividly shows why we take our nutritional supplements four times per day.

THE VITAMIN C CONTENT OF YOUR URINE TEST

Vitamin C, like other water-soluble vitamins, is rapidly excreted in the urine when taken in large doses. If vitamin C levels in your urine are kept high, your body and blood vitamin C levels will also be high. Elevated vitamin C levels in urine are of great importance to smokers and drinkers, since this can markedly reduce the risk of developing urinary bladder cancer.

You can easily measure your urine vitamin C concentration with C-Stix®, made by the Ames Division of Miles Laboratories and available from your pharmacist without a prescription. C-Strips, a similar product made by the Wholesale Nutrition Club in Sunnyvale, Ca., is less expensive but not as widely sold. The C-Stix® are chemical-impregnated plastic strips that turn color when dipped in urine containing vitamin C. The greater the C concentration, the darker the color. You simply compare the urine-dipped strip to the color chart on the bottle and read off your urine vitamin C concentration. C-Stix® are made to read vitamin C in the range of 0 to 40 milligrams per deciliter, which is the same as 0 to 400 milligrams per liter (a liter is about a quart). If your C level is higher than this, as ours is, simply dilute one part urine with

9 parts water and the C-Stix® will now measure 0 to 4,000 milligrams of vitamin C (in its desirable reduced form) per liter. Our urine C levels vary from a minimum of 500 milligrams per liter before our morning dose to over 2,000 milligrams per liter about three hours after a dose. Note how your urinary C levels vary during the day. What are your urinary vitamin C levels after a long party where you do a lot of smoking and drinking?

GASOLINE STORAGE AND BHT

If you have difficulty in starting your lawn mower, trail bike, outboard motor, or similar infrequently used gasoline engine, you will be interested in knowing the reason for this malfunction. Petroleum is subject to autoxidation, like oils in foods and in the human body. When gasoline is left for any long period (a few months or more), gums are formed by the reaction of oxygen with unsaturated components of the fuel. BHT (also known as 2, 6-ditertiary butyl p-cresol) is a U.S. Government approved additive to gasoline to meet military requirements for gasoline stability. A half pound of BHT added to 1,100 gallons of gasoline prevented gum formation when gasoline was stored in sealed (with standard rubber washers) 5-gallon cans for periods up to two years in the Mojave desert in full sunlight, compared to a storage life of only a few months for unprotected gasoline.

The amount currently recommended for military use is 1 pound BHT to 1,100 gallons of gasoline. For even longer storage, a chelating agent such as disodium EDTA, 100 milligrams per gallon, will chelate metal ions which would otherwise promote oxidation. BHT is effective in diesel fuel, lubrication oil, grease, and other fuels. You can add about ¼ teaspoon of BHT per gallon of fuel. Stir until it is dissolved.

BHT added to gasoline can solve the problem of gummed-up carburetors that make it difficult to start engines of lawn mowers, pleasure boats, campers, trail bikes, and generators. We included this information to demonstrate how the chemical mechanism underlying aging in biological organisms also cause preventable aging damage in fuels as well. Other materials besides fuels and plastics that are affected by similar aging mechanisms include plastics, rubber, paints, asphalt, and roofing shingles.

5
FDA's Recommended Daily Allowances

If you shut up truth and bury it under the ground, it will
but grow, and gather to itself such explosive power that
the day it bursts through it will blow up everything in its
way.

—Emile Zola

These humans are highly illogical.

—Mr. Spock, science officer, U.S.S. *Enterprise*

I'm not a bad man—I'm just a bad wizard.

—the Wizard of Oz

*The Recommended Daily Allowances (RDAs) of the Food and
Drug Administration have been promoted as the amount of
vitamins and minerals a normal person needs to ingest each
day. Recent research indicates that these recommended quantities of dietary nutrients are not a good guide to nutrition.
The RDAs were not determined by scientific studies (to find
out how much we should get) but instead were based on the
amount of these nutrients already present in the typical
American diet. The FDA's claim that all our nutritional needs
can be fulfilled with "a knife and fork" may not be valid for
many people, and for some individuals who smoke and drink
a great deal, the claim may be dangerous.*

Reprinted below are the FDA's current recommended
daily allowances for a number of vitamins and minerals. The

FDA says, "The U.S. RDAs are the amounts of protein, vitamins, and minerals people need each day to stay healthy. These allowances are set by the Food and Drug Administration. Set at generous levels, they provide a considerable margin of safety for most people above minimum body needs for most nutrients." The FDA booklet "Myths of Vitamins" (HEW Publication no. (FDA) 78-2047) states that, "Foods can and do supply most Americans with adequate nutrients."

But adequate for what?

In booklets about vitamin C ("What About Vitamin C?" publication no. 75-2015) and Vitamin E ("Vitamin E—Miracle or Myth?" publication no. 76-2011), the FDA claims that there is no evidence to support the idea that nutritional supplements in amounts larger than the RDA (60 milligrams of C and 30 I.U. of E per day) have any benefit. (These RDAs have recently been increased from 45 milligrams of vitamin C per day and 15 I.U. of E per day, apparently because these levels were not "generous" enough.) FDA rules absolutely forbid any nutrient manufacturer or distributor from making health claims. Furthermore, the FDA claims to have reviewed all pertinent scientific literature. This is nonsense. If they had spent $26 on a computerized literature search of the National Library of Medicine data base, they would have found the same papers that we have listed in Appendix K and hundreds more as well.

How did the FDA determine these RDA levels? These figures were created by determining how much Americans received in an average diet and adding what the FDA terms "a margin for safety." Thus the RDAs have little to do with a scientific standard determined by clinical studies in humans taking graded doses of these nutrients. Having thus fixed the RDAs, the FDA now spends your tax money to promote them as a guide to the health of Americans, with a threat of legal action if nutrient purveyors claim otherwise. Fortunately for us, we are scientists and not vitamin merchandisers.

In the early 1970s, the FDA expended considerable effort and taxpayers' money attempting to make a drug prescription necessary for the purchase of vitamins and minerals containing more than 1½ times their RDAs. Selling tablets of vitamin C containing more than 90 milligrams without a prescription would have become a criminal offense, and you would have had to get a prescription from your doctor in order to buy higher potency tablets at your drugstore. Happily,

Food and Nutrition Board, National Academy of Sciences—National Research Council

Designed for the maintenance of good nutrition of practically all healthy people in the U.S.A.

	Age (years)	Weight (kg) (lbs)		Height (cm) (in)		Protein (g)	Vitamin A (μg R.E.)[b]	Vitamin D (μg)[c]	Vitamin E (mg α T.E.)[d]
Infants	0.0-0.5	6	13	60	24	kg × 2.2	420	10	3
	0.5-1.0	9	20	71	28	kg × 2.0	400	10	4
Children	1-3	13	29	90	35	23	400	10	5
	4-6	20	44	112	44	30	500	10	6
	7-10	28	62	132	52	34	700	10	7
Males	11-14	45	99	157	62	45	1000	10	8
	15-18	66	145	176	69	56	1000	10	10
	19-22	70	154	177	70	56	1000	7.5	10
	23-50	70	154	178	70	56	1000	5	10
	51+	70	154	178	70	56	1000	5	10
Females	11-14	46	101	157	62	46	800	10	8
	15-18	55	120	163	64	46	800	10	8
	19-22	55	120	163	64	44	800	7.5	8
	23-50	55	120	163	64	44	800	5	8
	51+	55	120	163	64	44	800	5	8
						+30	+200	+5	+2
Lactating						+20	+400	+5	+3

Fat-Soluble Vitamins

a The allowances are intended to provide for individual variations among most normal persons as they live in the United States under usual environmental stresses. Diets should be based on a variety of common foods in order to provide other nutrients for which human requirements have been less well defined. See p. 23 for heights, weights and recommended intake.

b Retinol equivalents. 1 Retinol equivalent = 1 μg retinol or 6 μg β carotene. See text for calculation of vitamin A activity of diets as retinol equivalents.

c As cholecalciferol. 10 μg cholecalciferol = 400 I.U. vitamin D.

d α-tocopherol equivalents. 1 mg d-α-tocopherol = 1 α T.E. See text for variation in allowances and calculation of vitamin E activity of the diet as α-tocopherol equivalents.

e 1 N.E. (niacin equivalent) is equal to 1 mg of niacin or 60 mg of dietary tryptophan.

f The folacin allowances refer to dietary sources

Table 1. Recommended Daily Dietary Allowances,[a] Revised 1980

		Water-Soluble Vitamins							Minerals			
Vitamin C (mg)	Thiamin (mg)	Riboflavin (mg)	Niacin (mg N.E.)e	Vitamin B6 (mg)	Folacin f (µg)	Vitamin B12 (µg)	Calcium (mg)	Phosphorus (mg)	Magnesium (mg)	Iron (mg)	Zinc (mg)	Iodine (µg)
35	0.3	0.4	6	0.3	30	0.5g	360	240	50	10	3	40
35	0.5	0.6	8	0.6	45	1.5	540	360	70	15	5	50
45	0.7	0.8	9	0.9	100	2.0	800	800	150	15	10	70
45	0.9	1.0	11	1.3	200	2.5	800	800	200	10	10	90
45	1.2	1.4	16	1.6	300	3.0	800	800	250	10	10	120
50	1.4	1.6	18	1.8	400	3.0	1200	1200	350	18	15	150
60	1.4	1.7	18	2.0	400	3.0	1200	1200	400	18	15	150
60	1.5	1.7	19	2.2	400	3.0	800	800	350	10	15	150
60	1.4	1.6	18	2.2	400	3.0	800	800	350	10	15	150
60	1.2	1.4	16	2.2	400	3.0	800	800	350	10	15	150
50	1.1	1.3	15	1.8	400	3.0	1200	1200	300	18	15	150
60	1.1	1.3	14	2.0	400	3.0	1200	1200	300	18	15	150
60	1.1	1.3	14	2.0	400	3.0	800	800	300	18	15	150
60	1.0	1.2	13	2.0	400	3.0	800	800	300	18	15	150
60	1.0	1.2	13	2.0	400	3.0	800	800	300	10	15	150
+20	+0.4	+0.3	+2	+0.6	+400	+1.0	+400	+400	+150	h	+5	+25
+40	+0.5	+0.5	+5	+0.5	+100	+1.0	+400	+400	+150	h	+10	+50

as determined by *Lactobacillus casei* assay after treatment with enzymes ("conjugases") to make polyglutamyl forms of the vitamin available to the test organism.

g The RDA for vitamin B12 in infants is based on average concentration of the vitamin in human milk. The allowances after weaning are based on energy intake (as recommended by the American Academy of Pediatrics) and consideration of other factors such as intestinal absorption; see text.

h The increased requirement during pregnancy cannot be met by the iron content of habitual American diets nor by the existing iron stores of many women; therefore the use of 30-60 mg of supplemental iron is recommended. Iron needs during lactation are not substantially different from those of non-pregnant women, but continued supplementation of the mother for 2-3 months after parturition is advisable in order to replenish stores depleted by pregnancy.

Food and Nutrition Board, National Academy of Sciences—

*Estimated Safe and Adequate Daily Dietary Intakes of Selected Vitamins and Minerals[a]

| | | | | Vitamins | | Trace Elements[b] | | |
	Age (years)	Vitamin K (µg)	Biotin (µg)	Pantothenic Acid (mg)	Copper (mg)	Manganese (mg)	Fluoride (mg)
Infants	0-0.5	12	35	2	0.5-0.7	0.5-0.7	0.1-0.5
	0.5-1	10-20	50	3	0.7-1.0	0.7-1.0	0.2-1.0
Children	1-3	15-30	65	3	1.0-1.5	1.0-1.5	0.5-1.5
and	4-6	20-40	85	3-4	1.5-2.0	1.5-2.0	1.0-2.5
Adolescents	7-10	30-60	120	4-5	2.0-2.5	2.0-3.0	1.5-2.5
	11+	50-100	100-200	4-7	2.0-3.0	2.5-5.0	1.5-2.5
Adults		70-140	100-200	4-7	2.0-3.0	2.5-5.0	1.5-4.0

Table II. Recommended Dietary Allowances, Revised 1980.

Category	Age (years)	Weight (kg)	Weight (lb)	Height (cm)	Height (in)
Infants	0.0-0.5	6	13	60	24
	0.5-1.0	9	20	71	28
Children	1-3	13	29	90	35
	4-6	20	44	112	44
	7-10	28	62	132	52
Males	11-14	45	99	157	62
	15-18	66	145	176	69
	19-22	70	154	177	70
	23-50	70	154	178	70
	51-75	70	154	178	70
	76+	70	154	178	70
Females	11-14	46	101	157	62
	15-18	55	120	163	64
	19-22	55	120	163	64
	23-50	55	120	163	64
	51-75	55	120	163	64
	76+	55	120	163	64
Pregnancy					
Lactation					

Table III. Mean Heights and Weights and Recommended Energy Intake

			Electrolytes		
Chromium (mg)	Selenium (mg)	Molybdenum (mg)	Sodium (mg)	Potassium (mg)	Chloride (mg)
0.01-0.04	0.01-0.04	0.03-0.06	115-350	350-925	275-700
0.02-0.06	0.02-0.06	0.04-0.08	250-750	425-1275	400-1200
0.02-0.08	0.02-0.08	0.05-0.1	325-975	550-1650	500-1500
0.03-0.12	0.03-0.12	0.06-0.15	450-1350	775-2325	700-2100
0.05-0.2	0.05-0.2	0.1 - 0.3	600-1800	1000-3000	925-2775
0.05-0.2	0.05-0.2	0.15-0.5	900-2700	1525-4575	1400-4200
0.05-0.2	0.05-0.2	0.15-0.5	1100-3300	1875-5625	1700-5100

Energy Needs (with range) (kcal)	(MJ)
kg × 115 (95-145)	kg × .48
kg × 105 (80-135)	kg × .44
1300 (900-1800)	5.5
1700 (1300-2300)	7.1
2400 (1650-3300)	10.1
2700 (2000-3700)	11.3
2800 (2100-3900)	11.8
2900 (2500-3300)	12.2
2700 (2300-3100)	11.3
2400 (2000-2800)	10.1
2050 (1650-2450)	8.6
2200 (1500-3000)	9.2
2100 (1200-3000)	8.8
2100 (1700-2500)	8.8
2000 (1600-2400)	8.4
1800 (1400-2200)	7.6
1600 (1200-2000)	6.7
+300	
+500	

a Because there is less information on which to base allowances, these figures are not given in the main table of the RDA and are provided here in the form of ranges of recommended intakes.

b Since the toxic levels for many trace elements may be only several times usual intakes, the upper levels for the trace elements given in this table should not be habitually exceeded.

a The data in this table have been assembled from the observed median heights and weights of children shown in Table 1, together with desirable weights for adults given in Table 2 for the mean heights of men (70 inches) and women (64 inches) between the ages of 18 and 34 years as surveyed in the U.S. population (HEW/NCHS data).

The energy allowances for the young adults are for men and women doing light work. The allowances for the two older groups represent mean energy needs over these age spans, allowing for a 2% decrease in basal (resting) metabolic rate per decade and a reduction in activity of 200 kcal/day for men and women between 51 and 75 years, 500 kcal for men over 75 years and 400 kcal for women over 75 (see text). The customary range of daily energy output is shown for adults in parentheses, and is based on a variation in energy needs of ± 400 kcal at any one age (see text and Garrow, 1978), emphasizing the wide range of energy intakes appropriate for any group of people.

Energy allowances for children through age 18 are based on median energy intakes of children of these ages followed in longitudinal growth studies. The values in parentheses are 10th and 90th percentiles of energy intake, to indicate the range of energy consumption among children of these ages (see text).

a Recommended Dietary Allowances. Revised 1980

a massive number of protest letters reached Congress (more than for the Vietnam war, Watergate, the JFK assassination, or any previous issue), which then wisely denied FDA the power to control nutrients. Below is one protest message sent to Congress by many concerned people. It is ironic to read in FDA's booklet "A Primer on Dietary Minerals" (HEW publication no. 77-2070), "The increasing sales of vitamin-mineral supplements and the considerable interest shown in new FDA regulations on these products attest to this awareness [of vitamins and minerals]."

For the sake of comparison, consider these estimated nutrient requirements for laboratory animals, as provided by the National Research Council:

1. Nonhuman primates (monkeys and apes) should have 100 milligrams of vitamin C per kilogram of diet. This is about twice the currently recommended RDA for humans. (pg. 19, "Nutrient Requirements of Nonhuman Primates," no. 14, 1978.)

2. Guinea pigs (which are, like man, unable to make vitamin C in their bodies) are suggested to eat a diet containing 200 milligrams of C per kilogram of food. This is four times the RDA for humans (pg. 65, "Nutrient Requirments of Laboratory Animals," no. 10, 1978.)

3. Consider that the Ralston Purina lab chow for monkeys (a standard diet for lab monkeys which is designed for maintaining normal health, not for extending life span) contains 750 milligrams of vitamin C per kilogram of diet. This is about thirteen times as much as the RDA for humans! The Ralston Purina guinea pig chow contains 1 gram of C per kilogram of diet, or eighteen times the human RDA.

What is going on here? Is FDA unaware of the immense scientific literature concerning health benefits of many nutrients? We can't be sure. All we can really say is that they are a very poor source of information about these nutrients. A possible motive for the FDA's stand on RDAs may be that a scientific study would indicate deficiencies in several vitamins and minerals in the U.S. population, which could be useful propaganda in such hostile nations as the U.S.S.R. and might be embarrassing to the FDA, the self-proclaimed "protector" of the health of Americans.

One of the latest efforts to come from the FDA is their attempt to block the vitamin and mineral fortification of snack and other "junk" foods. How can these foods ever be anything more than "junk" foods if they cannot be improved nutritionally? The FDA clearly has no respect for the choices of others, if they differ from their own. We would much rather see people drinking soft drinks containing vitamin C than with no vitamin C. There is little indication that the popularity of these types of foods is declining. The FDA's recent "Notice of Proposed Rule Making" would make it a crime to put vitamin C in a soft drink. Although not junk food, popular vitamin-and-mineral-fortified breakfast cereals are also having their problems because of the FDA. The FDA does not approve of these high levels of fortification (100 percent of their RDA in some cases) and has put considerable pressure on companies like Kellogg (Total cereal) and General Mills (Most cereal) to reduce or eliminate their vitamin/mineral fortification. Fortunately for us, these companies have so far resisted the FDA's efforts, at substantial legal and managerial cost. In general, we have found that the large food processing companies (such as General Mills, General Foods, Kellogg, and Post) take their share of responsibility for good nutrition very seriously, even when they have to fight the FDA to do it. Free from FDA harassment, these companies would eagerly compete for a new market: heavily fortified, highly nutritious items that look like junk food, taste like junk food, and are as convenient as junk food. Unlike the FDA, these companies are extremely responsive to customers' letters. (They have to be. If they aren't, their customers will buy from their competitors.) If you want to write to one of these large processed food manufacturers, address your letter to the president of the company. Explain that you want and are willing to pay for nutritious junk foods, heavily fortified with vitamins, minerals, fiber, and protein. They will not be able to market such foods without a long and very expensive legal battle with the FDA that acts as if it wants junk-food eaters (the majority of our population—especially children) to eat only junk. They will need your encouragement if they are to fight this battle for better nutrition, so do write them.

400 Part IV: Nutrition and Life Extension

When the FDA proposed making high potency vitamins into prescription drugs in the early 1970s, there was strong negative public response, resulting in millions of cards and letters like this one sent to Congress.

YOUR NUTRITIONAL RIGHTS ARE UP FOR GRABS IN CONGRESS!

The struggle for *your* nutritional freedom is still going on. We have won a few important battles—but we can still lose the war!

A Federal court has made a number of rulings favorable to this freedom, and has temporarily blocked the proposed F.D.A. restrictions on nutritional supplements—at least until July 1, 1975. But Congressional action is still uncertain. So Congress is the battleground where *your* support is needed to strengthen and reinforce the fighters who are protecting your nutritional freedom.

The Proxmire Bill, designed to make sure that your nutritional supplements continue to be safe, wholesome, and accurately labeled...while preserving your right to continue buying and using the supplements that you feel contribute to your personal nutrition...passed the Senate by a vote of 81 to 10, as an amendment to the Kennedy Health Bill. (In good part, this was thanks to the cards and letters many of us sent our Senators.) This was a great victory for nutritional freedom. But it can be undone—unless you help protect what you have won!

Right now, the House of Representatives Committee on Interstate and Foreign Commerce is considering the Kyros Vitamin Bill (H.R. 16317). This bill contains a number of provisions that would be most damaging to your right of nutritional choice—the right to buy and use the vitamins and food supplements you feel contribute to your personal nutrition! It must not be allowed to pass!

The names of the members of the House Committee considering the Kyros Bill are listed on the reverse side. You will find the name of *your* local Congressman among them.

To help protect *your* nutritional rights, by helping the Proxmire Bill become law, send the postcard below to your local Congressman. Be sure to sign it. Have your spouse...any other member of your family...or any friend who is a registered voter in your district send one also.

Dear Congressman:

I urge you, as a member of the House Committee on Interstate and Foreign Commerce, to help prevent the erosion of my personal freedoms, by voting against the Kyros Vitamin Bill in Committee.

I want to be able to continue buying and using the vitamin, mineral and food supplements that I feel contribute to my personal nutrition. Unfortunately, the Kyros Bill contains provisions which would interfere with my freedom to do so.

While I oppose this sort of arbitrary action, I do favor legislation that would make sure that my supplements continue to be safe, wholesome and accurately labeled. That is why I urge you to support a bill containing all the provisions of the Proxmire Vitamin Bill as passed by the Senate—both by voting for it in Committee and by working and voting for it on the floor. Please let me know how you stand on this issue.

Sincerely,_____

My address is_____

_____

_____

6
Vitamin E, the Lipid Antioxidant

A theory is the more impressive the greater is the simplicity of its premises, the more different are the kinds of things it relates, and the more extended is its range of applicability.

—Albert Einstein

It's not easy to summarize in a paragraph the properties and uses of this remarkable substance, vitamin E. Vitamin E is the body's most important nutrient lipid (fat) soluble antioxidant. It protects fats in our bodies from the damaging effects of uncontrolled oxidation and free radicals. These uncontrolled oxidations can cause cancer, induce abormal blood clots resulting in stroke or heart attack, and damage the DNA in our cells which controls growth, development, and programmed aging. Large doses of vitamin E have been shown to increase resistance to cancer, bacterial and viral infections, stroke, arthritis, heart attack, and even smog.

All animals (except for a few anaerobic—non-oxygen requiring—bacteria) metabolize oxygen to obtain energy. Plants obtain their energy from the sun by photosynthesis, but this involves oxidation reactions as well. (Oxidation is not confined only to reactions by oxygen but refers to all reactions in which a compound—the oxidizer—attacks another compound by removing an electron from it.) The process of lipid (fat or oil) oxidation in plants and animals results in the generation of free radicals, dangerously promiscuous chemically reactive atoms or molecules with an unpaired electron. In order to survive the damage done by these free radicals, plants and animals have evolved protective mechanisms. One of the most important of these protective substances is vitamin E, an antioxidant which dissolves in body fats or plant oils. Wheat germ oil contains vitamin E, not as a favor to humanity but because otherwise these oils would become rancid (peroxidized), damaging the plant's seed embryo. In fact, seeds are particularly sensitive to peroxidation (oxidation by or to peroxides) owing to their high lipid (fat and oil) content. The higher the level of peroxidized lipids, the smaller the likelihood that a seed will be capable of germinating. Thus, wheat germ, the seed embryo of wheat, contains large quantities of vitamin E to prevent this peroxidation. Seeds can retain their full potency essentially indefinitely if they are stored under inert nitrogen gas, without exposure to any oxygen.

Peroxidation of animal lipids is a very significant source of damage which, according to substantial evidence, is a major contributor to the aging process. Dr. A. L. Tappel, a well known food and nutrition scientist at the University of California at Davis who has been studying peroxidation and vitamin E for many years, says, "Lipid peroxidation of membranes of cells and subcellular particles can be very damaging. . . . Damage to membranes may be simple, as in the case of a membrane breaking, which allows contents to leak out, or complex, as in the case of a membrane containing integrated enzyme systems. Hemolysis (rupture) of red blood cells is an example of relatively simple membrane breaking. Tsen and Collier (1960) found that hemolysis of red blood cells is concurrent with lipid peroxidation." In fact the most common test for serum vitamin E level is to measure how much nasty treatment a test tube of the blood will tolerate before the red cells break down. The higher the E level, the harder it is to damage the red blood cells. Vitamin E is one of the most important of the natural lipid antioxidants.

Vitamin E is anti-thrombic (prevents formation of abnormal blood clots) and anti-proteolytic (protects proteins from enzymatic destruction). It prolongs the clotting time of recalcified human plasma and in rats when injected into their intestinal cavity (interperitoneally). In doses of 800 I.U. per day, it has been used effectively to prevent the formation of deep vein thrombosis (clots) in bedridden postoperative patients.

As we mentioned earlier, scientists Vane and Moncada recently discovered the body's natural anti-clotting hormone, prostacyclin (also called PGI_2), which lines the walls of healthy arteries. Vitamin E helps the body in the manufacture of prostacyclin by preventing the formation of peroxides which inhibit the formation of prostacyclin. For more about prostacyclin and how it prevents clots, see Part III, Chapters 16, 17, and 18.

Vitamin E feeding experiments in animals for life span effects have only been modestly effective in increasing life span. Fruit flies' average life span was extended by 8 to 15 percent and their maximum life span by 12 percent by eating a diet containing 0.25 percent vitamin E, but in other studies there were no improvements in life span. Both humans and flies suffer from similar aging mechanisms, such as lipid peroxidation. Vitamin E is not a particularly strong antioxidant. Other stronger antioxidants (such as BHT, NDGA, BHA, and ethoxyquin) have increased the life span of mice, other animals, and insects.

Vitamin E is a very effective protectant against ozone toxicity. When rats were exposed continuously to 1 part per million of ozone, they lived only 8.2 days. When a similar group of rats was fed a diet containing 100 milligrams (about 100 units) of vitamin E acetate per kilogram of diet, they lived for 18.5 days, over twice as long. The vitamin E prevents the ozone from oxidizing the lung lipids by being oxidized itself. The E acts as a sacrificial target, is used up, and must be replaced in order for protection to be maintained. Dr. Tappel showed in human subjects that vitamin E protects the lungs against ozone found in smog. When ozone attacks lipids (fat) in the lungs, hydrocarbon fragments of the lipids are broken off. Some of these are gases, such as ethane and pentane, that are breathed out and can be measured. Dr. Tappel found, by measuring these fragments in the breath of the human subjects, that lipid damage to the lungs was greatly decreased by a few hundred units of vitamin E.

Free radicals are so promiscuous in their chemical reactions that they frequently damage DNA, causing mutations and cancer. Since vitamin E is an antioxidant (a free radical destroyer), it should be capable of preventing some mutations and cancer. Experiments have shown this to be true. If free radical carcinogens and mutagens such as are contained in cigarette smoke are added to cell cultures, the DNA of some of these cells is damaged and detectable mutations are produced. Vitamin E, as well as other antioxidants, reduces the mutation rate significantly. Vitamin E has also been shown in Irish wolfhounds to reduce the rate of spontaneous deaths from cancer from nearly 100 percent to nearly zero. Animals given injections of cancer cells live longer and are more likely to survive when given vitamin E in doses of 200 to 2,000 I.U. per kilogram of food. These effects on injected cancer cells may be due to stimulation of the immune system, possibly because vitamin E maintains the white blood cell and thymic cell membranes in a normal molecular configuration by preventing peroxidation. The immune system depends on intact membranes for its complex interactions. It was recently reported that vitamin E is an effective treatment for fibrocystic breast disease (a noncancerous lumpy breast tissue) that occurs in about 20 percent of American woman. (In many conditions, fibrosis is caused by free radical induced crosslinking.) In this report, 26 patients and 8 control subjects were given a placebo for four weeks followed by 600 I.U. of vitamin E a day for eight weeks. There was a regression of the disease observed in 22 of the 26 patients. The development of fibrocystic breast disease is thought to indicate a higher risk of developing breast cancer.

It has recently been reported that vitamin E (as vitamin E acetate) exerted a significant stimulatory effect on the immune system of several studied animals: rats, chickens, lambs, and turkeys. Both B- (bone-marrow-derived antibody-making white blood cells) and T-cells (several types of thymus-derived white blood cells which kill and eat invaders and give orders to B-cells) were stimulated in response to challenges by bacteria, viruses, and tumor cells when fed doses of 200 to 2,000 I.U. of vitamin E per kilogram of food daily. The control animals received a diet adequate in E (40 to 60 I.U. per kilogram of food), already about four times the average dietary human consumption. We expect similar effects on the human immune system. See Part II, Chapter 5, and Part III, Chapters 14 and 19, on the immune system for further information.

The Shute Clinic in Canada has achieved impressive results in treating cardiovascular diseases with vitamin E over the past thirty years in more than 35,000 patients. Experimental animals given vitamin E can survive longer and in better condition when they are subjected to a dangerously low oxygen environment. Therefore, heart patients with insufficient circulation should take vitamin E supplements (but see cautions in the following paragraph). In tissues with low but non-zero oxygen availability, free radical activity is greatly increased, according to Dr. Harry Demopoulos, because oxygen gas is itself a free radical scavenger, and also because normally occurring electron transport free radicals, such as coenzyme Q, get out of control. Electron transport is a step-wise system of carrying out controlled combustion in mitochondria, the cell's energy producers. Vitamin E's free radical scavenging activity is the mechanism of its protective effects in cardiovascular disease. There are other age-related problems that involve poor circulation, including atherosclerosis, cerebral vascular insufficiency (poor blood circulation in the brain), and intermittent claudication (circulatory failure in the limbs). Vitamin E and other antioxidants (such as C and selenium) will help provide worthwhile protection from the cumulative free radical damage which would otherwise occur. Smokers, particularly, should remember that carbon monoxide in their smoke destroys the oxygen-carrying capacity of the hemoglobin in their blood, making the above problems even worse and the use of antioxidant supplements even more vital. Free radicals cause cross-linking, the same process that causes skin wrinkles and loss of lung tissue elasticity (as in emphysema). This damage can be slowed with free radical scavengers such as vitamin E. High doses of E—in excess of 1,000 I.U. daily—frequently cause a dramatic improvement in skin appearance. This difference is sometimes noticeable in a few days, but a month is a more usual period over which to notice these results. See Part III, Chapter 1, "Some Immediate Benefits of Life Extension Measures."

Vitamin E has no known toxic side effects. **CAUTION:** Some people experience a temporary rise in blood pressure when they first begin using it. Heart disease patients should begin with low doses of E, perhaps 100 I.U. a day, and work up to a higher dose slowly. Dr. Shute's book *Vitamin E for Ailing and Healthy Hearts* has explicit instructions for vitamin E use by patients with active heart disease. We strongly recommend following them.

There are several different forms of vitamin E. The alcohol, alpha tocopherol, is much less stable in the presence of oxygen than the ester forms of vitamin E; vitamin E acetate (alpha tocopherol acetate) and vitamin E phosphate (alpha tocopherol phosphate) are the most common esters. These ester forms will remain potent in storage for far longer than the alcohol form. Vitamin E, like many biochemicals, occurs in two mirror-image forms: D-alpha tocopherol (which is the right-handed natural form) and L-alpha tocopherol (which is left-handed). Synthetic vitamin E is a 50/50 mixture of the D and L forms and is labeled DL-alpha tocopherol. The I.U. or international unit of vitamin E potency is a measure of E's biological activity, so 1,000 I.U. of the DL form is exactly as active in tests of biological activity as 1,000 I.U. of the D form. We and other biochemically oriented gerontologists usually use DL-alpha tocopherol acetate in our experiments; this form of E is generally the least expensive and is the most stable form readily available. Vacuum distilled natural vitamin E esters are satisfactory, though usually more expensive, but avoid taking megadoses of vitamin E in the form of cold pressed wheat germ oil because wheat germ oil processed in this way contains significant quantities of plant-produced estrogens (female sex hormones). See Part I, Chapter 14, for further details.

CAUTION: Be particularly wary of vitamin E esters in oil-filled gelatin capsules. Many vitamin packagers add oil to their capsules to make them larger. Tocopherol (vitamin E) esters are not good antioxidants until they are de-esterified in your body. Hence, the accompanying oil is often autoxidized (rancid). One way to minimize this problem is to buy the vitamin E capsules which are the smallest for their particular dose of the various brands offered. We use vitamin E acetate (an ester) on a dry, powdered, hydrolyzed protein carrier designed for direct compression tabletting from Roche. It contains no oil fillers.

7
Vitamin C

We were all hearty seamen, no colds did we fear,
And we have from all sickness entirely kept clear
Thanks be to the Captain, he has proved so good
Amongst all the Islands to give us fresh food.

—200-year-old sailor's song referring to the protective
effects of fresh food (contains vitamin C) against colds and
other disease (quoted in Pauling's *Vitamin C, the Common
Cold, and the Flu)*

. . . synthetic ascorbic acid is natural ascorbic acid, identical
with the vitamin C in oranges and other foods.

—Dr. Linus Pauling

*People used to believe (many still do) that vitamin C is only
good for curing scurvy. But vitamin C is good for* much *more
than just that. It's useful in so many different ways that it
seems like a miracle drug. Vitamin C stimulates your immune
system so that you can resist disease better—including bacteria, viruses, and even atherosclerotic plaques and cancer cells.
The survival time of terminal cancer patients taking 10 grams
of Vitamin C per day was quadrupled in one study! And 13
percent of the terminal cancer patients in the study were reportedly "cured." Vitamin C is required for wound healing.
By taking enough vitamin C, the time required for healing of
a fractured bone can, in some instances, be cut in half. Vitamin C can also reduce serum cholesterol in some people by 35
to 40 percent. It protects against the effects of many pollutants. These and other uses are described in this chapter.*

All animals require vitamin C to survive. The vitamin is needed to protect the brain and spinal cord from free radicals, for collagen (connective tissue) synthesis, in lipid (fat) and carbohydrate metabolism, to manufacture neurotransmitters, and for the proper maintenance of the immune system. All except man, apes, guinea pigs, and a fruit-eating bat and bird make vitamin C in their liver or adrenals from glucose (a sugar). Man and the other non-C producers lack an enzyme required in the C manufacture process. When you look at the amounts of vitamin C produced by some of these animals, particularly the ones of similar size to man (e.g., goat, cow, sheep, and dog), you find that they make roughly 10 grams per day for a 70-kilogram (154-pound) body weight. Under stressful conditions, they may make several times as much. The nutritional recommendation for the monkey (from the Committee on Animal Nutrition's "Nutrient Requirements of Laboratory Animals," 1962) is 55 milligrams of C per kilogram of body weight, or 3,830 milligrams (3.83 grams) of vitamin C per day based on the weight of an average adult human. Yet the FDA's Recommended Daily Allowance of vitamin C for people is only 60 milligrams (.06 gram)!

Man and the other non-makers of vitamin C must get their supplies daily (vitamin C isn't stored in large amounts) from their diet or (in the case of man) from dietary supplements. Gorillas can get up to about 3 grams a day of vitamin C from their diet. But people who want to take that amount, or more, cannot hope to get that much from diet alone.

In one study by Pelletier and Keith (1974), the relative bioavailability (availability to the body for use) of ascorbic acid in synthetic form was compared to ascorbic acid as part of orange juice in human subjects. Vitamin C was measured in serum, leucocytes (white cells), and urine. Synthetic C was given with and without rutin, a bioflavonoid. The dose was 75 milligrams of ascorbic acid, either as contained in orange juice or as the synthetic (with or without 400 milligrams of rutin). Measurements were made after two hours (at about the peak serum concentration). The results: synthetic ascorbic acid without rutin resulted in the greatest increase in serum ascorbic acid level and lower urinary excretion, indicating a slightly greater bioavailability with the synthetic vitamin C.

Some "experts" have claimed that it is a waste of money to take large doses of C (greater than about 100 milligrams per day) because this results in tissue saturation, so that most of the C is excreted and wasted. This is not true. The steady state level of vitamin C in blood plasma results from the difference between the rate of input of vitamin C and its rate of removal by the kidneys and use in the body. A sufficient rate of intake can raise the steady state level of vitamin C in plasma despite the loss of C through urination. The raised levels of C in plasma result from a dynamic interchange between C in plasma, lymph, and tissues, and the kidney excretion.

Dr. Feigan at Stanford has done oral-dose versus serum-level response measurements on C with both guinea pigs and humans. He found that you have to increase the oral dose by a factor of ten to increase the serum C level by a factor of two. For example, going from 50 to 500 milligrams per day doubles serum levels. Going from 500 milligrams to 5 grams (5,000 milligrams) per day doubles the serum level again so that it is four times that obtained with 50 milligrams a day. This is known as a logarithmic dose-response relationship. (When injected intravenously, however, the serum levels are directly proportional to the dose, which is why intravenous ascorbate salts are sometimes used for cancer therapy and in other very serious conditions.)

Vitamin C has more uses than the prevention of scurvy, although many doctors still believe that that is its only use. C has been successfully used in the treatment of a number of conditions in humans and animals. Vitamin C supplements can even provide dramatic benefits to animals already making large quantities of the vitamin in their bodies. Vitamin C has been used in such conditions as:

• To prevent the formation of carcinogenic nitrosamines from nitrites and nitrates in foods and amines found in the same food. These carcinogen-forming reactions also occur in your gut even if you eat no nitrites or nitrates. Lots of vitamin C in your gut will block these dangerous reactions. The feces of normal humans contain mutagenic (mutation causing) substances, which may be N-nitroso derivatives of intestinal lipids. Bruce and associates fed vitamin C and vitamin E to human volunteers and found the level of fecal mutagens reduced by the vitamins to about 25 percent of that of control (no supplemental vitamins given) subjects.

• To stimulate the activity of phagocytes (white cells which identify, kill, and eat unwanted invaders such as bacteria, viruses, and cancer cells). In one study, human volunteers taking 2 or 3 grams of ascorbate per day showed stimulation in some measures of cellular immunity. Their white cells were stimulated to mature and transform into fully functional types. And neutrophils, a type of mobile white cell, became more active in seeking out sources of bacterial toxins.

• To reduce serum cholesterol. A dose of 0.5 gram three times a day orally in atherosclerotic patients reduced blood cholesterol levels by 35 to 40 percent. Vitamin C controls the rate of destruction of cholesterol by transformation to its main metabolic product, bile acids (for fat digestion) in the liver.

• To reduce deposits of lipids in arteries.

• As an anti-cancer therapy. At a dose of 10 grams a day, 100 terminal cancer patients lived an average of over 200 days compared to only 50 days for the control terminal cancer patients in the study (Cameron and Pauling). Some patients in the 10-grams-per-day vitamin C supplemented group were reportedly "cured" of their cancer (13 out of 100 terminal patients). All the controls died. In a recent study, scientists found that vitamin C is directly toxic to a number of types of cancer cells, especially melanoma, in concentrations within reach by using very large vitamin C supplements.

• As a general immune stimulant, vitamin C has been effective in heightening the immune response to many viral and bacterial infections. At least part of this effect is because vitamin C stimulates the production of interferon (a potent anti-cancer, anti-virus chemical made in the body by lymphocytes—white blood cells—and fibroblasts—connective tissue cells).

In one study of the effect of vitamin C on viral infections, a combination of 600 milligrams of water-soluble bioflavonoids and 600 milligrams of ascorbic acid was given three times a day to a group of patients with recurrent oral cold sores (herpes type 1 or herpes labialis) less than forty-eight hours after the cold sores appeared. A control group of similar patients received a placebo (lactose, milk sugar). The interval from initial onset of the herpes attack to complete remission was reduced from 9.7 plus or minus 2.8 days in the lactose placebo group to 4.2 plus or minus 1.7 days in the ascorbate-bioflavonoid group.

Vitamin C in repeated intravenous or intramuscular doses of 500 to 1,000 milligrams has been reported to successfully treat tuberculosis, scarlet fever, pelvic infections, septicemia, and virus diseases (polio, encephalitis, measles, herpes zoster, viral pneumonia, and others). It has also been used to treat rattlesnake bite in dogs, rabies, scorpion sting, lead poisoning, and other conditions. Dr. Robert F. Cathcart III, a physician practicing medicine in Incline Village, Nevada, has treated over 7,000 patients with megadoses of vitamin C in cases of mononucleosis, pneumonia, influenza, hepatitis, and other conditions.

Vitamin C was used in rabies treatment of experimental animals (100 milligrams per kilogram twice a day for seven days after inoculation with rabies virus). The treated animals reportedly had a 35.42 percent mortality rate, while the controls (received a salt-water injection rather than vitamin C) had a 70 percent mortality rate. The results were statistically significant at $p < 0.01$. (This means that the probability of getting these results by chance alone is less than 1 percent.)

• Vitamin C is required for collagen synthesis and, therefore, for wound healing. Dr. G. H. Bourne did a study of the effects in guinea pigs of different doses of vitamin C on the formation and tensile strength of collagen fibers in healing wounds. The guinea pigs were given a diet containing no vitamin C and daily supplements of either 0, 0.25, 0.5, 1, or 2 milligrams daily dose of pure synthetic C. After a week on the diet, two cuts ¼-inch deep were made on the back of each anesthetized animal. Seven days later (still on the diet), the animals were killed and the strength of the healing wounds tested by cutting out the pieces of skin with the wounds and hanging weights of various sizes from the skin to see how much it would take to tear them open. The results were:

Tensile Strength of Wounds in Guinea Pigs Given Graded Doses of Vitamin C

Daily dose of C in milligrams	Weight at which scar broke in grams
2.0	338.6 (+or− 26.8)
1.0	137.7 (+or− 13.9)
0.5	118.5 (+or− 19.0)
0.25	79.3 (+or− 10.4)
0	25.3 (+or− 7.4)

Dr. Bourne also did an experiment with groups of guinea pigs all fed the same diet, with each group given a daily supplement of either 4.0, 2.0, 1.0, 0.5, 0.25, or 0 milligrams of vi-

tamin C. A similar result was obtained with the healing of
fractured bone: The formation of the collagenous material of
the bone was speeded up with C. The 2 milligram dose was
optimal.

• The importance of vitamin C to recovery from heart attack damage is illustrated by the fact that, after a heart attack,
leukocytes (white blood cells) carry vitamin C to the heart
from other areas of the body, even when this means reducing
the supply to these other areas to a vitamin C–deficient state.
After a heart attack, so much vitamin C may be removed
from the rest of the body and transported to the damaged
heart that serum levels of C drop by a factor of two. The vitamin C helps protect the hypoxic (not enough oxygen present) area (infarct) in the heart from further free radical
damage.

• Vivid proof of the importance of vitamin C in protecting
the body's fats is that our brains have special transport systems that increase the concentration of C to 100 times more
than that which is present in the circulating blood. The brain
and spinal cord have the highest levels of C, along with the
adrenal glands. These amazingly high C levels are maintained
by two sets of vitamin C pumps, one in the blood-brain barrier (a very selective membrane surrounding the brain and
spinal cord), and the other in the nerve cell membrane itself.
The brain, spinal cord, and many sensory nerves contain a
great deal of the extremely polyunsaturated and easily autoxidized lipid known as docosahexanoic acid. Without the presence of very large amounts of vitamin C, severe nerve
damage occurs almost immediately.

• Vitamin C can prevent toxic effects due to histamine release in stressful situations.

• Vitamin C, B-1, and cysteine (a sulfur-containing amino
acid) form an oxidation-reduction system which is very effective in preventing damage due to aldehydes.

• Experiments have shown that vitamin C can provide
substantial protection against the effects of seven damaging
chemicals associated with drinking and smoking: acetaldehyde, nicotine, carbon monoxide (a major poison in cigarette
smoke), N-nitroso compounds, NOx (nitrogen oxides, nitric
acid gas), cadmium, and polynuclear aromatic hydrocarbons.
Vitamin C is used up in destroying these noxious substances,
so it is not surprising that smokers and alcohol drinkers have
much lower vitamin C serum levels than those who abstain

from these practices. These low serum levels can be promptly corrected with 1 gram or more of C taken three or four times per day.

• Vitamin C plays a key role in catecholamine (dopamine and norepinephrine, neurotransmitters in the brain) production and release. Some evidence suggests that C may help maintain normal or increased levels of tissue catecholamines as a factor in their synthesis by enzymes, by inhibiting their inactivation, by preventing excessive buildup of tissue catecholamines, and by protecting the activity of monamine oxidase (an enzyme which breaks down the catecholamines).

• Vitamin C can reduce the amount required for effective use of some powerful drugs, such as L-Dopa (4 grams a day of C permitted the use of reduced doses of L-Dopa, 2 grams per day, in successful treatment of Parkinson's disease). C has been able to reduce the requirements of cancer patients for painkillers. One way that it does this is understood: Vitamin C inhibits the enzymes that break down the brain's natural painkilling compounds, the enkephalins.

• Vitamin C has a powerful synergistic effect with other water-soluble antioxidants found in the body, such as cysteine and calcium pantothenate (a form of vitamin B-5). It is thought that C helps maintain the proper state of reduction and oxidation in many metabolic reactions. For example, it helps keep sulfhydryl compounds such as cysteine in the reduced state. Aging may be due, in part, to the decrease in blood and tissue levels of antioxidants that occur in aging. In one long-term study on humans, the best single predictor of continued survival was serum vitamin C. High serum C was more closely associated with long life than any other single factor, including whether a person was obese, smoked, or drank alcohol.

• Ascorbyl palmitate, a lipid-soluble form of vitamin C used as a food, vitamin, and drug preservative, is a powerful antioxidant synergist with other fat-soluble antioxidants, such as vitamin E.

• Vitamin C has been shown to provide substantial protection against experimental traumatic shock (weights dropped on the legs of anesthetized guinea pigs, mice, and rats) when administered very soon (within fifteen minutes to one hour) after the injury. The extra C doubled the crushing energy required to inflict a fatal injury. The minimum effective dose was 100 milligrams per kilogram of body weight. Note that rats and mice make their own vitamin C (equivalent to several grams a day for a human), yet they were helped by additional C added to their diets.

· Vitamin C has been shown to reduce the risk of abnormal blood clots. In one study, 1 gram daily of vitamin C in patients vulnerable to deep vein clots reduced the incidence of clots to half that of control patients (no supplemental C). In another study, 200 milligrams of C per day provided no protection against clots, suggesting that a greater dose of C must be taken to achieve this effect.

Side effects of vitamin C are few and generally minor. Diarrhea, acid indigestion, or nausea can occur as a result of its acidity. This can be minimized by neutralizing the acid with sodium bicarbonate (ordinary baking soda—should not be used by those on a low-sodium diet) or commercial antacids. Neutralizing ascorbic acid with baking soda results in the formation of sodium ascorbate; commercially produced sodium ascorbate is also made by neutralizing ascorbic acid. Powdered limestone plus ascorbic acid yields calcium ascorbate. Milk of magnesia plus ascorbic acid yields magnesium ascorbate. Very large doses of ascorbates, even sodium ascorbate, can cause diarrhea, particularly if the dose is increased more rapidly than your body can adapt.

Vitamin C remains at a higher serum level when it is protected by other stronger antioxidants, such as selenium, cysteine, and vitamin B-1, and works in conjunction with them. Linus Pauling suggests that it is the lowest daily serum level of C, rather than the highest level, which determines how much benefits we can get from taking vitamin C. Therefore, it is important to spread the vitamin C out over the day to maintain a high constant serum level. Vitamin C is water soluble and, consequently, is rapidly excreted. In humans after an oral dose it reaches peak serum concentration in about $2\frac{1}{2}$ hours and has dropped to half of the peak value in about $5\frac{1}{2}$ hours. It should probably be taken every four hours or so.

Some claim that vitamin C increases the probability of formation of oxalate or uric acid kidney stones, but extensive observations in people using multigram doses of C for many years has not resulted in discovery of such stones, nor are such stones a general problem in animals which manufacture large amounts of vitamin C. **CAUTION:** One side effect of megadoses of C is that glucose tolerance or blood sugar tests can give false positives (indicative of diabetes) because high C intake results in excretion of xylulose, a sugar. To the most common glucose tolerance test, this sugar appears to be glucose in the urine, a symptom of diabetes. C itself looks like sugar to the very commonly used orthotoluidine blood sugar test. Another commonly used blood sugar test, the glucose oxidase test, gives false abnormally-low readings in the presence of high concentrations of antioxidants such as C. Hence, high vitamin C dose users should ask for the very specific hexokinase test for blood sugar or glucose tolerance measurements.

Another possible problem with megadose use of C is that if C intake is suddenly lowered or eliminated, some symptoms of scurvy can develop. The body becomes used to a large supply of C and uses this chemical in a variety of ways which it could not if the supply were much lower (as, for example, in a natural diet). Therefore, when the C intake is reduced, it should be done slowly to give the body time to adjust.

It is very difficult to say how much optimum vitamin C could increase human life span. Vitamin C has been used alone in a few life span studies in experimental animals without impressive results. However, the difficulties of administering C to experimental animals, as discussed below, makes interpretation of such studies difficult. In addition, C alone is not a powerful antioxidant, but it is a powerful synergist with other antioxidants (synergy means that the effects are greater than additive). We infer, from its positive effects on the immune system, healing, stress resistance, and collagen synthesis, that it can increase the quality and perhaps the quantity of life. Twice–Nobel-laureate Linus Pauling estimates that the human life extension for optimal C intake is twelve to eighteen years.

The U.S. RDA is currently set at 60 milligrams per day, a low dose. The National Research Council recommends 200 milligrams of vitamin C for each kilogram (2.2 pounds) of food for guinea pigs, which, like man, cannot make their own C. This recommendation is almost five times the RDA for people on a percent-of-food basis.

As we explained in Part IV, Chapter 5, the reason the dose for C was set so low is that the Food and Drug Administration found out that the average diet supplies only this much. They do not want people to think they need to take supplemental C ("useless," according to them). Thus, the present U.S. RDA for C is purely political and certainly has nothing to do with what would promote optimal health. A few years ago, the FDA lowered the recommended daily dose from 60 milligrams to 45 milligrams. They have subsequently had to increase it back again due to the political fuss—they still haven't performed any experiments.

Vitamin C is an antioxidant, sensitive to air (oxygen), water, heat, and light. For longest storage life, therefore, it should be stored in a cool, dry, dark place in a tightly closed container. When vitamin C degrades, it turns darker, eventually becoming brownish and smelling burnt. Oxidized vitamin C is called dehydroascorbic acid, DHA, which has very different properties from vitamin C. In some respects, DHA is the opposite of vitamin C and has adverse effects on health. It is an oxidant and promotes free radical damage. Patterson (1950) reported that DHA can cause the development of diabetes. The easy conversion of vitamin C to DHA, especially when it is added to water or food for experimental animals' diets, may explain a few negative results with vitamin C in animal studies. Animals which have been given high doses of DHA can develop scurvy, even though they are able to make vitamin C.

Ascorbic acid   Dehydroascorbic
                                    acid

Vitamin C added to water is reduced to half the original concentration in 2 to 4 hours, the remainder having been oxidized to DHA. As a chemical naturally contained in some foods, the vitamin C may not be so accessible to air, being protected by cellular membranes (which are broken down in cooking or by mechanical means). However, the iron and copper in food stimulate oxidation reactions and thus cause C to be destroyed. Vitamin C in pills is far more stable than C in foods. But animals will not usually take tablets. In order to avoid the problems of DHA in experimental studies, vitamin C solutions could be prepared by:

1. Removing air from water by bubbling nitrogen through it, before adding the C, and

2. Having an air-tight valve on the C solution container which is operated by the animal to release drinking water (containing C) drop by drop, or

3. Adding the dry C powder to carefully dried feed powder, and changing the food very frequently.

Vitamin C in solid acidic form can be stored for years in a dry, dark place at temperatures below 86 degrees Fahrenheit.

There is a lot more to be said about vitamin C. You will find scores of other references to it in this book. We could write a whole book about C—but fortunately for us, Drs. Linus Pauling and Irwin Stone have already written four fine vitamin C books for the layman which are available in inexpensive paperback editions that are listed in Appendix A. They are a *must* for any serious life extension effort. You will be amazed and delighted with what you learn about vitamin C from these easy-to-read books.

8
Vitamin A

The formulation of a problem is often more essential than
its solution, which may be merely a matter of
mathematical or experimental skill.

—Albert Einstein

*Vitamin A does not have the romantic reputation that vita-
mins E and C have for being miracle workers. Yet vitamin A
can do many amazing things of which few people are aware.
Vitamin A is a powerful immune system stimulant, which increases the size of the thymus gland (the master gland of the
immune system) and boosts its functional capacity. Vitamin
A can prevent the decrease in size of the thymus which normally occurs after injuries. Vitamin A decreases the development of cancer in epithelial tissues (which include skin,
mucous membranes, lung and intestinal lining) in animals
exposed to cancer-causing chemicals. Vitamin A can also improve the appearance of your skin and help protect you from
viral and bacterial disease. Adequate vitamin A can apparently prevent some serious birth defects, such as spina bifida.
It is possible to take excessive amounts of vitamin A that can
cause damage, so it is a good idea to know the symptoms of
hypervitaminosis A given in this chapter. And do take a chelated zinc supplement if you take vitamin A. Zinc is required
for the liver to move vitamin A out of its storage depots.*

Vitamin A is a fat-soluble antioxidant vitamin which can
be toxic in excessively large quantities. However, there is a
wide range between the maximum physiological requirement

419

and the toxic dose. The initial symptoms of overdose (see below) disappear within one to four weeks after stopping vitamin A supplementation. This vitamin is required for vision, as part of photosensitive pigments. Inadequate vitamin A leads initially to reduced visual dark adaptation and eventually to retinal degeneration and blindness. It is also required for healing and epithelial cell (skin, mucous membrane, internal organs) growth and maintenance, helps stabilize cellular membranes, retards development of cancer in epithelial tissues (including the most common types, skin and lung cancer) and other functions. Beta carotene is pro-vitamin A, a yellow dye found in carrots and other plants. Each molecule of beta carotene is converted to two molecules of vitamin A in the body on demand. Because beta carotene is not converted to vitamin A except as the body requires it, you cannot get toxic levels of vitamin A (hypervitaminosis A) from it. Diabetics, cats, and certain other carnivores cannot convert beta carotene to vitamin A and must get A directly from their diet.

CAUTION: Excessive intake of vitamin A may result from either a chronic excessive ingestion or an acute overdose. Some arctic explorers developed hypervitaminosis A from eating polar bear or seal liver, which contained about 100 million units of vitamin A. They experienced drowsiness, irritability, headache, and vomiting a few hours later, followed by peeling of the skin. One polar explorer died from the vitamin A overdose. In children, a single dose of several hundred thousand USP units has resulted in increased intracranial pressure and vomiting, but no fatalities have been reported. Chronic poisoning may occur with doses of greater than 100,000 USP units per day for many months. (Infants may require doses of only 20,000 to 60,000 I.U. per day to develop symptoms of poisoning.) Early symptoms are: sparse coarse hair, loss of hair on the eyebrows, dry rough skin, and cracked lips (particularly at the corners). Later, severe headache and generalized weakness develop. Enlargement of spleen, liver, and kidneys may occur. Excess serum calcium is a common diagnostic indicator of hypervitaminosis A.

Vitamin A is stored primarily in the liver, but also in kidneys, lungs, gonads, and adrenals, from where it is released when needed. In order for vitamin A to be transported from the liver and other stores to the rest of the body, zinc is required. Therefore, if you intend to take vitamin A supplements, be sure to take a zinc supplement too. A dose of 50 milligrams of chelated zinc per day should be adequate. There is significant reason to believe that you require less vitamin A when you are also taking large supplements of other antioxidants, like vitamins E and C and selenium. The reason for this is that these other antioxidants can protect the vitamin A from oxidation, which is the primary reason that vitamin A disappears from circulation. You should be alert to the signs of vitamin A overdosage, even if you are not taking the huge doses of A mentioned in the preceding paragraph. Neither of the authors can take more than 15,000 to 25,000 I.U. of A per day due to the A-sparing effect of other antioxidant supplements. Before adding the other antioxidants to our diet, we could take 50,000 I.U. of vitamin A per day without problems. We now have just as much A in our systems but only need 15,000 to 25,000 I.U. per day to achieve this level.

Vitamin A is a very effective protectant of epithelial tissues like skin, gut, and lung lining from development of cancer. Retinoids, analogs of vitamin A, have been used to prevent cancer of the skin, lung, bladder, and breast in experimental animals. Vitamin A is important in controlling the differentiation (programmed development) of cells; carcinogenesis seems to involve a de-differentiation of the cells which become "transformed" (that is, become cancerous). Vitamin A has been used successfully to prevent cancer formation by certain chemical carcinogens (such as N-methyl-N-nitrosurea, as reported by Dr. Thompson and his associates; this material induces mammary cancer at high levels in animals unprotected by vitamin A).

Vitamin A is an important immune system stimulant. In vitamin A deficiency, Dr. Nauss and his co-workers reported that there was a reduced T-cell immune response. In mice inoculated with a cancer virus called Moloney Murine Sarcoma Virus, vitamin A prevented a sharp fall in numbers of white cells in the thymus gland and a rise in numbers of white blood cells in comparison with those of the control animals given a normal amount of vitamin A (in their lab chow). The thymus gland, the master gland of the immune system, drops in weight after injuries; Nauss and his associates found that vitamin A can prevent this decrease (in injury, serum may lose 5 to 10 percent of its vitamin A, liver may lose 5 percent of its A, and the thymus gland may lose 90 to 95 percent of its vitamin A content). This may be one reason why serious physical injury is so often followed by serious infection.

Beta carotene, though it is converted to vitamin A, has some unique properties of its own. A particularly activated form of oxygen, singlet oxygen, is formed in metabolism and as a result of exposure to sunlight or ozone, for example. This singlet oxygen can do considerable damage, especially to lipids (fats) and the nucleic acids DNA and RNA. Beta carotene is a quencher of singlet oxygen; that is, it reacts with the singlet oxygen, deactivating it without destruction of the beta carotene itself. Thus it can continue to react with other atoms of singlet oxygen. The specific part that singlet oxygen may play in aging has yet to be determined. However, it seems likely that it is another factor to add to the list of damaging oxidant mechanisms that contribute to aging. Beta carotene is now approved as a prescription drug for people who are abnormally photosensitive. These people have a defect in their ability to prevent and repair ultraviolet light damage to their skin; even fifteen minutes of sunlight can cause a burn or blistering. Repeated sunburns can lead to skin cancer, so this isn't merely a matter of comfort. If you sunburn easily, beta carotene (250,000 I.U. per day) plus vitamins C, E, PABA, and B-5 will probably lessen your problem. We are about three times as resistant to sunburn as we were before taking antioxidant supplements, including all of the above.

The use of very high doses of beta carotene to reduce photosensitivity does have a cosmetic drawback, however. The beta carotene will color your skin yellow (which can also occur if you eat a great many carrots), making you look jaundiced. Of course, it isn't really jaundice (caused by liver failure), and your doctor will realize it immediately when he sees that the whites of your eyes have not turned yellow. Nevertheless, you may not want to be carrot-colored. There is another carotenoid, canthaxanthin, which is very closely related to beta carotene. This is the material that makes flamingos and certain shellfish pink. We think it provides even better protection from ultraviolet light and singlet oxygen than beta carotene, and it colors the skin a beautiful natural-looking golden-copper tan when taken orally. It is currently available as Orobronze® (Rorer) in Canada for this purpose; however, it has long been used in the United States as an FDA-approved food color. We typically take our Orobronze® (brought in from Canada) with the meal having the highest fat content each day. Absorption is quite poor, and the feces will be colored bright tomato red. It literally works beautifully, but remember that this application is still experimental even though the carotenoids have a very low toxicity and are ubiquitous in plants. Acute overdose is likely to cause gastric upset, and chronic overdose will color you orange or red. This will fade away over a few weeks after discontinuing the use of Orobronze®

Any plant containing chlorophyll but no carotenoids will be killed by a few minutes of exposure to sunlight, since about one photosynthetic reaction in a thousand allows a dangerous molecule of singlet oxygen to escape. Like plants, we can protect ourselves from sunlight with carotenoids. Moreover, in some very recent reports, carotenoids appear to be remarkably effective inhibitors of carcinogenesis in humans.

9
Niacin (Vitamin B-3)

The experiment serves two purposes, often independent
one from the other: it allows the observation of new facts,
hitherto either unsuspected, or not yet well defined; and it
determines whether a working hypothesis fits the world of
observable facts.

—Rene J. Dubos

Niacin is widely used in the body as part of the natural an-
tioxidant (made in the body) called NADPH (reduced nicotin-
amide adenine dinucleotide). Without NADPH, for example,
it would be impossible for us to metabolize our food to gen-
erate the universally used energy-containing ATP molecule.
Niacin can also lower total serum cholesterol in humans (by
25 percent within two weeks on 3 grams per day), lowers se-
rum triglycerides (by 30 percent in the same study) and it re-
duces very low density lipoproteins (VLDL, associated with
increased risks of heart disease and possibly cancer). Niacin
is useful to smokers because many of its effects (widening
blood vessels, reduction of fat synthesis in the walls of arter-
ies) are just the opposite of nicotine. Niacin also provides
some protection from the free radical toxicity of the herbicide
paraquat.

Niacin (vitamin B-3), also called nicotinic acid, has wide
utilization throughout the body as part of normal metabolism.
It forms part of an important hydrogen transfer system, nicotinamide adenine dinucleotide phosphate (NADP is convert-

ed to NADPH, the hydrogenated form, and back again; in the process it transfers a hydrogen to another molecule). This biochemical is a major part of many metabolic reactions, such as the citric acid cycle which generates the universally used energy-containing ATP molecule. It also reduces and restores protective enzymes that have become oxidized in the process of destroying a dangerous oxidant, such as organic peroxides.

Niacin plays an important role in several processes essential to the maintenance of health and may have life extension effects.

Niacin is effective in reducing serum cholesterol and other lipids. In one study, 14 hypercholesteremic patients were treated with niacin as follows: 1 gram on the first day, 2 grams on the second day, and then 1 gram three times daily. Within two weeks, serum cholesterol was reduced by an average of 25 percent and triglycerides by 30 percent. In other studies, similar results were obtained over a year with 3 grams a day. Results were maintained as long as niacin was taken (for at least eight years). Niacin also reduces the VLDL, the very-low-density lipoproteins which have been associated with increased risks of cardiovascular disease and, probably, cancer. On page 768 of the standard medical text *The Pharmacological Basis of Therapeutics*, it says that "this agent [nicotinic acid] has its greatest usefulness in the treatment of patients with elevated very-low-density lipoproteins and a lesser or limited usefulness in the treatment of those with elevated low-density lipoproteins."

Niacin can be a valuable adjunct in weight reduction because it elevates and stabilizes blood sugar levels, thus mitigating the gnawing hunger and craving for sweets that can make dieting so difficult. Although niacin does raise blood sugar (by reducing glucose tolerance), it does not seem to pose a danger for diabetics. Niacin can be of benefit in cases of hypoglycemia by helping to keep blood sugar up.

Niacin has some properties which are the opposite of those of nicotine. Whereas nicotine is a vasoconstrictor (narrows blood vessels), niacin is a vasodilator (widens blood vessels). Where nicotine causes lipids (fats) to be deposited in arterial walls, niacin helps remove lipids from arteries. Thus, smokers should consider niacin as a way to help protect themselves from some of the damage smoking inflicts upon them.

Niacin has been found to reduce fluid loss in cases of severe burns.

We take over 3 grams per day of niacin primarily for psychochemical reasons. Niacin is intimately involved in brain metabolism. Large dosages of niacin, C, and B-6 have been effective in the treatment of some schizophrenics. Niacin can be used as a safe treatment for bad drug trips with LSD and other psychedelics and possibly PCP. About one hour after a dose of niacin (which may range from 1 to several grams), a hallucinating and frightened tripper may be calm and communicating. For many people, niacin can induce sleep and calm. See Part III, Chapter 4, on sleep and aging for how niacin does this.

CAUTION: Niacin has some uncomfortable, although not dangerous, side effects. It causes the skin to flush red, itch, and feel hot. This effect may last ten or twenty minutes and begin shortly after taking a dose of as little as 100 milligrams on an empty stomach. These effects are caused by dilation (widening) of blood vessels and by the release of histamine caused by niacin. Some people can become frightened, thinking they are having a stroke or heart attack. Fortunately, these side effects are not harmful. They can be reduced by taking niacin only on a full stomach and by starting with very small doses, building up the dose slowly. Tolerance usually develops to the flushing after consistently using niacin for a week or so. Although niacinamide does not cause nearly as much flushing as niacin, it also does not reduce serum lipids.

Because niacin is an acid, and because it releases gastric histamine which in turn releases stomach acid, it is important to neutralize this acidity. In some research studies with human subjects using large doses of niacin, neutralization was ignored, resulting in a few people developing ulcers from the excess acidity. This can be entirely avoided by taking the niacin *immediately* after a meal, or by taking an antacid along with it (baking soda will do a good job, but it should not be used by people on a low sodium diet or those who have essential hypertension).

As we explained previously, niacin or niacinamide may induce a temporary state of drowsiness. Adjustment of the dose or the development of a degree of tolerance after regular niacin or niacinamide use may mitigate this side effect. For further information on the use of niacin and niacinamide to replace Valium®, Librium®, Dalmane®, and other benzodiazepine anti-anxiety tranquilizers, see Part III, Chapters 2, 3, and 4, and Part II, Chapter 9.

PART V
YOUR PERSONALIZED LIFE EXTENSION PROGRAM

I
Your Biochemical Individuality

Discovery consists in seeing what everybody else has seen and thinking what nobody has thought.

—Albert Szent-Gyorgyi, Nobel laureate
who first isolated vitamin C from plants

We are all biochemically different. If we were all the same, it would be possible to take the same nutrients in the same doses and get exactly the same results. But we aren't all the same. Durk can't take RNA because he has inherited a tendency for gout. Sandy is able to use RNA because she doesn't have this problem. It is essential for you to take the time to get to know your own body and its special qualities. Talk to your relatives to find out about your heredity, conditions you may be subject to, the sorts of diseases that have killed your kin. Forewarned is forearmed. This information will help you to plan your own custom-made life extension program.

In biochemical terms, all men are created unequal. Our bodies are as different from one another as our fingerprints. The only exceptions are identical twins, who have the same genetic blueprints (DNA) and, consequently, are biochemically the same, at least in terms of their condition at birth.

Because we are all biochemically distinct, we have, among other things, different nutritional requirements, different rates of drug metabolism, and varying rates of aging. We all suffer from the same aging mechanisms but each of us has a somewhat different "blend" of aging factors that add up to our total aging rate.

429

In order to plan your own experimental life extension formula rationally, you'll want to learn as much as possible about your own physiology. For example, Dr. Clifford Odens used RNA to double the life spans of a small group of rats. But before you use it, you need to know whether your serum urate level is high. High urates (uric acid, sodium urate, sodium hydrogen urate) can be deposited as crystals in joints and kidneys in the painful and damaging disorder known as gout. Excessive RNA intake can precipitate attacks of gout, but only in susceptible individuals like Durk, particularly in males of families where gout occurs. A simple inexpensive clinical laboratory test for serum urate will tell you whether you are at risk for gout. **CAUTION:** In a well-planned human life extension experiment, it is important that you arrange for regular clinical laboratory tests, as suggested in Part V, Chapter 4. *With the help of your doctor,* you don't have to spend a lot of money to obtain useful data for monitoring your body's individual biochemical functions. An excellent book for the layman on the subject of biochemical individuality is *Biochemical Individuality,* written by the renowned biochemist Roger J. Williams, who discovered pantothenic acid (Vitamin B-5) and its life extension capability, and has been an outstanding pioneer in nutrition and vitamin research.

There are many significant biochemical differences between older and younger persons. A major difference, as discovered by Adelman, is that older people have a much slower rate of adaptability. That means that in many physiological situations requiring fast response, such as stress, it takes an older person much longer to react to the environment. As you become older (in the absence of successful intervention), your body's ability to respond to environmental stimuli becomes slower until, at some point, it is overwhelmed by a stress and you die.

The significance of the older person's slower adaptability is that a life extension nutrient program designed for a young individual would not be suitable for an older one. A young person might be able to start taking 10 grams of vitamin C a day without difficulty. An older person should begin with much smaller amounts, say a gram a day, and build up the dose little by little over a period of several weeks. This gives his or her body the opportunity to adapt gradually to the increased vitamin C levels.

Older persons often have a very different response pattern to a drug than a young person. This should be considered carefully before embarking on any type of drug-use program. For example, older people can usually tolerate a much larger dose of the prescription drug Deaner® (which increases the brain's acetylcholine) than young people, because of any or all of these factors: their lower brain levels of acetylcholine, their reduced receptor sensitivity to acetylcholine, or altered feedback in brain metabolism.

Pregnancy is a particular state of biochemical individuality. Because fetuses respond so differently to drugs than do adults, it is not yet advisable to take life extension drugs during pregnancy, except for normal doses of vitamins, minerals, and other nutrients. A simple multivitamin tablet designed for prenatal use poses no hazards to the unborn child and can help prevent some birth defects (spina bifida, for example). Vitamin B-6 has been used with success in the treatment of early-morning nausea in pregnancy. **WARNING: THIS BOOK IS NOT TO BE APPLIED TO PREGNANT WOMEN AND CHILDREN. SUBSTANCES THAT ARE SAFE FOR ADULTS CAN ADVERSELY AFFECT DEVELOPMENTAL PROGRAMS, PARTICULARLY IN A FETUS.**

Another common biochemical modification is caused by taking birth-control pills. This can result in vitamin B-6 and vitamin C depletion. The irritability and depression that sometimes occurs in women taking birth-control pills may often be mitigated by taking B-6 and C supplements.

CAUTION: People who are taking L-Dopa for Parkinson's Disease should *not* take vitamin B-6 supplements unless advised to do so by their physician. Vitamin B-6 helps convert the amino acid L-Dopa to the neurotransmitter dopamine in the brain, where such conversion is desired, but it also helps to convert L-Dopa to dopamine peripherally (outside of the brain) in the remainder of the body. If a Parkinson's patient takes large doses of vitamin B-6, so much L-Dopa may be converted peripherally that there may be undesired peripheral side effects while, at the same time, not enough L-Dopa may be available to adequately elevate dopamine levels in the brain. (L-Dopa crosses the blood-brain barrier, the selective membrane surrounding the brain and spinal cord, but dopamine does not.) This can result in a temporary worsening of Parkinsonism symptoms.

Most of the persons we know who are currently participating in life extension experiments do not have Parkinson's Disease, and many of these non-Parkinsonism patients have had a good response to ¼ to ½ gram of L-Dopa at bedtime (as indicated by fat loss and muscle buildup resulting from L-Dopa's stimulation of pituitary gland growth hormone release), even though they were also taking large doses of vitamin B-6 at the same time as they were taking L-Dopa.

WARNING: Because it takes the body time to adapt to increased intake of nutrients, it is always best to add only one new supplement at a time to your experimental life extension regimen. Remember that older people require longer to adapt. Start at low doses and work your way up over a period of at least one or two weeks for the young, several weeks for the old. Don't try to rush this process. If you do, you may have unpleasant side effects or even harm yourself.

Because of your biochemical individuality, an experimental life extension program will be most effective when it is designed for you personally. You can do that for yourself with the information in this book and the help of your doctor. Remember, there is no single "answer" to aging that fits the requirements of all people, because people are not identical and have different aging patterns.

2
How You Can Find the Right Dose for You

GROUCHO: You know what a lot is?
CHICO: Yeah, it's too much.
GROUCHO: I don't mean a whole lot, just a little lot with nothing on it.
CHICO: Every time you gotta too much, you gotta whole lot. Let me explain it to you. Sometimes you don't have a lot. Sometimes you got a little bit but somebody else thinks it's a whole lot. A whole lot ... too much ... a whole lot ... it's the same thing.

—The Marx Brothers, *Cocoanuts* (1929)*

What is the right dose for you of the different nutrients and medications we have been discussing? Instead of trying to tell you (because we don't know enough about you to do that), we explain here how to adjust your own dose.

You may wonder why we don't provide suggested doses for all the nutrients we discuss rather than telling you what amounts have been effective in experimental animals and in clinical practice, as well as what we ourselves take. There are some good reasons for this:

· We are scientists, not physicians. We are not licensed to practice medicine, nor do we have the training to do so.

· People vary greatly in their requirements for nutrients, not only because they have individual and distinct biochemistries, but also because they have different lifestyles. Our own doses are probably roughly right for us. There is no single dose that is optimal for everyone, but each person can deter-

*Copyright © by Universal Pictures, a Division of Universal City Studios, Inc. Courtesy of MCA Publishing, a Division of MCA Inc.

mine this for himself or herself, by following the steps outlined below.

• By explaining *how* to find a dose that is right for you, you can apply the technique to any nutrients or low-toxicity drugs of interest to you, whereas if we just gave you our opinion of the right dose for you, you wouldn't be able to do this for yourself.

• There are usually at least a few people who are allergic to particular drugs and chemicals, or who have a biochemical defect which results in an untoward reaction. We can't foresee who might run into these problems, but a careful method for you to find your own dose will minimize the likelihood of dangerous or undesired side effects.

• People have different evaluations of the benefits and costs of nutrients and drugs. For example, nicotinic acid (vitamin B-3, also known as niacin) causes flushing, tingling, and skin reddening for about half an hour shortly after a dose of a few hundred milligrams or more, particularly on an empty stomach. Some people like these effects, while others don't. The effects are not harmful. We happen to like them, but it's strictly a matter of individual taste. Even if you dislike them, you may take 3 grams of niacin per day anyway because you dislike your high serum cholesterol and triglycerides even more, and this dose will result in about a 25 percent reduction in these lipids.

NINE RULES FOR DOSE DETERMINATION

1. It is very important to keep good records of the substances you use, your clinical laboratory test results, and so on. If you are not good at record-keeping, do the best you can. Some records are better than none. With records, you can follow the course of your experimental life extension program to determine how you have benefitted, to adjust dosages, and add new materials to your experiment, to avoid further use of materials to which you are sensitive, and so forth. Keep these notes and all your medical records together in a single folder. Be sure that your physician has a copy of these notes in his medical records on you as well.

2. Before you begin using any new nutrients or drugs, you should have a set of clinical laboratory tests run to establish the health of your blood (which comes from your bone

marrow), kidneys and liver (which have to carry, excrete and/or metabolize all these chemicals), base lines of functions which can be altered (serum cholesterol is lowered by vitamin C, niacin, and lecithin, for example) and other standard body metabolic parameters. Two sets of suggested tests are listed in Part V, Chapter 4, on clinical laboratory tests. Consult with your doctor.

3. One of the most important rules is that you should begin taking any nutrient at the *low* end of the expected therapeutic dose range and work your dose up *slowly*. If you have no idea how much this might be, you could start with 1/20th *or less* of the nutrient dose we use, note how you feel as you use this dose for a week to several weeks, depending on your age, and then increase the dose by 50 percent or so at a time, up to a dose that you feel comfortable with. Varying the dose of many prescription drugs could be potentially hazardous, so do not make any changes without discussing this with your physician. The prescription drugs we take for life extension are generally (for normal healthy persons) without serious toxic effects at the usual dose range used. L-Dopa, at dose levels used in Parkinsonism, for example, would be much too high a dose for our life extension purposes; most people we know who use it take only ¼ to ½ gram per day (taken just before bed). Moreover, as we mentioned before, some nutrients, such as RNA, may be contraindicated, as RNA can cause gout attacks in those susceptible to it. The clinical laboratory test for serum uric acid will reveal whether you are susceptible.

4. Have clinical laboratory tests taken at intervals, such as once every three to six months, or at the very least once a year, though we would feel uneasy with this long a test interval.

5. Often a good way to find your proper dose is to continue increasing the dose *slowly* until you reach an unacceptable level of the type of harmless and reversible side effects you can get with megadoses of these low toxicity nutrients—such as diarrhea with vitamin C, intolerable flushing with niacin, tense muscles with Deaner ®, and nausea with L-Dopa. Reduce the dosage somewhat when you reach this point, until you do feel comfortable. This is often a good personalized *maximum* dosage.

6. *Don't forget to neutralize acidic vitamins* (especially C, PABA, and niacin) with antacids such as Maalox ®, common baking soda, powdered limestone (calcium carbonate), or do-

lomite. Baking soda should not be used by those who must have a low-sodium diet, such as essential hypertension patients. Take a simethicone (silicone compound) antifoam, such as GAS-X®, to break up uncomfortable carbon dioxide gas bubbles produced by the interaction of baking soda, dolomite, or calcium carbonate with the acids.

7. Under conditions of stress and/or illness, your requirements for many nutrients will be higher, including vitamins C, E, A, pantothenic acid, etc.

8. Above all, be patient. Don't try to establish your entire life extension program in one month. Don't risk impairing your health by being in a hurry. Add one new item to your regimen at a time. Change your dosage of one item at a time. Dosage increases should not exceed 50 percent at each step for nutrients and low toxicity prescription drugs. Keep your physician informed and be sure to discuss prescription dosages with him or her. Keep in mind that you are engaged in an ongoing long-term experiment. Life extension is a life-long process.

9. *How to reduce dosages.* Sometimes people want to reduce dosages of vitamins and nutrients they have been taking. Perhaps they have not received enough benefits to justify continuing to take nutrients at their original dosages. Perhaps they run into annoying or uncomfortable side effects, such as flushing with niacin. Whatever the reason, it is important to *taper off gradually* rather than stop all at once when reducing the dosages of water-soluble nutrients. That is because the body has to make metabolic adjustments to the presence of the high levels of vitamins and nutrients. It cannot adjust instantly to the lower levels that will result within hours if you stop taking these materials. For example, if a person were to suddenly discontinue taking vitamin C after using it at high doses (a gram per day or more), he might develop subclinical symptoms of vitamin C deficiency (scurvy). So, just as you should increase doses slowly over a period of time, which may amount to weeks or even months, you should usually also decrease water-soluble nutrient dosages over a period of a few days to a few weeks.

3
Sensible Medical Surveillance

According to Francis Bacon (1561–1626), the three duties of a physician are: ". . . first the preservation of health, second the cure of disease, and third the prolongation of life." ". . . [the] third part of medicine regarding the prolongation of life: this is a new part, and deficient, although the most noble of all."

Your doctor can be a great help to you in planning and carrying out your life extension program. He can prescribe useful drugs and order appropriate clinical laboratory tests for you. If your present doctor won't cooperate, you may have to "shop around" for another who will. This chapter will help you to obtain medical technology through your physician to help you stay healthy and live longer.

It is wise to have a minimum set of clinical tests performed at least once a year for vital indicators of body health such as kidney and liver function, comprehensive blood count (for possible anemia, chronic infections, bone marrow damage, or some cancers), and so on. In Part V, Chapter 4, we list a set of suggested tests for a low-cost check on general health. In addition, there are other tests you may wish to consider having done on a yearly (or more frequent) basis which include tests of immune function, also listed there. The results of these tests will help your doctor to monitor your general health and especially those conditions found in aging members of your family.

You should obtain and keep copies of all your medical tests together in one place for *your* own use. It is *not* enough that your doctor maintains a medical file of your records; you should have a copy of everything in that file. If your doctor believes that your file should be kept secret from you, we believe you should patronize another doctor.

Your doctor can be of great value in helping you be on the lookout for symptoms of conditions to which you may be more susceptible than others in your age group. You can make up a list of conditions which you may be likely to develop by finding out what medical problems your relatives have died or suffered from—information that may be hard to come by but is important because many serious but controllable diseases run in families, including diabetes, high blood pressure, hypercholesterolemia (high serum cholesterol) and related lipid metabolism defects, rheumatoid arthritis, and senility. Heredity is such an important factor in natural longevity that your life-extension program can benefit greatly if you know what types of conditions have developed in aging members of your family. If you do not have this information, ask questions until you do. Keep this information together with your other medical records, and make sure to give a copy of this list to your doctor.

The ideal doctor should not only be knowledgeable about medicine (particularly diagnosis and treatment—you will still become ill once in a while) but should carefully consider his or her patient's medical condition, as well as their level of drug knowledge when prescribing drugs. For example, your doctor should explain possible side effects of drugs prescribed. It is not necessary to find a doctor who is an expert in life-extension medications, nor are you likely to find such a doctor. What you bascially need is a doctor who is willing to consider evidence that a drug is of value for use in conditions not approved by the FDA, or at least that the drug will not harm you and may help if it is prescribed for you.

If you already have a family physician, he or she may be willing to consider new *scientific* information, even if he or she has quite properly rejected unsupported allegations of health faddists. If this is not the case, you may want to look for an open-minded doctor. First, get information from your local AMA or the state or county medical association on young doctors in your area—doctors who have been licensed recently and are, therefore, eager to build up their new practices.

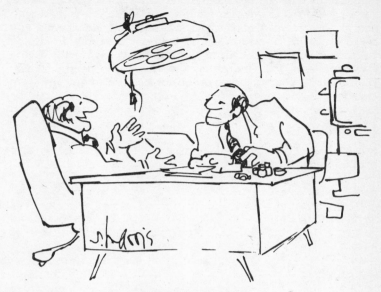

"But you can't sue me for malpractice. I'm not a doctor!"

The larger the license number, the newer the doctor. They are more likely to be flexible in considering your requests.

Next, make an appointment and visit one of these prospective doctors. Ask first for the services least likely to provoke objection, e.g., the clinical laboratory tests. Make sure that the doctor understands that you want a *copy of the test report the doctor gets from the laboratory*, not just the standard report to patients which generally contains little information beyond stating whether you had any clinical values outside the normal range. At this point, if the doctor refuses, you can leave his or her office without paying a fee since you have not received any advice.

A doctor who is willing to provide copies of your lab reports (as they are received directly from the lab) would probably be willing to consider prescribing low-toxicity prescription drugs, such as Diapid ® (vasopressin), Hydergine ®, and Deaner ® for general use, and Anturane ® for recent heart attacks, even though the official FDA indications for their use may not be met in your case. **WARNING:** Discuss your interests frankly with your prospective physician. Do not ever attempt to fool or deceive your physician; if you cannot get what you want from him or her honestly, you may be asking for the wrong thing, or simply asking the wrong doctor. Lying to your doctor isn't merely stupid—it can be deadly. If you plan to lie to your doctor, you better be sure to get burial insurance.

4
Clinical Laboratory Tests: Testing the Safety and Efficacy of Your Nutrient Supplements

Be careful about reading health books. You might die of a misprint.

—Mark Twain

Anybody who takes large doses of nutritional supplements is experimenting on himself and is a damn fool if he doesn't have regular clinical laboratory tests! Remember that nothing is absolutely safe. We don't know everything yet about the effects of taking large doses of nutrient supplements. We are pioneers in life extension and, thus, guinea pigs in a new frontier. Besides, if you want to know whether you are benefitting from your nutritional supplements, clinical laboratory tests can be of help. You should not judge your state of health by your feelings alone. Ten dollars of timely prevention can be worth more than a thousand dollars of belated cure.

People have not had the opportunity to attempt to extend their life spans by deliberate intervention in basic biochemical aging mechanisms until very recently. Knowledge of the chemical details of these mechanisms is expanding rapidly. But there is still a great deal to know before we are able to control all aspects of the aging process. The effects of any formula for life extension, no matter how safe its individual components may be for most people, should be carefully monitored by frequent clinical laboratory testing for possible toxic effects. You should have clinical laboratory tests because of individual variations between people in their responses to drugs—and don't kid yourself by thinking that large doses of vitamins and other nutrients are not drugs. In high doses, they can have additional biochemical effects beyond those at the low doses you might get in foods or even in a high potency multivitamin tablet. You should also have clinical laboratory tests because there is still much unknown about the biochemical events in aging and in normal metabolism. Moreover, your body has to adjust to the large doses of nutrients you may be taking for life extension. Clinical laboratory tests can be a great help in following this adjustment.

WARNING: In our opinion, anyone who tries to biochemically intervene in his own aging processes without adequate tests is a damn fool! *Much* more research on safety and efficacy must be done before it will be reasonable to approach biochemical life extension with the casual confidence with which you drink a glass of milk. We are looking forward to this day, but in the meantime, don't neglect clinical laboratory tests!

Following this introduction are two sets of clinical laboratory tests. One is a short and relatively inexpensive set designed by a doctor as a usually reasonably adequate screen for toxic effects. The other list contains most of the tests in the first set plus other tests for toxicity and tests which help you to see how your life extension regimen is affecting important metabolic indicators, such as serum cholesterol and lipid levels. The normal range of values is shown for all tests. These normal values are usually printed out on the laboratory test results report form and, because of variations in test procedures, may differ from those we show here. In this case, the normal values shown on the test results form should be used.

New clinical laboratory tests are being devised all the time, so these lists should be considered expandable. We have carefully considered the nutrients we use for possible chemical interference with the clinical laboratory test readings. For example, high vitamin C (and some other antioxidants, too) serum levels give false high or low sugar readings on the most widely used blood sugar and glucose tolerance tests. Once, when one of the authors (Sandy) had some clinical tests run, the printout came back and informed her that she was in a coma due to diabetic shock! In another case, the printout told her that she had died from insulin overdose. In both cases, antioxidants invalidated the blood sugar tests that were used.

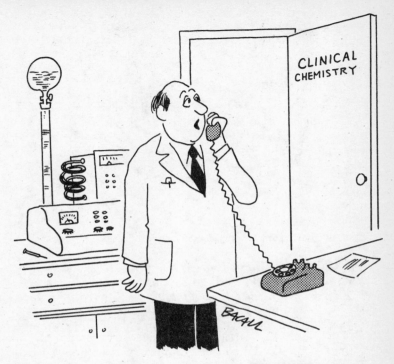

"No! I said my name is Dr. Gofman. G as in Glucose, O as in Ornithine, F as in Ferritin, M as in Methionine, A as in Acetylcholinesterase, N as in Nitrogen."

© Aaron Bacall 1981

Sandy was actually healthy, with normal blood sugar and insulin. We recommend an enzyme-based test, the hexokinase glucose determination, which is not affected by vitamin C or other antioxidants (this test is somewhat more expensive than the other more commonly used glucose tests). Do not trust the orthotoluidine or glucose oxidase blood sugar tests if you are taking megavitamins or other antioxidants.

There are a great many interactions between drugs and the chemicals measured or used in these clinical laboratory tests, far too many for us to list here. If you would like to find out more about these (you'll be better able to interpret your test results with this knowledge), you can consult:

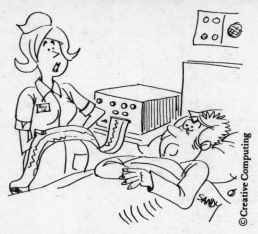

"Well, you can see right here the computer says that you're dead."

1. *Clinical Guide to Undesirable Drug Interactions and Interferences*, Solomon Garb, M.D., Springer Publ. Co., 1970

2. *Laboratory Tests in Common Use*, 5th ed., Solomon Garb, M.D., Springer Publ. Co., 1971

3. *Drug Interactions* ($3.95 each), Medical Economics Book Div., Box 149, Westwood, NJ 07675

Six other tools you can use to monitor your body's physiological condition include:

1. Blood pressure gauge. In a recent study, high blood pressure patients reduced their blood pressure by just checking their blood pressure twice a day. Forty-three percent showed a drop of at least 10 points in systolic (maximum pressure) and/or in diastolic (minimum pressure). This effect is probably due to biofeedback. A blood pressure gauge can help you assess your degree of conditioning. If you are exercising for better physical conditioning (especially cardiovascular), you can follow your progress by measuring your blood pressure. As you get into better condition, your pulse rate and blood pressure will fall, and the time required for them to return to normal after exercise will decrease. The lowest priced instruments require a fair amount of skill to use; your physician can help you. The higher priced ($100 to $200) instruments include a microprocessor which automates the process and makes it much easier to get consistently valid readings.

Extended Lifespan

JS&A was destined for failure when we introduced our first electronic blood pressure unit. But then a miracle happened.

Model 310

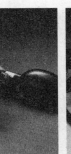

Model 410

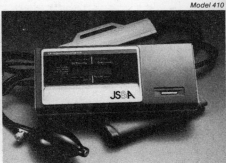

Advertisements were starting to appear everywhere. JS&A had just introduced the world's first home electronic blood pressure unit in a massive national advertising campaign.

But something was strange. JS&A often tests its products in its catalog first before they are nationally advertised. If they sell well, we then start a national magazine advertising campaign. The blood pressure unit sold well in our catalog, but for some strange reason, it wasn't selling well in magazines.

SHOCKING DISCOVERY

And then we found the answer. A few months earlier after our blood pressure unit appeared in our catalog, our computer manager (let us call him Ralph to protect his identity) handed us a computer printout of the catalog sales results.

Scanning the results, we discovered that the blood pressure unit was the best-selling product in our catalog—far exceeding every other product by five times.

The results were so positive that we immediately placed hundreds of thousands of dollars in an advertising campaign launched in early 1978.

Just as the advertisements were starting to appear, Ralph walked into our president's office with some startling news. "There's been a mistake," Ralph said. "The computer print-out was wrong. The blood pressure unit is actually our worst selling product but a computer error gave us the wrong information." -

And so our president sat back and watched JS&A advertisements appearing everywhere, knowing full well that the campaign would cost his company almost the price of a new computer.

Then came the miracle. As if by plan, the American Medical Association came out with

an advertising campaign urging consumers to take their blood pressure regularly to combat hypertension or high blood pressure. Ads appeared everywhere.

The campaign revealed that there may be as many as 25 million Americans who have high blood pressure and don't know it. Simply by taking their own blood pressure and discovering hypertension early enough, Americans could be saving their lives and reducing the chances of heart attacks. Suddenly our campaign started to sell blood pressure units by the thousands.

AWARD RECEIVED

This year JS&A's president received the Extended Lifespan award for "pioneering in the distribution of home health electronic devices" by the Committee for an Extended Lifespan. In accepting the award, our president made it very clear that the award was earned as a result of a computer error and not as a result of his brilliance.

This story is painfully true. And although it may be a slight embarrassment to us, there is one aspect that is not. JS&A was indeed the company that pioneered the electronic blood pressure units and has always selected the very best units available to offer at the very lowest prices possible.

NEWEST UNIT

Our newest unit shown above is another example. The model 310 sells for only **$69.95** plus $2.50 for postage and handling (Illinois residents, please add 6% sales tax.) You simply wrap the velcro cuff around your arm (you can even keep your shirt on) and inflate the cuff. Both an audible tone and a visible red light will indicate your systolic and diastolic readings. The system is extremely accurate, comes with a self-bleeding air valve and can be stored in a convenient carrying case that

comes with each unit.

The deluxe model 410 functions similar to the first system except that the readings are displayed in digits, and the unit also displays your pulse reading. It sells for **$139.95** plus $2.50 per unit for postage, insurance and handling. If for any reason you are not completely satisfied with either unit, you may return it within 30 days for a prompt and courteous refund including your $2.50 postage and handling. To order either unit, credit card buyers may call our toll-free number, or you may send your check or money order to the address below.

Both units use solid-state components, come complete with instructions and a one-year limited warranty, and should give you years of trouble-free service. If service should be required, we maintain a service-by-mail center as close as your mailbox. JS&A is America's largest single source of space-age products—further assurance that your modest investment is well protected.

If you are concerned about your blood pressure or know somebody who is concerned about monitoring his or hers, we recommend JS&A's latest units.

Incidentally, Ralph left JS&A on his own accord and bought a farm in another state. There were no hard feelings when he left. How could there be? Order your blood pressure unit at no obligation, today.

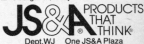

JS&A PRODUCTS THAT THINK®

Dept.WJ   One JS&A Plaza
Northbrook, Ill. 60062   (312) 564-7000
Call TOLL-FREE **800 323-6400**
In Illinois Call .... **(312) 564-7000**
©JS&A Group, Inc.,1980

2. Electronic pulse rate counters are readily available from the same vendors as blood pressure gauges (Sears, Montgomery Ward, and J S & A mail order sales). These devices are usually shirt-pocket-sized or smaller, and can be used during vigorous exercise, such as the excellent Morehouse high peak effort system (see Part III, Chapter 8). Like a blood pressure gauge, they can be used for biofeedback control of what is normally an autonomic (involuntary) function. When you lower your pulse rate by this method, you will also generally lower your blood pressure. The two of us have found that very little practice is required to will our pulse rate lower by as much as twenty beats per minute.

3. Urine densimeter—for detecting changes in specific gravity of urine. In diabetes, for example urine density is higher than normal. Kidney diseases can cause abnormally high or low urine density. We purchased a suitable device (constructed like an automobile battery acid hygrometer) for $4.95 from Amar, Inc., 1415 Highland Drive, Logan, Utah 84321.

4. Clinistrips® (available at drugstores) for detection of blood, albumin, and sugar in urine, and hidden blood in feces.

5. C-Stix® (made by the Ames division of Miles Laboratories, sold at many drugstores) measure the amount of vitamin C in your urine. You simply wet the indicator strips with a little urine, and compare the color of the strip with a chart on the C-Stix® box. C-Stix® measure urine vitamin C in its reduced, that is, its active antioxidant form over a range of zero to forty milligrams of C per deciliter (one-tenth of a liter or about four ounces of urine). This is the same as 0 to 400 milligrams of C per liter of urine. If you take very large C supplements, you may, like us, have a higher concentration of C in your urine than these strips can measure directly. It is very easy to extend the range of this test. Simpy dilute an ounce of your urine with an ounce of tap water, and double the C concentration readings given on the color chart. If you are still off the top of the scale, add two more ounces of water to the measuring cup which already contained one ounce of urine and one ounce of water, to give you a total dilution of four. You now simply multiply the color chart figures by four. If you are still off the scale, add six more ounces of water, giving you a dilution and color chart multiplication factor of ten.

The test can now measure up to four grams of C per liter of urine. This is a rough test; it is probably accurate within a factor of two most of the time. The two of us usually have urine vitamin C concentrations between roughly two to four grams per liter. We suggest about one half gram of C per liter of urine as being a reasonable goal for would-be life-extenders who do not wish to take regular clinical laboratory tests. Do not attempt to achieve our levels unless you have regular clinical laboratory tests for possible toxicity.

    6. Hemastix® (available at drugstores) will detect blood in urine, which is often not visible to the eye. Blood in urine could indicate a number of conditions, including kidney disorders, urinary tract infections, or cancer.

CLINICAL LABORATORY TESTS

SHORT SCREEN FOR TOXIC EFFECTS

WHITE BLOOD CELL count with differential; also called CBC (complete blood count)
RED BLOOD CELL count, hemoglobin level

SERUM:
  SGOT
  SGPT
  urate (uric acid)
  glucose (by hexokinase method)
  sodium
  potassium
  bilirubin
  creatinine
  BUN (blood urea nitrogen)

URINARY:
  sodium
  potassium
  cystine
  oxalate
  urate (uric acid)
  albumin
  occult blood

OTHER:
  stool guaiac test
  bleeding time

CLINICAL LABORATORY TESTS FOR
TOXICITY AND METABOLIC EFFECTS OF
LIFE EXTENSION NUTRIENTS

SERUM:
  urate (uric acid)
  glucose (hexokinase method)
  sodium
  potassium
  cholesterol, total
  cholesterol, free
  cholesterol, esterified
  total lipids
  phospholipids
  triglycerides
  total fatty acids
  free fatty acids
  albumin
  alkaline phosphatase
  acid phosphatase
  amylase
  bilirubin, total and direct
  BUN (blood urea nitrogen)
  creatinine
  CPK
  immunoglobulin electrophoresis (expensive option which
    tests some immune functions)
  LDH
  lipoprotein electrophoresis (always desirable, and essential
    if lipids are too high; this test gives the relative amounts
    of VLDL, LDL, and HDL)
  PBI
  SGOT
  SGPT
  6-GPD
  T-3
  T-4
  TSH

URINE:
    sodium
    potassium
    cystine
    oxalate
    urate (uric acid)
    albumin
    occult blood

OTHER:
    stool guaiac test
    BSP
    complete blood count, with white cell differential
    hemoglobin level
    bleeding time
    ESR (erythrocyte sedimentation rate)
    red blood cell osmotic fragility
    pulmonary macrophage sputum test (an immune assay);
        your physician can obtain a special sample mailing kit
        from the following two laboratories: Micronetic Labora-
        tories, 1420 Koll Circle, San Jose, CA 95112, (408) 297-
        7711. (Micronetic Laboratories provides a photomicro-
        graph of the specimen as well as a pathologist's evalua-
        tion); and California Micropathology Associates, 16311
        Ventura Blvd., Suite 860, Encino, CA 91436, (213) 995-
        7787.

There are many additional tests for immune function; however, the availability of particular tests depends on the clinical testing laboratory patronized by your physician. Almost any lab can test for rheumatoid factor, antinuclear antigen, sheep red blood cell rossette test, etc., but many labs only report whether the response is normal or abnormal. While this is often adequate for confirming a diagnosis of disease, *quantitative* data is much more useful for your personal life extension experiment. It may be necessary for your physician to refer you to an immunologist for a research quality immunological assay panel.

CLINICAL TEST	WHAT IT MEASURES/ NORMAL VALUES (*note:* normal values differ, depending on the specific test procedure used)	REASON FOR TEST
URIC ACID	blood uric acid: 3 to 7 milligrams per 100 milliliters of serum	diagnosis of gout (check before using RNA)
GLUCOSE (hexokinase method)	glucose in serum: fasting: 70 to 100 milligrams per 100 milliliters of whole blood	check glucose metabolism—can detect diabetes, liver disease
CHOLESTEROL	fasting: total lipids: 400 to 800 milligrams per 100 milliliters phospholipids: 150 to 380 milligrams per 100 milliliters total cholesterol: 120 to 260 milligrams per 100 milliliters free cholesterol: up to 50 milligrams per 100 milliliters cholesterol esters: up to 210 milligrams per 100 milliliters triglycerides: 25 to 150 milligrams per 100 milliliters free fatty acids: 0.3 to 1.0 mEq per liter	check lipid metabolism
HDL (high-density lipoproteins) LDL (low-density lipoproteins)	fractions of serum lipids	HDL is protective: low ratio of HDL/LDL reveals high risk of heart disease; high LDL is associated with high risk of heart disease. See Appendix L.
ALBUMIN, SERUM	ordinarily, albumin does not pass from blood into the urine; 4 to 5 grams per 100 milliliters of serum is normal	detects kidney disease, hypertension, heart failure, liver damage

Test	Normal values	Description
SERUM ALKALINE PHOSPHATASE	normal values: *units* *adults* *children* King-Armstrong 4–13 15–30 Bodansky 1.5–4.5 5–14 Bessy-Lowry .8–2.3 2.8–6.7	large amounts of this enzyme may indicate bone or liver diseases, leukemia, rickets, or other condition; levels are also elevated during pregnancy
SERUM AMYLASE	amylase, an enzyme which breaks down starches into sugars; 4 to 25 units per milliliter	can detect pancreatic diseases, mumps, intestinal obstruction
SERUM BILIRUBIN (van den Bergh's test)	bilirubin is a yellow bile pigment (secreted by the liver) and normally not found in urine; normal serum values are 0.4 milligrams per 100 milliliters direct, 0.7 milligrams per 100 milliliters total	a liver function test: elevated levels of bilirubin indicate liver disease
BSP (bromsulphalein retention)	less than 0.4 milligrams of bromsulphalein per 100 cc. of serum; less than 5 percent retention	tests for liver function: the normal liver removes about 80 percent of an injected dose of bromsulphalein
BUN (blood urea nitrogen)	8 to 25 milligrams of urea nitrogen per 100 milliliters of blood	tests kidneys—blood urea concentration should be fairly low
CPK (creatine phosphokinase)	an enzyme found in cardiac and skeletal muscle; normal range is 5 to 25 units per milliliter of serum for females, 5 to 35 units per milliliter of serum for males	this enzyme rises in myocardial infarction (heart attack) and may be 300 to 400 times normal in early muscular dystrophy
LDH (lactic dehydrogenase)	enzymes found in serum and several organs, including the heart; 60 to 100 units per milliliter of serum	an aid in the diagnosis of myocardial infarction (heart attack). High levels are also found in leukemia, liver disease, and several types of cancer.

CLINICAL TEST	WHAT IT MEASURES/ NORMAL VALUES (*note:* normal values differ, depending on the specific test procedure used)	REASON FOR TEST
PBI (protein bound iodine)	3 to 8 micrograms per 100 cc. serum	a test of thyroid function: the thyroid gland binds iodine
SGOT (serum glutamic, oxaloacetic transaminase)	10 to 40 units per milliliter	in myocardial infarction, the enzyme GOT in heart muscle cells leaks out, elevating serum levels 4 to 10 times; in liver disease, serum levels may be 10 to 100 times normal
SGPT (serum glutamic pyruvic transaminase)	5 to 40 units	detects liver disease
BLOOD COUNT with WBC differential	counts total numbers of red and white blood cells and the proportions of particular types of white blood cells; normal ranges are: red cells, 4,200,000 to 5,900,000 per cubic millimeter; white cells, 4800 to 10,800 per cubic mm.; white blood cells types: neutrophiles 54 to 62% eosinophiles 1 to 3% basophiles 0 to 1% lymphocytes 25 to 33% monocytes 0 to 9%	red blood cells carry hemoglobin, the oxygen transporting substance; white blood cells are important parts of the immune system
BLEEDING TIME	skin is punctured and bleeding is timed; normal is 1 to 6 minutes	test for normal clotting

Test	Description	Clinical Significance
ESR (erythrocyte sedimentation rate)	measures the rate at which erythrocytes (red blood cells) settle to the bottom of a glass test tube; normal values (by Westergren's method): men 0 to 15 millimeters per hour, women 0 to 20 millimeters per hour	useful in diagnosing such illnesses as rheumatic fever, arthritis, and heart attack
HEMOGLOBIN LEVEL	hemoglobin is the oxygen carrier in red blood cells 12 to 18 grams per 100 cc. of blood	diagnosis of anemia
STOOL GUAIAC TEST		detects blood in feces
CREATININE	measurement of kidney function (vitamin C can cause false high readings); normal, 0.6 to 1.3 per 100 cc. of serum	elevation of creatinine level indicates kidney disorder
CYSTINE	test for excessive cystine, the oxidized form of the amino acid cysteine, in the urine	excessive cystine in urine can lead to kidney stones
OXALATE	test for excess oxalate in urine	excessive amounts of oxalate can lead to kidney stones
ACID PHOSPHATASE, SERUM		a nonspecific indicator of tissue damage, commonly used to detect metastic cancer of prostate in men
GLUCOSE-6-PHOSPHATE DEHYDROGENASE		nonspecific indicator of tissue damage; acute hemolytic anemia can develop in deficient patients

5
How to Ask Your Doctor for a Prescription

I would like to die as young as possible and as late as possible!

—La Rochefoucauld

Before your doctor can give you a prescription that may be needed for a non-FDA approved use, he or she must ascertain that recent research warrants it. You can help your physician and yourself by learning more about such uses.

First, let's consider some reasons doctors may have for denying you a prescription for a low toxicity drug. Then we can decide how best to rationally respond to these objections.

1. The doctor may be concerned about a malpractice lawsuit for prescribing a drug for a non-FDA-approved use. Such fears are all too well justified.

2. The doctor may be unwilling to consider a new use for a drug unless another doctor of greater authority says it's OK.

3. The doctor thinks you may be careless and ignorant of the drug's effects and possible side effects.

The best approach is to arm yourself with knowledge about the drugs you want that may be beneficial in order to handle these objections. Basically, the doctor is concerned that you will get yourself into medical trouble using the drug and perhaps also that he or she will be blamed and sued for malpractice.

Buy yourself a copy of the *Physician's Desk Reference* (see references list), which lists prescription drugs of the United States, along with information about drug safety, including contraindications, adverse drug interactions, toxicity, side effects, etc. Your doctor already has a copy of this book, and trusts it. However, the PDR does not contain information about non-FDA-approved uses of these drugs. If you want to obtain such information to convince your doctor to prescribe it for you, you'll need to look up some of the literature references given in the appendix of this book. You can get copies of these papers in any large medical or life sciences library. Also, you can write to the manufacturers of the drugs you're interested in, asking for reprints of research papers on their effects.

Don't expect your doctor to know about the life extension uses of prescription drugs approved for other uses or to be familiar with the research papers you may show him. The pharmaceutical companies are legally prohibited from informing physicians of such FDA-non-approved uses. Most doctors, moreover, are not scientists. With the information you have collected, however, you can demonstrate that 1. the drug you want is low in toxicity and you know how to use it, and 2. you intend to use the drugs in a responsible manner, having clinical laboratory tests run before and while using them to monitor for possible adverse side effects that you have read about in the PDR and research papers.

You are used to thinking of your doctor as an authority figure, rather than as an expert professional for hire that you patronize. But it's not too late to re-direct your thinking into the more productive latter channel. A good physician should be guided by scientists, his or her own clinical experience, and the laws of economics, not by bureaucrats.

Here is an example of the value of the PDR: Sandy's mother, who is 63, was having severe shoulder pains due to arthritis. Her doctor prescribed Butazolidin®. Shortly after starting on this drug, she found her shoulder pain lessened, but a new symptom had appeared—painful swelling (edema) in her arms and ankles. She did not know what was causing this and was very concerned. She couldn't sleep at night because of pain in her swollen arms. These symptoms vanished promptly after discontinuing this drug. Her doctor had failed to warn her of this side effect, which is potentially serious, even fatal (congestive heart failure can result). Sandy's father thought the swelling might be due to the vitamins her mother had recently started taking. In just a few minutes, Sandy discovered the cause of the problem using our PDR. The

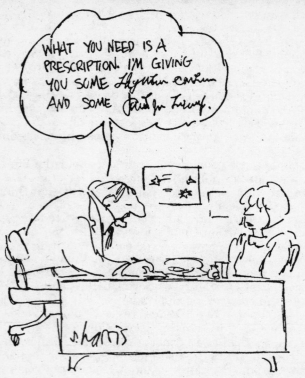

physician was notified, the offending medication was discontinued, and the edema promptly vanished, possibly saving her mother's life. Many people have safely used Butazolidin ® and benefited from doing so. The point of this story is that every person has individual biochemistry and therefore it is important to be aware of possible adverse reactions to any drug. With your own PDR, you'll know the side effects of medications you use. (If you tend toward hypochondria, you can have a friend read the section on a drug you're using and, if you begin to experience unusual symptoms, you can ask your friend whether this is one of the drug's side effects.) It is an unfortunate fact that doctors, in our experience, often do not provide data to patients about the possible side effects of the drugs they prescribe. The PDR, which contains this information, is a valuable reference work.

You may also want to buy a good medical dictionary—for example, *Dorland's Illustrated Medical Dictionary.*

If your physician says no to one of your prescription requests, you should be neither angry nor cowed. Ask for an explanation of the objections. In some cases, you will find that the objections are valid. In other cases, the objections will be based on lack of knowledge of the new non-FDA approved uses for old drugs. Then, you should give your doctor copies of the relevant papers. Your doctor is apt to be extremely busy, so don't just give him the literature citation (author, title, journal, page, date); it is your responsibility to provide full copies of these scientific papers. We tell you how to get these documents in Appendix B.

Keep the magnitude of your request within reason. You cannot expect physicians to ignore their other duties while they spend a full day reading a big stack of research papers on several different drugs. If there are objections to your request, limit your discussion and research literature substantiation to one drug at a time. You should make it clear that you recognize that your physician's time is valuable and that you are prepared to pay for it, even if it merely involves his or her reading a research paper. There is no such thing as a free lunch. Finally, if you find a physician with a personal interest in clinical research or life extension or free radical pathology, or simply new-but-non-FDA-approved uses for old familiar drugs, you will have found the best possible professional assistance for your personal experiment in life extension. It really pays to look around and make ceaseless inquiries until you find the help you need.

6
Keeping a File of Your Own Medical Records

Science is never merely knowledge; it is orderly knowledge.

—Josiah Royce

Documentation is essential, in any complex undertaking. It is through medical records and tests that you can map the alterations you are attempting to bring about in your body. You want to know where you started and enough details of the path you've followed to be able to assess your success in slowing your own aging. Enthusiasm is essential, but it is not a substitute for facts.

Aging, as we know, accelerates with time. Your utilization of effective life extension procedures should slow your rate of aging. In order to intelligently assess the benefits/costs ratio for particular life extension treatments, it is necessary that clinical laboratory tests be performed both BEFORE beginning any particular treatment or collection of treatments and DURING these treatments at regular intervals (at a very minimum, once a year when on a constant regimen, every 3 months during startup). Without such records, it is nearly impossible to know what is actually going on in your body, e.g., should you increase or decrease treatment A or treatment B and by how much?

In the chapter on clinical laboratory tests, we provide suggested test sequences for following particular life extension effects, checking for proper functioning of liver, kidneys, and other organs. We suggest both a low cost test combination and a more complex (and consequently, more expensive) set of tests you can consider for yourself. There is little point in embarking on an experimental life extension regimen that we have used on ourselves unless you are able to determine what it can do for YOU. The particular benefit/cost ratio for life extension therapies differs among individuals, as we point out in Part V, Chapter 1, "Your Biochemical Individuality."

Keep a diary of your mood changes (depression can cause immune system depression), increased stresses, illnesses, sleeping and eating habits, changes of diet or hazardous lifestyle activities (e.g., smoking, drinking), exercising, physical exams, medication and your personal experimental life extension regimen (vitamins, nutrients, and prescription drugs you take).

You should see to it that you receive a copy of all your medical records from your doctor. Many doctors are willing to cooperate in this respect. If yours won't, get another doctor. The data from clinical laboratory tests should be kept together in a single folder where you can consult them to assess your life extension experiment. Without these data, you don't know how much you are getting for your time and money or even whether you are getting benefit or harm. Your doctor is trained as a craftsman, not as a scientist, and it is very unlikely that he or she has any knowledge of or experience in anti-aging therapies. Some anti-aging substances, such as vitamin C, can affect certain clinical laboratory tests by chemically interacting with the constituents of the test, yielding a result that can be misinterpreted by physicians unfamiliar with these interactions. Some such clinical tests are described in our chapter on that subject. Hence, you cannot rely on an inexperienced opinion. Many doctors will be more than happy to order the tests for you and send along the results and their comments; you only need to make sure you have such a doctor.

Even if you don't plan to start a personal experimental life extension program immediately, it is a good idea to have a series of clinical laboratory tests done at least once a year and to keep all your medical records together. If you move, it will be more difficult to get your medical data from your old doctor (who may even throw out such records after a few years). Your medical history is every bit as much a part of your "roots" as a genealogical chart. How can you know where you are going if you don't know where you are or where you've been?

7
Our Current Personal Experimental Life Extension Formula

Aging and death do seem to be what Nature has planned for us. But what if we have other plans?

—Bernard Strehler, biological gerontologist

In this chapter, we examine a sophisticated experimental life extension formula—our own. The way we have developed this formula over twelve years—and it is still developing—is to study mechanisms of aging that exist in man and other animals, search the literature for successful methods of chemical intervention in each mechanism, then study the toxicology of possible life extension materials, and, finally, consider the physiological and economic expenses of the materials involved. We have put together an experimental multicomponent formulation active to varying degrees against all presently known mechanisms of aging, possibly even including some aging clocks.

We take most of our nutrients as powders, buying them directly from their manufacturers. The reason for this is, first, the doses of most components are large enough that using tablets would be inconvenient (perhaps even mechanically irritating) and require ingestion of a lot of unnecessary and potentially allergenic tablet fillers, and, second, powders are much less expensive than tablets. Be particularly wary of vitamin E esters in oil capsules. Many vitamin manufacturers add oil to their capsules to make them larger. Tocopherol (vitamin E) esters are not good antioxidants until they are de-esterified in your body. Hence, the accompanying oil is often autoxidized (rancid). We use vitamin E acetate (an ester) on a hydrolized protein carrier designed for direct compression tabletting from Roche. As we have warned repeatedly in earlier chapters, however, *no one should start their personal life extension experiment at our dose levels.*

Moreover, we have also warned that anyone embarking on a biochemical life extension experiment is a damn fool if he or she doesn't take regular clinical laboratory tests to monitor for possible toxic effects. (See Part V, Chapter 4.)

At lower dose levels, tablets may generally be used without difficulty, except in the case of allergies to fillers or binders and the case of vitamin C and niacin—doses as low as 500 milligrams can irritate the stomach (C and niacin are strong acids). We use vitamin C crystals and niacin powder because they dissolve quickly and do not sit in acid lumps on the stomach as tablets do. You can also neutralize acidity of vitamins like C and niacin with antacids (such as baking soda) or take the non-acidic sodium ascorbate form of vitamin C, especially if you use time-release capsules or tablets. **CAUTION:** People with essential hypertension or on a low sodium diet should not use baking soda or sodium ascorbate.

Following is our personal experimental life extension formula, including the reasons why we include each component, and, in Appendix K, references to primary scientific literature on effects of the nutrients. Most of the components of our formulation are available as tablets from health food stores and other vitamin vendors. A few of them are approved only as food additives at limited dosages but not as dietary supplements (for example, BHT, an antioxidant food additive). Yet others are prescription drugs (a good doctor can help you— see Part V, Chapter 5 on the subject). Quantitative data on our personal doses are given in Appendix G. Remember, these are doses which we have built up over the years, not doses for people just beginning their own life extension program. **WARNING:** Do not assume that because these huge doses seem to be safe for us that they are safe for you. Get regular clinical laboratory tests! Following the details of our formulation, we discuss what we would do if we wanted to start taking these materials as beginners (starting doses, precautions, etc.) We have also put together a second formulation of a less extreme nature which is more appropriate for the novice life extender.

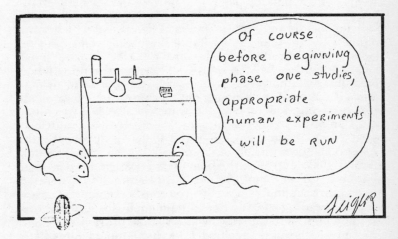

A word of explanation concerning our high vitamin B-3 (niacin, nicotinic acid) intake. Our dose is 11 grams per day, a dose few people will want to take. In our cases, the B-3 is being taken, in large part, for beneficial psychopharmacological effects, and also because B-3 reduces serum cholesterol and VLDL (very low density lipoproteins, a fraction of blood lipids associated with heart disease risk). At a dose of 3 grams per day in humans, serum cholesterol was reduced by 26 percent after a year. In another study, comparable results were obtained with doses of 3 grams per day after only 3 weeks. Many people dislike B-3's side effects—flushing, itching, and turning red—while others actually enjoy them. Although niacinamide has many of niacin's effects and the advantage of much less flushing, it does not reduce serum cholesterol, unlike niacin.

How long do we expect to live? We just don't know. Although we believe aging mechanisms to be essentially the same among all animals (and perhaps plants, too), the relative contributions of the mechanisms to each species' aging is still largely unknown. Therefore, while we expect to live well beyond the normal three score and ten, we can't really predict how long we'll live. Ask us again in 100 years!

We take the nutrient mix in 4 doses each day, one after each meal and one before bed. The reason that the doses are spread out through the day is that most of the nutrients in the mix are water soluble and, therefore, are excreted rapidly. You can do a simple demonstration of the rate at which water soluble vitamins (like the B vitamins) are excreted from your body. Take a 50 milligram vitamin B-2 tablet. In about a half hour, your urine will be bright yellow from elimination of some of the vitamin B-2. Note the color of your urine as time passes. In about 3 or 4 hours, your urine will be pale again, demonstrating how quickly the water soluble B-2 was eliminated. In order to keep serum levels elevated, you must take more. Linus Pauling has suggested that it is apparently the *lowest* daily serum levels of vitamin C (another water-soluble vitamin) that determine the benefits that can be derived from vitamin C, rather than the highest daily serum levels. In order to maximize vitamin C benefits, you must take vitamin C several times during the day to maintain adequate serum levels. This also applies to the other water soluble nutrients.

Unless otherwise specified, take supplements immediately after meals *only*, at least for the first few weeks. That fourth dose to be taken at bedtime on an empty stomach is likely to be rather upsetting until your body acclimates to the nutrients. By taking the nutrients with meals, their absorption will be initially retarded, thereby reducing acclimation problems such as gastro-intestinal upsets. When you do start taking the fourth (bedtime, empty stomach) dose, begin at about ¼ of your regular mealtime dose.

NOT RECOMMENDED FOR GENERAL USE
NOT FOR CHILDREN OR PREGNANT WOMEN

OUR PERSONAL EXPERIMENTAL LIFE EXTENSION FORMULA
(for amounts taken daily, see Appendix G)

mixed together as powders:
  vitamin E (dl-alpha tocopherol acetate)
  vitamin C (ascorbic acid)
  ascorbyl palmitate (lipid soluble form of vitamin C)
  beta carotene (pro vitamin A)
  vitamin B-1 (thiamine HCl)
  vitamin B-2 (riboflavin)
  vitamin B-3 (niacin)
  vitamin B-5 (calcium pantothenate)
  vitamin B-6 (pyridoxine HCl)
  vitamin B-12 (cyanocobalamin)
  PABA (p-aminobenzoic acid, a B vitamin)
  L-arginine (amino acid)
  L-cysteine (amino acid)
  hesperidin complex (bioflavonoid)
  rutin (bioflavonoid)
  zinc (chelated as the gluconate)
  selenium (as sodium selenite)
  dilauryl thiodipropionate (food additive antioxidant)
  thiodipropionic acid (food additive antioxidant)

taken separately:
  vitamin A
  inositol
  extra L-arginine or L-ornithine (amino acids, taken at bed-
    time)
  tryptophan (amino acid, bedtime)
  L-Dopa (prescription amino acid, bedtime)
  bromocriptine (Parlodel®, Sandoz)
  choline chloride (B vitamin)
  Deaner® (Riker)
  Hydergine® (Sandoz)
  vasopressin (Diapid® nasal spray, Sandoz)
  BHT (food additive antioxidant)
  RNA (not for those susceptible to gout)

If we were just beginning to take this formula, we would do so at a gradual rate. We would begin by taking the nutritional supplements, leaving the food additives for later experimentation. Before starting we would have a set of clinical laboratory tests run to determine the general condition of our bodies, including kidney, liver, and bone marrow function, serum lipids (cholesterol, HDL/LDL, etc.), immune function, etc. (See Part V, Chapter 4 on clinical laboratory tests for specific sets of tests and why.) We would start at a dose of about 1/20th (or less) of our present dose. The dosages could be increased slowly over a few weeks to a few months, taking longer for older persons. We would repeat clinical laboratory tests at regular intervals—preferably every six to ten weeks while increasing the dosage, and no fewer than once each year when on a constant regimen. A *minimum* goal for information could be obtained by having the clinical laboratory tests run just before beginning supplements, then a month later and again four to six months after starting the program, followed by tests once a year or so. This would provide a picture of what changes are taking place in those functions measured by the tests. For example, we expected our formula to greatly lower serum lipids, including cholesterol, on the basis of experiment and theory. This has been just what has occurred in ourselves and others using this mix. (An initial elevation of serum cholesterol may be noted while old deposits are dissolved and carried in the bloodstream for removal from the body).

Clinical laboratory tests can reveal tendencies toward metabolic defects or idiosyncrasies that limit use of some nutrients. For example, gout is a hereditary and painful disease affecting primarily males in which uric acid and its salts accumulate in serum and eventually deposits crystals in joints and kidneys. If you have such a tendency toward gout, you probably cannot take RNA supplements, because RNA is converted in the body to uric acid. The clinical laboratory test for serum urate will reveal whether you have this trait or not.

If you include clinical laboratory tests for serum levels of vitamins C, E, and thiamine, you can determine your own personal use pattern of these materials, that is, the serum levels you get for particular oral dose levels. Sometimes it is possible for scientists to get insights into your personal biochemical pathways from examination of such oral dose/serum level patterns. For example, some schizophrenics require far larger doses of niacin, B-6, and C to maintain normal serum levels compared to non-schizophrenics.

We didn't mention one further fact about our nutrient mix: it tastes awful! (We know of three people who liked the taste, two of whom were grossly vitamin C deficient.)

CAUTION: Persons with diabetes mellitus (sugar insulin diabetes) should use large doses of vitamins C and B-1 and the amino acid cysteine with caution and *only* under the supervision of their physician. This nutrient combination is capable of inactivating insulin by reducing some disulfide bonds, including one or more of the three disulfide bonds that determine insulin's tertiary (three-dimensional) structure. We have clinical laboratory serum glucose determinations—USE HEXOKINASE METHOD ONLY—on about two dozen nondiabetic adults using these nutrients, and all serum glucose levels have been normal, and all urine samples have been sugar free. We have *not* seen test results showing its effects on diabetics.

A PRELIMINARY EXPERIMENTAL LIFE EXTENSION FORMULA

Our personal experimental formula is definitely advanced—not for beginners; that is, there are few if any people taking larger doses of many of these materials. We are human guinea pigs, and we have ourselves tested as such. Below is a more moderate experimental formula. In most cases, a significant number of people have taken doses of these nutrients which are as large or larger for a year or more. Relatively few people, however, have taken a combination of this sort. **CAUTION:** Even with this moderate formula, you are still a self-selected guinea pig—so treat yourself accordingly and take the clinical laboratory tests regularly, along with your doctor's consultations. You are a damn fool if you don't. Do not start at these doses—work up to them slowly (see "How You Can Find the Right Dose for You," Part V, Chapter 2). We would be rather surprised if this formula would significantly increase maximum life span (110–120 for a human). We think it very plausible, however, that this formula would significantly extend the average human lifespan, especially the youthful and middle age portions, and that it would very significantly reduce the risks of cardiovascular disease (heart attack, atherosclerosis, and stroke), cancer, infection, autoimmune diseases (such as arthritis), senility, loss of vigor, strength, flexibility, and sexuality, and help prevent old age depression. This is a formula for helping to "square the survival curve" (see Part I, Chapter 2).

THIS EXPERIMENTAL FORMULA IS *NOT* FOR CHILDREN OR PREGNANT WOMEN. WE HAVE MADE NO ATTEMPT TO EVALUATE SAFETY FOR THEM

Once Per Day

vitamin A	10,000 to 20,000 I.U.
beta carotene (pro vitamin A)	25-100 milligrams
vitamin E acetate (dl-alpha tocopherol acetate)	500 I.U. to 2,000 I.U.
selenium	250 micrograms
zinc (chelated as the gluconate)	50 milligrams
L-arginine	3 grams at bedtime
tryptophan	2 grams at bedtime
L-Dopa (prescription)	¼ gram (middle aged) to ½ gram (older) at bedtime
Deaner ® (Riker) (prescription)	Up to 300 milligrams—must be individualized
choline chloride	1 to 3 grams
RNA	2 grams—not for people with elevated serum uric acid or urates
vitamin B-12	500 micrograms
High Potency Multivitamin with chelated minerals	1 per day (this will most likely supply the 10,000 to 20,000 I.U. of A listed above)

The following are total amounts taken per day. They should be divided into four doses; one taken after each meal, and one before bed. Remember to use antacids along with the acid vitamins, particularly when taken on an empty stomach.

vitamin B-1, thiamine HCl	250 to 500 milligrams
vitamin B-2, riboflavin	100 to 200 milligrams
vitamin B-3, nicotinic acid (niacin; not niacinamide)	3 grams
vitamin B-5, (calcium pantothenate)	1 gram to 2 grams
vitamin B-6, pyridoxine HCl	250 to 500 milligrams
rutin	500 milligrams to 2 grams
Hesperidin Complex	500 milligrams to 2 grams
PABA	1–2 grams (discontinue PABA while taking sulfa drugs; it nullifies their effectiveness)
L-cysteine (not cystine)	1 gram to 2 grams (take at least three times as much of vitamin C as you take of cysteine)
vitamin C	3 to 10 grams
inositol	1 to 3 grams
Hydergine ® (Sandoz) (prescription)	Individualized—up to 12 milligrams (Note: FDA says 3 milligrams). See Part V, Chapter 11 to avoid substitution.
Diapid ® (Sandoz, vasopressin) (prescription)	Individualized, 16 I.U./day generally safe except for angina sufferers, considerably more can usually be safely used. Note: This is primarily to improve cognitive performance although there is some evidence for life extension with this and oxytocin, a closely related polypeptide.
Sex hormone replacement (prescription—optional, but frequently desirable for post-menopausal women)	Must be individualized with the help of your doctor— see Part III, Chapter 5.

HOW TO REDUCE DOSAGES

Sometimes people want to reduce dosages of vitamins and nutrients they have been taking. Perhaps they have not received enough benefits to justify continuing to take nutrients at their original dosages. Perhaps they run into annoying or uncomfortable side effects, such as flushing with niacin. Whatever the reason, it is important to *taper off gradually* rather than stop all at once when reducing the dosages of water-soluble nutrients. That is because the body has to make metabolic adjustments to the presence of the high levels of vitamins and nutrients. It cannot adjust instantly to the lower levels that will result within hours if you stop taking these materials. For example, if a person were to suddenly discontinue taking vitamin C after using it at high doses (a gram per day or more), he might develop subclinical symptoms of vitamin C deficiency (scurvy). So, just as you should increase doses slowly over a period of time which may amount to weeks or even months, you should usually also decrease water-soluble nutrient dosages over a period of a few days to a few weeks.

ANNOTATIONS ON SOME FORMULA COMPONENTS

ZINC is required for growth and healing. It is part of the enzyme superoxide dismutase, which controls oxygen free radicals that form peroxides, and is required for mobilization of vitamin A from its stores in the liver.

Zinc's effects on the peroxidation of fats have been studied. Rats were fed zinc at levels of 40 and 1000 ppm (parts per million) in their diet and only half of the usual amount of vitamin E (5.5 grams of dl-alpha tocopherol per 100 kilograms of diet). The amount of malonaldehyde (formed during lipid peroxidation) and rupture of red blood cells (among other indicators of lipid peroxidation) were measured. Spontaneous rupture of red blood cells was inhibited in the rats fed 1,000 ppm zinc diet. The zinc, therefore, acts as a membrane stabilizer. The high zinc diet also resulted in significant inhibition of malonaldehyde formation in the liver. Zinc is a constituent of the enzyme superoxide dismutase (SOD), which reacts with superoxide radicals in your body to prevent their damaging cellular structures. Thus, zinc's effects on lipid peroxidation may be connected with its role as a part of SOD.

The antioxidant effects of zinc are probably why it is sometimes useful in preventing hair loss, dandruff (Head and Shoulders®), and loss of taste and smell.

PARLODEL® (bromocriptine), a prescription drug made by Sandoz, is a powerful but selective dopaminergic stimulant—it has fewer side effects than L-Dopa. It can often be used to replace about half of L-Dopa in those using L-Dopa for Parkinsonism and result in about as much benefit with fewer side effects and frequently with less long-term degeneration. Parlodel® stimulates release of growth hormone (GH) when there is too little GH, but normalizes GH levels when too high. It suppresses release of prolactin, a hormone which supports milk production in females and has a role in immune system inhibition. It has a demonstrated ability to reset some neuroendocrine aging clocks. **WARNING:** It is very important that women past menopause who take this drug use contraception since menstrual cycling may be restarted. Children conceived late in life have an extremely high incidence of genetic errors and birth defects.

SELENIUM is an important antioxidant mineral which forms part of your enzyme glutathione peroxidase. Each molecule of this enzyme must contain four atoms of the trace element selenium. This enzyme protects the body from peroxides by breaking them down without releasing uncontrolled free radicals. Tissues which contain high levels of polyunsaturated fats should also contain high levels of glutathione peroxidase.

Selenium has been shown to inhibit carcinogenesis (the production of cancer). It is synergistic with vitamin E (their combined effects are greater than additive) and sulfur-containing amino acids such as cysteine. Selenium should be taken as inorganic sodium selenite rather than as organic compounds such as selenocystine or selenomethionine. The reason for this is that the body cannot distinguish between selenocystine and sulfur-containing cysteine and could improperly substitute selenocysteine for cysteine in protein construction, and similarly for methionine and its seleno-analog. Such substituted proteins may not function properly due to the differing spatial electronic properties between normal sulfur-containing cysteine and selenocysteine. These substitutions do not occur with moderate doses of inorganic sodium selenite, as long as the animal does not have a severe sulfur amino acid (methionine and cysteine) deficiency. The usual early symptom of selenium toxicity is garlic breath, urine, and sweat. Selenium's antioxidant effects are probably why it is often useful in stopping hair loss and dandruff, both when taken internally and in selenium-containing shampoos (such as Selsun Blue ®). (See Appendix K for a selenium containing yeast that works as well as sodium selenite.)

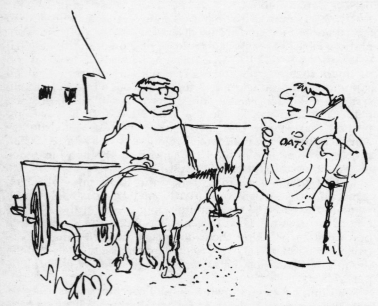

"With the new, vitamin-enriched formula, you'll get an additional five miles per feed bag."

VITAMIN B-2 is a yellow, water-soluble B vitamin which is essential in regulating oxidation of food in your body. In addition, it is required in the making of glutathione reductase, an enzyme which is used to recycle one of your body's important antioxidants, cysteine-containing reduced glutathione.

RNA, ribonucleic acid, is an important cellular macromolecule which exists as several distinct types to fulfill its many functions. One type of RNA carries genetic information from cellular DNA to cell polyribosomes, where proteins are manufactured. Many scientists think that RNA is the molecule on which memories are stored for long periods of time.

RNA is of value in a life extension program. It was discovered to increase the life span of white mice by about 16 percent when fed at a dose of 25 milligrams per day in an experiment by Robertson in 1928. In another experiment (Gardner, 1946), old mice already 600 days old received 2.5 milligrams per day of yeast RNA and lived 7–8 percent longer than untreated mice. The treated animals retained vigor longer, did not lose weight before death like the controls (no RNA supplements), and fewer treated mice went blind. RNA is an antioxidant and can, therefore, slow aging caused by free radicals and other oxidants.

The quantity of RNA in the brain decreases with age. This contributes to failing mental function, especially loss of memory. RNA has improved memory and learning in some mental function tests. Vitamin B-12 increases brain cell manufacture of RNA.

RNA breakdown can lead to uric acid, which is excreted from the body. Some people accumulate uric acid and its salts, which can crystallize out in joints and kidneys, sometimes causing permanent damage and considerable pain. When this condition, called gout, occurs, 95 times out of 100 it is in males and tends to run in families. You should have a uric acid (also called serum urate) test before using RNA and shortly after starting use (say, a month later). Durk has a genetic predisposition to gout and, consequently, cannot take RNA. He does, however, take vitamin B-12 without difficulty.

PABA, p-aminobenzoic acid, is a B vitamin you can make in your body. But even though you can make it, the doses required for some of its benefits would be too expensive to make in the body—it's cheaper from a bottle! PABA is an antioxidant and a membrane stabilizer. As a membrane stabilizer, PABA helps protect red blood cells from bursting (lysing) and lysosomal membranes from breaking and releasing lysosomal (tissue dissolving) enzymes which can damage tissues. In experiments with rats, PABA provided substantial protection against ozone toxicity. Assuming similar metabolism, the dose of PABA given the rats was equivalent to about 3 grams for a man. Therefore, for people living in smoggy areas, PABA is a protective dietary addition.

PABA can sometimes help prevent hair loss, probably due to its antioxidant and lysosomal membrane-stabilizing ability. Occasionally, PABA use causes gray or white hair to darken toward its original color. In our limited experience, this seems to occur to some extent in about ten percent of the cases.

PABA or one of its ester forms is found in many good sunblock preparations. The PABA absorbs ultraviolet energy, thus blocking its damaging effects—mutagenic and carcinogenic—to skin. PABA counteracts and nullifies the effects of sulfa drugs, so if your doctor gives you a sulfa drug, immediately discontinue PABA use for the duration of this treatment.

VITAMIN B-6 plays a role in many aspects of metabolism as an enzyme cofactor. It is required for proper utilization of proteins and amino acids and for growth. It is necessary for fatty acid synthesis and maintenance of the insulating myelin sheath around nerves. It is necessary for converting amino acids into neurotransmitters, the chemicals that brain cells use to communicate with each other. Vitamin B-6 deficiency in monkeys leads to development of atherosclerotic plaques; B-6 has been used successfully in combination with vitamin C to regress atherosclerotic plaques in rabbits. It has also been used in the clinical treatment of arthritis, with substantial reduction of swelling and pain reported. B-6 administration has been reported to relieve the nausea of radiation sickness and pregnancy (Goodman and Gilman)—both are free radical problems. MIT researchers Gruberg and Raymond have found that B-6 deficiency combined with a high protein diet can cause atherosclerosis. Your body converts the antioxidant amino acid methionine into the oxidant homocysteine which is converted with the help of B-6 into the antioxidant cystathione. If you have a lot of methionine and not enough B-6 (such as from an unsupplemented diet containing a lot of cooked meat), you could end up with excess oxidant, thereby promoting cardiovascular disease. B-6 is easily destroyed by cooking. The requirement for B-6 is increased by birth control pill use, pregnancy, smoking, and alcohol consumption.

WARNING: People who are taking L-Dopa for Parkinson's Disease should *not* take vitamin B-6 supplements unless advised to do so by their physician. Vitamin B-6 helps convert the amino acid L-Dopa to the neurotransmitter dopamine in the brain, where such conversion is desired, but it also helps to convert L-Dopa to dopamine peripherally (outside of the brain) in the remainder of the body. If a Parkinson's patient takes large doses of B-6, so much L-Dopa may be converted peripherally that there may be undesired peripheral side effects while, at the same time, not enough L-Dopa may be available to adequately elevate dopamine levels in the brain. (L-Dopa crosses the blood-brain barrier, the selective membrane surrounding the brain and spinal cord, but dopamine does not.) This can result in a temporary worsening of Parkinsonism symptoms.

Most of the persons we know who are currently participating in life extension experiments do not have Parkinson's Disease, and many of these non-Parkinsonism-patients have had a good response to $\frac{1}{4}$ to $\frac{1}{2}$ gram of L-Dopa at bedtime (as indicated by the fat loss and muscle buildup resulting from L-Dopa's stimulation of growth hormone release by the pituitary gland), even though they were also taking large doses of vitamin B-6 at the same time as they were taking L-Dopa.

VITAMIN B-1 is a sulfur-containing antioxidant compound. It is necessary for the formation of the enzyme acetyl-CoA, essential in the Krebs citric acid (energy producing) cycle and for conversion of choline to acetylcholine. Vitamin B-1 (thiamine) is required for lipid synthesis from carbohydrates. Thiamine, along with vitamin C and the amino acid cysteine, forms a potent antioxidant system (helps control free radicals) which can provide substantial protection against the cross-linker, free radical initiator, mutagen, and carcinogen acetaldehyde. This damaging chemical, a relative of formaldehyde, is formed in the liver from alcohol and is also found in cigarette smoke and smog. Acetaldehyde rapidly autoxidizes by a free radical route. Dr. Herbert Sprince fed a group of rats doses of acetaldehyde high enough to kill 90 percent of them. Another group of rats was fed the same amount of acetaldehyde, but were also given C, B-1, and cysteine—all of these rats survived. Since the chemical effects of other aldehydes are similar to acetaldehyde, there is reason to believe that C, B-1, and cysteine can protect against other aldehyde environmental free radical oxidants and cross-linkers.

Thiamine requirement is increased in smoking, pregnancy, and alcohol consumption.

ASCORBYL PALMITATE is a lipid soluble form of vitamin C. Ascorbic acid and its salts, such as sodium ascorbate, are water soluble forms of C, practically completely insoluble in fats (lipids). Thus, they cannot provide any direct benefits within fatty tissues. They do provide protection at the lipid-aqueous (fat-water) interface. Ascorbyl palmitate is an antioxidant and powerful synergist (the total effects are greater than the sum of the effects of the individual components in a mixture) in combination with other antioxidants. In addition, palmitate compounds are concentrated by the heart, so if ascorbyl is carried by the palmitate to the heart, this is an excellent way of increasing vitamin C in the lipids there.

BETA CAROTENE is pro-vitamin A (gives carrots their yellow color), converted in the body to vitamin A as it is needed, except in diabetics and carnivores, which cannot perform this conversion. No vitamin A overdose can occur with beta carotene. In addition, beta carotene can react with a powerful damaging species of activated oxygen called singlet oxygen and, by this interaction, prevent damage to DNA and other cellular constituents. Beta carotene is not destroyed in this interaction and can, therefore, quench many atoms of singlet oxygen. Vitamin A can quench singlet oxygen, too, but not nearly as well as beta carotene. Beta carotene is also an effective treatment for photosensitivity in humans (unusual vulnerability to damage by sunlight). Recent evidence indicates that beta carotene and other carotenoids are effective for preventing cancer in humans.

DILAURYL THIODIPROPIONATE and THIODIPROPIONIC ACID are FDA approved G.R.A.S. (Generally Recognized As Safe) food antioxidants. They are specifically sulfur-containing secondary antioxidants, which means they can not only prevent formation of peroxides in the body but can also degrade already formed peroxides into harmless products, as does your enzyme glutathione peroxidase. (Primary antioxidants such as C, E, B-5, BHT, etc. cannot break down already formed peroxides.) Though these chemicals are G.R.A.S., they are rarely used by the food industry because they impart an undesirable flavor to food in effective concentrations. We once added them in high concentrations to the butter used in a batch of brownies. The brownies ended up with an odd taste, so they weren't much fun to eat. However, they didn't go rancid for 6 months at room temperature and exposed to air! Butter is rather like human fat.

INOSITOL is a sugar found in muscles which does not stimulate the release of insulin when eaten. It is metabolized as a carbohydrate, like ordinary table sugar (sucrose), but more slowly.

Inositol-deficient mice develop baldness and this sugar seems to be of some value in reducing the rate of hair loss in human balding. It occasionally (about 10 percent of the time in our very small sample) causes graying hair to darken to-

ward its original color. This may be due to its membrane stabilizing properties. It is also a hydroxyl free radical scavenger,
as is DMSO, and may, therefore, be of value in arthritis and
in limiting the damage of crushing injuries. Inositol is required for the growth of muscle cells in tissue culture. It also
increases the binding of vitamin B-3 to the natural anti-anxiety (benzodiazepine) receptors in the brain to which Val-
ium ® and Librium ® also bind.

VITAMIN B-12 (cyanocobalmin) is a water soluble essential nutrient. Its absorption depends on the "intrinsic factor"
secreted in the stomach. Some people who lack intrinsic factor may have to take large doses of B-12 to prevent deficiency. Sorbitol, a carbohydrate, is effective in restoring proper
absorption of B-12 when taken with the vitamin and makes B-
12 injections unnecessary, even in most deficiency cases.

Vitamin B-12 increases RNA synthesis in rat brain neurons, and improves learning.

RUTIN and HESPERIDIN are bioflavonoids, membrane
stabilizers and antioxidants which have synergistic effects in
combination with vitamin C. The bioflavonoids decrease the
fragility and permeability of capillaries and protect experimental animals from radiation damage. A certain type of cataract (those caused by aldols) can be prevented by rutin.

L-ARGININE and L-ORNITHINE are amino acids, found
in milk products, chicken and other meat. They cause release
of growth hormone, an immune system stimulant. In animal
experiments, arginine and ornithine have improved immune
responses to bacteria, viruses, and tumor cells. Arginine and
ornithine are wound healing promoters and are involved in
regeneration of liver in rats. Ornithine is about twice as effective as arginine per gram but also costs about twice as much.

GROWTH HORMONE CAUTION: Inappropriate use of
GH releasers may have adverse consequences. They should
not be used by persons who have not completed their long-
bone growth (that is, who have not grown to their full height)
unless they have been advised to do so by their physician.
After full height is attained, GH will not cause further height
increases. Excess GH will cause the skin to grow so rapidly
that it becomes noticeably coarser and thicker; this effect is
reversible when excess GH is withdrawn. Very excessive GH
over an extended period of time can cause irreversible enlargement of joint diameter (which may be unsightly but is
usually not dangerous) and lowering of voice pitch due to lar-

ynx growth. The maintenance of extremely high levels of growth hormone (above normal teenage to young adult levels) for extended periods of time requires further safety research. In some GH releaser experiments on animals either previously or subsequently given cancer, the GH releasers usually caused an improvement. At Cornell University Medical Center, however, hypophysectomy (surgical removal of the hypothalamus) in women with advanced metastatic breast cancer has sometimes produced dramatic improvements. Since this procedure affects many other hormones besides GH, including LHRH, LH, FSH, TRF, TSH, thyroid prolactin, estrogens, progestins, endorphins, beta lipotropin, etc., it is not yet clear what is going on here.

BHT, BUTYLATED HYDROXYTOLUENE, is a powerful synthetic antioxidant, used as a food preservative (in cereals, potato chips, pork sausage, etc.). It is a very effective antioxidant, which has been extensively tested for toxicity. Rhesus monkeys fed BHT at levels of 500 milligrams per kilogram and 50 milligrams per kilogram had lowered cholesterol levels. BHT also lowered the susceptibility of the monkeys' liver lipids (fats) to peroxidation and increased levels of lipid phosphorus (phospholipids). Phospholipids are surfactants, that is, agents that lower the surface tension between fats and water, thereby promoting their emulsification and removal. In this respect, they resemble household detergents for grease removal. You are less likely to suffer from fat deposits in the arteries if a higher portion of your total lipids are phospholipids. The majority of our serum lipids are phospholipids. The investigator who performed this experiment noted that the observed decrease in serum cholesterol in the rhesus monkeys might indicate a therapeutic use for BHT in people with hypercholesterolemia (high serum cholesterol). Several animal life span experiments have been done with BHT. In one study, BHT was administered in a semi-synthetic diet to a mouse strain with a high natural tumor incidence, resulting in an increase of mean life span by about 45 percent at a dose of 0.50 percent of dry food intake. The differences between these species patterns of disease with age and that of people make quantitative prediction of life extension potential of BHT for people very difficult. BHT is a liver enzyme inducer, which means that it causes the liver to increase its production of certain enzymes and, at the very high doses sometimes fed to experimental animals, can cause a reversible increase in liver size.

BHT is a powerful inhibitor of viruses which are comprised of a lipid coat around a small diameter nucleic acid core. These include herpes viruses (which have been associated with some human cancers and many animal cancers) and some flu viruses. BHT is an effective and relatively non-toxic treatment for many lingering herpes infections which are now being treated with FDA approved dangerous and mutagenic compounds. BHT, in tissue culture, decreased mutations caused by PAH (polynuclear aromatic hydrocarbons), the carcinogens produced during the burning of fuels, tobacco, etc. BHT and BHA both inhibit the binding of the PAH metabolites to DNA, a critical step in the production of cancer by PAH. BHT in large quantities elevates liver enzymes (SGOT, SGPT, LDH, alkaline phosphatase) in both experimental animals and humans, since it is an enzyme inducer. Do not confuse these modest elevations due to enzyme induction with the large elevations that can occur when liver cells are seriously damaged by disease or poisons.

CALCIUM PANTOTHENATE is vitamin B-5, an antioxidant and antistress vitamin. In experiments with rats swimming in cold water, high B-5 doses resulted in greatly extended (twice or more) times to reach exhaustion. Frog muscle preparations perfused with a calcium pantothenate containing solution were able to do twice as much work before giving out. The increased stamina produced by B-5 stems from its central role as part of a key enzyme, acetyl CoA, in the energy producing Krebs or Citric Acid Cycle. B-5 is also required for fat synthesis. Many expensive "miracle" skin creams and scalp and hair tonics contain B-5 (usually as pantothenyl alcohol) as their principal active ingredient. The principal nutrient in royal jelly is vitamin B-5.

The discoverer of vitamin B-5, Roger J. Williams, increased the lifespan of rats by about 20 percent with a dose of B-5 of 12 milligrams/kilogram/day (about 0.2 percent of food intake).

L-DOPA, an amino acid, is used by the brain to make dopamine and NE (norepinephrine), the catecholamine neurotransmitters. (Neurotransmitters are chemicals which carry messages between nerve cells.) Male Swiss mice fed L-Dopa in life span experiments (Cotzias) had significant life extensions. At 18 months, the percentages of survivors were (1) no L-Dopa, 39 percent, (2) 1 milligram per gram of diet, 38 percent, (3) 40 milligram per gram of diet, 73 percent. However, in these mice, there was a high initial mortality among the animals given the highest dosage of L-Dopa (they were not given gradually increasing doses). Because L-Dopa is a catechol, it has antioxidant properties. It is a fairly good radiation protection drug, and some investigators believe that pigmented malignant melanomas (black cancer) are resistant to radiation, in part, because of their L-Dopa content. Vitamin C may work synergistically in L-Dopa metabolic pathways.

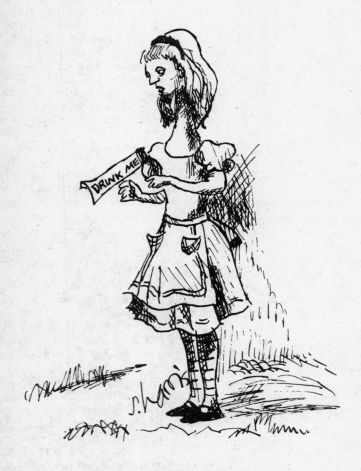

"Why, it must be somatotropin, the growth hormone!"

L-Dopa, a powerful dopaminergic stimulant, stimulates release of growth hormone (somatotropin), needed for growth and healing and proper immune system function. It is converted in the brain to an important neurotransmitter, dopamine. The dopaminergic nervous system is one of the brain's tracts showing the greatest decrease in activity with age. This can be countered by taking L-Dopa. The release of growth hormone and beta-lipotropin associated with L-Dopa use results in loss of weight or difficulty in gaining weight because of their lipolytic (burning fats for energy) effects. (See Part III, Chapter 2, and Part II, Chapter 7 for increased antioxidant requirement with L-Dopa.) Brain dopamine controls movement. In one fascinating experiment, aged rats given L-Dopa were able to swim in water as vigorously, successfully, and as long as young rats! Aged rats not given L-Dopa were able to swim only a short time and made less efficient use of their motions. (See Part III, Chapter 9.) L-Dopa may increase the requirements for other antioxidants.

WARNING: Patients with pigmented malignant melanomas should not take L-Dopa, tyrosine, or phenylalanine supplements because these nutrients are in particularly great demand as a metabolic energy source in this type of cancer.

L-CYSTEINE is an antioxidant sulfur-containing amino acid. It can protect animals from radiation and is an anti-cross linking agent. Aldehydes are a major source of cross-linking damage and combine with and reduce tissue levels of cysteine. Acetaldehyde is made by enzymes in the liver from alcohol. Another aldehyde, malonaldehyde, is a breakdown product of peroxidized fats in the body. Yet other aldehydes are found in smog and smoke. Aldehydes spontaneously oxidize via a free radical mechanism. The combination of vitamins C and B-1 and the amino acid cysteine is effective in protecting experimental animals from the toxic effects of acetaldehyde. In life extension experiments, cysteine extended the life spans of several species, including rats, mice, and guinea pigs.

Aging may, in part, be due to the decrease in blood and tissue levels of antioxidants that occurs in aging. Cysteine is itself an important antioxidant and is used in making reduced glutathione, one of your body's major antioxidants.

L-cysteine is an immune system stimulant. It was shown to maintain normal levels of bacterial ingestion by lung macrophages (white blood cells) during exposure to cigarette smoke, which normally decreases their activity. These macrophages have the important task of destroying cancer cells and invading bacteria and viruses.

Cysteine can also block the effects of insulin in the serum and, thereby, abort the hypoglycemic effects of insulin. It does this by reducing one or more of insulin's surface-exposed three disulfide bonds, thus altering the shape and function of the insulin molecule. **WARNING:** Diabetics should note the warning in "Sugar, Diet, and Longevity," Part IV, Chapter 2.

Hair is 8 percent by weight cysteine. Cysteine is uncommon in the diet. Eggs are the best natural source, containing about $\frac{1}{4}$ gram (250 milligrams) per egg. Hair growth can often be accelerated with cysteine supplements, whereas cysteine deficiency will speed the progress of male pattern baldness.

CAUTION: Do not take supplemental cysteine unless you take at least two to three times as much vitamin C supplement. While cysteine is quite water soluble, its oxidized form, cystine, is rather insoluble in water. If large amounts of cysteine are taken without other water soluble antioxidants such as C, cystine stone formation could conceivably occur in the kidneys and urinary bladder.

HYDERGINE® (SANDOZ) protects both brain and liver (and presumably other tissues) from free radical damage produced by oxidants like aldehydes and by hypoxia (low oxygen availability). It increases protein synthesis in the brain, which is required for learning. Evidence suggests that it stimulates the growth of neurites, small nerve fibers connecting nerve cells to one another. These neurites are required for learning. Hydergine® seems to stimulate neurite growth via the same mechanism as the natural hormone nerve growth factor. Hydergine® can reverse, at least in part, some brain damage resulting from stroke, infections, radiation, and even some birth defects. At 12 milligrams per day for two weeks, Hydergine® increased the intelligence of normal human subjects in a double blind study. Hydergine® has also been used successfully in the treatment of bronchial asthma and tardive dyskinesia. In a two year oral feeding of Hydergine® to rats (males received 6.2 milligrams per kilogram of food per day, while females received 3.1 milligrams per kilogram of food each day), there was a significant reduction (25 percent) in the cholesterol content of treated male rats' thoracic aorta compared to controls (received no supplementary Hydergine®). A similar trend oc-

REASON FOR INCLUDING THESE COMPONENTS

INGREDIENT	REASON FOR INCLUSION
vitamin C, PABA, vitamin E, calcium pantothenate, (vitamin B-5), beta carotene, cysteine, dilauryl thiodipropionate, thiodipropionic acid, ascorbyl palmitate, BHT, vitamin A, selenium, vitamin B-1, vitamin B-3 (niacin), vitamin B-6, Hydergine®, Deaner®, choline, L-Dopa, zinc, hesperidin complex, rutin, inositol, RNA, tryptophan	antioxidants, free radical scavengers
vitamin B-2	antioxidant co-factor
vitamin C, vitamin E, cysteine, L-Dopa, vitamin A, selenium, zinc, arginine, ornithine, Diapid® (vasopressin)	immune system stimulants
niacin, vitamin C, vitamin B-6, vitamin E, BHT, choline	reduce serum cholesterol; C and B-6 have regressed atherosclerotic plaques in rabbits
calcium pantothenate, cysteine, vitamin E, BHT, Deaner®, RNA, L-Dopa, selenium	increase life span of experimental animals
L-Dopa, bromocryptine (Parlodel®), phenylalanine	stimulate dopaminergic nervous system in brain; growth hormone releasers
arginine, tryptophan, ornithine, vasopressin (Diapid®)	growth hormone releasers
vitamin B-1, cysteine, thiodipropionates	sulfhydryl compound (contains reduced sulfur), anti-cross-linking agents; protect against acetaldehyde and other aldehydes
vitamin A, vitamin E, inositol, Deaner®, PABA, choline hesperidin complex, rutin, zinc, selenium	membrane stabilizers
hesperidin complex, rutin	synergists with vitamin C; decrease capillary fragility; rutin can prevent aldol-caused cataracts
Hydergine®, Deaner®, RNA, vasopressin (Diapid®), vitamin B-12, choline	improve memory and learning
Hydergine®	nerve-growth-factor-like effect

curred in triglycerides. Female rats had slight reductions in cholesterol and triglycerides. A human eats roughly a kilogram of food a day. The administration of a fat load (2 grams per kilogram of body weight of 98 percent butter and 2 percent cholesterol) to Hydergine® treated and control rats resulted in an inhibition of the normal increase in serum cholesterol and triglycerides in treated rats. This is consistent with our hypothesis that supplementary antioxidants can substitute in the bloodstream for the natural antioxidant cholesterol. Via a feedback mechanism, cholesterol may be synthesized and released at a reduced rate when adequate antioxidant protection already exists in the bloodstream. For more about Hydergine® see the subject index.

DEANER® (RIKER), DMAE BITARTRATE, and other DMAE salts and esters: Deaner® is dimethylaminoethanol p-acetamidobenzoate, a prescription drug. The bitartrate salt of dimethylaminoethanol has the same active constituent, DMAE. Both increase the level of acetylcholine in the brain and body, remove lipofuscin age pigment from cells in which it has accumulated, and are free radical chain transfer agents. This means that while alkylaminoalcohols such as DMAE are not antioxidants themselves, they can capture a free radical and transfer it to something else. In the presence of adequate antioxidants, they often improve the free radical scavenging ability of these other antioxidants. In an antioxidant-deficient pro-free-radical environment, they accelerate free radical reactions. For further information, see Part II, Chapters 7, 8, and 9; also see Part III, Chapters 2, 3, 4, 5, and 6.

DIAPID® (SANDOZ) is a prescription drug and is a synthetic version of a natural anterior pituitary hormone, vasopressin, which is also called ADH or antidiuretic hormone. This hormone is involved in water balance, memory, visualization, dreaming, sensory discrimination, reaction time and coordination, fat metabolism (via its action in causing the brain to release the fat-burning hormone beta lipotropin), and orgasm. Its effects on blood pressure are usually negligible, except in traumatic injuries and serious loss of blood, when large amounts of vasopressin may be released by the pituitary, and when large doses are given intravenously. A related hormone, oxytocin, has increased the life spans of experimental animals. For further information, see Part II, Chapter 9, and Part III, Chapters 2, 3, 4, 5, 9, 12, and 13.

POSSIBLE ALLERGIC REACTIONS TO TABLET BINDERS
AND FILLERS

Fillers and binders comprise the bulk of the contents in many vitamin tablets. We have seen people who exhibited adverse side effects (such as headaches, rashes, hives, itching, and upset stomach) to large doses of vitamin tablets who did *not* have these adverse reactions to the same vitamin doses taken as the pure vitamin powders in gelatin capsules.

Dr. Hunter Harang is an oral surgeon who uses megavitamins in his practice, and who does clinical research on allergies. He observed many such undesirable reactions (including headache, arthritis, joint pain, chronic fatigue, depression, personality changes, gout attacks, and even chronic earaches and infections in children), and, hence, he set out to find the source of the problem. He discovered that the allergic reactions are generally to tablet fillers and binders, not to the vitamins themselves. (Of course, even pure vitamins can cause trouble in excessive doses.) Dr. Harang found that 8 to 10 percent of his tested clinical population is allergic to cornstarch and other corn products and about another 10 percent to soy products. He has also noted frequent allergic reactions to yeast in B vitamin products, and sometimes even to the cod liver oil in vitamin A capsules. These allergies can be sufficiently severe to produce very unpleasant symptoms when megadoses of vitamins using these fillers and binders are taken. Dr. Harang uses vitamins from M Squared Ethical Pharmaceuticals, (P.O. Box 174, West Chicago, Illinois, 60185), which in his experience have been relatively free of allergic complications.

WARNING: *To keep your reading in perspective, it is a good idea to read the disclaimers in "The Engraved Invitation" at the beginning of this book, if you skimmed over them.*

8
Is There Anything Perfectly Safe?

NO.

(See Appendix K: References and Chapter Notes.)

9
Avoiding Problems with Acidic Vitamins

Those who fall in love with practice without science are
like a sailor who enters a ship without a helm or compass,
and who never can be certain whither he is going.

—Leonardo da Vinci

*Vitamins C (in its most common form, ascorbic acid) and nia-
cin are both acids. If you take large doses of these as supplements, you should neutralize their acidity. This chapter tells
you how to avoid acid problems like acid indigestion, diarrhea, or, in extreme cases, even a stomach ulcer.*

Most vitamin C is ascorbic *acid* and most vitamin B-3 is
nicotinic *acid*. It is very important to neutralize these acids,
especially if taken in large doses (a gram or more per day). If
you do not neutralize the acids, you can get acid indigestion
and heartburn, or, more seriously, ulcers. In addition, excess
acidity in the urine can promote the formation of uric acid
kidney stones in people susceptible to gout, as well as increase
tobacco consumption by smokers (see Part III, Chapter 10 on
smoking). There may not be any obvious early symptoms of
excess acid intake. You can demonstrate the irritating effects
of acidic vitamins by holding a tablet of ascorbic acid in your
cheek pouch, between your cheek and gum. Wait for the tablet to dissolve and notice that it burns while this is happening.

The digestive tract is not well equipped with pain nerves, so do not assume that your gut is tolerating acidic vitamins well just because you feel no pain. While the stomach is normally acidic, the degree of acidity at the surface of a dissolving ascorbic acid or nicotinic acid tablet is much greater. When the stomach is irritated, it attempts to get rid of the irritant either by vomiting or by passing its contents on to the duodenum. When the duodenum is irritated, it passes its contents on to the small intestine, which is supposed to be basic (alkaline), not acidic. An incompletely dissolved acidic tablet may be quite upsetting here, so the small intestine may quickly pass the problem along to the large intestine, which is also normally basic. The large intestine may respond to this irritating acidity with diarrhea, often accompanied by a burning sensation in the anus if the acid is particularly strong.

We take vitamin C and nicotinic acid as crystals and powder, respectively. (C crystals are widely available, but niacin powder is not.) In these forms, the acid vitamins are less likely to irritate the stomach because they go into solution immediately, rather than sitting in lumps against the stomach while the tablets dissolve (which may take considerable time, depending on the quality of the tablet).

There are several ways to minimize acid irritation or damage:

1. Take vitamins *immediately* following meals. The stomach detects the acid level of its contents and adjusts its own acid output accordingly.

2. Use vitamin C crystals rather than tablets. Or, use a good brand of tablet (try dissolving one in a glass of water to check its speed). Do *not* use time-delayed tablets, which take a very long time to dissolve, unless they are the non-acidic ascorbate salts such as sodium ascorbate.

3. You can neutralize acid vitamins with over-the-counter antacids such as Maalox®. Sodium bicarbonate (ordinary baking soda) is excellent, but should not be used by persons with essential hypertension (people on a low sodium diet for high blood pressure). Calcium carbonate (limestone powder) or dolomite powder plus the acidic vitamins yields the calcium salts or calcium plus magnesium salts of the vitamins. Calcium carbonate or dolomite can be used by people on a low sodium diet, as can any other low sodium antacid recommended by your physician.

4. The carbon dioxide gas formed in the interaction of the acid and some antacids (including baking soda, calcium carbonate, and dolomite) can be eliminated, avoiding the discomfort and even diarrhea caused by gas ballooning the gastrointestinal tract, by taking simethicone (a food grade silicone) antifoam (as in the over-the-counter Gas-X® tablets). This reduces the surface tension of the gas bubbles, causing them to break, allowing the gas to escape and the pressure to be relieved. Excessive flatus (intestinal gas escaping from the anus) will occur often if simethicone antifoam is not used.

If you would like to know whether you are placing an excessive acid load on your body, one way to find out is to measure the pH of your urine. Buy some litmus or pH papers at a pharmacy. Normal urine should have a pH of 4.6–8.0 (average 6.0). Neutral pH is 7.0. Numbers over 7.0 indicate an alkaline (basic) urine pH, while numbers less than 7.0 indicate an acid urine pH. You can also measure the pH of your feces with pH paper. If the pH is well below 7, you may need more antacid.

10
Nutrient Shopping Tips: Save 50 Percent

Chance favors only those who know how to court her.

—Charles Nicolle

You can easily save fifty percent on your nutritional supplements by following some of our suggestions. Sometimes the most expensive supplements are less safe and less effective than the cheapest. Sometimes supplement labels can be shamefully misleading. Caveat emptor: let the buyer beware. Here is knowledge you need to make wise, economical purchases and avoid costly—or even dangerous—ripoffs.

Like any other products, vitamins and other nutrients are generally available in a wide range of prices, sizes, dosages, quality, and forms. They are not necessarily equally good buys. Here are some factors to consider:

• Telephone around to several stores supplying vitamins and nutrients and compare prices. You may easily find a 50 percent or greater difference between the lowest and highest prices. Ask these stores for the prices of the largest bottle of the highest dosage available for each nutrient—this is likeliest to have the lowest cost per unit of dosage.

• It makes no difference biologically whether a nutrient is obtained from natural sources or is synthetic. Synthetics are usually by far the lowest priced. See Part I, Chapter 14 on synthetic versus natural vitamins.

• Vitamins C and E are sometimes sold as loss leaders to encourage buyers to come into a store and hopefully purchase other items with high markups. Even Sears and Ward's have half price C and E sales about twice a year. Keep bottles tightly closed in a cool, dry, dark place. If stored in this way, good quality vitamins will maintain potency for at least a year.

• No matter what form of vitamin E you buy, an I.U. (international unit) is the same standardized measure of biological activity. In other words, 100 I.U. of one form of vitamin E has the same biological effect as 100 I.U. of any other form of vitamin E, whether natural or synthetic, tocopherol or acetate; their biological activities are equal.

• If you buy very large jars of vitamins, transfer some to a smaller jar (jelly jars with metal lids are excellent) for day to day use. This keeps exposure to air and light at a minimum. Don't use unnecessarily large jars—the moisture and oxygen in the air that gets inside the jar every time you open it attacks many sensitive vitamins including C, E, B-1, and A.

• Vitamin C is particularly difficult to store. It is stable in water solution for only a few hours. Fruit juices fortified with vitamin C may lose their C content in a matter of hours after opening the can or bottle; a lot depends on the acidity—if the pH (a measure of acidity) is very low, the vitamin C content will not fall as rapidly. Even some scientists are not aware of the instability of C in solution. In some experiments where vitamin C has been given to animals in their drinking water or in moist food prepared long in advance, no benefits or in some cases even toxic effects have been reported for this form of vitamin C supplementation. This is because the oxidized form of vitamin C, toxic dehydroascorbic acid, is formed when moist vitamin C is exposed to oxygen in the air. These toxic effects can be countered by giving the animals even larger doses of ascorbic acid, a non-oxidized form of vitamin C.

• Some forms of vitamins are much more stable than are other forms. The most stable forms of vitamin E are called esters and include vitamin E acetate, vitamin E succinate, and vitamin E palmitate. Vitamin E in its unesterified form (as alpha tocopherol) is very sensitive to oxygen in air, light, and heat and does not remain at full potency as long as the above mentioned vitamin E esters under similar storage conditions (unless stored under inert dry nitrogen gas, which is the way the manufacturers of alpha tocopherol store and ship it). Vitamin E esters are not good antioxidants until they are de-esterified in your body and, consequently, vitamin E esters do not protect oils from oxidation that are added to the capsule to make it look larger. Avoid vitamin E esters in oil fillers, particularly polyunsaturated oil fillers. Dry vitamin E acetate tablets do not have this problem. In a similar way, the most stable forms of vitamin A are its esters: vitamin A palmitate, vitamin A acetate, and vitamin A succinate. Calcium pantothenate is far more stable than the acid form of the same vitamin, pantothenic acid.

· For fresher vitamins, shop at a store where there is a fast turnover of vitamin stocks. Under conditions of storage at some low volume retail vitamin outlets, you may not be getting full potency at time of purchase, and filler oils may be rancid (peroxidized).

· TAX DEDUCTIONS: If your doctor prescribes medications, even vitamins, you can deduct them as a medical expense on your income taxes. See a professional tax advisor for further details. Keep your receipts and copies of the prescriptions in case of a tax audit to prove your purchases.

· *Drug Topics Red Book: The Pharmacist's Guide to Products and Prices* is a huge catalog listing most prescription drugs and their wholesale prices to your druggist. This book will greatly help you in locating a good price when you shop around for prescription drugs. (Published annually with updates by Medical Economics Co., Div. of Litton, Oradell, NJ 07649.) Don't expect to purchase drugs at near wholesale cost, however; pharmacies are usually high-overhead operations. Their markup has to cover the usual rent and utilities, the pharmacist's professional fees, the cost of maintaining an expensive inventory of drugs, and the cost of discarding overage pharmaceuticals.

· Ask the company nurse where you work if they offer vitamins for sale. If not, contact Vitamins for Industry (2716 E. Florence, Huntington Park, CA 90255) and ask them to help you get prepaid sales of low cost vitamins established at your place of employment. Many employers are willing to cooperate, due to the lower sick pay and absenteeism costs which usually result.

· GENERICS: See the comments on generic drugs, particularly generic imitators of Hydergine® in Part V, Chapter 11.

11
Caveat Emptor: Faking It, Mistaking It, and Raking It In

"In my youth." said the sage, as he shook his grey locks,
    "I kept all my limbs very supple
By the use of this ointment—one shilling the box—
    Allow me to sell you a couple?"

—Lewis Carroll, *Alice in Wonderland*

And many have made a trade in deceits and feigned
miracles, cozening the foolish herd, and if no one showed
himself cognizant of their deceits they would impose them
upon all.

—Leonardo da Vinci

In nearly every magazine and newspaper, you see products advertised for promoting youthfulness, from cosmetics to alleged anti-aging therapies. Many of these advertisements make false claims, either deliberately or in error. It's not always easy to tell a mistake from a fake, but at least we can point out bad information. We do that here, giving examples of products you may be considering buying. Read this before investing a lot of money in possibly useless youth formulas.

There are countless unsupported hypotheses about aging presented to the public, and treatments claimed to restore youth. It is important to be able to decide which treatments are likely to be effective and which are errors or fakes. In this chapter, we'll describe some things to watch out for, including a sample case of either a very careless mistake or perhaps

493

a potential fraud and what aroused our suspicions. In our original version of the book manuscript, we had included actual names of persons and magazines and specific page numbers and dates. However, we have been told by Warner's lawyers that referring to these specific entities, no matter how much evidence we feel supports our interpretations, we might still have to face expensive and time-consuming litigation. Although we could prove our case in court, we would rather spend our time on science than on lawsuits, so we have deleted such names.

Recently we saw a copy of an article from a popular tabloid in which a Dr. X (actual name withheld) claimed to have invented a life extending and youth restoring pill. He refused to divulge the formula's contents to the writer of the article, except to say that it contained dozens of ingredients, including sex hormones, vitamins, enzymes, iron, cobalt, minerals, calcium, protein, sulfur, and others. The fact that he wouldn't reveal the contents of the formula is not necessarily an indication of fraud because he intended at that time to market the pill in South America. However, Dr. X also declined to reveal whether or not *he* was taking the pill or to give his age. Although the article's writer stated that Dr. X looked "fit as a fiddle," the photograph of his face accompanying the article appeared old, with sagging neck and face tissues and heavy facial wrinkling.

The photographs showing "before" and "after" for 3 old persons using Dr. X's formula were particularly revealing. All three "before" pictures were taken with lighting falling from above, creating shadows that highlighted and accentuated wrinkles and facial folds (such as bags under the eyes). The "after" photos were all taken with lighting from directly in front (there were no shadows). The probability of this set of lighting conditions being random chance is less than 1 in 64.

It is possible, of course, that Dr. X did not know about standard lighting procedures for medical photography. (See Kodak publication N-3 "Clinical Photography" on lighting in medical photography.) The lighting in *all* three "before" photos makes the face appear older and in *all* three "after" photos makes the face appear younger. This set of conditions is improbable by chance alone. We found this to be rather suspicious. The results depicted could have been obtained by carefully contrived photography alone. The "amazing" sexual rejuvenation mentioned as an effect of Dr. X's pills is anything but amazing. It has been known for decades that treatment with sex hormones, which he acknowledged were constituents of the pills, can sometimes restore a more youthful sex drive in older persons. But, of course, we have not had access to the data to check these claims. All in all, we would definitely not purchase Dr. X's formula.

The "proof of rejuvenation" photos from Dr. Ana Aslan's Rumanian clinic for GH-3 (Gerovital, a procaine compound) are also taken under such variable lighting conditions that they prove very difficult to evaluate. In the case of Aslan's photos, however, the lighting changes are random rather than consistently emphasizing age in the before shots and youth in the after shots. Although we consider Dr. Aslan to be a legitimate gerontologist, her case would be much more convincing (we hope) with standard photographic records.

There are periodicals for lay persons in which a good deal of information is provided about aging and therapies that have been tried for the slowing, prevention, or reversal of aging. The purpose of some such magazines seems to be the sale of a large number of in-house purported anti-aging remedies. Even when most of the information contained in these magazines' articles are reasonably accurate, which is rare, we suggest that the purchase of the products they promote be approached with extreme caution. A number of disturbing elements in products' advertisements point to some deliberate deceptions.

For example, products we've seen advertised as procaine vitamins and creams contained no procaine at all. They did contain the B vitamin PABA, which is an active ingredient in Aslan's Rumanian GH-3 procaine preparation. However, there is no evidence (contrary to their product implication) that PABA is the *only* active ingredient in this procaine formulation. Even if PABA were the only active ingredient, PABA is not procaine. Many scientists, including the two of us, consider the diethylaminoethanol (DEAE) part of the procaine molecule to be active as well. Like the dimethylaminoethanol (DMAE) in Deaner ®, DEAE is a free radical chain transfer agent, and also forms alkanolamine detergents with free fatty acids of the sort potentially useful for lipofuscin removal. The DEAE is also a mild, reversible monamine oxidase inhibitor that provides the mood elevation one obtains with procaine or GH-3. And, finally, GH-3 contains other antioxidants such as sodium bisulfite, not found in these imposters.

Another product aggressively advertised in some health-oriented magazines is superoxide dismutase (SOD) tablets. While the enzyme SOD has been found to have powerful beneficial effects in conditions where superoxide radicals are causative factors, as in arthritis and cataracts, for example (see Part II, Chapter 7 on the free radical theory of aging), all experiments of which we are aware involved SOD administered by injection. Less than one part in 10,000 of SOD administered orally survives processing in the stomach and reaches the bloodstream. In addition, the SOD oral tablets being sold contain a very small dose of the material to begin with. In our opinion, the suggested dose is at least 1000 times too small to produce a detectable non-placebo effect in humans when given orally, as is claimed for it. In one SOD product, the amount is far too small to beneficially affect a mouse, even if the whole bottle were given by intravenous injection. Remember that SOD is the fifth most common protein in the human body. Systemic microgram doses are not effective.

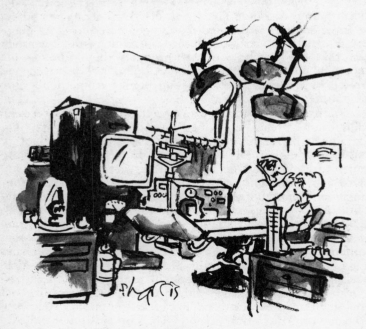

"This is all just a front. Actually, I'm a faith healer."

At the end of one ad for an alleged breast size-increase product was a statement that they couldn't have said what they did in the ad if it weren't true. This is a chilling claim because it simply isn't so, and we don't think the advertisers saying this believed it either. Who would stop these claims if they weren't true? Not the Federal Trade Commission (FTC) or the Food and Drug Administration (FDA). Many, if not most, of the health claims made for anti-aging therapies and treatments run counter to FDA pronouncements on these substances. Yet, neither the FDA nor other government agencies have stopped the ads. Dr. Frederick J. Stare, professor and founder of the Harvard Department of Nutrition, says that the FDA is helpless to stop this type of advertising because ". . . misrepresenting nutritional information is legal as long as it does not appear on the actual label." The organizations selling these products are generally considered too small to merit the attention of the giant government agencies. More scientific research will eventually resolve disputes over hypotheses and interpretations of experimental data. But there will continue to be people willing to buy health products based on a wide variety of untested hypotheses and claims, many not scientifically justifiable on the basis of experiments reported in the scientific literature. In a healthy marketplace, people have many alternatives available to them. So remember: CAVEAT EMPTOR: LET THE BUYER BEWARE! There is no government agency with the magical power to ban all lying! (Indeed, we would not welcome such a dangerously powerful entity.)

We have stated elsewhere in this book that we have found in reading lay nutrition magazines that in many cases much of the information they contain is incorrect. Here are some actual examples taken from a recent issue of a popular lay health magazine, a nutritional educational magazine also offering various alleged health-promoting products. In an article on losing weight, the author states that phenylpropanolamine, unlike the amphetamines commonly prescribed as appetite suppressants, affects the lateral hypothalamus rather than the central nervous system. Unfortunately for readers seeking accurate information in this article, the lateral portion of the hypothalamus in the brain (as well as the rest of this structure) is an essential *part* of the central nervous system, contrary to the claim made here. On the same page, the author stated that it is not necessary to take increasingly large doses to maintain phenylpropanolamine's effectiveness. But it IS necessary to take increasingly large doses of this chemical because it causes the brain to use up its stores of NE (norepinephrine) without causing the brain to make more of it. As the supply of NE (a neurotransmitter in the brain which regulates appetite, among other functions) falls, users must take more and more phenylpropanolamine to get the same appetite reducing effect as previously. In the same issue of the magazine, an advertisement on the inside front cover for a weight control product containing phenylpropanolamine as the active ingredient ("the most effective appetite suppressant available anywhere without a prescription"), claims that this product does not affect the central nervous system, causing you to lose sleep and feel disoriented, and that it produces none of the irritability and "wired" feeling that are common side effects of caffeine. People who believe these claims and actually shell out the asking price ($8.99 for 40 tablets) will receive a product that acts directly on the central nervous system, may frequently cause side effects such as insomnia and irritability, and becomes less effective over a few weeks of continuous use (depending on the individual's response), and users often suffer a letdown and rebound eating binge after discontinuing use. The wholesale cost of phenylpropanolamine is $8.85 per pound. The retail cost at $8.99 for 40 tablets, each containing 100 milligrams, is $1,000 per pound. Phenylpropanolamine is, however, a big improvement over the use of amphetamines for appetite inhibition because phenylpropanolamine does not cause as severe a depletion of NE. On another page in the same magazine, a "natural sweetening" product is promoted that contains 100 percent crystalline xylitol, a natural sugar. The advertisement mentions research with xylitol, indicating that it does not promote cavities, but also that it may have a cavity retarding property. There is evidence in support of these claims. The ad goes on to state that xylitol may be better than artificial sweeteners because some of the leading artificial sweeteners (no names are mentioned) "may be quite unhealthy." What this ad fails to mention is that the same charges leveled against saccharin have also been leveled against xylitol. Xylitol, too, in extremely high doses (much higher dose levels than actual levels used in foods) produced tumors in special sensitive tumor-prone experimental animals. That is why Wrigley's removed xylitol from a chewing gum product (Orbit): they were concerned over public response to this news. Personally, we have used cyclamate, saccharin, and xylitol and will continue to do so, as we do not consider them to be a significant hazard. However, we try to avoid the first two because, to us, they have an unsatisfactory flavor. Taste perception for cyclamates and saccharin varies from individual to individual, another example of biochemical individuality. We would like to impress upon you how important it is that you check out your nutritional sources of information (see Part I, Chapter 13 on how to do this).

In another popular health education magazine which sells in-house products alleged to retard aging or promote health, many products are advertised in large color layouts that do not provide the ingredients in the product or the dosages of these substances. The magazine's attitude toward food preservatives, artificial vitamins, and antioxidants is schizophrenic. In one issue, for example, there are warnings about food preservatives on one page; artificial vitamins are treated with alarm on another page; and the inclusion of antioxidants in ice cream is deplored. But then on a later page, antioxidants are promoted for health. The issue also contains an advertisement for a product which contains artificial chemicals (a temporary wrinkle "remover," actually a coverup cosmetic), although artificial chemicals are deplored in most articles. Artificial vitamins are the same molecules as their natural counterparts. Hence, their fear of artificial vitamins is not warranted. See Part I, Chapter 14.

Many unfortunate advertising practices are a direct result of government agency policies concerning advertising claims. Since they will not allow claims which are scientifically justifiable, based on experiments reported in reputable scientific literature, they have reduced the incentive to make truthful claims since the possible legal penalties are essentially the same for both reasonable and unreasonable claims.

In contrast to the questionable treatments for restoring youth discussed in this chapter, we would like to mention plastic surgery as a valid means for improvement of appearance. We do not consider facial surgery and wrinkle removal by collagen injections to be a form of fakery. Our reasons for that judgment are:

• The skin continues to grow throughout life, so no matter how youthful you may be, eventually the skin will become slack due to this growth. It is not unreasonable or fraudulent

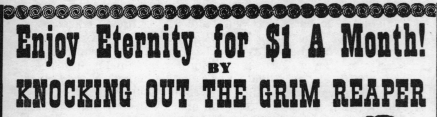
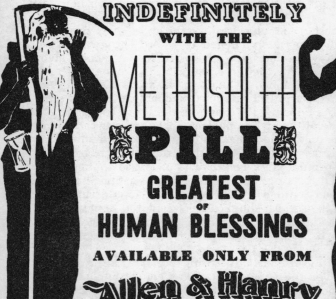

to remove this excess skin. The flattening out of wrinkles caused by cross-linking by excessively tightening the facial skin should be avoided, however. This excessive skin tension temporarily conceals the underlying pathology and stimulates more rapid sideways skin growth resulting in the need for frequent repeated facelifts.

• The nose and ear cartilage continues to grow throughout life so that eventually a person develops a prominent "hook" nose and enlarged ears. Again, we see no fraud in correcting this excessive growth.

• Cosmetic surgery does not cover up a dysfunction. The excess skin is perfectly normal. A person of 20 who could remain at that age for 150 years might end up with a nose like Pinocchio! It is even possible that the skin and cartilage in age-retarded people might have a higher growth rate than normal.

It would be a fraud to have cosmetic surgery and then claim you hadn't. But, in the absence of such misrepresentations, facelifts and other types of cosmetic surgery are no more fraudulent than removing a wart. Although neither of us has had any cosmetic surgery, in 15 years or so it may be a good idea.

GENERICS

An additional source of confusion arises from the existence of name brand prescription drugs with available generic versions (usually less expensive). This is *not* a matter of fraud, but in some cases can involve "mistaking it." It is unfortunately the case that generics are, in a few instances, not therapeutically equivalent to their better known brand product. See "Approved Drug Products with Proposed Therapeutic Equivalence Evaluations," U.S. Dept. of HEW, Public Health Service, FDA Bureau of Drugs, January 1979. In these cases, it may be a mistake to expect the less expensive generic drug to do the same thing as the name brand pharmaceutical. An important example is Hydergine ® (made by Sandoz). Hydergine ® (dihydroergotoxine mesylate) is composed of equal quantities of three ergot alkaloids. One of these, dihydroergocryptine mesylate, occurs in two forms, alpha and beta, in the ratio of 2 to 1. This distinction is biochemically meaningful. No generic version of Hydergine ® at the time of this report had the same ratio of alpha to beta and, therefore, are *not* considered pharmaceutical equivalents of Hydergine®. When you ask your doctor for Hydergine®, we suggest that you ask him to specify the Sandoz product and to write *"no substitutes"* on the prescription. Otherwise, you may be given a generic without realizing it, even if your doctor writes "Hydergine." The pharmaceutical firms marketing these generics are ethical companies, not frauds. We are not saying that the Hydergine® imitators are ineffective. We do know that they are biochemically different. We do know that authentic Hydergine® does many remarkable things because of the 3,300 experiments in the scientific literature that used Hydergine®, not a generic look-alike. Sandoz has spent a lot of money on this published scientific research, while their thoroughly reputable generic competitors have not published this sort of research. Hence, we just don't know how effective the generics might be. We purchase several money-saving generic drugs which work quite well. But with our present state of knowledge, we choose to use only Sandoz Hydergine®.

We strongly urge the manufacturers of the generic versions of Hydergine® to fund the scientific research necessary to determine whether their products are as effective as Hydergine®, both in vitro (outside the body) and in vivo (in the body), as antioxidant free radical modulating agents, as NGF (nerve growth factor)-like agents, as c-AMP (cyclic AMP) elevators and stabilizers, as protectants of membrane-dependent enzyme function during hypoxia (low oxygen availability), as anticarcinogens, and as intelligence increasers in both animals and humans. It will take courage on the part of the corporate management to fund such research because the results pertain to non-FDA-approved uses—uses that may never be FDA approved. We believe, however, that such research would be quite profitable in terms of increased sales and would certainly be an important contribution to the science and technology of life extension. Sandoz has quite a big head start—about 3,300 research papers on Hydergine® so far—and they are hard at work spending an astounding 40 percent of their pharmaceutical research budget on Hydergine®, in spite of the fact that the patents have expired. This policy has been rewarded with worldwide Hydergine® sales of approximately $300,000,000 per year. We expect a very dramatic increase in sales as Americans in particular become aware of Hydergine®'s non-FDA-approved uses. Until the generic manufacturers (who are reputable and ethical firms) do this research on their chemically nonidentical generic versions of Hydergine®—Caveat Emptor.

Finally, we cannot refrain from mentioning the deceptive effects of some government labelling requirements. These rules are put forth by bureaucrats at the FDA who were not elected by anyone and yet have the power to seize products, fine, and even imprison persons responsible for manufacture and sale of foods and drugs. As a consequence of the FDA's Standards of Identity (their definitions of specific types of foods, such as mayonnaise or canned tuna), traditional foods in which variations in the ingredients are desired must often be labelled as "imitation." For example, a tasty Kraft mayonnaise product containing only half the fat required by the FDA's Standard of Identity for mayonnaise is required by FDA regulations to be labelled as "imitation mayonnaise." It would be a crime for the manufacturer to call their product mayonnaise, even though that's what it is. When Kraft told their customers the facts about their low-fat mayonnaise in a TV commercial, they said, "We have to call it imitation, but you don't." The FDA was enraged and threatened Kraft with legal action, forcing these commercials off the air even though they were entirely truthful. In another case, Hain Pure Food Company decided to make a catsup containing honey instead of sugar. They have to label their catsup as "natural imitation catsup"! You can imagine what this did to sales in the targeted premium natural food market! The FDA requires it—or else! We can think of a lot more important things to do with our money than to support an FDA oriented toward counter-productive regulation rather than toward the public dissemination of scientifically sound information.

12
Epilogue
What Is Coming?

When I examine myself and my methods of thought, I
come to the conclusion that the gift of fantasy has
meant more to me than my talent for absorbing positive
knowledge.

> Albert Einstein, from *Einstein, the Life and Times* by
> Ronald W. Clark

In times to come it will often be difficult, perhaps, to
decide whether an advance in knowledge represents a
step forward in physics, information theory, or philosophy,
whether physics is expanding into biology or whether
biology is employing physical methods and approaches to
an ever greater extent.

> —Werner Heisenberg, Nobel laureate

Onward, and forever onward, mightier and forever
mightier, rolls this wondrous tide of discovery ...

> —George Henry Lewes (1845)

*What kind of world will we be extending our lives to live in?
In the coming years, many amazing new developments will
enrich our lives. Here we make a few forecasts for the near-
term future. We have a lot more but this is a book on life extension, not futurology!*

It takes about 5 to 10 years for the amount of knowledge
in the biological and physical sciences to double. By the turn
of this century, the amount of knowledge we have about aging will be between 4 and 16 times as much as we now know.

Predicting the future of science and technology is a very challenging mental exercise due to the accelerating pace of new discoveries and knowledge. Nearly 500 years ago, if Leonardo da Vinci, the great Renaissance genius, attempted to forecast what our present-day world was like, he would have had to stretch his imagination across about 6 to 8 doubling times. In da Vinci's time, change was much slower than now. The time it took for knowledge to double was around 100 years. It is as difficult for us in 1981 to see ahead 50 years as it was for him to see ahead 500 years! As much innovation and discovery will take place in the next few decades as happened in the previous 500 years.

Da Vinci invented a number of devices which have only recently become practical reality: the helicopter, glider, parachute, submarine, scuba diving, torpedos, mines, machine guns, automatic cannon, the tank, hydraulic mining, perhaps the reflecting telescope (he experimented with curved mirrors), and the "exploded" view of mechanical devices. He also discovered atherosclerosis in cadavers he dissected (which may explain why he became a vegetarian: he hoped to avoid the buildup of fats he observed in the arteries of these corpses). Three oft repeated questions which da Vinci tried but failed to answer remained enigmas for long after his death:

1. Why is the sky blue?—this question was answered by Nobelist John W. S. Rayleigh in the late 19th century. Oxygen molecules scatter blue light more effectively than longer wavelengths due to their electronic structure.

2. Why are offspring like their parents? This was answered with the discovery of the DNA structure and function by Crick and Watson in mid-20th century.

3. Why do people grow old and die? This question is only now becoming answered.

The pace of change in our time has radically accelerated from the time of da Vinci and even in our own lives. It is only since 1952 that tractors have outnumbered plow horses, mules, and oxen on American farms! In the authors' own childhood, gas lights were used on urban American streets and horse drawn carts were still used in large American cities. (Indeed, Durk clearly remembers the gas lamps illuminating the Chicago street of his childhood, and the lamplighter with his Model T Ford.) What will happen by the year 2000? Here are some predictions and guesses:

1. Human DNA will be entirely decoded, making possible genetic engineering for elimination of genetic diseases, selection of offspring inheritance, control of aging inherent in genetic programming (aging clocks), etc.

A quote from the editorial in the May 8, 1980 *Nature* (a leading scientific journal) gives an idea how close we are:

"Mount Everest, as we all know, was first climbed 'because it was there.' The Everest of those scientists who are devoted to the sequencing of DNA is the complete human genome, a peak that cannot yet be conquered. Nevertheless it seems not out of the question, even now, to attempt to sequence a single chromosome from man or *Drosophila* [fruit fly]; or at least to tackle a substantial fragment of one such chromosome. And certainly some of the more ambitious sequencers would no longer consider the complete genome of the bacterium *Escherichia coli* to be a sufficient challenge to their skills.

"The reasons why grandiose sequencing can now be contemplated are technical."

Less than one year later (April 9, 1981), fourteen research scientists reported in *Nature* the sequence and organization of the human mitochondrial genome! (Mitochondria are energy factories in cells.)

Dr. Martin Cline of UCLA has already started genetic engineering experiments on humans suffering from a terminal genetic blood disease.

2. Regeneration of amputated and lost limbs and organs will be routine. This capability is under active investigation now. Crude regeneration of part of amputated limbs has already been achieved in adult rats.

3. Cloning of mammals will be available. Its first non-research users will be in animal husbandry, for duplication of exceptional breeders. Human use may be fraught with emotional considerations but it will be done by some people no matter how much it is frowned upon. Keep in mind that identical twins are clones of each other, and that cloning of humans is simply the artificial production of identical twins which may have different birth dates. We do not consider this to be sinister or even unnatural.

Potential cloning applications go far beyond the controversial cloning of human beings. Cloned animals will become very useful in aging research because it will be possible to easily compare results for groups of clones given various anti-aging treatments. Moreover, cloning can produce genetically identical animals of widely differing ages, permitting the isolation of biochemical changes involved in aging. Using clones can avoid the complications introduced by the large variations among individuals in a normal population. Scientists will be able to substitute individual chromosomes or even genes into animals of otherwise identical genetic makeup to map out genetic controls of life span, development, sexuality, reproduction, and so on.

Organisms which have already been used in successful nuclear transplant (cloning) experiments include mice, salamanders, frogs, toads, amoeba, honeybees, fruit flies, and protozoans (single celled animals). In terms of technical—but not economic or legal—difficulty, cloning humans is very similar to cloning mice.

4. Space colonization in high orbit will begin. (There is a lot more that we could add about this subject—we are both professional futurologists—but this is a book on life extension, not on previewing the future).

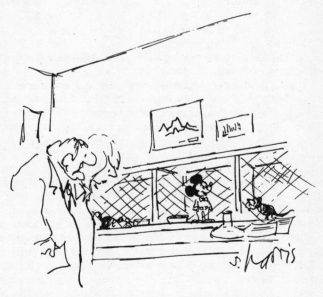

"Somehow I was hoping genetic engineering would take a different turn."

5. Thermonuclear powered spaceships using inertial confinement fusion (a now widely known "secret" of the H bomb) will be available to wealthy individuals, as well as institutions, corporations, and governments. Unlimited thermonuclear industrial heat and electric power will be nearing commercialization.

6. Lunar and asteroid mining will be taking place on a commercial, profit-making basis.

7. Human life spans of 150–200 years may be possible, but not yet reached by 2000—because only about 50 years will have passed since the beginning of serious life extension science and technology. But some people alive now may eventually reach this age. By the year 2000, even greater potential life span would not surprise us.

8. Communication with dolphins on their own terms may be achieved.

9. There will be man-computer direct linkup by implantation. You'll be able to "remember" any data in the Library of Congress as easily as remembering your own address!

10. Tests will be developed to disqualify cyborgs (mechanically augmented humans) and genetically engineered superhumans at the Olympics!

11. Computer teacher-babysitters, responsive to the infant or child, will be in wide use.

12. There will be an equal rights movement for self-aware computers and robots.

13. Politically created energy crises will no longer occur due to widespread understanding of their political causes and a greater public understanding of economics. (Frankly, this is our most uncertain prediction, more a hope than a prediction. Our present energy problems are purely political; there is no natural shortage of energy.)

14. There will be development of the true "feelies," movies which are designed to stimulate the senses or brain sensory projection areas, so that they are perceived like reality through the use of a sophisticated helmet. Such technology would be a great boon for the blind and the deaf who probably do not provide a large enough potential market by themselves to justify the extremely expensive long-term developmental program which would be necessary for such a complex project.

15. There will be a growth-hormone-releaser scandal in the bodybuilding business and in the Olympics. Although officials may bar the use of L-Dopa, they can't do anything about the use of tryptophan, arginine, ornithine, phenylalanine, tyrosine, and other nutrients to boost growth hormone release and stimulate muscular growth. Nor is there anything they can do about the natural hormone vasopressin.

16. Monsanto has already entered the gene-splicing business. It is developing genetically engineered microbes to produce bovine (cattle) growth hormone by the pound for use as a growth augmentor and feed-to-meat conversion efficiency enhancer for the beef industry. Since bovine GH has no activity in humans, there should be no concern about possible residues in the meat. Similar species-specific growth hormones will undoubtedly be manufactured for other domestic food animals. Of course, human growth hormone can and will be produced inexpensively and in unlimited quantities by these techniques. In addition to its obvious medical uses for tissue repair and immune system enhancement, we expect its extensive use in athletics. Following the Olympic GH releaser scandal, there will be an Olympic GH use scandal. Since GH occurs naturally in the human body, and since it has a short biological half life, prohibitions against its use will be unenforceable.

17. Ballet dancers and other professional athletes will be able to add 20 to 40 years to their professional careers. We would be delighted if they would contact us through our publisher. In particular, we invite three of our favorites, Rudolf Nureyev, Mikhail Baryshnikov, and Anthony Dowell to contact us; it would give us the greatest pleasure to be able to do something for these wonderful artists, who have given us so many hours of excitement and inspiration.

18. Data encryption (secret codes or, more properly, ciphers) technology will be available for individuals owning personal computers. These unbreakable encryption methods will give these individuals the ability to keep their records and communications secret, an ability now possessed by only a few government agencies, such as the National Security Agency and the Soviet KGB. Privacy maintained by mathematical law rather than by force will then be widely available.

MORE ON LIFE EXTENSION FROM DURK AND SANDY

Some time this summer, we are going to use one of our computers to construct a complete and comprehensive cross-index for this book, employing a fairly extensive hierarchy of subheadings. This index will list every single appearance of each vitamin, mineral, amino acid, other nutrients, food additives, chemicals, drugs, hormones, neurotransmitters, aging mechanisms, diseases, technical terms, warnings, research scientists, physicians—indeed, everything except common non-technical English words. Due to the convenient use of subheadings, sub-subheadings, etc., each entry will appear in numerous places. As a result, we anticipate that our "Researcher's Index to *Life Extension: A Practical Scientific Approach*" will be somewhere around 100 pages long, which is much too long to be included in this book. If you send us a stamped, self-addressed envelope, we will inform you of the price and length when it is ready, at which time you can decide whether you really wish to order it. Please also tell us if you would like to purchase annual updates to our *Life Extension*. What would you be willing to pay for such periodic updates? If there is a large enough demand for these, we'll write them. Send your stamped, self-addressed envelope to: Durk Pearson and Sandy Shaw, P.O. Box 835, Hawthorne, CA 90250. Do not expect a prompt response or answers to individual questions. Remember that we are research scientists, not physicians, and are neither professionally nor legally equipped to diagnose or treat diseases, so do not ask us to do so!

We will also be substantially expanding our already long list of references and reorganizing it to make it more convenient to use in our own research projects. In addition, we will be establishing our own elaborate computerized data base management and literature search and retrieval system for life extension research information. If there is sufficient demand, we will make these systems generally available. If you are also interested in the "Researcher's Expanded Reference List for *Life Extension: A Practical Scientific Approach*," in either printed form or on a computer readable magnetic disc, include a *second* stamped, self-addressed envelope so that we can notify you of the price and contents when it is ready (probably early in 1983).

SOME AGING RESEARCH TO COME—AN OVERVIEW

Biologically oriented gerontologists, including ourselves, have a lot of exciting research to perform in the near future. We are briefly outlining some of *our* areas of greatest personal interest below; this should *not* be taken as some sort of proposed master plan for gerontology research. Beware of "master plans" in research; only a bureaucrat, idiot, or madman would be deluded enough to believe that anyone can be a master of the not-yet known. We intend to use nearly all of the proceeds from this book and our media appearances to fund these (and other) research and development programs. Do not make the mistake, however, of thinking that we are altruists. Exploring, mapping, and understanding the unknown is our greatest pleasure in life.

1. Our first major research area involves R&D on improved quantitative instrumentation and systems characterization techniques for measuring aging and age-related phenomena in biological systems ranging in complexity from isolated bacteria and human red and white blood cells to adult human beings and other long-lived animals. Much more accurate and meaningful (of known relation to the basic underlying physical and chemical mechanisms) quantitative data is required. The experiment time and influence of uncontrolled variables must be greatly reduced compared to animal life span studies.

2. Our second major research area is the use of some of the above instruments and techniques for the ultra-low cost, ultra-low sample size, very rapid, completely automated quantitative screening of candidate free radical modulating agents, including a rough screen for toxicity.

3. Our third major research area is to use the instrumentation and systems characterization techniques to measure the rate of aging and repair of various physiological subsystems in a time period *very* short compared to the species life span. In particular, we have very good reason to believe that by using a complex but exceedingly powerful non-linear systems characterization tool called Wiener Analysis (invented by Norbert Wiener of MIT, the father of cybernetics), that we will be able to measure age-related degradation (and the extent of its reversibility) of a variety of human subsytems over a period of a year, and possibly over a period of a few months.

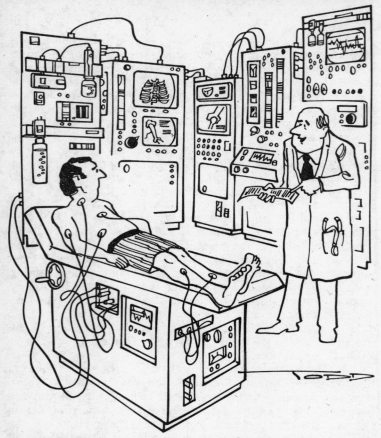

"Thanks to advanced technology we can start treating you immediately . . . for either one of five things!"

Wiener Analysis is well suited to dealing with the extremely high noise levels so common in biological measurements. Wiener Analysis has received very little notice in spite of its immense power for two reasons: The mathematics are conceptually rather complex (plenty of MIT mathematics graduate students had trouble with Wiener's courses) and the number of computations required for the practical analysis of a complex system may easily exceed a billion. Inexpensive powerful number crunching computers have eliminated the latter objection.

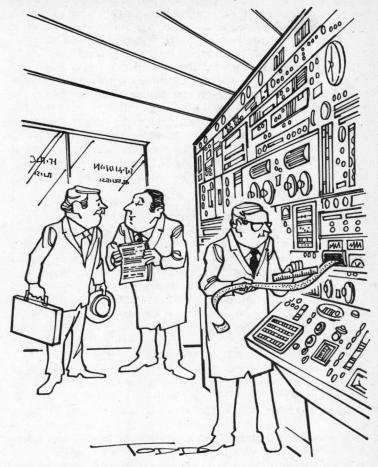

"No charge at all to process these questions, ... the answers will be $850 an inch, though!"

4. Our fourth major research area is the truly rational formulation of free radical modulating regimens. The experimental formulations given in this book are unquestionably far from optimum, both in terms of contents and in terms of the relative amounts of different ingredients. In developing the experimental formulas in this book, we selected materials whose mode of action was roughly understood, and which

should be effective at sub-toxic levels on the basis of animal experiments and subsequent self-experimentation. This gives us a starting point, not an optimized formulation. The quantitative instrumentation techniques referred to above will be used to provide the data for the construction and validation of computer models of the damaging and protective processes, and for the computerized non-linear optimization of the multicomponent free radical modulating formulas.

5. Our fifth major research area is to help fund much more detailed safety studies by professional pathologists and toxicologists. These studies will be practically oriented and no attempt will be made to satisfy FDA criteria for new drugs. We have no interest in commercializing any such formulations.

6. Our sixth major research area is double blind placebo controlled clinical studies on humans and other long lived animals. Of particular interest are studies on persons exhibiting moderate amounts of age or free radical related progressive deterioration in the circulatory, respiratory, and especially the central nervous system. The instrumentation techniques referred to above are essential if these studies are to yield useful, accurate, meaningful, quantitative data in a period of time very short compared to the person's or animal's life span.

7. Our seventh major research area is to explore the utility of computerized quantum chemistry calculations for the modeling of the interactions between free radicals and free radical modulating agents, both to suggest compounds for screening tests and to aid in rational formula optimization. Calculations of this type often require literally billions of computations and have only recently become economically feasible.

8. Our eighth major research area is to explore aging clocks further, both from the point of view of biochemistry and from the viewpoint of cybernetics and information theory. The complete sequence of a human's DNA blueprints does not immediately tell you how the entire system works. When sequenced, the human genome will be like a program in computer machine language (object code), not in human readable source code. We will almost immediately know what parts of the genome specify which known proteins, but what we really need is intricate details of the control system. Computer systems programmers—especially those who delight in penetrating, exploring, modifying, and playing pranks on

very large protected software systems for the fun of it, will play a large part in this task. Computer software hackers arise—you have nothing to lose but your death clocks! *Experienced* computer hackers are invited to write to us, describing their professional experience: DNA Software Project, Box 758, Redondo Beach, CA 90277. Of course, death clocks are a subset of developmental clocks in general, hence progress in death clock control software will inevitably mean parallel progress in developmental clock control software. When the developmental clocks are understood, they can be reprogrammed to give humans the ability to regrow a missing limb, kidney, eye, etc.

9. Our ninth major research area is to do more research and development on the human biological control systems for fat synthesis, storage, and consumption; muscle growth, cardiovascular conditioning, etc. Sandy's experience with growth hormone releasers where she gained about 5 pounds of muscle and lost about 25 pounds of fat while doing exercise sufficient to burn the calories in only *one ounce* of fat vividly demonstrates the naivete of current diet and athletic conditioning concepts. The remarkable effectiveness of Dr. Morehouse's 30 minute per week cardiovascular conditioning program further underscores the importance of working smart rather than merely working hard. This is an area in which we intend to become a lot smarter. Will Rudolf Nureyev still be a ballet star at 70? His spirit is certainly willing, and we would love to have a chance to do something about the age-related progressive weakening of the flesh. We would like to run a sports medicine research institute dedicated to this type of research.

10. Our tenth major research area involves the controlled induction of protective enzymes. Why do your eyes stop burning after a few days of exposure to downtown Los Angeles smog? Because the eye irritant peroxyacetylnitrile in smog induces the increased production of peroxidases in the tears, which then destroy this irritating organic peroxide. Why do farmers and ranchers who are exposed to solar ultraviolet radiation every day get fewer skin cancers than the golfing doctor or bank officer who is exposed only once a week? Again, this is widely thought to be due to the induction of protective and/or DNA repair enzymes. Why is the population (age distribution-corrected) incidence of cancer higher in relatively clean San Francisco than in dirty Newark, New

Jersey? Quite possibly, this is due to the greater induction of protective enzymes by some of the Newark pollutants. Small negative air ions produce superoxide free radicals on contact with water. Is the induction of SOD (superoxide dismutase, an enzyme that destroys superoxide free radicals) a cause of some of the beneficial effects of moderate levels of small negative air ions? Is induction of protective enzymes a reason for the sometimes beneficial effects of periodic exposure to hyperbaric oxygen? And, finally, is induction of protective enzymes the reason why experimental small mammals have had a longer life span and lower cancer incidence when experimentally exposed to about 10 times the normal background level of high energy radiation? (These experiments were the basis for Dr. Edward Teller's oft maligned remark that a little bit of radiation might be good for you.)

Wiener Analysis is very well suited to the characterization of these non-linear protective enzyme induction control systems. Too much of the inducer (a damaging agent such as ozone or x-rays), or exposure with the wrong schedule will result in more damage rather than more protection. We have already acquired an accurately calibrated laboratory ozone generator, a secondary standard ozone analyzer, a quantitative Scott NO_x (nitrogen oxides) analysis system, and a secondary standard x-ray dosimeter for these studies, and we will be constructing a similar controlled small air negative ion source. These and other inducers will be used to characterize our own human protective enzyme induction control systems, and to determine what factors can augment this process.

11. Our eleventh major research area involves extensive further studies on the psychobiochemical aspects of both youthful function and aging in the neuroendocrine system. In particular, we are interested in the psychobiochemical events involved in love, limerance, pair-bonding, and lust, and their interaction with mental parameters such as personal and sexual self-image and individual values. We are also particularly interested in sexual chauvinism and its sociobiological underpinnings, psychobiochemical mode of operation, and its possible psychopharmacological correction. The importance of body image is underscored by the fact that, among the more than 100,000 letters sent to Durk after his Merv Griffin TV Show appearances, over a third were sent in by men and some women desperately seeking a remedy for their balding or thinning hair. It must be emphasized that the emotional tone of many of these letters was indistinguishable from that

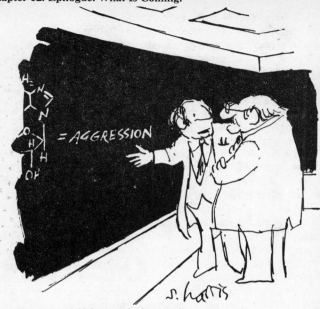

"The answer to sociobiology: sociochemistry."
© 1981 by Sidney Harris/American Scientist Magazine

of thousands of letters written by terminal cancer patients! An adequate understanding of these systems in human beings will require that attention be paid to human software (such as values and self-image), firmware (genetic read only memories, or GROMS) mediating instinctual behavior, and hardware (psychobiochemistry, etc.). In some experimental animals, including mammals, some important aging clocks seem to be linked closely with reproductive behavior and the biological clocks governing it. The central importance of self-image software, particularly in the area of sexual activity, extends far beyond humans and even mammals in general. The sexual behavior and neuroendocrine psychobiochemistry of a bullfrog with a territory is quite different from that of a bullfrog without a territory. We doubt very much that fantasy plays a part in the life of a bullfrog, but is is a very important software element in mediating human neuroendocrine sexual and emotional responses. To ignore these factors is to ignore an essential part of the system, and to deal with the magnificent complexity of the human mind as if it were that of a bullfrog.

SOME AGING RESEARCH TO COME—A FEW DETAILS

Further remarks concerning research areas 1, 4, and 6:

Find out the optimal mixture of antioxidants for free radical protection using a red blood cell hemolysis model. Red blood cell membranes can be protected from free radical damage with antioxidants and can be used to help discover the optimal proportions of a mixture of antioxidants. This technique would be suitable for low cost mass screenings requiring small sample size.

One cubic millimeter of blood (far less than one drop) contains millions of very simple experimental "animals," red blood cells. Various damaging agents cause hemolysis, the breakdown of the red cell membrane and leakage of hemoglobin, a rather readily automated measurement. A standard assay for vitamin E status is the degree of red blood cell hemolysis in salt-water solutions of varying osmotic stress. Other readily applied membrane damage agents include a variety of oxidants and free radicals: hydrogen peroxide, ozone, singlet oxygen produced photochemically via rose bengal dye, ultraviolet light, x-rays, hypochlorite, and a host of specific chemically or electrochemically produced free radicals.

For initial screening, candidate free radical modulation agents and other protective substances can be added directly to the cubic millimeter (one milligram) of blood. A material (not requiring metabolic activation) active at 50 grams per day in an adult human should usually produce effects at less than one microgram in this assay. This permits the screening of minute specimens produced by the separation (by high pressure liquid chromatography, gell electrophoresis, etc.) of natural materials. What is it in bristle cone pine trees that enables them to live for thousands of years? What, besides huge amounts of superoxide dismutase, catalase, and peroxidase, enables the bacterium *radiodurans* to live in operating nuclear reactors? Why do some species of parrots live so long?

Further tests can be performed on the red blood cells of species of animals having differing life spans, and on the red blood cells from people with high versus low family incidence of cancer, cardiovascular disease, progerias (premature aging), drinking, smoking, etc.

Finally, in vivo experiments can be done by giving animals—and our favorite guinea pigs, ourselves—varying types, amounts, and ratios of potential protective substances, and observing the response of our experimentally protected red blood cells to the applied stressing agents. In conjunction with a non-linear optimization computer program, we can then rationally adjust the ratios of the protective substances in our experimental life extension formulation.

Similar, even more informative (but more complex to interpret) experiments can be done using white blood cells as an experimental animal. A cubic millimeter of blood contains thousands of them. Unlike red blood cells, the white blood cells have a nucleus with the same genes as the rest of the nucleated cells in one's body. They are much longer lived, much more complex, must function in a free radical-rich environment, have much more mammalian like protective mechanisms and damage targets, and play a very central and direct role in the aging process.

Human white cells often live a couple of years in the body and make excellent experimental animals. According to Dr. Harry Demopoulos, white cells suspended in serum and exposed to x-rays, dramatically, suddenly, and reproducibly explode after receiving a particular dosage. By varying our antioxidant mix, we can use our own serum and white cells and quantitatively measure their resistance to x-rays (free radicals), thereby allowing us to rationally optimize the free radical modulating properties of our experimental formula. Many extremely effective non-linear computer optimization programs exist for this purpose. This technique is very well suited for low cost mass screening of potential antioxidants. It requires very small quantities of materials, is readily automated, and provides some toxicity information as well, since anything that kills the white blood cells will be quite obvious.

We want to screen all available ergot compounds for free radical modulating activity. Many ergot compounds have been relegated to the chemical storage room because they show no noticeable physiological activity in standard assay tests (such as making a strip of rat intestine contract); something with negligible physiological activity on these tests may be a far more powerful free radical modulator than Hydergine®. Remember that Hydergine® was not developed or assayed for this purpose. There are almost certainly even more potent compounds sitting on the shelf right now! Note that Hydergine® will probably be active in this test (on one cubic millimeter of white blood cell-containing serum) at a sample size of less than 10^{-10} gram (1/10,000,000,000 of a gram).

We have fairly good experimental reasons to believe that ergot compounds exist which are over 1000 times as potent as Hydergine® in free radical modulating activity; that is, compounds that would be effective in an adult human at a dose of a few micrograms per day. Such compounds are not yet being produced as free radical modulating agents, but are now being tested for other purposes.

Further remarks on research areas 1, 4, and 6:

Optimization of the experimental protective formulations can also be done on a chemical macroscopic scale. For example, the ability of one's serum to destroy hydrogen peroxide can be measured by a modified version of the glucose oxidase clinical laboratory method for measuring blood sugar. This became obvious when we both received glucose oxidase assayed blood sugars so low that we "should" be dead. In reality, our blood sugars were normal. The test works by enzymatically oxidizing glucose, to produce hydrogen peroxide which is coupled with the enzyme peroxidase to a colorless dye precursor, o-dianisidine, which when oxidized turns brown. The brown dye is measured by a spectrophotometer and is normally proportional to the amount of glucose present. In this test, our serums were over 10 times as active as normal in destroying the hydrogen peroxide produced in the first step, hence little brown dye was produced, hence the false, seemingly fatally-low blood sugar reading.

This assay can be readily modified to measure the ability of serum to destroy hydrogen peroxide, and this test can easily be run on standard automated clinical laboratory analysis equipment. In the modified assay, the enzyme glucose oxidase is left out, and instead, a known amount of hydrogen peroxide is added. The test tube of serum is then incubated for several minutes at body temperature, and the remainder of the assay run as normal. The less brown dye produced, the greater is one's ability to destroy hydrogen peroxide. Analagous measurements can be made of other protective enzymes such as SOD, etc.

Experiments involving research areas 1 and 4:

Quantum electronic instrumentation—the electron spin resonance spectrometer (ESR) also called the electron paramagnetic resonance spectrometer (EPR)—is capable of identifying different free radicals, counting each type, measuring their lifetimes, and characterizing their interactions with each other, with free radical modulating agents, and with molecules found in cells. Most free radicals are very short lived in water-rich biological systems and they exist in very low concentrations. This requires the use of special ESR equipment involving high magnetic fields and radio waves only a fraction of an inch long. If this book sells enough copies, we will be purchasing a $150,000 Varian Q-band ESR spectrometer to perform this research.

Experiments involving research areas 1, 3, 4, 6, and 9:

Wiener Analysis will permit the measurement of both age related damage and treatment-accelerated repair in biological systems in a time period very short compared to the average life span of the animals involved. Calculations indicate that it should be possible to measure biological system function degradations of 0.1 percent or so, even in the presence of a great deal of random noise. For those human functions that degrade at a rate of about 1 percent per year, a good clinical experiment on human aging could be performed in a year or two, with greater quantitative accuracy than the usual type of experiment which might well require 25 years or more.

Wiener Analysis is an extraordinarily powerful and general mathematical technique for relating the output response of an arbitrarily complex non-linear memory-containing experimental system to a set of input stimuli. It is necessary that the tested system's output be integratable (which is generally true of physically realizable systems) but it does not have to be continuous. Wiener Analysis works very well on noisy discontinuous systems such as multi-neuron chains.

What stimuli should one use for exciting the system to be tested? Information theory shows that the most general possible stimulus is white noise having a bandwidth a few times wider than the tested system passband. (Any signal can be derived by subtracting components from [simplifying] white noise.) Hence white noise is used to stimulate the system.

The output of the noise-stimulated experimental system is then cross-correlated with the input stimulus for delay times ranging from zero to a few times as long as the system memory. This yields a quantitative set of response functions called Wiener kernels. Using these Wiener kernels, it is possible to predict the experimental system's output response sequence to any arbitrary input stimulus sequence. In practice, the three lowest order kernels do a remarkably good job of characterizing a complex non-linear system such as a chain of three different types of neurons. Quantitative changes in these Wiener kernels, not in the raw system output, are the measures of changes—such as age damage and repair—in the system.

Here is a concrete example. A person may easily lose half of his or her visual acuity before realizing that something is wrong. An ophthalmologist is doing fairly well to reliably measure a 25 percent loss in acuity. Dr. Derek Fender at Cal Tech has applied Wiener Analysis to this problem. The subject stares at a television screen filled with pseudorandom noise; this looks rather like the "snow" that you can see on an unused TV channel. Electrodes around the eyes pick up the electrical signals generated in the retina. Wiener Analysis is then used to relate the retinal output to the light-pattern input. Fender can detect a $\frac{1}{2}$ percent change in visual acuity with about 30 seconds of testing. Since the signal-to-noise ratio improves with the square root of the test time, a $12\frac{1}{2}$ minute test period should suffice, even with present equipment, to measure a 0.1 percent change reliably.

Wiener Analysis can be used on a host of physiological stimulus-response sets. The pupil servomechanism has already been analyzed. Spinal reflex arcs would be simple to characterize. Analysis could be performed on EEG signals from the auditory and visual projection areas. The motor servo loops in health, Parkinsonism, and in multiple sclerosis, etc., could be characterized, as could the viscoelastic physical properties of the vascular system. In general, just about any input/output relation of a living system could be characterized by Wiener Analysis. We will be doing a lot in this area. See the chapter notes for a list of references.

More research projects involving areas 1, 3, 4, 6, and 9:

Ballistocardiography has already been mentioned in Part III, Chapter 16. When a person's heart beats, a pressure wave travels through the vascular system which makes the person's body shake like a bowl of Jell-O®. If the person lies on a table which is isolated from environmental vibrations and is instrumented with accelerometers, this pulse-induced shaking can be characterized, and the viscoelastic physical properties of the vascular system determined. Such a system requires low drift, low frequency, high sensitivity sensors and amplifiers, a decent viscoelastic pulse wave analysis computer program, and lots of cheap computer time. None of these were available when this technique was invented in the early 1950s. Thanks to aerospace R&D, all are now readily available and far less expensive. This technique should be very valuable for measuring hardening—and unhardening—of the arteries in a safe, comfortable, quick, convenient, inexpensive (on a large scale) non-invasive manner.

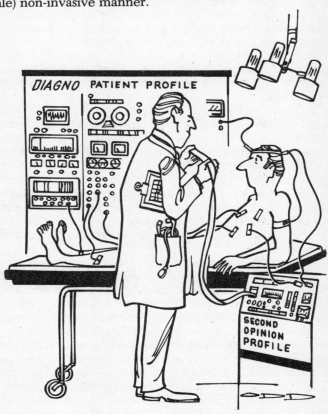

MORE AGING RESEARCH TO COME

Investigate the effects of dehydroepiandrosterone on various aging parameters in animals and humans. This hormone declines in quantity between the ages of 20 and 30 in humans by a greater amount than any other known substance in the human body. When Dr. Arthur Schwartz of Temple University gave mice dehydroepiandrosterone in an experiment, the mice lived 50 percent longer, ate normally but didn't become obese (although they had a genetic predisposition to obesity), and had a reduced susceptibility to breast cancer. Preliminary human clinical experiments have already commenced.

Use ESR to produce three dimensional pictures of free radical activity over the whole human body. This may be a useful technique for quantifying changes in free radical activity due to aging or for detecting many pathological conditions (hypoxic areas in arteries, for example). The improved signal-to-noise ratio required for this task may be obtainable by using coherent demodulation as does the Dicke radiometer used in radio astronomy.

Use Wiener Analysis to study the brain functions of people with unsuspected hydrocephaly, which has been discovered during CAT scans recently. Some of these brains contain as little as 50 to 100 grams of nerve tissue but some of these individuals are reported to behave normally. One such person has an IQ of 126. This was reported in *Science* (12 December 1980). We would like to investigate whether these brains can really perform normal simultaneous processing functions and, if they can, how they are able to do so.

Develop computer software for modeling aging and biochemical processes.

Test a possible new emergency procedure for victims of carbon monoxide poisoning and mine fires, for example, which result in hypoxic conditions. Part of the victim's blood could be replaced with fluorocarbon blood substitute. This would make oxygen available to the victim's tissues rapidly and avoid the many safety hazards of blood transfusions.

Measure the quantitative effect of Hydergine® and its chemical cousins on neurite growth in animals.

Determine the extent of protection offered by Hydergine® in cases of sickle cell anemia and emphysema (damage largely due to free radicals produced under the hypoxic conditions). Many victims of serious, repeated sickle cell crises suffer progressive brain damage due to the hypoxia produced when sickled red blood cells cannot pass through the small capillaries. It may be possible to prevent much of this damage by using Hydergine®, a powerful antioxidant and free radical scavenger.

Conduct a clinical trial of the antioxidant combination vitamins B-1 and C and the amino acid cysteine in alcoholics, to determine their effects on serum acetaldehyde, and to determine if an alcoholic can be biochemically and behaviorally converted to a social drinker.

Investigate the use of Hydergine®, particularly the injectable form, in hypoxic emergencies such as heart attack, strokes, drowning, and crushing blows, particularly to the brain and spinal cord. Paramedics could carry the Hydergine® injectable for immediate use in such conditions.

Investigate DMSO-based antioxidant formulations for the above emergencies.

Investigate the use of free radical-modulating agents in autoimmune diseases of the nervous system, such as multiple sclerosis. A physician we know has used large doses of antioxidants in such patients and reports good results.

Afterword
The Laugh That Lasts—For the Life Extenders

No great discovery is ever made without a bold guess.

—Newton

The existence and potential of life extension research is just beginning to become familiar to the public. Articles have been appearing in many magazines, newspapers, and even on television about this fascinating subject. On the other hand, practical applications of life extension technology have not been receiving as much publicity for several reasons.

• Most people are afraid to be among the early users of new technologies, they prefer to "wait and see."

• Government policies, as we have shown, greatly discourage applications of medical research findings. Manufacturers of vitamins, nutrients, and prescription drugs cannot legally make life extension claims, even if well supported by the scientific literature.

• Many people are hoping for eventual development of a definitive anti-aging pill which not only will eliminate aging entirely but also will be approved by medical authorities and the government. They will do nothing until that day arrives. We think that may be a very long time indeed.

• People are not used to acting on their own judgment in health matters.

• Most popular writers about life extension research are doing little or nothing about their own aging. They write about life extension research, but they don't apply the findings to themselves. It makes you wonder if they themselves really believe what they say!

We're laughing because the hard job of presenting our ideas to you is nearly over. We can sit back, relax, and dream about new research projects made possible by this book. With the proceeds from this book, we plan to buy more scientific

526

books and journals (our last year's outlay for these was about $20,000), a peptide synthesizer, a Varian Q-band ESR (electron spin resonance spectrometer) for measuring and identifying free radicals, a scanning electron microscope, a flame ionization and electron-capture detector gas chromatograph, a Zeiss Axiomat® microscope with phase contrast, a Normanskii interferometer, fluorescent illuminator and television and photographic camera ports, a Waters high pressure liquid chromatograph, a pseudo-random pulsed field emission X-ray machine for Wiener analysis of free radical mechanisms in lymphocytes and other cells, a Tissuemat® (for preparing specimens), several more computers, including an elaborate hard-disc relational data base management system (derived from that used by NASA on Project Viking) linked directly to the National Library of Medicine database, Comtel computerized image analysis equipment (as was used in NASA's Project Viking), a Unimate Puma® laboratory robot, a large building to put the equipment and ourselves in (we have literally lived in our own laboratories for over a decade and intend to continue doing so—for us, science is a way of life, not just a way to earn a living), and, if there is anything left, a vacation (we need one after our three years of work on this book!), a lot more fine art, a good astronomical telescope, a set of seismographs, 2 small sportscars, a Cessna 185® light plane, and perhaps even a powered sailplane like the Caproni AJ-21!!

You may be laughing, too, because now you know that aging need not be as inevitable and certainly doesn't have to be as unpleasant as it has been in the past. You know of many ways to slow your aging and improve health and performance—starting right now. The rapid increase in scientific knowledge offers the promise of continuing development of better methods for the control of aging. We plan to continue studying aging (among other things) and applying new knowledge (carefully!) to our own life spans. Some of these new findings will appear in our next book, too. We'll be laughing often and hope you will, too. Because, after all, isn't that what makes life worth living?

LIVE LONG AND PROSPER!

Durk

and

Sandy

Los Angeles, May 1981

PART VI
APPENDICES, CHAPTER NOTES, AND LITERATURE REFERENCES

APPENDIX A:
Source Information for the Interested Lay Person

All men naturally desire to know.

—Aristotle

It is a great thing to start life with a small number of really good books which are your very own.

—Sherlock Holmes

SECONDARY SOURCES: BOOKS

Physicians Desk Reference, Medical Economics Company, annual

Physicians Desk Reference for Nonprescription Drugs, Medical Economics Company, annual

Handbook of Drug Interactions, Gerald Swidler, Wiley-Interscience, 1971

Vitamin C, the Common Cold, and the Flu, Linus Pauling, Freeman, 1976, $3.45 pb

Cancer and Vitamin C, Cameron and Pauling, Pauling Institute of Science and Medicine, 1979, $9.95 in hardback

Pro-Longevity, Albert Rosenfeld, Knopf, 1976, $8.95 pb

Mental Alertness, Sandy Shakocius (now Shaw) and Durk Pearson, and Kurt W. Donsbach, published by Donsbach University, PO Box 5550, Huntington Beach, CA 92647, $1.00 (contains some of the material on improvement of brain function as Part III, Chapter 2).

Good News for Smokers, Durk Pearson and Sandy Shaw, published by Donsbach University as above, $1.00 (almost the same as Part III, Chapter 10).

You Can Enjoy Alcohol and Good Health, Too!, Durk Pearson and Sandy Shaw, published by Donsbach University as above, $1.00 (almost the same as Part III, Chapter 12).

Slowing Down the Aging Process, Kugler, Pyramid, $1.50 pb

The Healing Factor: Vitamin C Against Disease, Irwin Stone, Grosset and Dunlap, $1.95 pb

Vitamin E for Ailing and Healthy Hearts, Shute, Pyramid, 1972, $1.65 pb

Total Fitness in 30 Minutes a Week, Morehouse, Simon and Schuster, 1975, avail. in pb.

The Life-Extension Revolution, Saul Kent, Morrow, 1980

Secrets of Life Extension, A Practical Guide for the Use of Life-Extension Therapies, John A. Mann, Harbor Publishing, Inc., And/Or Press, Inc., 1980

Vitamin B-6, the Doctor's Report, Ellis and Presley, Harper and Row, 1973

Vitamins and You, Benowicz, Grosset & Dunlap, 1979

Supernutrition, Richard Passwater, Dial Press, 1975

Supernutrition for Healthy Hearts, Richard Passwater, Dial Press, 1977

Regulation of Pharmaceutical Innovation, Sam Peltzman, American Enterprise Institute for Public Policy Research, Washington, D.C., 1974, $3.00

Friedman, Milton (Nobel laureate, economics) & Rose, *Free To Choose,* Harcourt Brace Jovanovich, 1980

An Introduction to Scientific Research, E. Bright Wilson, McGraw-Hill, 1952

Licit and Illicit Drugs, Consumer's Union, 1972

SECONDARY SOURCES: GENERAL SCIENCE PERIODICALS

Scientific American $21/year (12 issues), subscription address: PO Box 5919, New York, NY 10017

Science News, $12.50/year (52 issues), subscription address: 231 West Center St., Subscription Dept., Marion, Ohio 43302

American Scientist, $15/year (12 issues), 345 Whitney Ave., New Haven, CT 06511

Science Digest, PO Box 10076, Des Moines, IA 50306, $11.97/10 issues

Omni (science fact and fiction; medical data sometimes good, sometimes poor—they need good science advisers or to make better use of science advisers they may have), 909 Third Ave., New York, NY 10022, $24/year

Scientific American Offprints (article reprints) Published by W. H. Freeman and Co., 660 Market St., San Francisco, CA 94104, excellent content and style of presentation. An inexpensive education at only $.40 per offprint ($5 minimum order). Send for a free catalog of hundreds of offprints. Selections of interest might include:

Number	Title and Author
1351	"The Origin of Atherosclerosis," Benditt
1103	"Human Cells and Aging," L. Hayflick
155	"The Aging of Collagen," Verzar
335	"Free Radicals in Biological Systems," Pryor
1256	"Cyclic AMP," Pastan
1260	"The Hormones of the Hypothalamus," Guillemin and Burgus
138	"The Thymus Gland," Burnet
1061	"The Repair of DNA," Hanawalt and Haynes
1074	"Gene Structure and Protein Structure," Yanofsky
1013	"Hormones and Genes," Davidson
123	"The Genetic Code," Francis Crick
78	"The Mechanism of Immunity," Burnet
57	"Ionizing Radiation and the Cell," Hollaender and Stapleton
1085	"Lysosomes and Disease," Allison
1291	"Nutrition and the Brain," Fernstrom and Wurtman

Scientific American article collections, including:
The Chemical Basis of Life, 405 pp., $7.95 pb

SECONDARY SOURCES: LIFE EXTENSION PUBLICATIONS

You can read Durk and Sandy's regular health column, including new research findings, in *Claustrophobia, Anti-Aging News, Reason,* and *Health Express; Reason* is a twelve-year-old publication about individual liberty and libertarianism, $11.99/12 issues, subscription address: Box 40105, Santa Barbara, CA 93103; *Health Express,* $10/year bimonthly, Donsbach University, 7422 Mountjoy Drive, Huntington Beach, CA 92648; *Claustrophobia* is a combination magazine including publications on life extension, commercial development of space (including the L-5 Society News), and libertarianism, $30/12 issues (1 year), $2 for a sample package—subscription address: The Howard Foundation, 5047 SW 26th Dr., Portland, OR 97201); see *Anti-Aging News* below.

Anti-Aging News, $27/yr., published by Life Extension, Box 1067, Hollywood, FL 33022; includes a regular health and nutrition column by Durk and Sandy

Medical Hotline, 119 W. 57th St., New York, NY 10019, $24/year
   Telephone orders to: (212) 977-9585
Highly recommended. Excellent source for latest research findings regarding new unapproved uses for old drugs, plus new drug research data. Useful to both layperson and doctor, although aimed at doctors. The publisher contributes 3 percent of this gross business to non-profit charitable research foundations dedicated to biological aging research and intervention. We exercise no control over these foundations, and we have never received and will not receive any grants from them, so as to avoid a potential conflict of interest.

"Mind Food" (May 1979 *OMNI,* pg. 54) by Sandy Shakocius (now Shaw) and Durk Pearson (article on how to increase intelligence and memory with nutrients and prescription drugs which, according to *OMNI* editor Ben Bova, is the most popular single article to appear in *OMNI* to date; much of this material is also in Part III, Chapter 2). Send $1.00 and a stamped, self-addressed envelope to *OMNI* for a reprint.

LIFE-EXTENSION ASSOCIATIONS

Our listing of these institutions does not imply their approval of our work. We receive no support from these institutions and have no control over their funding practices. Send stamped self-addressed envelope for further data:

The American Aging Association, Inc. (AGE)
Attn: Denham Harman, M.D.
University of Nebraska Medical Center
Omaha, Nebr. 68105

AGE publishes *AGE News,* a newsletter on aging research written for both scientists and interested laymen. Membership is $20 per year. Very highly recommended! Dr. Harman is the originator of the free-radical theory of aging. Donations are tax deductible.

FIBER
Fund for Integrative Biomedical Research
1742 N Street, NW
Washington, DC 20036
Attn.: Aging Research Information Service
(202) 293-7660

FIBER is a non-profit foundation dedicated to prolonging the prime of life through research. Tax deductible contributions are accepted. Contributors of $20 or more become Sustaining Members of FIBER and receive quarterly reports on the latest biomedical advances in extending human life. Donations and bequests may be made for research work in specific areas, such as "research on biological aging mechanisms and means of intervention." If no designation is made, funds will be used for interdisciplinary biomedical research in a wide range of fields.

Foundation for Experimental Ageing Research
Felix Platter-Spital
4055 Basel, Switzerland
061 / 440031
Attn.: Dr. Marco Ermini

The Linus Pauling Institute of Science and Medicine
2700 Sand Hill Road
Menlo Park, CA 94025

The Pauling Institute publishes a very interesting Newsletter with emphasis on research with vitamin C. Donations are tax deductible and you may specify areas in which to use the money, such as research on biological aging mechanisms.

To get on the mailing lists of the Pauling Institute, AGE, FIBER, and the Foundation for Experimental Ageing Research and receive a life-extension reading list, send a stamped self-addressed envelope to:

Life Extension, PO Box 1067, Hollywood, FL 33022
24 hour toll free number: 1-800-327-9009 x47
24 hour toll free number for Florida residents: 1-800-432-7999 x47
This is a non-profit organization, donations are IRS approved for tax deduction.

SECONDARY SOURCES: TELEVISION

NOVA: Public Broadcasting System, often has excellent to outstanding life sciences material on these one hour weekly shows. Some of these programs have unstated ideological biases, especially in programs concerning environmental issues.

Time-Life and National Geographic TV specials: These shows are sometimes on the life sciences and usually have outstanding photography and production values and usually rate good to very good on information content.

Durk and Sandy appear frequently on television, particularly on the *Merv Griffin Show, Tomorrow* (Tom Snyder) Show, and the NBC *Everywhere* show. Our own 1½ to 2 minute news spots (à la "The Pharmacist," "The Baby Doctor," "The Green Grocer," etc.) and 4 to 5 minute news specials, both features called "Science on Our Side," are currently appearing on television and will be syndicated to many other stations after publication of this book. These spots and short specials have a heavy emphasis on nutrition, preventive medicine, brain function, and life extension, and nearly all of them provide specific how-to-do-it-right-now instructions. We are producing these specials ourselves in our own facilities.

We currently have serious offers from five TV producers to do our own ½ to 1 hour weekly TV show (each show will be edited to be available in both time lengths). A pilot will be available soon after this book is on sale. Again, we will be stressing interesting, useful, practical, and entertaining science and technology. Producers, TV and radio station programming managers are invited to write on their letterhead to one of our attorneys: Scott Tips, Esq., Box 835, Hawthorne, CA 90250.

STANDARD REFERENCE TEXTS USEFUL TO LAYPER-SONS WITH SOME LIFE SCIENCES TRAINING:

The Pharmacological Basis of Therapeutics, Goodman and Gilman eds., Macmillan, 1975, (occasional new editions)

Remington's Pharmaceutical Sciences, Osol and Hoover eds., Mack Publishing Co., 1975, (occasional new editions)

The Merck Manual, Berkow ed., Merck Sharp & Dohme Research Laboratories, Rahway, N.J., 1977, (frequent new editions)

The Merck Index, Windholtz ed., Merck Sharp & Dohme Research Laboratories, Rahway, N.J., 1976, (occasional new editions)

DATA FOR PHYSICIANS: The following two publications contain information on new FDA-unapproved uses for old drugs:

Medical Hotline, 119 W. 57th St., New York, NY 10019, $24/year
   Telephone orders to (212) 977-9585

This is one of the few publications we read cover to cover; contains many valuable leads, particularly concerning new unapproved uses for old drugs and latest research findings in medicine. Highly recommended. The publisher contributes 3 percent of this gross business to non-profit charitable research foundations dedicated to biological aging research and intervention. We exercise no control over these foundations, and we have never received and will not receive any grants from them, so as to avoid a potential conflict of interest.

Trends in Pharmacological Sciences, Elsevier/North-Holland, Inc., 52 Vanderbilt Ave., New York, NY 10164, $42.50/12 issues.

Highly recommended. Aimed toward the research scientist rather than the medical practitioner; excessively technical for laypersons. This publication is very useful to the clinical research oriented physician.

APPENDIX B:
How to Find Research References

Knowledge is of two kinds. We know a subject ourselves or we know where we can find information upon it.
   —*Samuel Johnson, from Boswell,* Life of Johnson *(Spring, 1772)*

The primary sources of scientific information are the scientific journals in which research reports are first published. You may or may not wish to consult scientific journals, but it is always wise to buy nutrition books and magazines that refer to these journals, rather than to lay publications or newspapers, as information sources. You may also need this information to convince your doctor to give you a prescription for a non-FDA-approved use of an FDA approved drug. Here we tell you how to find a scientific reference.

The use of libraries is a grossly underrated skill that is almost entirely ignored in education. Yet much of available human knowledge can be found in the large libraries associated with educational institutions, if we know how to use them.

In science, it is essential that the chain of reason and experiment be carefully documented because a cornerstone of science is the reproducibility of research findings. That means that if scientist A specifies carefully the conditions of his or her experiment (what type and strain of animals used, the temperature at which bacterial cultures are grown, what companies supplied the chemicals used, etc.), then any other scientist should get the same results as scientist A. Many promising experiments have not been reproducible. (Of course, even in such cases, much may be learned by tracing back to find out what factors were not taken into account.)

539

References are points on a map. By following them back in time, we can see the evolution of ideas. We can find out how present thinking came about. References can be primary, being taken from original scientific papers, or they can be secondary, coming from magazine and book interpretations of scientific papers. Most nutrition and anti-aging books list only secondary references. Primary references are far better, however, because they provide the experimental evidence with at least one less layer of biases (those of the book or magazine writer and editor). We have provided many primary scientific references for this book in Appendix K, so that you can check our interpretations if you wish or follow up leads that interest you.

A reference is a standardized notation which tells you <u>who</u> wrote the paper, <u>what</u> the paper is about, <u>where</u> the paper was published, and <u>when</u> it appeared in the publication. A sample reference is:

Kormendy and Bender, "Chemical Interference with Aging," *Gerontologia* 17:52–64, 1971

The authors Kormendy and Bender wrote about chemical interference with aging. The paper appeared in the journal *Gerontologia,* volume 17, pages 52–64 in 1971. You can find the location of *Gerontologia* by looking under "G" in the periodical cardfile (ask the librarian where the file is located).

It is possible to do a great deal of your own personal research by searching for and studying already published papers. Some scientists have even been awarded Nobel Prizes for interpreting (in new ways!) other scientists' experimental work. You may not get a Nobel Prize, but you may be able to answer some of your own questions about aging and increase your healthy active life span!

The very useful MEDLARS Search Service is available in many medical university libraries. For a modest fee (as little as $10), you can specify any particular limited subject area—for example, the effect of vitamin A on cancer—the MEDLARS computerized data base management system will search its extensive data banks and send you a long print-out of references to scientific papers published on this subject. The service covers over 3000 different journals. There may be hundreds of references, many with abstracts (brief summaries of the paper's contents). You can then followup on the

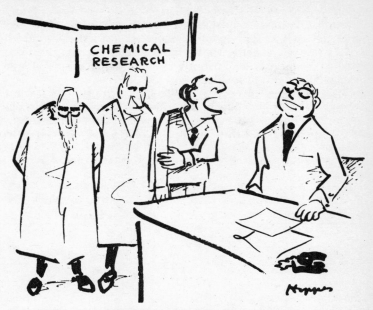

"Doctor Askin will explain his breakthrough to Doctor Bixter who'll give me his interpretation, which I'll interpret for you."

ones of greatest interest. See the next section, Appendix C, "Computerized Biomedical Literature Search Service."

In a large university or medical library, you'll find several indexes which list references by subject and author and supply the name and issue of the journal which contains the information you are looking for. *The Unabridged Index Medicus, Chemical Abstracts,* and *Biological Abstracts* are three particularly useful ones for finding data on biochemical-related topics. Ask the reference librarian to show you how to use them. In Appendix J, we've included a short (not comprehensive) list of journals which frequently publish information in the field of biological gerontology, and the abbreviations commonly used in place of their names. We've found these journals particularly helpful in our own literature searches.

Chapter 99, "Utilization and Evaluation of Clinical Drug Literature," in *Remington's Pharmaceutical Sciences,* (Mack Publishing Co., 1975) is a very handy guide to finding research references. You can find this standard reference in any university life science or medical library, and if you have become acquainted with your pharmacist (you should get to know your pharmacist; they are not sales clerks, they are health professionals who can give you valuable advice), he or she may allow you to look at a copy.

In a matter as important as life span extension, you want to have the best possible information. Primary scientific papers are the basis for the successful development of life-extension technology. And they are accessible to you, as well as to scientists.

APPENDIX C:
Computerized Biomedical Literature Search Service

The greatest desire of men is for eternal youth.
—*Alexis Carrel*, Man the Unknown *(1935)*

A professional medical information search service, MED-LARS, is available to scientists and to you, too, at many medical school libraries. For a reasonable fee, usually $10 to $26, you can obtain hundreds of references to original scientific papers covering your specified area of interest.

A very useful and inexpensive tool for persons wishing to search for scientific data on aging or other specific biomedical subjects is MEDLARS. MEDLARS, a bibliographic search service designed by the National Library of Medicine to provide health professionals with rapid access to current journal literature, is available to the general public as well. A companion search service, BACKFILES, contains literature references to past research (back to the early 1960s).

MEDLINE (as the computerized data base management system is called) and BACKFILES do not contain the actual research papers. They retrieve the references and, in the case of citations indexed since 1970, may include abstracts (summaries). You receive by mail a computer printout of these references. Complete papers can be obtained by going to a large medical or life sciences library and looking them up. Most such libraries have inexpensive photocopying machines available, and there are librarians to assist you. Search costs vary up to $26 for both MEDLINE and BACKFILES (early 1960s to date). You should first obtain a MEDLARS search request (a sample form is shown on pages 548–549) from the library. This form contains questions concerning the subject area to be searched, years to be included in the search, and some references to relevant papers, if you know of any (it is helpful for getting leads). Then mail in the form with your fee prepaid.

Chapter 99, "Utilization and Evaluation of Clinical Drug Literature" in *Remington's Pharmaceutical Sciences,* Osol and Hoover eds., (Mack Publishing Co., 1975, occasional new editions) provides a concise useful guide to this subject. This standard reference can be found in any university life sciences or medical library, and your pharmacist will also own a copy.

MEDLARS covers about 3,000 different publications in the biomedical field and can provide an excellent starting point for an individual wishing to do some research of his or her own.

REGIONAL MEDICAL LIBRARIES AND MEDLARS CENTERS

Regional Medical Libraries

(1) GREATER NORTHEASTERN REGIONAL MEDICAL LIBRARY PROGRAM
The New York Academy of Medicine
2 East 103rd Street
New York, New York 10029
Phone: 212-876-8763

States served: CT, DE, MA, ME, NH, NJ, NY, PA, RI, VT, and Puerto Rico

(2) SOUTHEASTERN/ ATLANTIC REGIONAL MEDICAL LIBRARY SERVICES (STARS)
University of Maryland
Health Sciences Library
111 South Greene Street
Baltimore, Maryland 21201
Phone: 301-528-7637

States served: AL, FL, GA, MD, MS, NC, SC, TN, VA, WV, and the District of Columbia

(3) REGION 3—REGIONAL MEDICAL LIBRARY
University of Illinois at Chicago
Library of the Health Sciences
Health Sciences Center
P. O. Box 7509
Chicago, Illinois 60680
Phone: 312-996-2464

States served: IA, IL, IN, KY, MI, MN, ND, OH, SD, WI

(4) MIDCONTINENTAL REGIONAL MEDICAL LIBRARY PROGRAM (MCRML)
University of Nebraska
Medical Center Library
42nd and Dewey Avenue
Omaha, Nebraska 68105
Phone: 402-559-4326

States served: CO, KS, MO, NE, UT, WY

(5) SOUTH CENTRAL REGIONAL MEDICAL LIBRARY PROGRAM (TALON)
University of Texas
Health Science Center at Dallas
5323 Harry Hines Blvd.
Dallas, Texas 75235
Phone: 214-688-2085

States served: AR, LA, NM, OK, TX

(6) PACIFIC NORTHWEST REGIONAL HEALTH SCIENCES LIBRARY SERVICE (PNRHSLS)
Health Sciences Library
University of Washington
Seattle, Washington 98195
Phone: 206-543-8262

States served: AK, ID, MT, OR, WA

(7) PACIFIC SOUTHWEST REGIONAL MEDICAL LIBRARY SERVICE (PSRMLS)
UCLA Biomedical Library
Center for the Health Sciences
Los Angeles, California 90024
Phone: 213-825-1200

States served: AZ, CA, HI, NV

MEDLARS Centers

Health Center Library
Ohio State University College
of Medicine
1645 Neil Ave.
Columbus, OH 43210
(614-422-6374)

University of Michigan
3490 Kresge Medical Research
Bldg.
Ann Arbor, MI 48104
(313-763-3136)

Lister Hill Library of the
Health Sciences
University of Alabama
1919 7th Ave. S.
Birmingham, AL 35233
(205-934-3613)

Denison Memorial Library
University of Colorado Medical
Center
4200 E. 9th Ave.
Denver, CO 80220
(303-394-7460)

Texas Medical Center
Jesse H. Jones Library Building
Houston, TX 77025
(713-529-0762)

Foreign MEDLARS Centers

National Library of Australia
Canberra, A.C.T. 2600
Australia

National Science Library
National Research Council of
Canada
100 Sussex Drive
Ottawa 7, Canada
(613-996-221)

National Lending Library for
Science and Technology
Boston Spa
Yorkshire, Great Britain
LS23 7BQ

Centre de Documentation de
l'INSERM
(Institut National de la Sante et
de la Recherche Medicale)
Centre Hospitalier de Bicetre
78 Avenue du General Leclerc
94 Kremlin-Bicetre
Paris 16e, France

DIMDI (Deutsches Institute für
medizinische Dokumen-
tation und Information)
5 Koln 41, Postfach 420580
Germany West

JICST, The Japan Information
Center of Science and
Technology
C.P.O. Box 1478
Tokyo, Japan
or
5-2 2-tyome, Nagatatyo
Tiyoda-ku, Tokyo, Japan

Biomedical Documentation
Center
Karolinska Institutet, Fack
S-104 01 Stockholm 60
Sweden

World Health Organization
Library
Avenue Appia
1211 Geneva 27
Switzerland

BIBLIOGRAPHIC SEARCH REQUEST

DATABASE(S)

YEARS

Name (Please Print) _____ Date_____

Mailing Address _____

   City_____ State_____ Zip _____

Position or Title _____Telephone _____

Department/Organization/School _____

Submitted by (if different from above)_____

Telephone _____

1. DETAILED STATEMENT OF QUESTION: Please describe your search topic as specifically as possible. Indicate any points NOT to be included.

2. ABSTRACTS: Do you want abstracts included with the citations? Yes_____ No_____

3. SCOPE OF SEARCH: Do you wish your search to be:
   _____ Comprehensive: include all articles discussing topic regardless of emphasis
   _____ Selective: limit to major articles

4. RETRIEVAL ESTIMATION: Please estimate the number of articles you expect to be retrieved in the last three years (e.g. 25, 100, 200). _____

5. DEADLINE: Please indicate if you have a deadline (it usually takes 7 to 10 working days after the search is run to receive the print-out). _____

OFFICE USE ONLY

Received	Disposition	Released
☐ Date _____	☐ Mail _____	☐ Mailed on _____
☐ Amount _____	☐ Pick up:	☐ Called for pick up:
☐ Payment mech. _____	☐ 1st 25 citations _____	☐ 1st 25 citations on
☐ Initials _____	☐ all citations _____	☐ all citations _____

6. SEARCH PURPOSE:

_____ patient care
_____ talk/grand rounds
_____ cancer therapy/
research
_____ clinical research
_____ teaching
_____ basic research

_____ book or journal
publication
_____ site review
_____ course assignment
_____ dissertation/thesis
_____ other (specify)
_____
_____

7. SEARCH SPECIFICATIONS:

Languages
_____ Accept English and foreign language articles with English summaries
_____ Accept only English
_____ Accept all languages
_____ Accept certain languages only (please specify): _____

Research subjects
_____ Human   _____ Female   _____ Male
_____ Animal experiments; if only certain animals or animal groups are of interest, please list these:

Age groups
_____ 0 to 1 month
_____ 1 to 23 months
_____ 2 to 5 years
_____ 6 to 12 years

_____ 13 to 18 years
_____ 19 to 44 years
_____ 45 to 64 years
_____ 65 years and over

8. COST LIMITATIONS:

_____ Maximum number without additional cost
_____ All citations, regardless of cost
_____ Limit to _____ citations or _____ dollars

9. KNOWN RELEVANT PAPERS PUBLISHED WITHIN THE LAST THREE YEARS:

I hereby authorize the _____ Library to perform the online search(es) specified on the reverse side and agree to pay the charges incurred for computer time, telecommunications, printing, and service fee (when applicable).

_____
Signature

APPENDIX D:
Becoming Involved in Aging Research

> *It's necessary to be slightly underemployed if you are to do something significant.*
> —James Watson (Nobel laureate, co-discoverer of the DNA double helix)

Intrigued by aging research? You don't have to be a scientist to contribute to this rapidly growing field. Here are a number of ways that you can become involved in aging research.

You may have become intrigued by reading this book and given some thought to the possibility of becoming personally involved in aging research. You need not be a full-time scientist or know much about biology, or even do any experiments! For example, Crick and Watson discovered the double-helix structure of DNA and won a Nobel Prize without doing any experiments of their own. These two geniuses built paper models based on other people's experimental data. Mostly, though, they <u>thought</u> about the problem. George Gamow, a physicist and science writer, first suggested the DNA triplet code (where three nucleotides of the DNA code for an amino acid in a protein). He thought of this without doing any experiments. And consider the fact that Einstein's general theory of relativity was conceived by Einstein as a *gedanken* or thought experiment years before he was able (with the help of a German mathematician) to produce the mathematical proofs for the theory. Einstein was stimulated by unexplained experimental results of others to develop first his special theory of relativity, followed by his general theory of relativity.

Areas that can make contributions to aging research include:

1. Science: physics, chemistry, biology, materials
2. Information theory—evolutionary theory, genetic coding, computer programming (e.g., aging model simulations and especially elucidating the aging and developmental clock control systems coded on the DNA). Information theory is a general body of laws governing any data processing, including biological data.
3. Economics—the process of making available aging-research applications, bottlenecks to drug innovation. Moreover, economics is very closely related to evolutionary theory.
4. Technician—lab, electronics, chemical, medical, etc. Aging research instrumentation is a newly developing field of great importance.
5. Engineering—they design and build a host of lifesaving biomedical hardware.
6. Law—pharmaceutical regulations, legal liability
7. Medicine—doctor—clinical research
8. Writers and journalists

There are several sources of funding for aging-research work. The first is you. Some research can be done with a small amount of money. When you fund your own research, you are free to work on problems that interest you and you needn't be concerned about brown-nosing or writing fancy reports for others. Some occupations offer opportunities to work on research related to aging, such as in the food and plastics industries (e.g., antioxidants are used widely as food and plastics preservatives).

Outside agencies are another source of funds: educational, medical, or governmental agencies (such as the National Institute of Aging). These institutions are not an easy way to acquire research funds. Besides being bureaucratic and sometimes intolerant of new ideas, they have control of which projects you can work on, and you have the problem of getting university tenure. The government hardly funds biological aging research at all, although the NIA makes some funds available. However, social gerontologists outnumber biological gerontologists by about 10 to 1, and are in control of NIA allocations. But if you don't mind working in the post office, you may not mind working for NIA. (After all, Einstein accomplished a great deal while working at the patent office!)

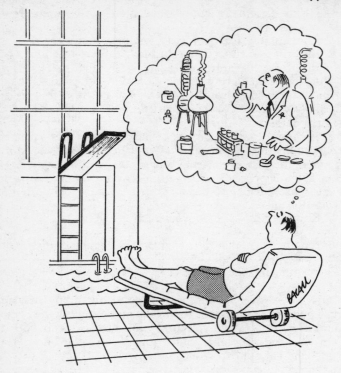

© 1981 Aaron Bacall

You can learn a lot and meet scientists working on biological aging research by attending some aging conferences
for professionals. At first, you won't understand much, but by
studying hard in advance, asking questions and persevering,
you can get right into the aging-research subculture. The
American Aging Association is a good place to start. This organization was set up for both scientists and interested lay
persons. (See Appendix A for membership information.)
These conferences are the best place to find out about private
funding, yet another source of research funds. There are some
private foundations and even some individuals who make
grants of up to a few hundred thousand dollars per year for
projects which offer good potential for practical application.
If you are interested in this approach, bring available information on your ideas and proposed experiments, if any.

Three books which you may find of value in planning the use of your resources to pursue aging research and other goals are:

1. Michael Phillips' *The Seven Laws of Money* (Random House, 1974) describes a world view relating money to the things you want to do. How <u>not</u> to end up losing your enthusiasm for projects because of money problems, and how not to lose sight of your original goals while making that money. Michael Phillips is an investment banker who, among other things, funded the *Whole Earth Catalog*

2. Don Lancaster's *The Incredible Secret Money Machine* contains a lot of practical information and good philosophy on how to do what you really want to do and how to make money doing it. This book is published by Howard W. Sams & Co., Inc., 4300 West 62nd St., Indianapolis, Ind. 46268

3. Alan Lakein's *How to Get Control of Your Time and Your Life,* Wyden, 1973

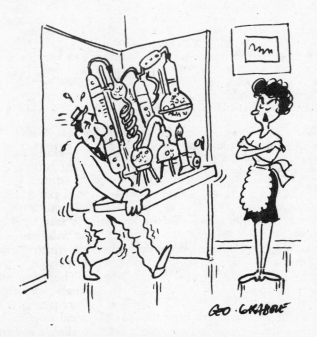

"Harold! Why can't you bring home . . . work . . . like other men?"

APPENDIX E:
What Is the Government Doing About Aging Research?

So long as a medical discovery remains in the laboratory stage, it is of little value to anyone. It cures no disease, saves no lives. It is a scientific curio. It is only when a manufacturing company starts producing the material in large quantity that the product can find its way into the stock rooms of hospitals and the handbags of physicians. No matter how brilliant the discovery, it doesn't begin to save lives until this step is taken. In giving our research men the great credit due them, we often forget to pay tribute to the manufacturers who make the fruits of this discovery available to all of us.
—*Ratcliff,* Yellow Magic: The Story of Penicillin *(1945)*

To consider any extension of the human life span without a serious effort to anticipate and plan for the impact of increased longevity on society would be entirely irresponsible.
—*Alexander Leaf, former head of the President's Special Commission on Aging,* Scientific American, *Sept. 1973*

Already it is complained that the burden of supporting old people is too heavy, and statesmen are perturbed by the enormous expense which will be entailed by State support of the aged.
—*Metchnikoff, "The Prolongation of Life" (1908)*

I'm not a bad man. I'm just a bad wizard.
—*Frank Baum,* Wizard of Oz

Government agencies have had a profound and generally negative impact on the progress of aging research and, especially, the application of that research to human aging problems. The FDA's regulatory policies have drastically reduced the amount of pharmaceutical innovation without a measurable increase in either drug safety or efficacy. The National Institute of Aging, which is supposed to be spending many millions each year on aging research, actually spends only a small part of their funds on studies of biological aging that are potentially useful for life extension; the rest is spent on psychological and social studies of the aged. The head of the National Institute of Aging has written that the NIA will not fund studies aimed specifically at extending human life span. He claims that there is no evidence that it can be done.

INTRODUCTION

This appendix is as much about individual values and personal moral choices as it is about facts. Facts alone do not cause a person to take action. We act as a result of choices based on the interaction between what we want (our values) and what we think we can achieve (our perception of reality). If you value **freedom of choice,** you will probably agree with most of this chapter. If you believe that responsibility must ultimately reside in the individual rather than with a collective, you are likely to applaud what we say here. But if your personal values are very different from ours, if you feel that responsibility must be a function of masses of people rather than the individual, if you insist that some adults must be protected by force from the opportunity to make mistakes, then you will disagree with most of what we say here. If the latter are your philosophical beliefs and personal values, this appendix may only make you angry.

The regulations of government agencies, particularly those of the Food and Drug Administration (FDA), have had a significant and generally negative effect on the development of life extension technology.

LIFE EXTENSION AND GOVERNMENT
CONFLICT OF INTEREST

The second epigraph given under the appendix title above is the response of Alexander Leaf, at the time the head of the President's Special Commission on Aging. With this philosophy, we may not be permitted to extend our lives beyond the traditional three score and ten until the government figures out how to handle all the expenses and changes arising from widespread life extension.

Is Leaf's comment merely an abstract point of no practical consequence? Already, Britain's socialized medical service generally refuses to provide expensive treatments such as dialysis to patients over 65. The U.S. government already legally limits the number of hospitals that may purchase expensive, high-technology, life-saving biomedical equipment such as CAT scanners and modern radiation therapy units, due to their impact on Medicare costs. As it happens, we agree with these decision-makers that spending Medicare funds for these purposes is not the most cost-effective method of saving lives with this tax money. As a matter of principle, however, we are opposed to all government attempts to limit access to life-saving biomedical technologies for patients able to pay for them (usually through insurance).

These decisions may, so far, represent no more than a well intentioned attempt to avoid wasting money on unnecessarily expensive (by their standards) treatments. But the people who made these decisions and the governments they work for face an inherent conflict of interest. These governments have colossal income-transfer programs, which take money from the young and transfer it to the old, for example, Social Security. These programs and growing public awareness of advances in life extension research require that choices be made between the extension of human life span and the expectations of the electorate for ever more services at tax rates that they can afford. Either electorate expectations for government services must decrease, or taxes (either direct or indirect, such as inflation) must increase, or the human life span must be held constant by government policy. One cannot simultaneously choose a longer average life span, lower taxes/inflation, and more government medical and old age services.

VETERANS ADMINISTRATION

The Veterans Administration has funded a small amount of excellent aging research. In terms of <u>medical</u> economics, it would probably be sensible for them to spend more money on basic and applied research in free radical pathology and its biochemical prevention. Most of the expensive chronic neurological damage and age-related diseases (whose treatment in veterans takes the bulk of the VA medical budget) are caused to a large extent by free radicals, and can be prevented and treated with free radical modulating agents. Diseases in which free radicals are implicated as causative agents include cancer, cardiovascular disease, autoimmune diseases (such as rheumatoid arthritis), and a variety of neurological problems, including paraplegia and quadraplegia caused by brain or spinal cord trauma, and senility. This research may not be funded, however, because the VA also has to pay veterans' retirement benefits. This is a clear conflict of interest; life extension for veterans means much higher retirement costs for the VA and the taxpayers.

NATIONAL INSTITUTE OF AGING

The National Institute of Aging appears to be spending many millions on aging, but most of their budget is allocated to grossly descriptive or psychological, psychiatric, psychosocial, and sociological studies of the elderly, rather than to real biological aging research. A minority of the NIA funds go for basic research on biological aging mechanisms. Some of this work has been outstanding. **No NIA money is being spent on applied research aimed specifically at extending the human life span.** In fact, Robert Butler, the head of the National Institute of Aging, has written that the NIA will not support studies aimed at increasing human life span because, he maintains, there is no evidence that it can be done. Since he has made it a point to attend several professional gerontology meetings at which biological aging data were discussed, one can only conclude that perhaps he didn't understand what he heard.

This funding disposition reflects a fundamental division among American gerontologists: only about 10 percent are biochemically oriented gerontologists, the remainder being interested in psychosocial gerontology. Since the problems studied by psychosocial gerontologists are nearly all caused by biochemical aging processes, a really satisfactory solution will not be forthcoming until we have a far greater understanding of these biological aging mechanisms. The psychosocial studies can, at best, provide only a relatively slight improvement in the quality of life for older persons, while they do little or nothing to prevent the severe deterioration in quality of life caused by aging itself. We would prefer to see the NIA spend its entire budget on biological studies aimed at both basic and applied research on aging mechanisms and the means for retarding and reversing these mechanisms. Perhaps the NIA should be given a new legislative charter by Congress as the National Institute for Research on Biological Aging Mechanisms.

A precaution is in order at this point. Nobel laureate economist Milton Friedman has pointed out that government research grants can be a two edged sword. Government grants can, if misguided, slow, rather than accelerate, progress by taking scarce resources, such as research scientists, away from more fruitful work. Lest we be considered ungrateful, however, we must credit the taxpayers for financing much of the research cited in this book. Under the present FDA regulatory charter, there is relatively little incentive for pharmaceuticals firms to invest heavily in either basic or applied aging research. It is our opinion that if the FDA regulatory barriers were eliminated, pharmaceutical firms would rapidly move into this field in a big way, creating a "golden age" for aging research and for those of us who intend to take advantage of the results of this research. The actual development and delivery of anti-aging technology can be performed most efficiently by the private sector. For this to occur, the FDA-imposed market barriers must be eliminated or drastically reduced.

NATIONAL CANCER INSTITUTE

The National Cancer Institute has spent billions of dollars in their "war on cancer" with varying degrees of wisdom. In our opinion (which we have held for a decade), a far larger portion of that research money should have been spent on biochemical studies involving free radicals, the chemoprevention of cancer (eg., the prophylactic use of selenium, other antioxidants, and protective enzyme inducers), and the natural immune system mechanisms which are normally almost completely effective in the prevention or self-curing of cancer in its earliest stages (including prophylactic immune system stimulation with low toxicity nutritional supplements). As the Nobel Prize winning tumor biologist P. B. Medawar has suggested, everyone probably gets cancer thousands or possibly even millions of times during their lives—and almost always cures themselves before it becomes noticeable. We think that these studies will be a much more cost-effective approach to the control of cancer.

The NCI has focused—apparently at the request of Congress—on curing relatively advanced cases of cancer, rather than on cancer's biochemical prevention, and its recognition and destruction or redifferentiation by the immune system. Our suggested approach is of limited value to people who already have advanced cancers, but it is of great importance to the roughly 75,000,000 living Americans who do not now have detectable cancer but who will eventually die from cancer if its incidence remains unchanged. Very similar comments can be made about the government's expensive "war on cardiovascular disease," conducted by another of the National Institutes of Health. Practically no money has been spent on free radical pathology research and effective biochemical prevention of the free radical induced development of cardiovascular disease.

NATIONAL INSTITUTES OF HEALTH

The National Institutes of Health (NIH) is the parent organization of the other biomedical National Institutes, such as the NIA and NCI. The NIH has had a 20-year-old policy which excludes scientists who work for profit-making companies from applying for competitive research grants. This policy is supposedly coming under scrutiny now and may be reversed, according to the 26 March 1981 issue of *Nature.* This is a disastrous policy if the goal of providing grants is to fund the best possible science. Rarely, however, is governmental policy so straightforward; clearly, there are ideological goals (someone's value choices) involved here, rather than a real search for excellence or cost effectiveness in science. We believe that it is time to examine these unstated value choices of bureaucrats that underlie government regulations and tax money giveaways.

AGING RESEARCH AT THE AEC?

The AEC (Atomic Energy Commission) no longer exists, having been gobbled up by the formation of Jimmy Carter's amazingly counterproductive, ill designed, and philosophically confused DOE (Department of Energy). The AEC lives on in the scientific literature, though, because of the thousands of research papers on the effects of radiation on biological systems (a type of free radical pathology) published under its auspices. The AEC spent very roughly $1,000,000,000 (a billion dollars) of taxpayers' money on this research over a period of about 30 years. This great body of free radical research represents a gold mine of underutilized information. A vast amount of antioxidant-oriented free radical research has also been performed and a great deal published by the food, animal feed, plastics, petroleum, and rubber industries. Very few gerontologists have been aware of these studies because they have generally not been cited in scientific journals publishing biomedical basic research, remaining confined to industry oriented research publications, and because the often practical nature of these studies has led many research scientists to believe incorrectly that they weren't relevant to basic research. For example, research into personnel safety in H-bomb fallout, breakfast cereals with a one-year shelf life, crazy chick disease in poultry, better refinery gasoline yields, and more durable vinyl tops and tires for automobiles appear to be so remote from the field of gerontology that they are usually ignored or unnoticed. But free radical damage is the underlying mechanism in all these processes and many scientists in these industries publish papers explicitly involving free radicals. The AEC, the food and feed, and petroleum-petrochemicals-plastics-rubber industries have each spent far more on free radical research than the NIA, NCI, and all the other National Institutes of Health combined!

EPA, NIOSH, OSHA, CPSC, ETC.

The EPA (Environmental Protection Agency), NIOSH (National Institute of Occupational Safety and Health), OSHA (Occupational Safety and Health Administration), the CPSC (Consumer Product Safety Commission), and a host of similar regulatory bureaucracies are infamous among scientists for basing multibillion dollar impact regulations on hopelessly inadequate scientific studies. Congress—or the agency itself—sets a regulatory deadline, and, by golly, they go right ahead and issue regulations that cost all of us billions of dollars, in spite of their ignorance of the basic mechanisms causing the problem. Inadequate scientific research guarantees bad regulations and bad regulations mean that scarce resources will be wasted on activities that do not yield benefits worth their cost and that the real problem remains unsolved, although possibly now concealed. Consider pollution regulations as an example. Environmental regulations are extremely expensive and have tied up resources that could be put into alternative uses such as research and development instead. If these agencies really know what they're doing, then why is it that relatively environmentally clean San Francisco has a higher (age adjusted) incidence of cancer than relatively environmentally dirty Newark, New Jersey; Pittsburgh, Pennsylvania; Cleveland, Ohio; Detroit, Michigan; or Los Angeles?

Does OSHA understand safety? There are many good reasons to doubt that they do, including the incredible number of OSHA safety violations recently discovered in OSHA's own Washington DC headquarters office building. The Council on Economic Priorities (CEP), a self-appointed pro-OSHA "public interest" organization, has stated that Du Pont had the worst OSHA compliance record (1,357 violations in the study period) as measured by four of OSHA's own health and safety criteria (such as the number of serious OSHA violations discovered per inspection) of the eight largest chemical producers. CEP said that the severity of the chemical industry OSHA violations "exceeded all other U.S. industries with the exception of mining." Since Du Pont has the worst OSHA health and safety regulation compliance record, Du Pont would be expected to have the worst accident and industrial illness record, right?

Wrong! According to both the U.S. Bureau of Labor Statistics and the National Safety Council records, Du Pont has the best health and safety record of any large chemical producer. Chemical manufacturing, moreover, is the second safest of the 42 major U.S. industries according to the National Safety Council. Clearly, the correlation between OSHA regulations and safety and health performance leaves much to be desired. In fact, Du Pont has such an outstanding safety reputation in the industry that they have set up a very successful division to market their safety expertise to industrial firms around the world. Durk (who has done extensive project safety work for the Space Shuttle's Materials Processing in Space laboratory system) has seen some of Du Pont's safety literature, and considered it excellent. The brutal truth is that your home is far more dangerous than your place of work, unless you are a professional race car driver or something of that sort.

We would like to see a constitutional amendment placing the scientific and legal burden of proof on the regulatory agencies; in order for a regulation to have the force of law, the agency would be required to reasonably prove that their proposed regulation would produce more benefits than costs.

Moreover, if subsequent events and information showed that a regulation was not cost-effective after all, that would be the constitutionally required end of the regulation. Congress passed the laws which explicitly instruct these agencies to regulate, **no matter how large the cost, no matter how small the benefits are in comparison, and no matter whether the susceptibility to damage from the other environmental factors is self-induced, as by smoking.** We cannot afford this immensely wasteful, ineffective, and arrogant philosophy of legislation and regulation.

It is always easy to find ways to spend other people's money. But there are limited resources available and a virtually unlimited number of problems to which they could be applied. For example, paramedic programs have a track record of saving human lives at a cost of under $100,000 per person. It is clearly more cost-effective (more lives saved for the dollars spent) to invest scarce resources in a program like this than in one that might save a few human lives at $100,000,000 per person (such as with the EPA's carbon monoxide auto emission standard and OSHA's benzene vapor exposure standard). Human life is an extremely important value, but there are not enough funds available (and never will be) to do everything. Money spent to save lives one way cannot be used to save lives in another way. Not taking costs into account is fine if you happen to be one of the people who might benefit from these price-is-no-object government-mandated programs, but what about the value judgments of the people who pay the bills? And who decides which people are to become more equal than the rest of us by becoming beneficiaries to such a free spending program?

BATF AND ALCOHOL AND TOBACCO RELATED DEATHS

The BATF is a major contributory factor in about 500,000 human deaths every year in the United States. The BATF, the Bureau of Alcohol, Tobacco, and Firearms, is an arm of the Treasury Department. The primary function of the BATF is to collect federal taxes on and regulate alcoholic beverages, tobacco, and certain types of firearms, such as machine guns. The BATF does a pretty good job of tax collecting. It makes no claims to any biomedical expertise, however, even though it has the job of regulating the two most widely used drugs in America, alcohol and tobacco. BATF is the agency that forbids the addition of antioxidant vitamins such as B-1 to booze, although medical experts familiar with some of the mechanisms of the biochemical actions of alcohol (such as free radicals formed in the autoxidation of acetaldehyde, the primary metabolite of alcohol formed in the liver) agree that such supplementation would significantly reduce alcohol-induced brain and liver damage. Many free radical pathologists also think that adding antioxidants to booze would reduce the dramatic multiplicative increase of cancer risk that occurs when alcohol and tobacco are used together.

The BATF also regulates tobacco. Their regulations preclude adding pure nicotine to a low tar cigarette to create a high nicotine and low carcinogen cigarette. We agree with Dr. Gio B. Gori (Deputy Director, Division of Cancer and Prevention, National Cancer Institute) and the medical staff of the Consumers Union that this simple, inexpensive type of cigarette could markedly reduce the cancer risk for tobacco use, perhaps by a factor of two or more. Congress wrote the BATF enabling legislation with tax collections and firearms control apparently in mind, but they also unintentionally handed out a charter with considerable power to regulate drugs as well. The BATF should be just a tax collector. We do not think that the BATF is competent to regulate drugs; these functions would be better transferred to an agency such as the Division of Cancer and Prevention of the National Cancer Institute.

If such a transfer of power is legislated by Congress, we hope they will explicitly write a charter to regulate in a way that minimizes legal roadblocks to producing and marketing alcohol and tobacco products and substitutes for them which are less hazardous than those currently on the market. We do not think that high tar cigarettes or booze without supplemental vitamins should be banned. We are simply suggesting that the regulating agencies for alcohol and tobacco should not discourage innovations which make these two popular, addicting, and frequently lethal recreational drugs less hazardous without impairing the pleasures they offer to users. The technology for creating such safer recreational drugs already exists. It is up to Congress to change the law so that we can start reducing the over 500,000 tobacco and alcohol-related deaths each year.

FOOD AND DRUG ADMINISTRATION

The FDA is by far the greatest roadblock to the rapid and efficient development of reasonably safe and effective life extension drugs and biomedical devices. Because of the great cost and delays involved in meeting FDA drug requirements of safety and efficacy, many useful drugs are never brought to market. Biomedical devices are now subject to similar FDA regulations, with roughly the same adverse effects. Under present FDA rules, it takes about 8–12 years and $56,000,000 on the average to take a basically new drug through research and development, toxicity tests, clinical tests, and the FDA's regulatory procedures, before you can market the drug and <u>begin</u> to recover your expenses. Your patent expires in 17 years. . . . For comparison, an estimate given in Milton and Rose Friedman's *Free to Choose* (page 206) for the same process in the 1950s and early 1960s is about $500,000 and about 25 months to develop a new drug and bring it to market. Allowing for subsequent inflation would raise the cost to about $2,000,000, only about 4 percent of what the same process costs today and in about 25 percent of the time required today. (The estimate was made by Wardell and Lasagna in *Regulation and Drug Development*, Washington, D.C.: American Enterprise Institute for Public Policy Research, 1975, p. 8.)

Dr. R. L. Landau, Professor of Medicine at the University of Chicago, and University of Chicago economist Margot Doyle maintain that:

"It should be emphasized that the investment in the identification of interesting new biological activity is minute in comparison with the very high cost of clinical testing. Thus, the discovery phase of a new chemical entity is controlled by the cost of the clinical phase—and this is determined by the regulatory agency, which decides the amount and kind of data that must be available to justify the marketing of a drug." (From *Regulating New Drugs*, R. L. Landau, ed., pg. 281, The University of Chicago Center for Policy Study, 1973.)

An example of a useful drug that the FDA has kept off the market is thymosin, an extract 'of the thymus gland that is not only successful in treating some cancers, but which is far less toxic than such FDA-approved anti-cancer compounds as bleomycin. Thymosin has been used experimental-

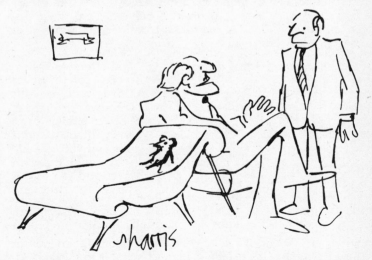

"I believe I have a new approach to psychotherapy, but, like everything else, the FDA tells me it first has to be tested on mice."

ly on a variety of life threatening diseases in human subjects since 1965, often with great success, but as yet this drug cannot be made available to the public due to the FDA's drug rules. The giant pharmaceutical company Hoffmann-La Roche, which probably made the vitamin C you took today, has developed a process for making thymosin and is ready to make it available. But they must wait for FDA approval. Genetically engineered bacteria can be developed that make low-cost thymosin. While the FDA delays and delays, cancer patients and their physicians must choose from the available FDA-approved medications. They cannot choose thymosin.

At the same time that the major drug and food companies are hampered in their efforts to offer innovative products in the U.S., small firms offering alleged anti-aging treatments are, in practice, able to make any claims they wish, whether truthful or not. As Dr. Frederick J. Stare, professor and founder of the Harvard Department of Nutrition, has said, ". . . misrepresenting nutritional information is legal as long as it does not appear on the actual label." (See Part V, Chapter 11, for more about frauds and mistakes in consumer nutrition products.)

You may wonder why the FDA has interfered so greatly in the marketing of new drugs. Consider it from the FDA's point of view. The FDA can make two different types of errors in passing judgment on new drugs:

I. It can pass a bad drug.

II. It can fail to pass a good drug.

As Dr. Louis Lasagna, then Professor of Pharmacology and Toxicology and of Medicine at Johns Hopkins University, said:

"It has been suggested that drug regulation would be better if it worried less about Type I errors than about Type II errors. A drug that is erroneously judged to be active may at least be correctly identified as ineffective ultimately by the test of performance in the marketplace. A drug that is kept off the market by the fallacious judgment that it is ineffective, however, will never have the chance to set its record straight." (From "Alternative Systems of New Drug Regulation," pg. 269, in *Regulating New Drugs*, R. L. Landau, editor.)

If the FDA passes a bad drug, it will soon be found out, damaging the FDA's reputation. The FDA—and the public—will always remember thalidomide. If the FDA fails to pass a good drug, it usually goes without notice because so few people know about it (other than the drug's developers). It is more costly to the FDA to pass a bad drug than it is to fail to pass a good drug. Therefore, the FDA's regulations make it very difficult for a drug to be passed. That is the situation today. A statement of a former FDA Commissioner, Dr. A. Schmidt, as reported in the *Chemical Marketing Reporter* of Nov. 4, 1974 is illustrative: "... in all of FDA's history, I am unable to find a single instance where a Congressional committee investigated the failure of FDA to approve a new drug. But the times when hearings have been held to criticize our approval of new drugs have been so frequent that we aren't able to count them." And as Dr. Schmidt also says, "... failure to approve an important new drug can be as detrimental to the public health as the approval of a potentially bad drug." Bravo! Perhaps this is one reason why Dr. Schmidt resigned as head of the FDA. When you have bad laws, good men who obey them are frustrated and paralyzed. This is not a problem that can be solved by simply "appointing the right man." In our opinion, it can be solved only by adopting a fundamentally different approach to assuring drug availability, safety, and effectiveness.

Economics professor Dr. Walter Oi has expressed the problem succinctly in his "Economics of Product Safety," in *The Bell Journal of Economics and Management Science*, pg. 27, Spring 1973:

"The goal of public policy toward product safety should not be the minimization of accident costs. If that were the goal, we should not permit any rotary lawnmowers but insist instead on the old-fashioned unpowered mowers or as a second-best, allow only reel-type power mowers since these restrictions would reduce home accidents. The appropriate goal should be the maximization of the economic welfare of consumers who, when given a choice, will choose that product grade which minimizes the sum of accident costs and accident prevention costs. Policies that give consumers greater freedom of choice and that place less reliance on direct government controls would seem to come closer to this goal."

Dr. Sam Peltzman, an outstanding economics professor who has done very extensive analysis of the costs and benefits of pharmaceutical regulations, has discussed this problem, too:

"A failure to recognize these facts will lead to a persistent intolerance of risk and a bias against innovation. Indeed, the least expensive way to assure that drugs will be safe and effective—measured by direct expense only—is to tolerate no innovation and rely completely on the tried and true. But in a wider perspective, any attempt to minimize risk in this area has costs which (according to the history of drug innovation) far exceed the benefits: those who will suffer death and disease while a potential drug therapy is evaluated will suffer no less than the victims of a drug disaster, but their number is likely to be much larger than the number of victims of the disaster. The case for present regulatory policy becomes highly dubious if the benefits of risk taking are given the same recognition as the potential costs.

"The unequal emphasis placed on the benefits and costs of risk taking may be explained, if not excused, by the contrast between the anonymity of the beneficiaries and the visibility of the victims." (From *Regulation of Pharmaceutical Innovation*, Sam Peltzman, pg. 88, American Enterprise Institute for Public Policy Research, 1974.)

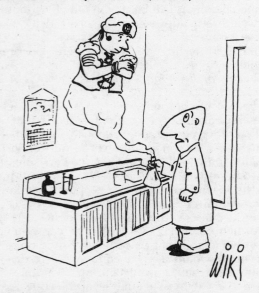

"Sure, I can see you're real, but what will I tell the NIH?"

No drug is risk-free. That's why the concept of benefits versus costs is gradually becoming a new way of looking at chemicals, food additives, drugs, pollution controls, safety regulations, etc. Each drug has its own benefits to costs ratio, which also depends on the personal values of the drug's user. For example, a terminal cancer patient might be a lot less concerned with costs (such as drug side effects) of a new cancer treatment than other people. In general, the benefits versus risks analysis depends on an individual's preferences and personal values. This seriously complicates these calculations since FDA's system allows only a single judgment of pass or no-pass for everybody. There is currently no way of opting out of the FDA's "protection," no matter who you are or what good reason you think you have for getting a new but unapproved drug. Even if your life may depend on it. . . .

As Professor of Law Dr. Guido Calabresi has said:

"I would argue that, on the whole, a system that puts the costs which arise from the introduction of new drugs on the drug company is less likely to create the kind of situation in which it can be said that some victims have clearly been sacrificed by our government, than does a system where the choice of allowing a new drug rests with a centralized government agency. A mistake by the FDA based on a wrong cost-benefit analysis is the same as the government saying that lives are not worth much. A mistake by a drug company for which it must pay compensation may be a tragedy, but it is not the equivalent to 'a judicial sentencing to death.' " (From "Preclinical and Clinical Problems of New Drug Development," pp. 58–9, in *Regulating New Drugs*, R. L. Landau, ed., The University of Chicago Center for Policy Study, 1973.)

Specific instances of poor scientific judgment in FDA decisions come readily to mind. For example, several years ago, the FDA tried to make vitamins in doses greater than $1\frac{1}{2}$ times their Recommended Daily Allowances (RDA) into prescription drugs. This would mean that 100-milligram vitamin C tablets could only be obtained with a doctor's prescription! Fortunately, there was a widespread public protest reflected in over a million letters written to congressmen, and the Congress would not allow the new regulations to take effect. The FDA, ignoring the expressed will of millions of people and the Congress, has repeatedly tried since then to make high-potency vitamins either unavailable or only obtainable with a doctor's prescription. The newest proposed regulation speaks of a "doctor's written permission" rather than of a prescription, in a bureaucratic attempt to blatantly evade an existing law passed by Congress which limits the FDA's power to regulate nutrients.

Another questionable FDA policy is based on a law known as the Delaney Amendment. The Delaney Amendment states that if a chemical added by man—BUT not by nature—causes cancer in any animal at any dose level, that chemical must be prohibited from food completely. This well intentioned law is unworkable because:

• There is great individual variation among humans in personal values, and this inevitably and quite properly results in great individual variation in benefit versus risk assessments.

• There is great individual variation among humans in response to various chemicals.

• Humans have many mechanisms for repair of damage. Significant damage may occur at high dosages of a chemical and not at a lower dosage. The Delaney Amendment denies the existence of thresholds for all significant hazardous effects. Moreover, humans are usually much more resistant to carcinogenesis than experimental animals with short life spans.

• The higher dosages at which an animal can get cancer may be thousands, millions, billions, or even trillions of times higher than any dosage a human may be exposed to.

• The Delaney Amendment does not apply to natural substances in foods, or the foods themselves which can contain a wide variety of cancer-causing substances. A good example is peanuts, which may contain aflatoxins, cancer-causing poisons made by a mold living on peanuts. (The mold makes the aflatoxins to kill off competing microorganisms.) Aflatoxins may cause thousands of cases of cancer a year in the U.S. In some areas of the world (such as parts of Africa), the number-one cause of death is aflatoxin-induced liver cancer.

• New analytical methods can find carcinogens almost anywhere. Under the Delaney Amendment, normal city tap water is technically illegal for use in foods since it contains minute amounts of detectable carcinogens produced by the germicidal water chlorination process. The Delaney amendment has cost American pharmaceutical companies many millions of dollars, and obese consumers the health advantages of improved low calorie sweeteners. The two compounds sodium cyclamate and sodium saccharin are examples of food additives attacked on the basis of this law. In both instances, the amounts required to produce a substantial risk of cancer in specially bred cancer-prone rats were 1000 times the doses used by humans. Quantities of sugar having far less sweetening power, or the same number of calories of fat added to the diets of these rats can cause a much higher incidence of cancer, but sugar and fat are natural, and hence the Delaney Amendment (fortunately) ignores them. Congress initially passed the Delaney Amendment into law and has the power to repeal it. As long as the law stands, the FDA is required to try to enforce it.

• It is, in effect, an attempt by Congress to repeal a law of nature, the Second Law of Thermodynamics in physics. Congress does not have the power to amend or repeal natural laws! (See the chapter notes for Part V, Chapter 8.)

As Dr. Sanford Miller, FDA Director of the Bureau of Foods has said, "My concern is not the cancer rate. My concern is protection of individual freedom. Each step of protection brings its own threat. And the increase in that threat with each decision is geometric not arithmetic. People have to decide how far they want to go with this protection." Dr. Miller seems to be acutely aware that the costs of poor regulations can far exceed their benefits, and that our fundamental concepts of individual freedom are seriously threatened, yet there is very little that he can do to solve the problem so long as the laws are unchanged. This is a problem of bad laws, not bad men.

Surprisingly, even the thalidomide ban reflects badly on the FDA's policies. For most people, thalidomide is an effective sleeping aid that is far safer than barbiturates which are widely abused, addictive, and hazardous. The exception is the case of unborn children during a short, critically sensitive period of development during which many substances can cause birth defects. (In rodents, these include reasonably normal scaled doses of caffeine, tobacco, and alcohol.) However, thalidomide poses no such hazards in men or in non-pregnant women, yet it was banned for everybody. Over a thousand people die each year from barbiturate overdoses or barbiturate-alcohol interactions who might have been alive using the safer drug thalidomide. The FDA's response to the thalidomide tragedy was not based on reason, but on the immediate hysteria of the poorly informed public. Thalidomide was a great public relations victory in the long run for the FDA, but as usual, we all get stuck with the hidden costs: continuing use of obsolete drugs which are more hazardous.

The FDA strictly controls what vendors and manufacturers of vitamins and prescription drugs can claim about their products. A major regulatory function of the FDA is to very narrowly limit the drug information available to physicians, pharmacists, and consumers. These regulations have little to do with the findings of legitimate scientific research. A drug company is not allowed to inform doctors about unapproved uses for their drugs, no matter how many scientific studies have been performed, no matter how successful new treatments may be, and no matter how many lives are lost because of the FDA's delays in approving new drugs and new uses for old drugs. This situation is reminiscent of the disaster that happened to biology in Russia under the rule of Lysenko. Or what happened to Galileo when he tried to communicate his "illegal" knowledge. This is "science" by edict—and "science" at the point of a gun.

An important part of the cost of FDA delays to drug approvals is that, even after a drug is finally approved for a specific therapeutic use in the United States, obtaining approval later for additionally discovered therapeutic uses of that drug is difficult. These delays for new uses of old drugs are far longer than in most other technically advanced countries, such as many western European nations. Trying to obtain approval for new uses of an already approved drug in the U.S. is so costly that drug manufacturers often seek approval only for those uses which are likely to receive easy approval, and/or which are for relatively common conditions, even when the drug may be helpful to patients with any of several other conditions.

The FDA's desire to suppress communication of "unauthorized" information, such as new uses for old drugs, is not shared by all national drug regulatory agencies. Sir Derrick Dunlop, physician to royalty and an expert on British drug regulation, has pointed out:

"In the United Kingdom the primary concern of the Authority has been to ensure the safety and quality of the medicines it licenses for the profession's use, and it is felt that opinion on efficacy per se should be left to the free processes of scientific publication, debate, and undergraduate and postgraduate education. The Licensing Authority does not deny a minority the right to use any medicine it desires provided it is reasonably safe for its intended purpose. Herbal and homeopathic remedies are examples of the principle involved.

There must be no chance of prejudiced individuals securing power to impose their ideas on the medical profession and community. It is considered that there is no safe depository of ultimate power in the use of medicines save the medical profession and, if doctors are thought to be insufficiently enlightened to exercise such power with a wholesome discretion, the remedy is not to take it away from them but to improve their discretion by education—particularly in clinical pharmacology." (From "The British System of Drug Regulation," pp. 236–7 in *Regulating New Drugs*, edited by Richard Landau.)

FREEDOM OF CHOICE—A NEW FDA CHARTER

There are many possibilities for solving this deadly problem. In our opinion, only one class of solutions will be effective: solutions which remove the legal barriers to **freedom of choice** for physicians, pharmacists, patients, and pharmaceutical manufacturers.

THE OPT-OUT FORM:

We would like to see legislation which makes it possible for adults to use unapproved prescription drugs and treatments by signing an "opt-out" form in which they may waive their FDA protection and accept the risks of using unapproved prescription drugs. Doctors are discouraged from using unapproved treatments now, no matter how much of an improvement they may be over approved treatments, because of the threat of malpractice suits.

For example, we know of a case where a doctor at the City of Hope (a research hospital in Duarte, California) wanted to try treating his patients who had persistent ocular herpes (a blinding and sometimes fatal viral infection) with BHT, a food additive with low toxicity which has powerful anti-herpes-virus effects. The FDA-approved treatment of choice for herpes, idoxuridine, is a very toxic compound, a mutagen, carcinogen, and an immune system T-cell suppressor. The Hospital Board would not allow the doctor to administer BHT to his herpes patients, however, because of their fear of malpractice suits, and due to the extensive, expensive, and extremely time-consuming New Drug Application procedure required by the FDA. Patients cannot usually effectively sue for malpractice when approved treatments are properly prescribed in approved quantities, no matter how nasty these materials may be. Yet these patients had no way of obtaining BHT treatment because they could not waive the protection of either the FDA or malpractice suits.

If an "opt-out" procedure were instituted, no one would be forced to waive his or her protection. Only adults who wished to use unapproved treatments and were willing to forego both FDA controls and protection would sign the "opt-out" form. Only those who wished to use a new, potentially risky procedure or drug would sign away their option to sue for malpractice. All those persons who want the controls, regulations, and sort of protection as at present, would automatically continue to have all such protections.

A good analogy to FDA "opt-out" is a Federal highway law recently passed that did not require motorcycle riders to use crash helmets. We personally consider it foolhardy to accept the risks of not using a helmet, but to some motorcycle riders the joys of feeling close to the environment, hair flying in the wind, and so on, are worth the danger. People have different value judgments of benefits and costs associated with their actions. We think a free society should allow an adult individual to choose levels of benefits and risks for himself, without forcing his choices for these levels on everyone else as well. This applies whether it is a judgment concerning whether to wear a crash helmet, or whether to use a non-FDA-approved drug. Freedom to choose does not guarantee that people will always make good decisions (nothing can guarantee that), but it does mean that they are free to make their own choices, and that they are not forced at gunpoint to accept the judgment of a bureaucrat who may be far more concerned with not passing a bad drug than in curing the diseases of those subject to his decisions.

THE SPLIT LABEL:

Another idea for increasing both physician and public access to new prescription drug information would be to have prescription drug labels, drug insert sheets, and advertisements in professional journals divided in half. The FDA could put whatever it wanted on its half, and the pharmaceutical manufacturer could put whatever it wanted on the other half.

Physicians and consumers could be guided entirely by the FDA's conclusions if they wished. Others may find the data supplied by the manufacturer to be of particular value in making a decision, especially when it is based on and refers to peer-reviewed scientific research studies. There are several advantages to this. Drugs that have already been approved are now limited to those uses the FDA specifies. Thus, if an old drug is found to have a new use, the manufacturer must obtain a New Drug Application and go through essentially the same procedure as he did when the drug was approved for earlier uses: spend millions of dollars and years of effort to demonstrate safety again and also efficacy for the new use. Manufacturers may not inform physicians of these new uses before they have received the FDA's permission which may or may not come after completing this very expensive, several year procedure. In the meantime, the public's knowledge about these potential applications of already available drugs is seriously restricted. Doctors increase their risk of malpractice suits by using approved drugs for unapproved uses, and patients cannot now waive either FDA or malpractice suit protection in order to obtain such unapproved treatments. (Although some doctors may not realize it, it is legal for them to prescribe any substance for any purpose, except for controlled "drugs of abuse" such as narcotics, stimulants, sedatives, etc, and specifically banned substances such as laetrile.)

For example, in one fairly large clinical study, Anturane® (Ciba-Geigy), a common gout medicine, reduced the risk in males of a second or subsequent fatal heart attack by 74 percent. The FDA didn't challenge the size of the study, the statistical significance, or the finding of a reduction in deaths, but argued that these deaths may not have all been due to heart attacks because not all these patients were examined by autopsy after death. However, all these patients had had a prior heart attack and all exhibited the symptoms of a heart attack before they died. This is a particularly important study since if first heart attack is not fatal, it is usually followed by a fatal heart attack within several years.

The FDA has already refused to approve Anturane® to reduce the risks of death from a second and subsequent heart attack. By the time this new use for Anturane® might receive FDA approval, the patent on the drug will probably have expired. This situation leaves little incentive for the manufacturer to spend millions of dollars and years of effort seeking

FDA approval when competitors will get as many benefits if approval is granted, without spending all that money. Competition will then prevent the manufacturer of Anturane® from charging a higher price in order to recover these costs. And it is not at all certain that the FDA will ever give its approval.

We have very roughly calculated the order of magnitude of the minimal monetary costs imposed on heart attack victims and their families by the failure of the FDA to approve Anturane® for the prevention of death from second and subsequent heart attacks. We have also used the figure of $250,000 as the value of a lost life (we realize that few friends or relatives of heart attack victims will agree with this figure, but in terms of the estimated production over a lost lifetime, it is a useful guide). If 250,000 heart attack victims, about half the total per year, could be saved with Anturane®, then each year the FDA fails to approve this use for the drug means a cost to the victims and those who would have interacted with them of about $62,500,000,000. Even if you calculate only the lost income as just $20,000 per year per human life unnecessarily lost to heart attacks for only 3 years before death from some other cause, the total annual cost of FDA non-approval of this one new use for one old drug is $15,000,000,000 per year—without even considering the emotional losses and medical costs. This astronomical cost to the health of many Americans is due to FDA failure to approve just one new use for one old drug! (We have assumed here that physicians are conforming to the FDA's edicts. Fortunately for their patients, many are not; currently 90 percent of new Anturane® prescriptions are for heart attack patients. Obviously, the FDA should not receive credit for the decisions of these independent-minded physicians.)

The Commissioners of the FDA have not been evil men. In general, they have been health professionals, mostly surgeons, who accepted a cut in pay and a career full of headaches because they sincerely wanted to protect and improve your health. We believe that the rapid resignations of recent FDA commissioners reflects their realization that they cannot improve your health in that position. As the Wizard of Oz said, after being uncovered as a humbug, "I'm not a bad man. I'm just a bad wizard." The philosophical premises upon which the FDA's enabling legislation are founded guarantee that the FDA Commissioner is doomed to be a bad wizard.

The problem is not in finding the right man or reorganizing the agency or even getting a bigger budget; the problem is built in by the underlying philosophical basis of the FDA's enabling legislation. Without fundamental changes here, all alterations will be merely cosmetic. As Nobel laureate economist Milton Friedman put it in his February 19, 1973 column in *Newsweek* entitled "Barking Cats":

"What would you think of someone who said, 'I would like to have a cat provided it barked'? Yet your statement that you favor an FDA provided it behaves as you believe desirable is precisely equivalent. The biological laws that specify the characteristics of cats are no more rigid than the political laws that specify the behavior of governmental agencies once they are established. The way the FDA now behaves, and the adverse consequences, are not an accident, not a result of some easily corrected human mistake, but a consequence of its constitution in precisely the same way that a meow is related to the constitution of a cat. As a natural scientist, you recognize that you cannot assign characteristics at will to chemical and biological entities, cannot demand that cats bark or water burn. Why do you suppose the situation is different in the social sciences?"*

When Congress set up the FDA, and when they have periodically amended this legislation, their intent was entirely laudable: to protect people from bad food and drugs. Unfortunately, the road to hell is paved with good intentions. Good intentions are no substitute for knowledge.

There are two fundamentally different approaches toward achieving the end of protecting people from bad food and drugs. The first is to pass and enforce more and more laws and regulations. If something has gone wrong, hire more bureaucrats, pass more laws, hire more policemen to enforce them, and build more jails to lock up offenders. With respect to pharmaceuticals, we now live in a totalitarian bureaucratized police state. People in many other technologically developed countries (such as some in western Europe) have far greater freedom than people in the United States in this area.

Our present legalistic approach to the social control of potentially voluntary interactions has great costs, both in terms of individual liberty and in terms of scientific and technological progress. Worse yet, this system fails to deliver the better drugs that it promised. Econometric studies by Dr. Peltzman and others have shown that our current regulatory approach greatly impairs the development of new drugs, yet provides no measurable improvement in either drug safety or efficacy over the far less stringent regulations of times past. (See the section in Appendix K, References and Chapter Notes for Appendix E for a startling look at how free the drug trade really was in the United States until 1938, the year the FDA was established by Congress.)

Dr. Sam Peltzman, Professor of Economics at the University of Chicago and also at UCLA, has been studying the effects of pharmaceutical regulation, particularly the 1962 Kefauver Amendments, for the past decade. This body of work is sufficiently long and detailed to make more than one book by itself. It will be possible to touch on only a few points of particular interest here; in the process, many methodological details must be omitted. We strongly recommend study of the complete papers so briefly cited here.

Dr. Peltzman's work is held in high regard by his professional peers. Dr. Yale Brozen, Professor of Economics at the University of Chicago, has said, in *Regulation of Pharmaceutical Innovation* (p. 1):

"How can anyone quarrel with a requirement that a new drug must be shown, to the satisfaction of a government agency, to have the curative powers its producer claims for it before it can be sold? But that is what this study does.

"Professor Peltzman did not set out to criticize this requirement when he undertook this study. He intended to measure the net benefits produced by the 1962 amendments to the Food, Drug and Cosmetic Act—the amendments that instituted the efficacy requirement. In order to produce a result as favorable as possible to the 1962 amendments, he has made assumptions, where assumptions are necessary, which result in an overstatement of benefits and an understatement of costs. He has assumed, for example, that unsafe drugs will be kept off the market by the added information required of manufacturers to prove efficacy but that they would not have been kept off by the pre-1962 requirements of the law. (Under the law before it was amended, a marketer of a new drug had to prove to the satisfaction of the Food and Drug Administration [FDA] that his proposed new drug was safe for human consumption.) Professor Peltzman has made this assumption despite the fact that drugs such as thalidomide, which is safe except for use by pregnant women, had in fact been kept from being marketed under the proof-of-safety requirements existing before the 1962 amendments were passed. By making this assumption, he has attributed to the amendments benefits that might have occurred without the amendments." (From *Regulation of Pharmaceutical Innovation*, pg. 1.)

Dr. Peltzman has been quite cautious; in making assumptions he consistently gives the benefit of the doubt to the regulators and their regulations, saying:

"These missed benefits will be assumed nonexistent, in part for procedural simplicity, but, also to impart a conservative (pro status quo) bias to the empirical results. I believe that, given the importance of the policy implications which might be suggested by the empirical results, such a conservative bias is not undesirable. And, wherever a choice of procedure may entail bias, I shall try to make a pro amendments-are-right choice." (Peltzman, "An Evaluation of Consumer Protection Legislation: the 1962 Drug Amendments" in *Journal of Political Economy*, pp. 1049–1091, Sept–Oct 1973.)

Lester G. Telser, Professor of Economics at the University of Chicago has said, in *Regulating New Drugs:*

"Professor Peltzman's study is a model of economic reasoning applied to a difficult subject. It is a comprehensive, imaginative, and laborious investigation of an important subject deserving of more attention by professional economists than it has so far received. Among the impressive achievements of Peltzman's work is the demonstration of the power of economic theory in predicting the outcome of the new drug regulations. As a result of this work we can reach certain definitive conclusions. First, there is now [1973] a two-year delay in the introduction of new drugs. Second, there is a reduction in the number of new drugs. Third, the risk involved in the use of new drugs prior to the new regulations is much exaggerated. Fourth, the losses imposed on the public, as the consequence of these new regulations, far outweigh the gains. It is implicit in Peltzman's results that the drug companies themselves have powerful incentives to exercise care in their introduction of new drugs, even in the absence of federal and state laws. At the outset, therefore, I wish to make it clear that Professor Peltzman's study is deserving of high praise.... [Telser, however, is uncomfortable with assigning any particular monetary value such as $250,000 to a human life.]

"In my opinion the most ingenious empirical analysis is contained in the subsection "Expert Drug Evaluations." These data show that boards of experts are far more conservative than private practitioners, yet, the data indicate that the market share of NCEs chosen by the experts eventually attains the same level as the private practitioners' shares. It would be useful for Peltzman to supply us with some calculations, using his analytical apparatus, giving his estimates of the cost to society of the delays in the acceptance of NCEs by the committees of experts who devise the formularies for hospitals and for state and federal agencies." (NCEs are new chemical entities, that is chemically novel drugs, not just a combination or reformulation of old drugs. From L. G. Telser, "The Legal and Economic Effects of Drug Regulatory Policies," in *Regulating New Drugs*, pp. 213–225.)

Professor Peltzman's analysis of the costs and benefits to the U.S. public of the FDA's regulations (particularly the 1962 Kefauver Amendments) and their impact on safety, efficacy, and new drug development and introduction can be found in *Regulation of Pharmaceutical Innovation* (American Enterprise Institute for Public Policy Research, Washington, D.C. $3, pb.), in *Regulating New Drugs*, R. L. Landau, ed. (The University of Chicago Center for Policy Studies, Chicago, Illinois, $5.25, pb.), and in the *Journal of Political Economy*, pp. 1049–1091, September–October 1973. Dr. Peltzman concluded that there is a <u>minimum</u> yearly net cost beyond benefits to Americans of between $250,000,000 and $350,000,000 (calculated in late 1960s dollars). That is, the cost of the FDA's policies is greater than the benefits of the FDA's policies by at least somewhere between these amounts. In calculating these costs, the following were among the <u>very</u> charitable assumptions made:

• FDA delays the introduction of new drugs by no more than 2 years.

• FDA does not prevent any useful drug from reaching market.

• FDA prevents all bad drugs from reaching market.

• FDA's policies do not discourage introduction of any useful new drugs.

None of these incredibly generous assumptions are true. The FDA performs far worse on all four counts. Dr. Peltzman used $250,000 as the value of a human life in making the calculations (for example, when estimating the costs of people dying of a disease during the period while FDA was deciding whether to pass a drug which could have saved their lives). A higher value placed on human lives would further increase the calculated FDA costs in excess of benefits.

*　　　*　　　*

The following material broadly describes Dr. Peltzman's econometric analysis. We have taken these extracts directly from his *Regulation of Pharmaceutical Innovation:*

"Chapter II attempts to establish the effect of the [1962 Kefauver] amendments on the flow of new drugs and their gestation period. These effects turn out to substantial: the new drug flow is shown to be more than halved and the gestation period more than doubled by the amendments.

"Chapter III outlines a method for measuring the net consumer benefit or cost of the amendments. The operating assumption is that the more effective a new drug, the more durable will be the demand for it—that is, the demand for ineffective drugs or drugs which do not live up to the claims made for them tends to decline in the light of cumulative physician-patient experience with them. On the basis of this assumption, economic theory is applied to provide a measure of the gains and losses yielded by any set of new drugs. For the sake of implementing this measure, the losses which arise from uninformed consumption of ineffective drugs are assumed to be eliminated by the amendments. While the same economic analysis is applicable to some aspects of drug safety, it is inadequate for unusually unsafe or unusually beneficial drugs. [p. 10]. . . .

"One way to do this, for a group of consumers, is to examine behavior at different points in time. If physicians persistently believe exaggerated claims of new drug efficacy, we should observe a heavy demand for new drugs immediately after the bulk of doctors have been exposed to the claims, and then a decline in demand. If the efficacy claims were in fact exaggerated, we would expect some physicians to learn this from their own practice, from that of colleagues, from the medical literature, and so on. Unless the majority of physicians were perverse, we would expect that this learning process would, over time, erode the demand for the new drug. Put differently, the quantities doctors would be willing to prescribe would be revised downward. Once this learning process is complete, a comparison of the resulting demand with the initially overoptimistic demand can be used to measure the gross loss from exaggerated efficacy claims. [pg. 23]. . . .

"The net benefits of the 1962 amendments are estimated in Chapter IV. These estimates indicate that consumer losses prior to 1962 were negligible. It follows, then, that little benefit has been produced by the amendments. It also follows that the severe decline in new drug flows produced by the amendments must result in a net loss to consumers. The loss is estimated at between \$300 and \$400 million annually as of 1970, or about 7 percent of total drug expenditures.

"The evaluations of pre- and post-1962 new drugs by some "expert" groups are then examined to see whether these groups differ from ordinary consumers and the physicians prescribing for them in their judgment about the incidence of ineffective drugs. In general, the "experts" seem to agree with ordinary consumers (doctors and patients) that there has been no substantial change in the efficacy of new drugs because of the amendments. [original emphasis] The conclusion that the decline in innovation has entailed a net loss to consumers is reinforced. An alternative measure of the loss resulting from ineffective new drugs is derived from one "expert" group's evaluations (the group being the AMA Council on Drugs): the estimate is that the loss amounts to at most 2 percent of total drug expenditures. [pp. 10–11]

". . . Thus the assertion by one expert group (the FDA) that post-1962 drugs are more effective than pre-1962 drugs is not corroborated by the action of another expert group (formulary committees). The inability of independent expert groups to improve on the consistency of a random number table might imply that inefficacy is too difficult to define or that it is empirically trivial. Neither circumstance would be conducive to a major reduction in the incidence of inefficacious drugs, and the data in Table 4 are in fact inconsistent with any such reduction. [pg. 43]

"Finally, it is shown that the barrier to entry created by the amendments has resulted in slightly higher prices for old drugs. The annual cost to consumers from the barrier to entry is about 1 percent of total consumer drug expenditures. Chapter IV concludes that the 1962 amendments impose a net cost on consumers in excess of 5 percent of their drug expenditures.

"Chapter V analyzes effects of the amendments on unusually harmful or beneficial new drugs. The analysis focuses on effects of these drugs on the earnings of those who use them and on costs of disease treatment. It is shown that a moderate increase in the gestation period for beneficial drugs costs far more than the savings from complete suppression of harmful drugs. This conclusion need not be modified even if it were assumed that a drug such as thalidomide would occasionally have been widely marketed in a pre-1962 environment, but would have been suppressed under the amendments (in fact, of course, thalidomide was suppressed in the pre-1962 environment). The specific costs and savings attributable to the amendments are uncertain. It is shown, however, that their potential cost is high. Had the amendments been passed a decade or two before 1962, the net cost of delayed marketing of new drugs would have been sufficient to double the total cost of the amendments as computed in Chapter IV—assuming that the drugs involved were not prevented from reaching the market eventually, that is, were not among those never developed because of the increased cost of meeting post-1962 FDA requirements. Similar potential costs are shown to be inherent in delay of innovations in health problems currently engaging pharmacological research [pg. 11]. . . .

"Chloramphenicol: Thalidomide-type products do not appear to have been introduced frequently in the years before 1962. Systematic data on their health effects are extremely rare. I will therefore have to rely for concrete data on the one case where these are available, and where adverse health effects of the type that the amendments might reasonably have been expected to reduce were present. The case is that of the drug chloramphenicol, marketed under the trade name Chloromycetin®.

"This antibiotic was introduced in 1949 and met with immediate market success. Within the next three years, however, the drug was implicated as a cause of a sometimes fatal blood disease, aplastic anemia. In 1952, the FDA temporarily halted sales of the drug. It permitted their resumption with the drug's indications limited to a few infections such as typhoid fever. It is reasonable to suppose that, had the 1962 amendments been law in 1949, the relationship between chloramphenicol and aplastic anemia would have been discovered before marketing. It may be less reasonable to suppose that all users of chloramphenicol who perished in ignorance of its relationship to aplastic anemia would have been spared by such a discovery. After a precipitous decline from 1952 to 1954, chloramphenicol sales—and aplastic anemia deaths—more than recovered their pre-1952 levels by 1960. Users of the drug, knowing the risks, found them outweighed by prospective benefits. This seems to imply that the initial market reaction to knowledge of chloramphenicol's adverse effects might have been smaller had the knowledge been conveyed in a less dramatic fashion than it was in 1952 [pp. 52–53].

". . . But, in fact, disasters are neither so frequent nor so severe as to begin to offset the gains from major innovations. To put the matter baldly, if generally greater risk taking had hastened the marketing of TB [tuberculosis] drugs by six months, the number of lives saved directly (that is, excluding the effects of reduced communication of TB and hastier diffusion of the drug) would have been three times as great as all those lost to the delayed discovery of the lethal effects of chloramphenicol.

"I am unaware of any data that shed light on the question whether the benefits from greater haste might in fact have been purchased at a cost smaller than tripled incidence of major drug disasters. However, if empirical support for the proposition that there was too little risk taking before 1962 is lacking, the data then available emphatically fail to support the contrary proposition embodied in the amendments. The amendments have produced less haste. Even if the future number of major therapeutic advances were unaffected, this change would be costly. It would, for example, require the prevention of more than one chloramphenicol incident annually to offset the direct cost in lives lost because of a two-year delay of a once-in-a-decade innovation like the TB drugs. A similar comparison between something like the tranquilizers and chloramphenicol cannot be this direct, since a tradeoff between lives and disability is involved. However, the more-than-fifthfold difference between the cost of two-year delay in introducing something like tranquilizers and the total cost of excess chloramphenicol deaths indicates how great the pessimism about safety of unregulated drugs or the nonmeasurable value of life must be for the prospective benefits of the amendments to offset their costs.

"These conclusions hold even when we consider the potential costs of a thalidomide tragedy in its most virulent form [the German disaster which was about 10 times as bad as in other European countries, which were in turn far worse than in the United States] and on the most extreme interpretation of its costs—that malformation is the equivalent of death. My high estimate of the economic cost (or cost in "lives" lost) of such a hypothetical tragedy is well below that of a one-year, let alone two-year, delay in marketing either the TB drugs or the phenothiazines [antipsychotic drugs, the major tranquilizers]. Moreover, it should be remembered that these do not nearly exhaust the major innovations of the pre-1962 period, while it would be difficult to expect anything like a thalidomide tragedy more than once in a decade. It is interesting in this connection that the high estimate of the cost of a hypothetical birth-defects outbreak is roughly equal to the benefit of a three-month speed-up in the introduction of the three beneficial innovations discussed here. If one views the outbreak of birth defects as the likely consequence of any relaxed (pre-1962) safety regulation which would permit the three-month speed-up to be attained for all drugs, it may be concluded that there was almost surely too little risk taking before 1962, not to mention since 1962.

"This conclusion is further reinforced when it is recalled that the measurable prospective benefit of eliminating all chloramphenicol and thalidomide tragedies falls well short of the measurable cost of the amendments in benefits forgone on the ordinary new drugs whose development they discourage. This net loss may be further exacerbated by modest delays in introducing unusually beneficial new drugs. It is worth emphasizing that such delay is intrinsic in the regulatory procedure required by the amendments. When one considers the prospective payoff for innovation in the treatment of something like heart disease or cancer, the potential cost of delay becomes awesome. Should only a moderately successful innovation in the treatment of either disease come within the ambit of the amendments, our estimate that their cost is something like a 5- to 10-percent drug excise tax will prove egregiously low. And even the data on innovations in the treatment of less widespread diseases will indicate how extravagant is the cost of reduced risk built into the amendments [pp. 72–73]. . . .

"The 1962 drug amendments sought to reduce consumer waste on ineffective new drugs. While this goal appears to have been attained the costs imposed on consumers in the process seem to have outweighed the benefits. The reason for this is that the benefits are largely a by-product of a reduction of consumer exposure to all types of new drugs. The incidence of ineffective new drugs does not appear to have been materially reduced. Even if it has been, the pre-1962 waste on ineffective new drugs that might now be prevented appears to have been too small to compensate for the benefits consumers have had to forgo because of reduced drug innovation. The largest estimate of this annual waste prevention, based on ungenerous interpretations of the drug evaluations by the AMA Council on Drugs and pessimistic assumptions about consumer behavior, is $100–$500 million: this must be reduced by more than half to take account of the loss of market share of ineffective drugs over time.

"In the present context, the forgone benefits of innovation show up as a decline in the demand for (and consequently the consumer surplus generated by) new drugs. In Chapter II, it was shown that essentially all the post-1962 decline in drug innovation—a reduction of over 50 percent in the number and output of new drugs—can be attributed to the 1962 amendments. This, combined with the absence of any increase in the relative price of new to old drugs, suggests a lower demand for new drugs. In part, this decline in demand simply reflects the fact that consumers cannot manifest a demand for products which are not marketed. However, the explicit restrictions on seller promotion of new drugs in the amendments and the reduced number of sellers who are informing consumers about new drug types have also contributed to this decline in demand.

"The bulk of the evidence indicates that the post-1962 decline in demand does not reflect a more realistic physician appraisal of the genuine worth of new drugs. The pre-1962 demand did not fall after doctors had time to learn the worth of new drugs from experience as it would have if they were initially overoptimistic. Since doctors did not act as if they regretted their initial evaluations of pre-amendment drugs, the lower post-1962 demand for new drugs resolves largely into reduced net benefits ($300–$400 million annually) to drug consumers from a reduced flow of new drugs and information about them (and an additional $50 million annual cost resulting from reduced price competition). This conclusion is verified by assessments of experts and sophisticated drug buyers. The probability that they will assess a new drug as being ineffective is about the same for the pre- and post-1962 sets of new drugs and any reduced losses from ineffective drugs post-1962 merely offset a part of the missed benefits [pp. 48–49].

". . . The actual post-1962 rate [of new chemical entity drug introductions] has been roughly 60 percent below that [pre-1962] average.

"For a decline of this magnitude to be regarded as "a good sign and ultimately of benefit to the American people," [as was claimed by FDA commissioner J. Richard Crout] we must believe that the pre-amendment regulatory environment produced substantial numbers of ineffective drugs and that the amendments have been highly selective in screening these out. Even if one assumes the selectivity, the belief in the substantial number of ineffective drugs is untenable. It is difficult to conclude that much more than 10 percent of pre-1962 drug purchases went for ineffective drugs. This figure is suggested by the sales of those drugs which the FDA itself has indicated it will remove from the market as a result of the drug-efficacy review conducted by the National Academy of Sciences-National Research Council. A similar estimate (9.4 percent) is obtained by Jondrow in his study of the NAS-NRC review [pg. 87]. . . ,

"If the Food, Drug and Cosmetics Act is intended to benefit consumers, the inescapable conclusion to which this study points is that the intent is better served by reversion to the status quo ante 1962. This conclusion follows directly from the size of the problem with which the 1962 amendments sought to cope. Consumer losses from purchases of ineffective drugs or hastily marketed unsafe drugs appear to have been trivial compared to gains from innovation. In this context, any perceptible deterrent to innovation was bound to impose net losses on consumers. The amendments clearly provided such a deterrent. Indeed, the conclusion can be put more strongly. If our estimates of the gains and loses from exceptionally beneficial and unsafe drugs, respectively, are at all reasonable, there was already a costly bias in the pre-1962 proof-of-safety requirement. If relaxation of that requirement would have compressed the new-drug development process only slightly, the resulting gains would have left a margin of lives saved and disability avoided that would more than have offset increased losses from unsafe drugs. The risk-return tradeoff was already biased against drug consumers in 1962. The amendments have simply exaggerated the bias.

"It is easier to state our conclusion than it is to be sanguine about the prospects for reduced regulation of drug innovation. Since the 1962 amendments do not appear to have benefitted any substantial group and have hurt some, one might question their political viability. However, the most important group that has been hurt, drug consumers, cannot be expected to offer effective pressure for change. The damage to each member of this group can be little more than a few dollars per year, so that the members of the group have little incentive to bear the costs of political organization. Moreover, reduced regulation of the quality of any consumer good sharply contradicts the thrust of most organized groups that today purport to promote the consumer interest. One organized group that might share in the gains from reduced regulation of drug innovation is the American Medical Association, but the AMA has not taken a strong position on the matter since the Kefauver hearings when it testified against requiring proof of efficacy for drug advertising. Finally, our results indicate that the producer group which has benefitted from the amendments may be at least as large as that which has been hurt: coherent support for reduced regulation cannot confidently be anticipated from producer groups.

"If there will be no substantial reduction of the formal restraints embodied in the amendments, it is unlikely any substantial reduction in the costs they have generated will be accomplished by purely administrative changes. The FDA is, after all, confronted by the same political forces that favor legislative inertia. In addition, the FDA can expect little of the reward for extremely successful innovations, but substantial cost for wrongly certifying an unsafe or ineffective drug. Surely, no FDA official who has assisted the speedy introduction of a highly beneficial drug has received anything remotely resembling the public accolades accorded the colleague who prevented marketing of thalidomide. Exhorting the FDA to speed up the NDA process or to reduce its information requirements is not likely to be very fruitful. And it would be misleading to seek the source of the inefficiency of drug regulation in the detail of FDA procedures. The important conclusions of this study are that, perhaps before and certainly after 1962, too many resources have been devoted to testing of drug safety and efficacy before marketing and that, unless the law requiring proof of efficacy is rescinded, continued resource waste is inevitable. A favorable change in FDA procedures could reduce, but could never eliminate, the waste commanded by the law [pp. 82–83]."

*　　*　　*

If a regulatory bureaucracy such as the FDA cannot protect us from bad drugs without an even greater cost in preventing the cure of disease, what are we to do? **The other approach to providing protection against bad drugs is based on maximizing** **informed freedom of choice**. In this approach, the FDA would function as a public advisory agency and provide information about prescription drugs. The FDA would have no powers to regulate prescription drugs, only to inform all interested parties of their opinions and scientific research findings. Much of the FDA's legal and regulatory budget might be given to their scientists, who would be able to perform far more safety research than their meager research budget allows at present. Although both approaches to providing safe and effective drugs share the same initial intent, the long-term consequences of these two viewpoints are very different, indeed. Many regulatory bureaucrats suffer from the delusion that you can control nature by regulating people. Scientists and engineers control nature directly by studying its mechanisms and applying this knowledge. Bad drugs can be eliminated by severe regulations but, unfortunately, this also eliminates good drugs, too; and regulations cannot eliminate the diseases. Bad drugs can be effectively eliminated by informed physicians who refuse to prescribe them, by informed pharmacists who refuse to sell them, by informed patients who refuse to buy them, and, most of all, by vigorous, unfettered, dog-eat-dog competition in the marketplace by responsible pharmaceuticals manufacturers who develop and market superior products. Moreover, these firms will not ignore the potential for another thalidomide, and the tragedy and publicity surrounding it.

The conventional objection to the **freedom of choice control system** is that the information is unavailable, too expensive, too hard to find, too hard to understand, or that nobody gives a damn about that information, and that we are all imbeciles, unable and unwilling to inform ourselves about the drugs that we pop into our mouths without question. We contend that if a legal system is based on the assumption that most people are uncaring unquestioning imbeciles, that you will have an imbecilic legal system fit only for uncaring, unquestioning imbeciles. This may or may not be good for the imbeciles, but what about the rest of us?

A FREEDOM OF CHOICE PROPOSAL

We propose the following **free market alternative** to the FDA for protecting and informing consumers, pharmacists, and physicians, while permitting pharmaceutical manufacturers to get on with development and promotion of new drugs, without excessive regulations.

The moral concept of **freedom of choice** is central to our proposal. We support this principle quite apart from any specific implementation of this principle in law.

In accord with these, our own personal values and moral principles, we would very much like to see the following **freedom of choice** legislation:

1.) Congress should rewrite the FDA enabling legislation to make the FDA an information-disseminating advisory agency, but not a regulatory agency for prescription drugs.

2.) Prescription drugs may be researched, developed, manufactured, prescribed, sold, and used without FDA approval provided that any such drugs are clearly marked "FDA: THIS DRUG IS NOT FDA APPROVED" on the package label, package insert, and in advertisements and other promotional materials.

3.) New non-FDA-approved uses for FDA approved drugs may be listed on the package label, package insert, and in marketing materials and advertisements, provided they are clearly marked "**FDA: THIS USE IS NOT FDA APPROVED**".

4.) Drugs and uses not approved by the FDA shall have **SPLIT LABELS**. The manufacturers and marketers shall give the FDA equal space on their drug package labels, package inserts, and advertisements and promotional material. This equal space provision only applies to "NOT FDA APPROVED DRUGS" or to that portion of the package labels, inserts, advertisements, etc. that refers to uses that are "NOT FDA APPROVED".

5.) In order to purchase a "NOT FDA APPROVED DRUG" or a drug for a "NOT FDA APPROVED USE", the purchaser would have to be an adult, and would have to sign an **OPT-OUT** form which explicitly and clearly waives FDA protection with regard to that purchase.

6.) Federal legislation should be passed to permit an adult to sign another **OPT-OUT** form which waives one's right to sue for malpractice or other civil damages with respect to a particular drug, drug use, or medical procedure. Of course, this would *not* waive one's right to recover damages for criminal fraud.

7.) Prescription biomedical instruments, devices, diagnostics, etc., should receive the same relief from FDA regulations as prescription drugs.

8.) The existing statutes dealing with criminal fraud would remain in force, but mere lack of FDA approval would not be grounds for a charge of fraud unless the warnings required above were not given.

9.) The FDA would be free to continue approving or disapproving drugs and their uses except that they could no longer enforce their opinions on everyone else at the point of a policeman's gun. FDA approvals and disapprovals would be advice—not orders—to pharmaceutical firms, physicians, pharmacists, and patients.

NOTE THAT AN INDIVIDUAL WOULD AUTOMATICALLY CONTINUE TO RECEIVE CURRENT FORMS OF FDA PROTECTION UNTIL HE OR SHE OPTED OUT OF THIS PROTECTION IN WRITING.

592
Appendices

Remember this: no one would have to use non-FDA-approved prescription drugs. Those who wanted the full protection of the FDA would still have it; they need only confine themselves to FDA approved drugs and uses. The FDA would still approve drugs and uses, just as they do now. But you, your physician, and your pharmacist would no longer be FORCED to support their decisions. You would have freedom of choice!

We definitely would like to see prescription drugs offered in the market that have not yet received FDA approval. They could be labelled with a large warning that "this drug has not been FDA approved." A useful symbol for such products would be the letters FDA with a slash across it, F̸D̸A̸, indicating non-FDA approved. Such a prescription drug could be purchased but would have no legal protection associated with it—you would use it at your own risk, with the advice and consent of your doctor, who prescribes it, and at least the consent of your pharmacist, who sells it. We can think of many drugs now trapped in the limbo of the FDA's approval process which may never receive approval, that we would like to buy and use right now. In order to provide opportunity for opposing comments, pharmaceutical manufacturers might be subject to a 3 month delay between the time that they publicly announce their intent to market a new non-FDA-approved drug, and the time that sales can commence.

A similar approach could deal with new non-FDA-approved uses for an old FDA-approved drug. In this case, only the non-FDA-approved uses proposed by the manufacturer would be marked with the non-FDA-approved symbol, rather than the name of the drug itself. Anturane®, for example, would remain an FDA approved prescription drug for gout and would continue to be marketed for this purpose. With this **freedom of choice** proposal, however, the FDA approved gout medicine Anturane® advertisements, package inserts, and bottle labels could legally inform you that: "F̸D̸A̸—THIS USE NOT FDA APPROVED! This drug has reduced the incidence of death from a second or subsequent heart attack in humans by 74 percent. See [references would be provided here]. Further information available on request." There would be no law requiring that the manufacturer provide scientific research literature references or further information, but few physicians or pharmacists are likely to believe unsupported assertions. The FDA would have an equal amount of space to state their opinions, to offer further information, and to give their scientific literature references, if any. Labeling and advertising of new non-FDA-approved uses for already marketed drugs could also be subject to a delay of perhaps 1 month after public announcement, again, to permit possible opposing comments.

The ordinary laws concerning criminal fraud would remain in force, however, and class action suits for recovery in such cases would be permitted. The burden of proof would be on those who allege that a fraud had occurred, just as in any other criminal fraud case. Under this **freedom of choice** proposal, the people bringing you a new non-FDA-approved drug or promoting a non-FDA-approved use for an FDA-approved drug would have the same legal rights as an accused murderer—that is, they would be legally assumed innocent of fraud or other crime until they are proven guilty beyond a reasonable doubt. In our view, there is something fundamentally wrong with our present legal system which treats the people who manufacture pharmaceuticals worse than accused murderers.

There is considerable evidence that the FDA is now subject to widespread criticism. The recently retired FDA Commissioner, Jere E. Goyan, made an appeal for a cease-fire of the drug industry's efforts to "shake the confidence of the American people in our system of drug regulation by the so-called drug lag campaign." Goyan would have liked the public to believe that there really is no drug lag caused by FDA policies. Goyan also said that "your [drug industry] ability to innovate, your incentive to innovate, owes a great deal to the integrity and effectiveness of the regulatory system." This statement is an example of Orwell's Doublethink. The problem of antibiotic-resistant microbes is a direct result of the FDA's regulatory policies that legally force the pharmaceutical manufacturers to be several years behind the microbes' development of resistance. The problem is not that biomedical knowledge cannot keep pace with microbial evolution. The REAL problem is the FDA-imposed lag in drug development and marketing. The FDA is responsible for reducing the amount of pharmaceutical innovation, though the agency is loved by the non-research oriented firms who would otherwise have to invest in new drug R & D to keep up with unfettered competitors.

As economist Dr. Peltzman has said,

"The effects we have traced to the 1962 amendments have conflicting implications for the wealth of drug producers. On the one hand, the amendments have raised the cost of innovation and reduced the demand for it. On the other hand, they have erected a barrier to new competition for producers of established drugs, and made the demand for the output of the established producers higher than it would otherwise be. The producer who specializes in new drugs will be hurt and the producer who specializes in old drugs will be helped. However, the typical drug firm produces both new and old drugs and the net effect of the amendments on this typical firm is ambiguous." [*Regulation of Pharmaceutical Innovation,* pg. 75].

A final remark by ex-FDA Commissioner Goyan is real food for thought: "If FDA tomorrow were to fall into some kind of black hole and disappear, it would be necessary for the continued health and existence of this industry to reinvent us as quickly as possible." Let's give it a try and find out. (See Chapter Notes and References for Appendix E for some details.)

We are not, and never have been, political activists; we prefer to spend our time and energy on science rather than lobbying for new legislation. This is not about to change. Moreover, as scientists, we have access to many drugs that are unavailable to pharmacists, physicians, and their patients due to FDA regulations. Without drastic changes to install **freedom of choice** legislation to make the FDA an advisory rather than a regulatory agency for prescription drugs, most of our readers will have to be satisfied with nothing more than benefitting from non-FDA-approved uses for FDA approved drugs—usually many years after these uses are first discovered.

Congress can be responsive to an aroused electorate. A few million letters asking Congress for **freedom of choice** legislation to make the FDA into an advisory—not regulatory—agency for prescription drugs would probably be very effective. Several years ago, public outrage at the FDA's proposal to make high potency vitamins into prescription drugs resulted in over a million letters to Congress, which then responded by passing legislation taking the control of nutrients away from the FDA. Further public outcries against a threatened FDA ban on saccharin resulted in Congressional action to block the ban. (There is no clear evidence that saccharin is more hazardous than sugar, and there is quite a lot of evidence that for the obese, sugar can be more hazardous than saccharin. The experimental rat strain that exhibited an increased incidence of cancer when given saccharin or cyclamate equivalent to thousands of cans of soft drinks per day also exhibits an increased incidence of cancer when given the calories equivalent to a dozen or so cans of sugar-sweetened pop a day. Incidentally, we both do eat moderate amounts of sugar.)

Congress is not likely to pass **freedom of choice** legislation for prescription drugs until they are sure that there is very broad public demand for it, and they are confident that the voters realize and accept that **freedom of choice** means that physicians, pharmacists, patients, and pharmaceuticals manufacturers will sometimes make unwise decisions which do more harm than good. No system can guarantee perfect safety, no matter what its supporters claim. An attempt to eliminate the risks from new drugs will inevitably eliminate the research, development, and introduction of new drugs. It will not eliminate the hazards of disease, to say nothing of aging.

Providing the public—physicians, pharmacists, and patients—with information from all interested parties on new prescription drugs and on new uses for old drugs is realistic and rational. We believe that physicians, pharmacists, and patients should be able to make their own free choices on prescription drugs, based on information provided by pharmaceutical manufacturers, the FDA, scientists, doctors, pharmacists, associations of health professionals (both the American Medical Association and the American Pharmaceutical Association have their own generally conservative drug evaluation boards), and even self-styled "public interest" groups, as well as those real public interest organizations which have actually achieved success in the marketplace by consumers voluntarily purchasing their information products, such as the usually excellent Consumers Union.

If the FDA continues to operate under their current legislative charter, we predict that FDA avoidance will become as popular as tax avoidance. (For example, even though not approved for this purpose, 90 percent of new Anturane® prescriptions are for heart attack patients.) The goals of safety and the accelerated development and marketing of more effective new drugs would be served better by a new charter for the FDA—a charter based on **freedom of choice** to provide information rather than regulation. Congress has the legal power to pass **freedom of choice** legislation, but whether it does or not depends very much on what <u>you</u> and other consumers do about it.

Although we do not have access to any drugs specifically approved by the FDA for life extension, there are many nutrients and drugs which may have life extension effects and some of them are even FDA approved for other uses. Those of us who want to start extending our lives now, rather than years from now at some indefinite time in the future, will have to carefully and intelligently approve drugs for ourselves.

Many useful drugs that are not available in the United States may be purchased in Canada, Mexico, and Western Europe.

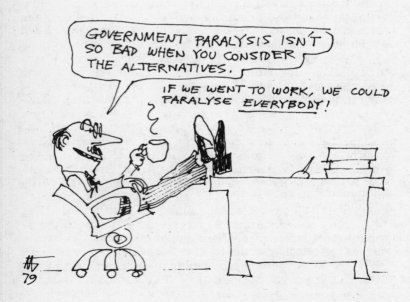

STATE OF CALIFORNIA—HEALTH AND WELFARE AGENCY / EDMUND G. BROWN JR., Governor

DEPARTMENT OF HEALTH SERVICES
714/744 P STREET
SACRAMENTO, CA 95814
(916) 445-2263

December 31, 1979

TO: MANUFACTURERS, DISTRIBUTORS, WHOLESALERS,
RETAILERS AND PHARMACIES

Recently there has been a proliferation of advertising by the vitamin and food supplement industry to promote products generally classified as foods for alleged therapeutic values. Commonly used wording includes, "Vitamin C aids in the healing of wounds and helps the body resist infections"; "Calcium....helps blood to clot and is also related to the proper functioning of the heart and nervous system." Catchy phrases such as "stress vitamins," "endurance vitamins," "vitamins for the hair," etc., have been noted not only in the ads, but on the product labels. Many more therapeutic claims of a similar nature could be cited, encompassing virtually every type of vitamin and food supplement available on the market.

Section 26460 of the California Health and Safety Code deems it unlawful for any person to disseminate any false advertisement of any food, drug, device or cosmetic. An advertisement is false if it is false or misleading in any way.

The Food and Drug Section, California Department of Health Services, considers many of these ads to be false and/or misleading within the meaning of the law, and stands ready through legal action (if necessary) to contest such claims.

The Health and Safety Code defines a drug, in part, as "any article which is used or intended for use in the diagnosis, cure, mitigation, treatment or prevention of disease in man or any other animal" and "any article other than food, which is used or intended to affect the structure or any function of the body of man or any other animal." Advertisement is defined as "any representations... disseminated in any manner or by any means, for the purpose of inducing, or which is likely to induce, directly or indirectly, the purchase or use of any food, drug, device or cosmetic."

A study of the code sections and corresponding federal and state case law suggests that many manufacturers and distributors have statutorily reclassified their vitamins and food supplements as drugs by the very nature of their advertisements and that they are inducing sales of their merchandise as drugs, by means of their promotional materials.

It is the opinion of this Section that where claims are made as to a product's therapeutic value, the labeler could be required to be licensed as a drug manufacturer within the State of California, and, if necessary, be required to prove the safety and efficacy of his product pursuant to the "new drug" section of the Health and Safety Code. In addition, all product labels, labeling and advertising would be required to be legally correct within the meaning of state and federal drug labeling laws and regulations.

This letter is being distributed on an industry-wide basis to place those affected on notice that the Food and Drug Section of the California Department of Health Services is actively monitoring vitamin and food supplement advertising and stands ready, where it deems necessary, to initiate corrective action.

Sincerely,

C.F. Bryson, Chief
Food and Drug Section

This is an example of alleged "protection" by regulation rather than by information. The well intentioned author of this document hopes to protect you by threatening to legally prosecute some of the people who would like to give you information—whether that information is true or not! You have read our book. You are capable of deciding the merits of his statement for yourself. Note that this bureaucrat has provided NO scientific literature references in support of his official I'm-going-to-put-you-in-prison-if-you-disagree position. Instead, he has cited a regulation. He has legal power, so therefore he doesn't have to bother giving you information to convince you that he is correct.

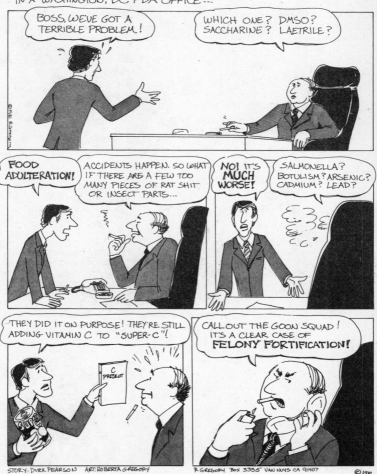

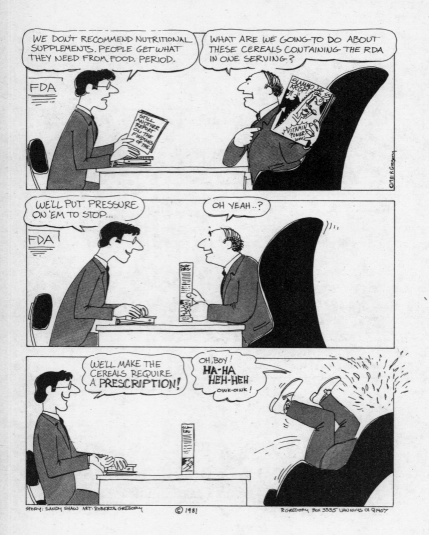

Story: Sandy Shaw Art: Roberta Gregory   © 1981   R.Gregory Box 3535 Van Nuys Ca 91407

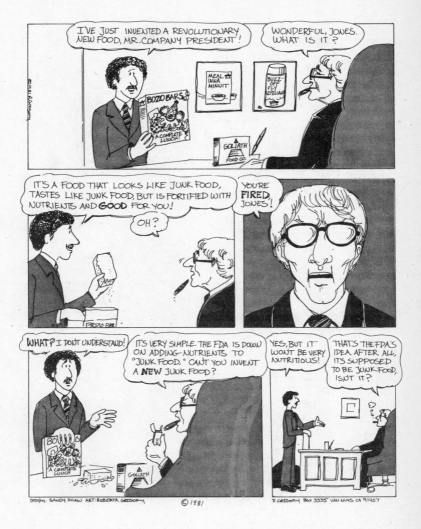

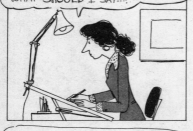

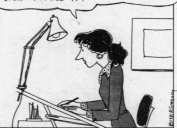

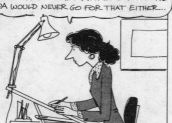

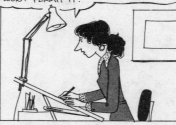

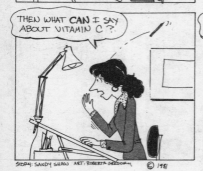

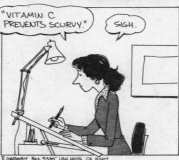

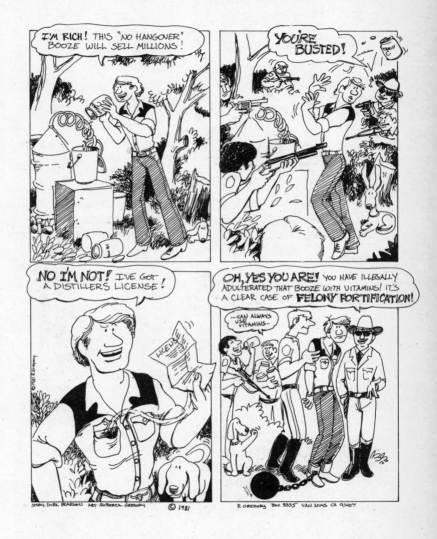

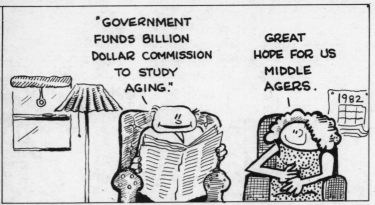

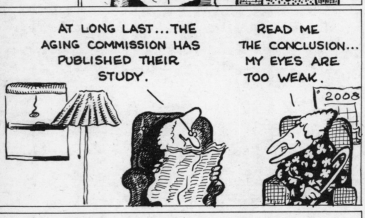

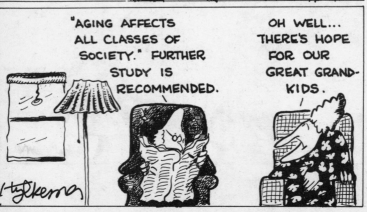

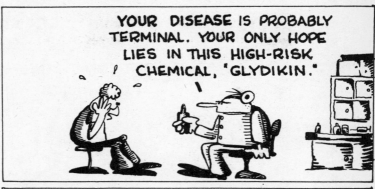

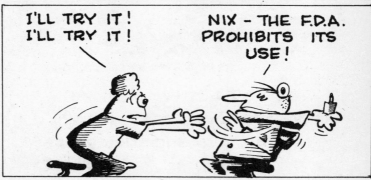

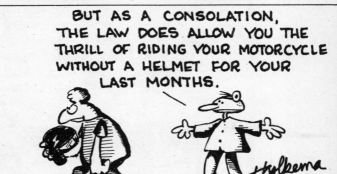

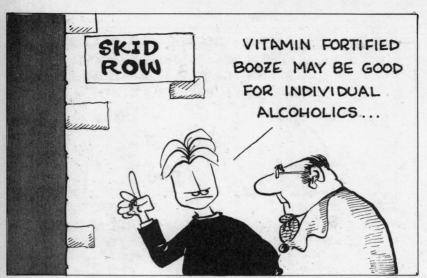

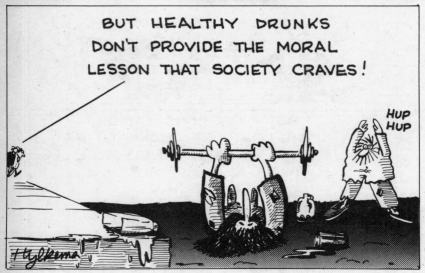

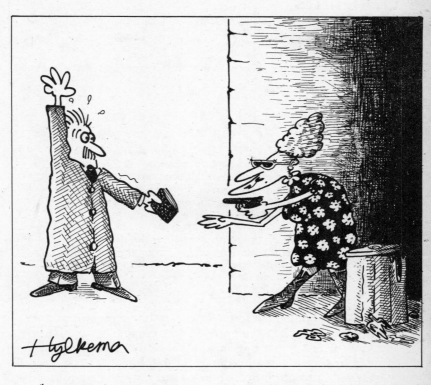

"SORRY, SONNY... BUT UNTIL THE F.D.A. APPROVES MY ARTHRITIS DRUG, I NEED $500 A DAY FOR MY BLACK MARKET SUPPLY."

APPENDIX F:
Cryonics

*I wish it were possible from this instance, to invent a
method of embalming drowned persons, in such a manner
that they may be recalled to life at any period, however
distant; for having a very ardent desire to see and observe
the state of America a hundred years hence, I should
prefer to any ordinary death, the being immersed in a
cask of Madeira wine, with a few friends, till that time, to
be recalled to life by the solar warmth of my dear
country. . . . in all probability we live in an age too early
and too near the infancy of science, to hope to see an art
brought in our time to its perfection . . .*
            —from a letter of Benjamin Franklin

**Cryonics (the immediate freezing at very low temperatures of
newly dead persons in the hope of thawing and revival later)
is a kind of last-resort option available now. It offers more
hope of further life than ordinary burial, but it is expensive
and carried out only by small, new, and untested companies
with little capital.**

We have not said anything in the foregoing chapters of
this book about cryonics, the prompt freezing of dead individuals treated with antifreeze materials at liquid-nitrogen temperature, to halt the biochemical degradation following death
(chemical reactions proceed very slowly at this temperature).

It may be possible at some future time to repair the damage of whatever killed the frozen dead, as well as the further
damage of being frozen and thawed. Present capabilities
toward reaching this goal are crude, but progress is being
made—animals as large as dogs have been cooled without

freezing to 0 degrees C (the freezing point of water) and revived after several hours without noticeable harm. At present, cryonics constitutes an improvement in cemetery design. It is difficult to evaluate the likelihood of revival on both technological and economic grounds, though this does not mean that it cannot or will not be done some day.

The economic questions stem from the present limited number of small inexperienced firms with little capital that are actually involved in cryonics suspensions. Only a few persons have actually been suspended. The $75,000 trust fund required for suspension provides only for maintenance at liquid-nitrogen temperature, but none of this is available for revival. Assuming that a successful revival might some day cost in the same ballpark as a heart-transplant operation, it will require another $100,000 or so. In addition, more money will be required to cure the fatal disease. Unless this money is provided by the suspendee, it is difficult to see why he or she will be revived except, perhaps, as a guinea pig for revival techniques. There are very little performance data to go on in evaluating the reliability of these cryonics firms. One firm has already gone bankrupt, having commingled the trust

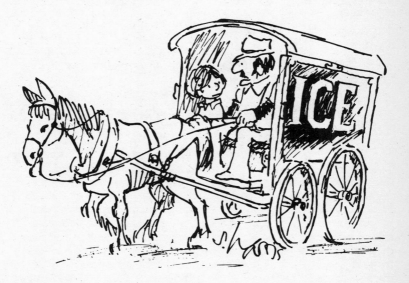

Stick to it. There's a future in cryogenics.

funds; all suspendees thawed out and had to be buried, even those who had paid $50,000 for a perpetual trust fund for liquid nitrogen plus storage space and security. The company's operators do not seem to have been bad men, only bad businessmen.

There is no question that cryonics suspension offers more hope than being buried in the ground. If death is imminent, it may be the most cost-effective course of action. Under such circumstances, we would take this option. But cryonics suspension is expensive and, hence, not for everyone. Whatever else may be said of it, it is a long shot, a gamble which depends upon technology not yet available, in contrast to life extension which has considerable resources in already available technology.

APPENDIX G:
Our Current Personal Experimental Life Extension Formula—Quantitative Data

THE INFORMATION CONTAINED
IN THIS APPENDIX
IS STRICTLY FOR USE BY
RESEARCH SCIENTISTS

THIS FORMULA IS STRICTLY EXPERIMENTAL. IT IS NOT RECOMMENDED FOR ANYONE OTHER THAN OURSELVES. THESE SUBSTANCES IN THESE DOSES REQUIRE FURTHER SAFETY TESTING. PREGNANT WOMEN AND CHILDREN MUST NOT USE THIS FORMULA. PERSONS WITH LIVER OR KIDNEY DAMAGE MUST NOT USE THIS FORMULA. EXTENSIVE FREQUENT CLINICAL LABORATORY TESTS MONITORED BY A RESEARCH-ORIENTED PHYSICIAN ARE NECESSARY, EVEN IF ONE IS IN PERFECT HEALTH.

OUR PERSONAL EXPERIMENTAL
LIFE EXTENSION FORMULA

(total amounts taken each day)

powder mixture, taken in 4 divided daily doses:

vitamin E (dl-alpha tocopherol acetate	6 grams (3,000 I.U., Roche 50 percent dry powder)
vitamin C (ascorbic acid)	20 grams

ascorbyl palmitate (lipid soluble form of vitamin C)	3 grams
beta carotene (pro vitamin A)	50-100 milligrams
vitamin B-1 (thiamine HC1)	2 grams
vitamin B-2 (riboflavin)	100 milligrams (Sandy)
	400 milligrams (Durk)
vitamin B-3 (niacin)	11 grams
vitamin B-5 (calcium pantothenate)	3 grams
vitamin B-6 (pyridoxine HC1)	1.75 grams
vitamin B-12 (cyanocobalamin)	500 micrograms
PABA (p-aminobenzoic acid, a B vitamin)	2 grams
L-arginine (amino acid)	3 grams
L-cysteine (amino acid)	2 grams
hesperidin complex (bioflavonoid)	500 milligrams
rutin (bioflavonoid)	500 milligrams
zinc (chelated as the gluconate)	60 milligrams
selenium (as sodium selenite)	1 milligram (1000 micrograms)
dilauryl thiodipropionate	200 milligrams
thiodipropionic acid	200 milligrams

taken separately, per day:

vitamin A	15,000–20,000 I.U.
inositol	10–20 grams (Durk)
extra L-arginine	17 grams (Sandy)
	5 grams (Durk)
or alternatively L-ornithine	3 grams (Durk)

tryptophan (amino acid, bedtime)	2 grams
L-Dopa (prescription amino acid)	250 milligrams at bedtime (Durk)
bromocriptine (Parlodel®, Sandoz)	3 milligrams (Durk) 1.25 milligrams (Sandy)
choline chloride (B vitamin)	1 to 3 grams
Deaner® (Riker)	200 to 300 milligrams
Hydergine® (Sandoz)	about 20 milligrams
Hydergine® (Sandoz)	about 20 milligrams
vasopressin (Diapid® nasal spray, Sandoz)	varies, 20–40 I.U. (Sandy) about 80 I.U. (Durk); (see Appendix L)
BHT (food additive antioxidant)	2 grams
RNA	1 gram, occasionally (Sandy)
thyroid extract	1 grain, in the morning (see Appendix L)
Orobronze® (canthaxanthin)	60 milligrams (Durk) (dose varies to maintain the degree of skin tan desired)
antacids (usually baking soda and glycine)	as required

1 ounce = 28.35 grams
1 pound = 453.59 grams
1 milligram = 1/1,000th of a gram
1 microgram = 1/1,000,000th of a gram
I.U. = international unit (a measure of biological activity)

APPENDIX H:
How Long Do Humans and Other Animals Live?

Would it be absurd then to suppose that this perfection of the human species might be capable of indefinite progress; that the day will come when death will be due only to extraordinary accidents or to the decay of the vital forces, and that ultimately the average span between birth and decay will have no assignable value? Certainly man will not become immortal, but will not the interval between the first breath that he draws and the time when in the natural course of events, without disease or accident, he expires, increase indefinitely?
—*Antoine Nicholas Marquis de Condorcet*, Sketch for a Historical Picture of the Progress of the Human Mind *(1794)*

Men do not live long enough; they are, for the purposes of high civilization, mere children when they die. . . . Life has lengthened considerably since I was born; and there is no reason why it should not lengthen ten times as much after my death.
—*George Bernard Shaw*, Back to Methuselah

If you read popular newspapers, magazines, or lay books on aging, you have read that there are magic areas of the world where people somehow live twice as long as here. Are there human beings alive today who are over 150 years old? You may be surprised by the findings of investigators into the claims of extreme old age in humans. People are a particularly long-lived species. We outlive most other animals. We do live longer than any other mammal. Here we compare natural longevity for people and other animals. Once we understand why we live twice as long as a chimpanzee or 30 times as long as a mouse, we will be able to live even longer.

614

Humans have been known to live for 110 years or so, but there have been no authenticated cases above 113 years. There have been persistent rumors, however, that people living in some areas of the world, notably the Hunzas in Kashmir, the Abkhazia villagers in Soviet Georgia, and the Vilcabamba villagers of Ecuador, have a far higher percentage of their populations reaching 100 years, with several villagers claiming to be 150 years of age and more. Unfortunately for these claims, investigations have revealed no evidence to substantiate them. In fact, several investigators who conducted careful examination of these claims concluded that many of the oldsters had taken their grandfather's name to avoid compulsory military service (they would then be too old for induction into the military!). The high altitude and clear, dry air result in lots of ultraviolet light which prematurely wrinkles (cross-links) the skin of these peasants, making visual age judgments difficult.

There is now a new technique available for helping to determine a person's chronological age: the racemization of aspartic acid (an amino acid) in the teeth. Amino acids come in two versions: left-handed and right-handed molecules, which are mirror images of each other. The right-handed molecule, known as D-aspartic acid, rotates polarized light to the right, while the left-handed version, known as L-aspartic acid, rotates polarized light to the left. The L-aspartic acid molecules are incorporated into the structure of the teeth when they first develop in the child. The body makes or uses only the L-aspartic acid. However, as soon as the L-aspartic acid is made, a process called racemization occurs, in which L-aspartic acid is gradually converted to D-aspartic acid at a certain rate (which is dependent on temperature, the conversion rate increasing rapidly as the temperature increases). The mouth temperature is nearly constant. By measuring the ratio of L-aspartic acid to D-aspartic acid, it is possible to determine with some accuracy the age of the tooth and, therefore, of the person. Serious attempts have been made by some researchers to get samples of teeth from the claimants of great age in Soviet Georgia, but the Soviet authorities have not been cooperative. The one specimen which they provided after years of repeated requests was determined to be from a 93 year old person. We are currently looking into the possibility of obtaining samples of tooth from the Hunzas and/or Vilcabamba. Preliminary Vilcabamba data from other researchers have found no one beyond the 80s in spite of claims to the contrary.

Listed below are life spans for various animals, as compiled by Marvin L. Jones from records of over 100 zoos throughout the world. Since these life spans reflect a life in captivity, it seems likely that animals in the wild do not live this long due to the predation and disease that they would normally encounter in their environments.

Indian fruit bat	31 yrs. 5 mos.
white faced capuchin monkey	46 yrs. 11 mos.
giant anteater	25 yrs. 10 mos.
chimpanzee	48 yrs., 47 yrs. 6 mos.
gorilla (western lowland)	47 yrs. 6 mos. (estimated)
Sumatran orangutan	49 yrs., 59 yrs. (estimated)
slender-tailed cloud rat	13 yrs. 7 mos.
mountain chinchilla	19 yrs. 6 mos.
coyote	21 yrs. 10 mos.
grizzly bear	35 yrs. 11 mos.
spotted hyena	33 yrs.
bobcat	32 yrs. 4 mos.
lion	24 yrs., 25 yrs.
elephant (Asian)	57 yrs., 69 yrs. (estimated)
great Indian rhinoceros	40 yrs. 4 mos., 38 yrs. 8 mos.
Syrian wild horse	32 yrs. 10 mos.
river hippopotamus	49 yrs. 6 mos.
Cape giraffe	36 yrs. 2 mos.

The Galapagos turtle lives well beyond 100 years, perhaps beyond 200 years. The life span of the cetaceans (dolphins, whales, and porpoises) has not yet been determined, although captive living whales and dolphins were recorded by Jones. An Atlantic bottle-nosed dolphin, still alive in 1978, was 25 years of age.

Although none of the other mammals seem to live as long as man, we can learn a great deal about genetic control of aging by finding out <u>why</u> man is able to outlive these other animals. By studying longer living animals, such as the Galapagos turtle, and even very long lived plants, such as the bristlecone pine that can live for a few <u>thousand</u> years, we can learn what protective and repair enzymes and what genetic mechanisms allow these organisms to reach these life spans. Genetic engineering experiments will probably be very informative; for example, a proposed aging control gene could be removed from the white footed mouse (which has about an 8 year life span) and installed in a common laboratory mouse (about $2\frac{1}{2}$ years life span), and the aging of the gene-spliced lab mouse closely observed. We expect that aging mechanisms are much alike between all living entities (on the Earth, at any rate), but the relative importance of these mechanisms' contribution to the aging of organisms must be quite different when large life span differences are involved.

APPENDIX I:
A Few Suppliers

Note: We have no financial involvement in any of the following companies or their offered products or in any other pharmaceutical or nutritional supplement firms. We assume no responsibility for any dealings with these firms.

Readers are urged to make their own careful decisions and comparisons with respect to price, quality, availability, and delivery time in purchasing from any supplier, including any of those listed in this book. We do not intend our listing them to be a recommendation or endorsement of them. Similarly, the listing of these organizations does not necessarily mean an endorsement by them of particular ideas in this book. There are many fine suppliers that are not listed here; our not listing certain suppliers here does not necessarily mean that we don't recommend them.

*   *   *

NUTRIENT SUPPLIERS:

HEALTH MAINTENANCE PROGRAMS, INC.
503 Grasslands Rd.
PO Box 252
Valhalla, NY 10595
914-592-3155

The owners of this business have stated that they intend to make generous donations to biomedical research on aging to avoid a possible conflict of interest, however, we will not be receiving any of these funds.

This firm supplies vitamins and very high potency vitamin mixtures as pure nutrients. The dl-alpha tocopherol acetate contains no easily peroxidized oil fillers. Dry nutrients are supplied in gelatin capsules without potentially allergenic fillers and binders such as corn starch, soy products, or yeast. These supplements are essentially sodium-free, for use by essential hypertension patients on low sodium diets.

This firm is run by a health professional rather than a businessman experienced in mail order marketing; there have been severe delivery delays reported. We suggest you check product availability before you order.

* * *

NUTRIENT SUPPLIERS:

Advanced Research Health
  Products Corp.
Box R
Summit, NJ 07901
Telephone orders to:
(212) 977-9579

PRODUCTS OFFERED:

Phylan 100 (100 milligram tablets of phenylalanine); AN-83 (antioxidant nutrients, 1983, an extremely potent formula of our design which is very similar to our own personal mixture, supplied in gelatin capsules with no binders or fillers)

The above manufacturer has a policy of donating a substantial portion of the profits of this business to legitimate non-profit charitable research foundations for research on biological aging mechanisms and means of intervention. We have no control over these foundations, and have never received grants from them, nor will we ever do so, thereby avoiding a potential conflict of interest.

* * *

NUTRIENT SUPPLIERS:

PRODUCTS OFFERED:

Bronson Pharmaceuticals
4526 Rinetti Lane
La Canada, CA 91011

Vitamin C crystals, both ascorbic acid and sodium ascorbate; intravenous ascorbate solution

*　　*　　*

Pure Planet Products
1025 N. 48th St.
Phoenix, AZ 85008

empty gelatin capsules (This is a very small company but we have received prompt and efficient service in buying small orders of empty gelatin capsules during the past few years.)

*　　*　　*

Vitamin Research Products
   Incorporated
1961-D Old Middlefield Way
Mountain View, CA 94043

(415) 967-7770

vitamins and amino acids including phenylalanine, cysteine, arginine; also BHT and other food additives; capsule filling plates; Na-PCA; carotenoids; custom nutrient mixes

The above firm offers powdered and crystalline nutrients for manufacturing, processing, or repacking. Vitamin Research Products Incorporated offers small quantities of the less well-known nutrients and food additives, and has pure bulk vitamins and nutrients available, without fillers and binders. (Many people are allergic to fillers and binders when taken in the quantities involved in very large doses of tableted vitamins; and even if there is no allergic reaction, mechanical irritation often results when taking dozens of tablets.) This firm has a policy of donating 3 percent of the gross of this business to legitimate non-profit charitable research foundations for research on biological aging mechanisms and means of intervention. As mentioned above, we have no control over these foundations, and have never received grants from them, nor will we ever do so, thereby avoiding a potential conflict of interest.

*   *   *

Wholesale Nutrition Club
PO Box 1113, Dept. Z
Sunnyvale, CA 94086

This firm offers a number of nutritional supplement tablets formulated without fillers, corn syrup, dyes, etc., and with minimal binders and lubricants. They will donate 3 percent of gross orders to the above address to the independent non-profit American Aging Association, AGE. (We receive no funds either from this company or from AGE.)

Three of this company's products are of special interest: C-STRIPS ($3.00 for 300) are for measuring vitamin C concentration in the urine. Their vitamin C based Drug Rehabilitation Kit for $40 (with a money-back guarantee which has never been requested, as of July 1981) will get a heroin, morphine, or meperidine addict off of these narcotics with no withdrawal symptoms. Methadone withdrawal is somewhat more difficult, with diarrhea being a problem. They also sell a book by Dr. A. Kalokerinos entitled *Every Second Child,* about the author-physician's use of vitamin C to prevent SIDS, sudden infant death syndrome (also called crib death).

*   *   *

M Squared Ethicals, Inc. (M² Ethicals, Inc.)
P.O. Box 174
West Chicago, IL 60185

The above firm supplies vitamins with no corn or soy products as binders or fillers.

NUTRIENT MANUFACTURERS

The following offer powdered and crystalline nutrients for manufacturing, processing, or repacking; relatively large minimum orders to commercial customers only.

Hoffmann-La Roche
Nutley, NJ 07110
(201) 235-3381

vitamins, carotenoids, ascorbyl palmitate

*   *   *

Ajinomoto Co., Inc.
9 West 57th St.
New York, NY 10019
(212) 688-8360

Na-PCA; amino acids including arginine, cysteine, phenylalanine, L-Dopa, tryptophan; vitamins

*   *   *

Takeda, Inc.
400 Park Avenue
New York, NY 10022
(212) 421-6950

vitamins and amino acids

*   *   *

Chemical Dynamics Corp.
P.O. Box 395
So. Plainfield, NJ 07080
(201) 753-5000

amino acids, vitamins

*   *   *

Eastman Chemical Products, Inc.
Kingsport, TN 37662
800-251-0351

food grade antioxidants

*   *   *

NUTRIENT MANUFACTURERS

Pfizer, Inc.   vitamins
Chemicals Div.
235 East 42nd St.
New York, NY 10017
(201) 546-7712

*   *   *

BASF Wyandotte Corp.   vitamins
Wyandotte, MI 48192
(313) 282-3300

*   *   *

Merck & Co., Inc.   vitamins and amino acids
Merck Chemical Div.
126 E. Lincoln Ave.
Rahway, NJ 07065
(201) 574-4000

*   *   *

Research Plus, Inc.   steroid hormones (avail-
P.O. Box 324   able to scientific and med-
Bayonne, NJ 07002   ical professionals only!)
(201) 823-3592

*   *   *

EM Chemicals   vitamins, minerals, amino
5 Skyline Drive   acids
Hawthorne, NY 10532
(914) 592-4660

*   *   *

William H. Rorer (Canada)   canthaxanthin (Orobronze®,
   Ltd.   30 milligram tablets)
Bramalea, Ontario

*   *   *

DEVICES:

Medical devices such as blood pressure gauges, pulse rate counters, etc., are readily available from Sears, Roebuck, Montgomery Ward, and by mail order from JS&A Sales, 1 JS&A Plaza, Northbrook, Ill, 60062 (800-323-6400), as well as from some drugstores and discount stores. The Consumer's Union annual *Consumer Reports Buying Guide Issue* has useful independent evaluations of some of these devices.

*   *   *

Peptide synthesizers are offered by:

Peninsula Laboratories, Inc.
PO Box 1111
San Carlos, CA 94070
(415) 592-5392

The Peptider: a manual solid-phase peptide synthesizer: $2,450 complete

*   *   *

Vega Biochemicals
420 E. Columbia
Tucson, AZ 85714
(602) 746-1401

Model 50 Peptide Synthesizer, $9,750; Model 105 Peptide Synthesizer, $85,000 (reaction vessels have capacities of 6 to 25 liters; solvents and reagents can be drawn from 55 gallon drums)

*   *   *

A gene synthesizing machine is available from:

Bio Logicals
Toronto, Ontario, Canada

gene synthesizing machine, $19,500

*   *   *

To purchase an air cleaner:

HEPA filter type: Alpaire, Inc., 4880 Havana St., Denver, Colorado 80239 (sizes available for both homes and businesses)

DEVICES:

electrostatic precipitator type:
for homes: Sears & Roebuck or Montgomery Ward's
for businesses: Minneapolis Honeywell Co., Minneapolis, Minnesota

        *   *   *

The company below is a reliable source for computer systems configuration, integration, sales and service for both software and hardware. See the "Special Thanks" in Part V, Chapter 12, for our system description.

> AEI, Automated Equipment Inc.
> 18430 Ward Street
> Fountain Valley, CA 92708
> Attn: Tom Dodge
> 1-(800)-854-7635, (714)-963-1414

        *   *   *

The following company is the manufacturer of the Osborne-1, an integrated portable computer system which includes the Wordstar® word processing software that we used to write this book. You will also need an NEC 5510 printer, or a similar letter quality printer. For light duty use, the inexpensive Epson MX-80 does a remarkably clear job for a dot matrix printer. The Osborne-1 software is already integrated for this printer.

> Osborne Computer Corp.
> 26500 Corporate Ave.
> Hayward, CA 94545
> Attn.: Lynn Hagen
> (415)-887-8080

APPENDIX J:
Some Journals Publishing Aging Research Data

JOURNAL	ABBREVIATION USUALLY USED IN REFERENCES
AGE Journal	AGE Journal
American Journal of Clinical Nutrition	Am. J. Clin. Nutr.
American Journal of Physiology	Am. J. Physiol.
Archives of Environmental Health	Arch. Environ. Health
Biochimica et Biophysica Acta	Biochim. Biophys. Acta
Brain	Brain
Brain Research	Brain Res.
Cancer	Cancer
Clinical Toxicology	Clin. Toxicol.
Endocrinology	Endocrinology
Experimental Cellular Research	Exp. Cell. Res.
Experimental Gerontology	Exp. Gerontol.
Federation Proceedings	Fed. Proc.
Food and Cosmetic Toxicology	Food Cosmet. Toxicol.

JOURNAL	ABBREVIATION USUALLY USED IN REFERENCES
Gerontologia	*Gerontologia*
Gerontology	*Gerontology*
Journal of Allergy and Clinical Immunology	*J. Allergy Clin. Immunol.*
Journal of the American Geriatric Society	*J. Am. Geriatr. Soc.*
Journal of the American Oil Chemists Society	*JAOCS*
Journal of Biological Chemistry	*J. Biol. Chem.*
Journal of Clinical Endocrinological Metabolism	*J. Clin. Endocrinol. Metab.*
Journal of Clinical Investigation	*J. Clin. Invest.*
Journal of Clinical Pathology	*J. Clin. Pathol.*
Journal of Experimental Medicine	*J. Exp. Med.*
Journal of Gerontology	*J. Gerontol.*
Journal of Immunology	*J. Immunol.*
Journal of Investigative Dermatology	*J. Invest. Dermatol.*
Journal of Nutrition	*J. Nutr.*
Journal of Pharmaceutical Sciences	*J. Pharm. Sci.*
Journal of the Society of Cosmetic Chemists	*J. Soc. Cosmet. Chem.*
The Lancet	*Lancet*
Life Sciences	*Life Sci.*
Mechanisms of Ageing and Development	*Mech. Ageing Dev.*
Molecular Biology	*Molec. Biol.*
Nature	*Nature*

JOURNAL	ABBREVIATION USUALLY USED IN REFERENCES
New England Journal of Medicine	*N. Engl. J. Med.*
Pharmacology	*Pharmacology*
Proceedings of the National Academy of Sciences	*Proc. Natl. Acad. Sci. USA*
Proceedings of the Nutrition Society	*Proc. Nutr. Soc.*
Radiation Research	*Radiat. Res.*
Science	*Science*
Toxicology and Applied Pharmacology	*Toxicol. Appl. Pharmacol.*
Trends in Pharmacological Sciences	*Trends Pharmacol. Sci.*
Vitamins and Hormones	*Vitam. Horm.*

Chapter 99 of *Remington's Pharmaceutical Sciences* has a fairly comprehensive list of journals which frequently publish scientific papers on the clinical use of drugs. This standard reference can be found in any biomedical library.

APPENDIX K:
References to *Life Extension: A Practical Scientific Approach* by Durk Pearson and Sandy Shaw

Part I Chapter 1: The Psychology of Life Extension

Wheeler, *The Adventurer's Guide*, David McKay Co., New York, 1976 (popular media)

Part I Chapter 2: It's a New Age

Robinson, "Molecular Clocks, Molecular Profiles, and Optimum Diets: Three Approaches to the Problem of Aging," *Mech. Ageing Dev.* 9: 226, 1979

Strehler, *Time, Cells, and Aging*, 2nd edition, Academic Press, 1977

Part I Chapter 5: The Evolution of Aging

Richard Cutler, "Evolution of Human Longevity," in *Advances in Pathobiology: Aging, Cancer, and Cell Membranes*, ed. Borek, Fenoglio, King, publ. Georg Thieme Verlag, 1980

Richard Cutler, "Evolution of Human Longevity and the Genetic Complexity Governing Aging Rate," *Proc. Nat. Acad. Sci. USA* 72(11): 4664–4668, 1975

Sacher, "Longevity and Aging in Vertebrate Evolution," *Bioscience* 28(8): 497–501, Aug. 1978

Hirsch, "Spontaneous Mutations Balance Reproductive Selective Advantage and Genetically Determined Longevity," *Mech. Aging Dev.* 9:355–367, 1979

Hirshleifer, Jack, "Economics from a Biological Viewpoint," *The Journal of Law & Economics* XX (1): 1–52, April 1977 (As the author says, the study of biology can be regarded as "Nature's economy." "Fundamental concepts like scarcity, competition, equilibrium, and specialization play similar roles in both spheres of inquiry." Highly recommended.)

Dawkins, *The Selfish Gene*, Oxford Univ. Press, 1976

Kirkwood and Holliday, "The Evolution of Ageing and Longevity," *Proc. R. Soc. Lond.* B205: 531–46, 1979

Kirkwood, "Evolution of Ageing," *Nature* 270: 301–304, 1977

Wilson, E. O., *Sociobiology: The New Synthesis*, Harvard University Press, 1975

Part I Chapter 7: Benefits Versus Costs of Aging Intervention

Schwing, "Longevity Benefits and Costs of Reducing Various Risks," *Technol. Forecasting and Soc. Change* 13:333–345, 1979

Part I Chapter 9: Doubling Time for Knowledge

Ziman, "The Proliferation of Scientific Literature: A Natural Process," *Science* 208:369, 25 Apr. 1980

Institute for Scientific Information, 3501 Market Street, University City Science Center, Philadelphia, PA 19104

"I don't think we're in Kansas anymore, Toto."
—Dorothy, Wizard of Oz

Part I Chapter 13: How Do You Know Who's Right?

Dixon and Massey, *Introduction to Statistical Analysis*, 3rd ed., McGraw-Hill, 1969

Cox, *Planning of Experiments,* Wiley, 1958

Hicks, *Fundamental Concepts in the Design of Experiments,* *2nd edition,* Holt, Rinehart, and Winston, 1973

Peng, *The Design and Analysis of Scientific Experiments,* Addison Wesley, 1967

Fisher and Yates, *Statistical Tables for Biological, Agricultural, and Medical Research* (New York: Hafner Press, 1953)

Wadsworth and Bryan, *Introduction to Probability and Random Variables* (New York: McGraw-Hill, 1960)

Eric Hoffer, *The True Believer,* Mentor, 1951 (popular media)

McCoy, *How to Organize and Manage Your Own Religious Cult,* Loompanics Unlimited, 1980 (popular media)

Singer and Benassi, "Occult Beliefs," *American Scientist,* pp. 49–55, Jan.–Feb. 1981

Strategy of Experimentation, 3 day course, Du Pont Corp., Applied Technology Division

Andrew Weil, *The Natural Mind,* Houghton Mifflin, 1972

E. Bright Wilson, *An Introduction to Scientific Research,* McGraw-Hill, 1952

deBono, Edward, *Lateral Thinking, Creativity Step by Step,* Harper Colophon Books, 1973

Part I Chapter 14: Synthetic versus Natural Controversy

There are many other examples of human illness and death resulting from eating plants containing natural toxins. According to the *Cecil Textbook of Medicine, 15th edition* (edited by Beeson, McDermott, and Wyngaarden, W. B. Saunders Co., 1979), antithyroid compounds in plants, particularly *Brassica* species, are thought to account for 4 percent of the world incidence of goiter. According to the same source, in 1973, 7719 accidental poisonings by eating plants were reported to the National Clearinghouse for Poison Information Centers (6210 of these were children under 5). One can only wonder how many other poisonings by natural plant toxins went unreported or even unrecognized.

Today's Food and Additives, General Foods Corp. (for a free copy, write to General Foods Consumer Center, 250 North St., White Plains, NY 10625) (popular media)

Gregory and Kirk, "The Bioavailability of Vitamin B-6 in Foods," *Nutr. Rev.* 39 (1):1–8, 1981

Laden and Spitzer, "Identification of a natural moisturizing agent in skin": *J. Soc. Cosmet. Chemists* 18:351–360, 1967

Pelletier and Keith, "Bioavailability of synthetic and natural ascorbic acid," *J. Am. Diet. Assoc.* 64:271–275, 1974

Part II Chapter 1: The Many Mechanisms of Aging

Mazess and Forman, "Longevity and Age Exaggeration in Vilcabamba, Ecuador," *J. Geront.* 34(1): 94–98 (1979)

Part II Chapter 3: How Aging Kills

Adelman and Britton, "The Impaired Capability for Biochemical Adaptation During Aging," *Bioscience* 25(10): 639–643, Oct. 1975

Roth and Adelman, "Age Related Changes in Hormone Binding by Target Cells and Tissues; Possible Role in Altered Adaptive Responsiveness," *Exp. Geront.* 10: 1–11, 1975

Denckla, "A Time to Die," *Life Sciences* 16:31–44, 1975b

Part II Chapter 4: Molecules of Life and Life Extension

Crick, "The Genetic Code," *Sci. Amer.* offprint 123, Oct. 1962

Lehninger, "How Cells Transform Energy," *Sci. Amer.* offprint 91, Sept. 1961

Nicholson, *Metabolic Pathways 1977,* (a wall chart) 11″ × 14″, $.80; 30″ × 40″, $4.00; Grand Island Biological, 3175 Staley Rd., Grand Island, NY 14072

Nicholson, *A Guide to Metabolic Pathways and Co-enzymes,* $.80 Grand Island Biological, 3175 Staley Rd., Grand Island, NY 14072

Pike and Brown, *Nutrition, an Integrated Approach,* Wiley, 1975

James D. Watson, *The Double Helix,* Signet, 1968

Part II Chapter 5: Aging and the Immune System

Adams and Bell, *Slow Viruses,* Addison-Wesley, 1976

Anderson, et al, "The effects of increasing weekly doses of ascorbate on certain cellular and humoral immune functions in normal volunteers," *Am. J. Clin. Nutr.* 33:71–76, Jan 1980

Greeder and Milner, "Factors Influencing the Inhibitory Effect of Selenium on Mice Inoculated with Ehrlich Ascites Tumor Cells," *Science* 209: 825–827, 1980

Barbul et al, "Arginine: A Thymotropic and Wound-Healing Promoting Agent," *Surgical Forum* 28:101–103, 1977

Bjelke, "Dietary Vitamin A and Human Lung Cancer", *Int. J. Cancer:* 15:561–565 (1975)

Brown and Reichlin, "Psychologic and Neural Regulation of Growth Hormone Secretion," *Psychosom. Med.* 34 (1): 45–61, 1972

Burnet, *Immunology, Aging, and Cancer,* Freeman, 1976

Burnet, "The Mechanism of Immunity," *Sci. Amer.* offprint 78, Jan. 1961

Cameron and Pauling, "Supplemental Ascorbate in the Supportive Treatment of Cancer: Prolongation of Survival Times in Terminal Human Cancer," *Proc. Nat. Acad. Sci. USA* 73(10):3685–89, Oct. 1976

Campbell, Reade, Radden, "Effect of cysteine on the survival of mice with transplanted malignant thymoma," *Nature* 251: 158–159, 1974

Catt, "Growth Hormone," *The Lancet,* pp. 933–939, 2 May 1970

"Symposium focuses on immune system," *Chem. Eng. News,* 18 March 1974, pg. 16

Goetzl et al, "Enhancement of random migration and chemotactic response of human leukocytes by ascorbic acid," *J. Clin. Invest.* 53:813–818, 1974

Goldstein, "Mode of Action of Levamisole," *Jour. of Rheumatology* Suppl. No. 4: 143–147, 1978

Goldstein, "Thymosin: Basic Properties and Clinical Potential in the Treatment of Patients with Immunodeficiency Diseases and Cancer," *Appl. Cancer Chemother. Antiobiot. Chemother.* 24:47–59, 1978

Walford, "Immunologic theory of aging: Current Status," *Fed. Proc.* 33(9): 2020–2027, 1974

Weksler et al, "Immunological Studies of Aging," *J. Exp. Med.* 148:996–1006, Oct. 1978

Spallholz, et al, "Immunologic Responses of Mice Fed Diets Supplemented with Selenite Selenium," *Proc. Soc. Exp. Med. Biol.* 143:685–689, 1973

Linus Pauling, *Vitamin C, the Common Cold, and the Flu,* Freeman, 1976 (popular media)

Nockels, "Protective Effects of Supplemental Vitamin E Against Infection," paper presented at 62nd annual scientific meeting (Apr. 9–14, 1978) of FASEB

Jerne, "The Immune System," *Sci. Amer.* offprint 1276, July 1973

Meites, "Role of Biogenic Amines in the Control of Prolactin and Growth Hormone Secretion," *Psychopharm. Bull.,* Oct. 1976, pp. 120–121

Khandwala and Gee, "Linoleic acid hydroperoxide: impaired bacterial uptake by alveolar macrophages, a mechanism of oxidant lung injury," *Science* 182: 1364–1365, 1973

Threatt, et al, "Brain reactive antibodies in serum of old mice demonstrated by immunofluorescence," *J. Geront.* 26(3):316–323, 1971

Jean L. Marx, "Thymic Hormones: Inducers of T Cell Maturation," *Science* 187:1183, 1975

Wood, "White Blood Cells v. Bacteria," *Scientific Amer.,* February 1951

Riley, Vernon, "Psychoneuroendocrine Influences on Immunocompetence and Neoplasia," *Science* 212: 1100–1109, 5 June 1981 [Emotional, psychosocial, or anxiety-caused stresses increase plasma concentration of adrenal corticoids and other hormones. A direct result of this is impairment of some parts of the immune system.]

Pecile and Muller, eds., "Growth and Growth Hormone," *Excerpta Medica*, 1972

Part II Chapter 6: Cross-linked Molecules and Aging

Some people who contract skin cancer during the period when canthaxanthin is available in Canada but not available in the United States may be able to sue the FDA for nonfeasance; consult your attorney.

Tanzer, "Cross-Linking of Collagen," *Science* 180:561–566, 1973

Verzar, "The Aging of Collagen," *Sci. Amer.*, April 1963

Bellows and Bellows, "Crosslinkage Theory of Senile Cataracts," *Annals of Ophthalmology*, pp. 129–135, Feb. 1976

Deyl et al, "Aging of the Connective Tissue: Collagen Cross Linking in Animals of Different Species and Equal Age," *Exp. Geront.* 6: 227–233, 1971

Bjorksten, "The Crosslinkage Theory of Aging," *J. Am. Geriatr. Soc.* 16: 408–427, 1968

Bjorksten, "A Unifying Concept for Degenerative Diseases," *Comp. Therapy* 4(1): 44–52, Jan. 1978

Bjorksten, "Pathways to the Decisive Extension of the Human Specific Lifespan," *J. Am. Geriatr. Soc.* 25 (9): 396–399, 1977

Bjorksten, "The Crosslinkage Theory of Aging as a Predictive Indicator," *Rejuvenation* 8 (3): 59–66, 1980

Kirk and Chieffi, "Variation with Age in Elasticity of Skin and Subcutaneous Tissue in Human Individuals," *Jour. Derm.* 17:373–380, 1962

Part II Chapter 7: Our Subversive Free Radicals

Kellogg et al, "Superoxide involvement in the bactericidal effects of negative air ions on *Staphylococcus albus*," *Nature* 281: 400–401, 1979

Shamberger et al, "Carcinogen-induced Chromosomal Breakage Decreased by Antioxidants," *Proc. Nat. Acad. Sci.* 70 (5): 1461–63, May 1973

Lundberg, ed. *Autoxidation and Antioxidants, Vols. I and II,* Wiley Interscience, 1961

Swern, ed. *Organic Peroxides, vols. 1,2,3,* Wiley Interscience, 1970

Khandwala and Gee, "Linoleic acid hydroperoxide: impaired bacterial uptake by alveolar macrophages, a mechanism of oxidant lung injury," *Science* 182: 1364–65, 1973

Georgieff, "Free radical inhibitory effect of some anticancer compounds," *Science* 173: 537–39, 1971

Pryor, "Free Radical Pathology," *Chemical and Engineering News,* 7 June 1971, pp. 34–51

Harman, Eddy, and Noffsinger, "Free radical theory of aging: inhibition of amyloidosis in mice by antioxidants; possible mechanism," *J. Am. Geriat. Soc.* 34(5): 203–209, 1976

Tappel, "Biological Antioxidant Protection Against Lipid Peroxidation Damage," *Amer. J. Clin. Nutr.* 23(8):1137–1139, 1970

Harman and Mattick, "Association of lipid oxidation with seed aging and death," *Nature* 260: 323–324, 1976

"Santoquin antioxidant: can it actually slow the process of aging," advertisement, *Monsanto Report No. 6 on Current Technology* (popular media)

Roehm, et al, "The influence of vitamin E on the lung fatty acids of rats exposed to ozone," *Arch. Environ. Health* 24: April 1972

Ranney, *Antioxidants—Recent Developments,* Noyes Data Corp., 1979

Nockels, "Protective Effects of Supplemental Vitamin E Against Infection," paper presented at 62nd annual meeting (Apr. 9–14, 1978) of FASEB

Comfort et al, "Effect of ethoxyquin on the longevity of C3H mice," *Nature* 229: 254–255, 22 Jan. 1971

Sincock, "Life extension in the rotifer Mytilina Brevispina var Redunca by the application of chelating agents," *J. Geron.* 30(3): 289–293, 1975

Sunde and Hoekstra, "Structure, Synthesis, and Function of Glutathione Peroxidase," *Nutrition Reviews* 38(8): 265–273, 1980

Tappel, "Vitamin E as the biological lipid antioxidant," *Vit. Horm.* 20:493–510, 1962

Sherwin, "Antioxidants for food fats and oils," *J. Amer. Oil Chem. Soc.* 49(8):468–472, 1972

Pryor, "Free Radicals in Biological Systems," *Sci. Amer.*, August 1970

Cort, "Antioxidant activity of tocopherols, ascorbyl palmitate, and ascorbic acid and their mode of action," *J. Amer. Oil Chem. Soc.* 51(7):321–325, 1974

Fridovich, "Oxygen: Boon and Bane," *Amer. Scientist* 63:54–59, 1975

Harman, "Free Radical Theory of Aging: Nutritional Implications," *AGE* 1(4):145–152, 1978

Harman, "Free Radical Theory of Aging," *J. Geront.* 23(4), Oct. 1968

Black and Chan, "Suppression of Ultraviolet Light induced Tumor formation by dietary antioxidants," *J. Inv. Derm.* 65:412–414, 1975

Harman, "Role of Free Radicals in Mutation, Cancer, Aging, and the Maintenance of Life," *Rad. Res.* 16:753–764, 1962

Kormendy and Bender, "Chemical Interference with Aging," *Gerontologia* 17: 52–64, 1971

Bender, Kormendy, Powell, "Pharmacological Control of Aging," *Exp. Geront.* 5(22):97–129, 1970

Thompson and Sherwin, "Investigation of antioxidants for polyunsaturated edible oils," *J. Amer. Oil Chem. Soc.* 43(12): 683–686, 1965

Pryor et al, "Autoxidation of Polyunsaturated Fatty Acids," *Arch. Environ. Health,* pp. 201–210, July/August 1976

Steiner and Anastasi, "Vitamin E: An Inhibitor of the Platelet Release Reaction," *J. Clin. Invest.* 57:732–737, 1976

Harman, et al, "Free Radical Theory of Aging: Effect of Dietary Fat on Central Nervous System Function," *J. Am. Geriat. Soc.* 24(7):301–307, 1976

McCord, "Superoxide radical may play a role in arthritis," paper presented at the Third Biennial Conference on Chemical Education, Pennsylvania State Univ., Aug. 1, 1974

Harman, "Free radical theory of aging: effect of adding antioxidants to maternal mouse diets on the lifespan of their offspring—second experiment," paper presented at the 8th Annual Meeting of the American Aging Association, Oct. 5–7, 1978

Simic and Karel, eds., *Autoxidation in Food and Biological Systems,* Plenum Press, 1980

Coker, Parratt, Ledingham, Zeitlin, "Thromboxane and prostacyclin release from ischaemic myocardium in relation to arrhythmias," *Nature* 291: 323–324, 28 May 1981 [Both thromboxane and prostacyclin are released from acutely ischaemic myocardium in dogs with coronary artery ligation. The ratio between these two prostaglandins determines susceptibility to post-infarct arrhythmias.]

Demopoulos, Pietronigro, Flamm, Seligman, "The Possible Role of Free Radical Reactions in Carcinogenesis," *J. Environ Pathol Toxicol* 3(4): 273–303, 1980

Demopoulos et al, "The free radical pathology and the microcirculation in the major central nervous system disorders," *Acta Physiol Scand* Suppl 492: 91–119, 1980

Kontos et al, "Prostaglandins in physiological and in certain pathological responses of the cerebral circulation," *Fed. Proc.* 40(8): 2326–2330, June 1981 ["These findings show that prostaglandins are mediators of the cerebral arteriolar damage due to brain injury and that their mechanism of action is dependent on the generation of free oxygen radicals."]

Hall and Braughler, "Acute Effects of Intravenous Glucocorticoid Pretreatment of in Vitro Peroxidation of Cat Spinal Cord Tissue," *Exptl. Neurol.* 72, June 1981

Young, Flamm, Demopoulos et al, "Effect of Naloxone on Post Traumatic Ischemia in Experimental Spinal Contusion," *J. Neurosurgery,* Sept. 1981

Spector, "Vitamin Homeostasis in the Central Nervous System," *New Engl. J. Med.* 296: 1393-, 1977 [vitamin C pumps in blood-brain barrier and in neuronal membranes maintains C levels about 100 times as high in brain neurons as in bloodstream]

Bracco, Loliger, Viret, "Production and Use of Natural Antioxidants," *JAOCS* 58 (6): 686–690, 1981

Mickel, "Peroxidized Arachidonic Acid Effects on Human Platelets and Its Proposed Role in the Induction of Damage to White Matter" in Kabara, ed., *The Pharmacological Effect of Lipids,* The American Oil Chemists' Society, 1978

Lewis and Del Maestro, editors, "Free Radicals in Medicine and Biology" Supplementum 492 of *Acta Physiologica Scandinavica,* Almquist & Wiksell, Uppsala, 1980 (168 pp., over a dozen papers; highly recommended)

Part II Chapter 8: Accumulated Wastes

Brody, Harman, Ordy, eds., *Aging: Clinical, Morphologic, and Neurochemical Aspects in the Aging Central Nervous System: Vol. I,* Raven, New York, 1975

Nanda et al, *Aging Pigment, Current Research: I,* MSS Information Corp., 1974

Reichel, "Lipid Pigment Formation as a Function of Age, Disease, and Vitamin E Deficiency," International Symposium on Vitamin E, Hakone, 1970

Harman, Eddy, and Noffsinger, "Free radical theory of aging: inhibition of amyloidosis in mice by antioxidants; possible mechanism," *J. Am. Geriat. Soc.* 34(5): 203–209, 1976

Mann and Yates, "Lipoprotein Pigments—their relationship to ageing in the human nervous system: the lipofuscin content of nerve cells," *Brain* 97:481–488, 1974

Nandy and Bourne, "Effect of Centrophenoxine (dimethyla-minoethanol p-chlorophenoxyacetate) on the lipofuscin pigments in the neurons of senile guinea pigs," *Nature* 210:313–314, 1966

Shakocius and Pearson, "Mind Food," *OMNI,* pp. 54–57, May 1979 (popular media)

Nandy and Schneider, "Effects of dihydroergotoxine mesylate on aging neurons in vitro," *Gerontology* 24 (suppl. 1): 66–70, 1978

Miquel, Lundgren, Johnson, "Spectrophotofluorometric and Electron Microscope Study of Lipofuscin Accumulation in the Testis of Aging Mice," *J. Gerontol.* 33(1): 5–19, 1978

"The Older You Grow, the More You Glow," *Aminco Laboratory News* 31(3): 1–5, Fall 1975

Part II Chapter 9: Decline of the Brain's Chemical Messengers

CAUTION: Schizophrenics should use growth hormone (GH) releasers with caution since they <u>may</u> increase the severity of symptoms. GH releasers include L-Dopa, arginine and ornithine (some schizophrenics may experience worsening symptoms, possibly due to the effects of methyl donation by polyamines made from these amino acids in the body), and bromocriptine (in doses over 30 milligrams a day, adverse effects on schizophrenic symptomology may occur in some people). If this occurs, discontinue use of the GH releasers.

Brain Information Service, University of California at Los Angeles, Los Angeles, CA 90024 (current alerting services and bibliographies concerning memory, learning, sleep, etc.)

Sitaram et al, "Choline: Selective Enhancement of Serial Learning and Encoding of Low Imagery Words in Man," *Life Sci.* 22: 1555–1560, 1978

Goldstein et al, eds., *Ergot Compounds and Brain Function,* Raven Press, 1980

Berde and Schild, eds., *Ergot Alkaloids and Related Compounds,* Springer-Verlag, 1978

Meites, "Role of Biogenic Amines in the Control of Prolactin and Growth Hormone Secretion," *Psychopharm. Bull.*, Oct. 1976, pp. 120–121

Boyd et al, "Stimulation of Human-Growth-Hormone Secretion by L-Dopa," *New Engl. J. Med.* 283(26): 1425–1429, 1970

Levi-Montalcini and Angeletti, "Nerve Growth Factor," *Physiol. Rev.* 48(3): 534–569, 1968

Guillemin and Burgus, "The Hormones of the Hypothalamus," *Sci. Amer.* offprint 1260, Nov. 1972

Pfeiffer et al, "Stimulant Effect of 2-Dimethylaminoethanol—Possible Precursor of Brain Acetylcholine," *Science* 126: 610–611, 1957

Bartus et al, "Age-related changes in passive avoidance retention: modulation with dietary choline," *Science* (Washington, DC) 209 (4453): 301–3, 1980

Myers, *Handbook of Drug and Chemical Stimulation of the Brain*, Van Nostrand Reinhold, 1974

Seiden and Dykstra, *Psychopharmacology, A Biochemical and Behavioral Approach*, Van Nostrand Reinhold, 1977

Fernstrom and Wurtman, "Nutrition and the Brain," *Sci. Amer.*, Feb. 1974

Cotzias, et al, "Prolongation of the Life-Span in Mice Adapted to Large Amounts of L-Dopa," *Proc. Nat. Acad. Sci. USA* 71(6):2466–2469, June 1974

Emmenegger and Meier-Ruge, "The Actions of Hydergine on the Brain," *Pharmacology* 1:65–78, 1968

Stein, et al, "Memory Enhancement by Central Administration of Norpinephrine," *Brain Res.* 84: 329–335, 1975

Finch, "Catecholamine metabolism in the brains of ageing male mice," *Brain Res.* 52: 261–276, 1973

Shakocius and Pearson, "Mind Food," *OMNI*, pp. 54–57, May 1979 (popular media)

"Workshop on Advances in Experimental Pharmacology of Hydergine," *Gerontology* 24 (Suppl. 1):1–154, 1978

Drachman and Leavitt, "Human Memory and the Cholinergic System," *Arch. Neurol.* 30:113, 1974

Sitaram, Weingartner, and Gillin, "Human Serial Learning: Enhancement with Arecholine and Choline and Impairment with Scopolamine Correlate with Performance on Placebo," *Science* 201:274–276, 1978

Legros et al, "Influence of Vasopressin on Memory and Learning," *Lancet*, 7 Jan. 1978, pg. 41

Oliveros et al, "Vasopressin in Amnesia," *Lancet*, 7 Jan. 1978, pg. 42

"Dopamine and age: Turning back the Clock" *Science* News, Nov. 10, 1979

Marshall and Berrios, "Movement Disorders of Aged Rats: Reversal by Dopamine Receptor Stimulation," *Science* 206: 477–479, 1979

Bodanszky, [life extension in rats with oxytocin], *Nature* 210: 751, 1966

Wheeler and Benolken, "Visual Membranes: Specificity of Fatty Acid Precursors for the Electrical Response to Illumination," *Science* 188: 1312–1314, 1975

Seil and Blank, "Myelination of Central Nervous System Axons in Tissue Culture by Transplanted Oligodendrocytes," *Science* 212: 1407, 1981

Dr. Nicolas Bazan, a neurochemist, has recently shown that arachidonic acid and other precursors of prostaglandins (and also of thromboxanes and leukotrienes) are released into the brain in large amounts in his rat model of epilepsy. Free radical autoxidation of arachidonic acid and similar polyunsaturated lipids can produce potentially damaging prostaglandins, thromboxanes (clotting hormones) and leukotrienes. Free radical damage to the membrane-bound enzymes which produce protective prostaglandins and related compounds (such as prostacyclin) makes the problem even worse. Dr. Bazan's hypothesis of epilepsy's cause suggests that free radical scavengers may help epileptics. In fact, we knew of two such cases before hearing of Dr. Bazan's work. A simplified version of our nutrient mixture taken at about ¼ of our doses has resulted in two (out of two) remarkable remissions. Both cases were chronic long-term (several years or more) focal epileptics with clear gross EEG abnormalities. These cases were not satisfactorily controlled by diphenylhydantoin and phenobarbitol, even in very heavy doses. Within a few days after the start of nutrient therapy, the epilepsy and the EEG abnormalities had vanished. The patients, who are under the continuous close care of a research-oriented physician, are now being <u>slowly</u> withdrawn from their conventional medications. As of June 1981, one patient was 90 percent withdrawn and the other was 80 percent withdrawn with no signs of epileptiform EEG pathology. Current plans are to complete the withdrawal from the barbiturates and diphenylhydantoin, and to continue the antioxidant nutrients indefinitely. At least some epilepsy is caused by free radical pathology, and at least some can be cured with free radical modulating agents.

Kontos, Wei, Ellis, Dietrich, Povlishock, "Prostaglandins in physiological and in certain pathological responses of the cerebral circulation," *Fed. Proc.* 40(8): 2326–2330, 1981 ["These findings show that prostaglandins are mediators of the cerebral arterial damage due to brain injury and that their mechanism of action is dependent on the generation of free oxygen radicals."]

Pfeiffer, Ward, El-Meligi, Cott, *The Schizophrenias, Yours and Mine.* Pyramid Books, 1970 (popular book)

Pfeiffer and Bacchi, "Copper, Zinc, Manganese, Niacin, and Pyridoxine in the Schizophrenias," *J. Appl. Nutr.* 27 (2,3): 11–39, 1975

Hazum et al, "Morphine in Cow and Human Milk: Could Dietary Morphine Constitute a Ligand for Specific Morphine Receptors?" *Science* 213: 1010–12, 28 Aug. 1981
     The unexpected finding of morphine in cow and human milk, in alfalfa, lettuce, and other plants, leads one to wonder whether morphine plays a more prominent role in behavior than has been previously thought. And what are those plants doing with it?

Part II Chapter 10: Turning Back Aging Clocks

Debono et al, "Bromocriptine and Dopamine Receptor Stimulation," *Brit. J. Clin. Pharmacol.* 3:977–982, 1976

Gay Gaer Luce, *Body Time,* Pantheon, 1971 (a popular book about physiological rhythms and social stress)

Robertson, et al, "Physiological changes occurring in the blood of the Pacific Salmon accompanying sexual maturation and spawning," *Endocrinology* 68(5):733–746, 1961

Robertson, "Prolongation of the Life span of Kokanee Salmon by castration before beginning of gonad development," *Proc. NAS* 47:609–621, 1961

Beck and Bharadwaj, "Reversed development and cellular aging in an insect," *Science* 178:1210–1211, 1972

Pengelley and Asmundson, "Annual Biological Clocks," *Sci. Amer.* offprint 1219, Apr. 1971

Winfree, "Resetting Biological Clocks," *Physics Today,* pp. 34–39, March 1975

Winfree, *The Geometry of Biological Time,* Springer-Verlag, 1980

Rheinwald and Green, "Epidermal Growth Factor and the Multiplication of Cultured Human Epidermal Keratinocytes," *Nature* 265: 421–424, 1977

Robinson, "Molecular Clocks, Molecular Profiles, and Optimum Diets: Three Approaches to the Problem of Aging," *Mech. Ageing Dev.* 9: 226, 1979

Denckla, "A Time to Die," *Life Sciences* 16:31–44, 1975b

Kohn, "Aging and Cell Division," *Science* 188:203–4, 1975

Hayflick, "Human Cells and Aging," *Sci. Amer.,* March 1968

Huang et al, "Induction of Estrous Cycles in Old Non-cyclic Rats by Progesterone, ACTH, Ether Stress, or L-Dopa," *Neuroendocrin.* 20:21–34, 1976

Miquel, Lundgren, Johnson, "Spectrophotofluorometric and Electron Microscopic Study of Lipofuscin Accumulation in the Testis of Aging Mice," *J. Gerontol.* 33(1): 5–19, 1978

Edmunds and Adams, "Clocked Cell Cycle Clocks," *Science* 211: 1002–1013, 1981

Aldridge and Pavlidis, "Clocklike behavior of biological clocks," *Nature* 259: 343–344, 1976

Holliday, Huschtscha, Tarrant, Kirkwood, "Testing the Commitment Theory of Cellular Aging," *Science* 198:366–372, 1977

Bell, Marek, Levinstone, Merrill, Sher, Young, Eden, "Loss of Division Potential in vitro: Aging or Differentiation?" *Science* 202:1158–1163, 1978

Hornsby, Gill, "Loss of Division Potential in Culture: Aging or Differentiation?" *Science* 208:1482–83, 1980

Part II Chapter 11: Factors Which Correlate with Natural Longevity

Richard Cutler, "Evolution of Human Longevity," in *Advances in Pathobiology: Aging, Cancer, and Cell Membranes*, ed. Borek, Fenoglio, King, publ. Georg Thieme Verlag, 1980

Schwartz, "Correlation between species life span and capacity to activate 7, 12-dimethylbenz(a)anthracene to a form mutagenic to a mammalian cell," *Expt. Cell Res.* 94:445–447, 1975

Sacher, "Longevity and Aging in Vertebrate Evolution," *Bioscience* 28(8):497–501, Aug. 1978

Little, "Relationship Between DNA Repair Capacity and Cellular Aging," *Gerontology* 22:28–55, 1976

Tolmasoff, Ono, Cutler, "Superoxide Dismutase: Correlation with life-span and specific metabolic rate in primate species," *Proc. Nat'l. Acad. Sci. USA* 77(5):2777–2781, May 1980

Harman, "Role of Free Radicals in Mutation, Cancer, Aging, and the Maintenance of Life," *Rad. Res.* 16:753–764, 1962

Daniel Hershey, *Lifespan and Factors Affecting It*, Charles C. Thomas, Springfield, IL, 1974

Hart and Setlow, "Correlation Between DNA Excision-Repair and Lifespan in a Number of Mammalian Species," *Proc. Nat. Acad. Sci.* 71(6): 2169–2173, 1974

Part II Chapter 12: Regeneration: Born-Again Limbs and Organs

Rose, *Regeneration*, Appleton Century Crofts, 1970

Bassett, C. A. L., and Becker, R. O., "Generation of Electric Potentials by Bone in Response to Mechanical Stress," *Science* 137:1063–1064, 1962

Bassett, Pawluk, and Becker, "Effects of Electric Currents on Bones in Vivo," *Nature*, 204:652–654, 1964

Bassett et al, "Acceleration of Fracture Repair by Electromagnetic fields: A Surgically Non-Invasive Method," *Ann. NY Acad. Sci.* 238:242–262, 1974

Bassett, Pawluk, and Pilla, "Augmentation of Bone Repair by Inductively Coupled Electromagnetic Fields," *Science,* 184:575–577, 1974

Becker, "Stimulation of Partial Limb Regeneration in Rats," *Nature* 235:109–111, 1972

Cone, C. D., and Cone, C. M., "Induction of Mitosis in Mature Neurons in Central Nervous System by Sustained Depolarization," *Science,* 192:155–158, 1976

Fausto, "Studies on Ornithine Decarboxylase Activity in Normal and Regenerating Livers," *Biochimica et Biophysica Acta* 190:193–201, 1969

Lavins, L. S. et al, "Electric Enhancement of Bone Healing," *Science,* 175:1118–1121, 1972

Levy, D. D., "Induced Osteogenesis by Electrical Stimulation," *J. Electrochem. Soc.: Electrochemical Science,* 118:1438–1442, 1971

Maass, J. A. and Maxim, M., "Contactless Nerve Stimulation and Signal Detection by Inductive Transducer," *IEEE Transactions on Magnetics,* 322–326, 1970

Schiefelbein, "The Miracle of Regeneration: Can Human Limbs Grow Back?," *Saturday Review,* 8–11, 7–8–1978 (popular media)

Stastny and Cohen, "Epidermal Growth Factor: Induction of Ornithine Decarboxylase," *Biochim. Biophys. Acta* 204: 578–589, 1970

Seil and Blank, "Myelination of Central Nervous System Axons in Tissue Culture by Transplanted Oligodendrocytes," *Science* 212:1407, 1981

Part II Chapter 13: Aging Theories Revisited

Strehler, *Time, Cells, and Aging,* 2nd ed., Academic Press, 1977

Roberts, Adelman, Cristofalo, eds., *Pharmacological Intervention in the Aging Process,* Plenum, 1978

Finch and Hayflick, eds., *Handbook of the Biology of Aging,* Van Nostrand Reinhold, 1977

Falzone, Samis, Wulff, "Cellular Compensations and Controls in the Aging Process," *J. Geront.* 22:42, 1967

Cutler, "Nature of Aging and Life Maintenance Processes," *Interdiscipl. Topics Geront.* 9:83–133, 1976

Kormendy and Bender, "Chemical Interference with Aging," *Gerontologia* 17:52–64, 1971

Bender et al, "Pharmacological Control of Aging," *Exp. Geront.* 5(22):97–129, 1970

Comfort, "Test-battery to measure ageing-rate in man," *Lancet,* pg. 1411, 27 Dec. 1969

Part III Chapter 1: Some Immediate Benefits

Jetten, "Retinoids specifically enhance the number of epidermal growth factor receptors," *Nature* 284:626–631, 17 April 1980

Sprince, Parker, Smith, "L-ascorbic acid in alcoholism and smoking: protection against acetaldehyde toxicity as an experimental model," *Int. J. Vit. Nutr. Res.* 47 (Suppl. 1G):185–212, Nov. 1977

Sitaram et al, "Choline: Selective Enhancement of Serial Learning and Encoding of Low Imagery Words in Man," *Life Sci.* 22:1555–1560, 1978

Drachman and Leavitt, "Human Memory and the Cholinergic System," *Arch. Neurol.* 30: 113, 1974

Sitaram, Weingartner, and Gillin, "Human Serial Learning: Enhancement with Arecholine and Choline and Impairment with Scopolamine Correlate with Performance on Placebo," *Science* 201:274–276, 1978

Legros et al, "Influence of Vasopressin on Memory and Learning," *Lancet,* 7 Jan. 1978, pg. 41

Ralli and Dumm, "Relation of Pantothenic Acid to Adrenal Cortical Fuction," *Vit. Horm.* 11:133–158, 1953

Laden & Spitzer, "Identification of a Natural Moisturizing Agent in skin," *J. Soc. Cosm. Chem.* 18:351–360, 1967

The Salts of PCA and their Moisturizing Effects, Technical Bulletin, Ajinomoto Company (with 8 references)

Part III Chapter 2: Revitalizing Your Brain Power

Odens, "RNA Effects on Memory," Lecture read at the 16th Convention on Civilisation Diseases, Nutrition, and Living Conditions, 14–20 Sept. 1970, in Treves and Luxembourg

Levi-Montalcini and Calissano, "The Nerve Growth Factor," *Sci. Amer.*, June 1979

Mellini, [Hydergine, tinnitus, visual disorders, etc.], Minerva med. 64:1844–1853 (1973)

Hindmarch et al, "The effects of an ergot alkaloid derivative (Hydergine) on aspects of psychomotor performance, arousal, and cognitive processing ability," *J. Clin. Pharmacol.* 19 (11–12):726–732, 1979

Richardson, "A two year oral study with Hydergine in rats," *Action on Ageing,* Proceedings of a Symposium held at Basle 20th/21st May, 1976 (published by MCS Consultants, England, for Sandoz Corp.)

Brody, Harman, Ordy, eds., *Aging: Clinical, Morphologic and Neurochemical Aspects in the Aging Central Nervous system: Vol. I.* Raven, New York, 1975

Wheeler, Benolken, Anderson, [polyunsaturated fatty acids are important functional components controlling electrical response of photoreceptor cell membranes] *Science* 188:1312–1314, 1975

Myers, *Handbook of Drug and Chemical Stimulation of the Brain,* Van Nostrand Reinhold, 1974

Seiden and Dykstra, *Psychopharmacology, A Biochemical and Behavioral Approach,* Van Nostrand Reinhold, 1977

Nanda et al, *Aging Pigment, Current Research:I,* MSS Information Corp., 1974

Enesco, "Effect of vitamin B-12 on Neuronal RNA and on Instrumental conditioning in the Rat," from Ch. 11 in *Recent Advances in Biological Psychiatry,* Vol. X, Plenum, 1968

Gene Bylinsky, *Mood Control,* Scribner's, 1978 (popular media)

Schubert et al, "Alterations in the surface properties of cells responsive to nerve growth factor," *Nature,* 273:718–723, 1978

Fernstrom and Wurtman, "Nutrition and the Brain," *Sci. Amer.*, Feb. 1974

Mann and Yates, "Lipoprotein pigments—their relationship to ageing in the human nervous system: the lipofuscin content of nerve cells," *Brain* 97:481–488, 1974

Stein, et al, "Memory Enhancement by Central Administration of Norepinephrine," *Brain Res.* 84:329–335, 1975

Finch, "Catecholamine metabolism in the brains of ageing male mice," *Brain Res.* 52: 261–276, 1973

Rawls, "Diet can Influence Functioning of the Brain," *Chem. Eng.* News, 23 Jan. 1978

Borison, et al, "Metabolism of an Antidepressant Amino Acid," presented in poster session at April 9–14, 1978 FASEB, Atlantic City, NJ [about use of L-phenylalanine in depression]

Drachman and Leavitt, "Human Memory and the Cholinergic system" *Arch. Neurol.* 30:113, 1974

Sitaram, Weingartner, and Gillin, "Human Serial Learning: Enhancement with Arecholine and Choline and Impairment with Scopolamine Correlate with Performance on Placebo," *Science* 201:274–276, 1978

Sitaram, Weingartner, Caine, Gillin, "Choline: Selective Enhancement of Serial Learning and Encoding of Low Imagery, Words in Man," *Life Sci.*, 22:1555–1560, 1978

Hirsh and Wurtman, "Lecithin Consumption Increases Acetylocholine Concentrations in Rat Brain and Adrenal Gland," *Science*, 202:223–225, 1978

Ferris et al, "Senile Dementia: Treatment with Deanol," *J. Am. Geriat. Soc.*, pp. 241–244, June 1977

Nandy and Bourne, "Effect of Centrophenoxine (dimethylaminoethanol p-chlorophenoxyacetate) on the lipofuscin pigments in the neurons of senile guinea pigs," *Nature*, 210:313–314, 1966

Legros et al, "Influence of Vasopressin on Memory and Learning," *Lancet*, 7 Jan. 1978, pg. 41

Oliveros et al, "Vasopressin in Amnesia," *Lancet*, 7 Jan. 1978, pg. 42

Shakocius and Pearson, "Mind Food," *OMNI,* pp. 54–57, May 1979 (popular media)

Pastan, "Cyclic AMP," *Sci. Amer.* offpr. 1256, Aug. 1972

Axelrod, "Neurotransmitters," *Sci. Amer.* offpr. 1297, June 1974

Nathanson and Greengard, "Second Messengers in the Brain," *Sci. Amer.,* pp. 108–119, Aug. 1977

Emmenegger and Meier-Ruge, "The Actions of Hydergine on the Brain," *Pharmacology,* 1:65–78, 1968

Marshall and Berrios, "Movement Disorders of Aged Rats: Reversal by Dopamine Receptor Stimulation," *Science,* 206:477–479, 1979

Harman et al, "Free Radical Theory of Aging: Effect of Dietary Fat on Central nervous system Function," *J. Am. Geriat. Soc.* 24(7):301–307, 1976

Pfeiffer et al, "Stimulant Effect of 2-Dimethylaminoethanol—possible precursor of brain acetylcholine," *Science,* 126: 610–611, 1957

Dr. Oliver W. Sacks, *Awakenings,* Doubleday, 1973

Goodman and Gilman, *The Pharmacological Basis of Therapeutics,* 4th ed., Macmillan, 1970

HOW SANDY MET DR. ALBERT HOFMANN, INVENTOR OF HYDERGINE® AND OTHER WONDER DRUGS

In the late 1970's, Sandy and Durk attended the 3rd International Scientific Conference on Native American Shamanism and Sacred Mushrooms. At this interesting event, we had the opportunity to meet and talk with Dr. Albert Hofmann, a legendary pharmaceuticals' chemist. Sandy decided to ask Dr. Hofmann about his Hydergine® consumption. (She and Durk were taking about 8 milligrams a day of Hydergine® at that time.)

SANDY: Dr. Hofmann, I am curious. How much Hydergine® per day do you use?

HOFMANN: Why, I don't use any at all. I don't need to. I'm not senile yet.

Sandy was very surprised. She doesn't remember the exact words of the rest of the conversation. She told Dr. Hofmann that we were using Hydergine® because we thought the evidence indicated that the use of Hydergine® in adequate doses could retard aging in the brain of young people, as well as help improve function in those who have already suffered damage from age, neurological diseases, or accidents. It can act as a prophylactic as well as a treatment of old age mental degeneration. Dr. Hofmann was under the misconception that Hydergine® was only for the already old and senile. He was not familiar at that time with the scientific literature about Hydergine® because he had retired from his position as head of research at Sandoz Pharmaceuticals in Switzerland. In addition, the antioxidant properties of Hydergine® had not yet been reported. (This data in our book is the first report, to our knowledge.) We have since sent him some of the interesting papers about Hydergine®. We hope Dr. Hofmann can now appreciate the value of his wonder child, Hydergine®.

Part III Chapter 3: Depression, Helplessness, and Aging

Anisman, et al, "Effect of Inescapable Shock on Subsequent Escape Performance: Catecholaminergic and Cholinergic Mediation of Response Initiation and Maintenance," *Psychopharmacology* 61:107–124 (1979)

Whelan, *Preventing Cancer: What You Can Do to Cut Your Risks by Up to 50 Percent,* pp. 202–207, Norton & Co. Publ., 1977 (popular media)

Seligman, *Helplessness,* Freeman, 1975

MacFarlane, "Procaine HC1 (Gerovital H3): A weak reversible fully competitive inhibitor of monoamine oxidase," *Fed. Proc.* 34(1):108–110, 1975

Borison et al, "Metabolism of an Antidepressant Amino Acid," presented in poster session at April 9–14, 1978 FASEB, Atlantic City, NJ (about use of L-phenylalanine in depression)

Gelenberg et al, "Tyrosine for the Treatment of Depression," *Am. J. Psychiatry* 137(5):622–623, 1980

Sachar et al, "Growth hormone responses to L-Dopa in depressed Patients," *Science* 178:1304–1305, 1972

Kiev, ed., *Somatic Manifestations of Depressive Disorders,* Excerpta Medica, 1974

Riley, Vernon, "Psychoneuroendocrine Influences on Immunocompetence and Neoplasia," *Science* 212:1100–1109, 5 June 1981 [Emotional, psychosocial, or anxiety-caused stresses increase plasma concentration of adrenal corticoids and other hormones. A direct result of this is impairment of some parts of the immune system.]

Part III Chapter 4: Sleep and Aging

Seiden and Dykstra, *Psychopharmacology, A Biochemical and Behavioral Approach,* Van Nostrand Reinhold, 1977

Prinz, et al, "Growth Hormone Levels During Sleep in Elderly Males," Presented at the 29th annual Gerontological Society Conference, Oct. 13, 1976

Brain Information Service, University of California, Los Angeles, CA 90024 (current alerting services and bibliographies on sleep, learning, memory, etc.)

Boyd, et al, "Stimulation of Human-Growth-Hormone Secretion by L-Dopa," *New Engl. J. Med.* 283(26):1425–1429, 1970

Wurtman and Wurtman, eds., *Nutrition and the Brain, vol. 3,* Raven Press, 1979 [see Growdon, pp. 117–181, "Neurotransmitter Precursors in the Diet: Their Use in the Treatment of Brain Diseases"]

Dement, *Some Must Watch While Some Must Sleep,* Freeman, 1972

Part III Chapter 5: Life Extenders Do It Longer

"Come up and see me sometime."
—Mae West

One's perception of oneself as an erotic being plays a very important role in one's neuroendocrine function and sexuality, and the way in which one integrates that sexuality with his or her larger world view and sense of life. For the theoretical basis for this research on the interaction of the neuroendocrine system, developmental and aging clocks, sexual and reproductive behavior, and sexual self image, see our comments on our major research area number 11 in Part V Chapter 12.

Mae West is a sexual self image hero and role model for both of us. Others whom we both admire include Grace Slick, Rudolf Nureyev, Diana Rigg, David Bowie, Mikhail Baryshnikov, Jim Morrison (Doors), Ted Nugent, Billie Jean King, Paul Stanley (KISS), Nijinsky, Rudolf Valentino, Anthony Dowell, and many other rock stars and ballet dancers.

Further insight into our sexual self images can be found in our love for art. We both derive a great deal of sensual and even erotic pleasure from our collection of fine art originals and reproductions. Sculpture is particularly potent due to its tactile three dimensional nature. Familiar sculpture that really turns us on includes Verrocchio's David (Leonardo da Vinci may have been the model); Donatello's David; Michelangelo's David, Bacchus, and Dying Captive; Bologna's Mercury and Apollo; our entire collection of Tibetan and Nepalese erotic bronzes and erotic Indian temple carvings; and a host of classical Greek statues and their Roman copies. Durk even has some favorite classical mythical beasts which include centaurs, satyrs, nymphs, and fauns.

Bahr, R., *The Virility Factor*, Putnam, 1976 (popular media)

Branen, "Lipid and enzyme changes to organs of monkeys fed BHA and BHT," *Food Product Development*, April 1973

Brecher, E. M., *The Sex Researchers*, Little, Brown, 1969 (popular media)

Boardman, J., and LaRocca, E., *Eros in Greece*, The Erotic Art Book Society, 1975 (popular media)

Bylinsky, *Mood Control*, Scribners, 1978 (popular media)

Hormones and Sexual Behavior, ed. by Carter, C. S.; Dowden, Hutchinson, & Ross Inc., 1974

Clark, Kenneth, *The Nude—A Study in Ideal Form*, Princeton University Press, 1953

Coffin, T. P., *The Female Hero in Folklore and Legend*, The Seabury Press, 1975 (popular media)

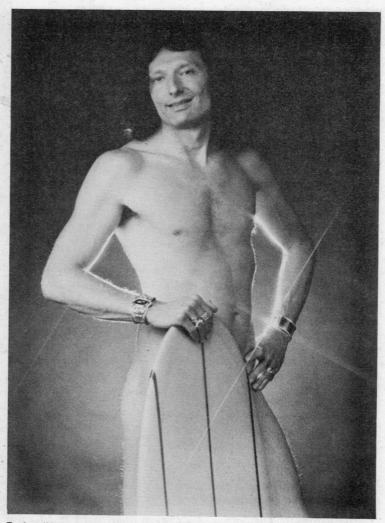

Erotic self-image plays a major role in neuroendocrine function. (Youthful erotic stimulation has been shown to alter the neuroendocrine systems of old male and female rats

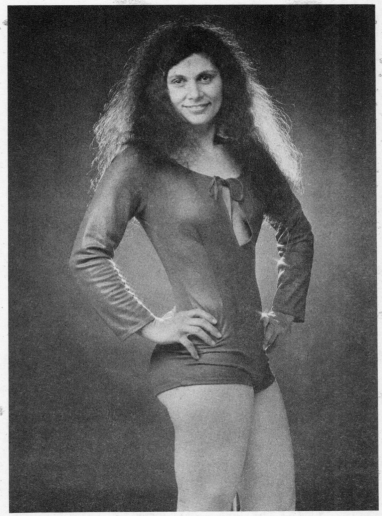

and rhesus monkeys toward more youthful function.) Not only is staying young good for your sex life, a good sex life can help you stay young.

Debono et al, "Bromocriptine and Dopamine Receptor Stimulation," *Brit. J. Clin. Pharmacol.* 3:977–982, 1976

DeMartino, M. F., *Sex and the Intelligent Woman,* Springer Publishing Co, 1974

Djerassi, *The Politics of Contraception,* Stanford Alumni Association, 1979

Adrenal Androgens, eds. Genazzani, Thijssen, and Siiteri; Raven Press, 1980

The Pharmacological Basis of Therapeutics, 4th ed., eds. Goodman, L. S., and Gilman, A., Macmillan, 1970, especially chapters 68, 69, and 70

Grant, M., and Mulas, A., *Eros in Pompey,* William Morrow & Co. 1975 (popular media)

Hormones in Development, eds. Hambrugh and Barrington, Appleton-Century-Crofts, 1971

Orthomolecular Psychiatry, Ch. 23, eds. Hawkins and Pauling, Freeman, 1973

Kinsey, Pomeroy, Martin, and Gebhard, *Sexual Behavior in the Human Female,* Saunders, 1953

Kinsey, Pomeroy, Martin, and Gebhard, *Sexual Behavior in the Human Male,* Saunders, 1948

Lal, Kanwar, *The Cult of Desire: An Interpretation of Erotic Sculpture of India,* University Books, 1967

Malitz, ed., *L-Dopa and Behavior,* Raven Press, 1972

Masters, W. H., and Johnson, V. E., *Human Sexual Response,* Little, Brown, & Co., 1966

Masters, W. H., and Johnson, V. E., *Human Sexual Inadequacy,* Little, Brown, and Co., 1970

Masters, W. H., *The Pleasure Bond,* Bantam, 1976 (popular media)

Melville, R., *Erotic Art of the West,* Putnam, 1973 (popular media)

Money, "Components of Eroticism in Man: I. The Hormones In Relation to Sexual Morphology and Sexual Desire," *J. Nerv. Ment. Dis.* 132:239–248, 1961

Kim, Moon, Sapienza, Pularkat, *J. Infect. Dis.* 138:91–94, 1978 [This paper is about BHT and cytomegalovirus. Cytomegalovirus may play a role in AIDS.]

Cupp, Wanda, Keith, Snipes, *Antimicrob. Agents Chemother.* 8:698–706, 1975

Wanda, Cupp, Snipes, Keith, Rucinsky, Polish, Sands, *Antimicrob. Agents Chemother.* 10:96–101, 1976

Money, *Love & Love Sickness, The Science of Sex, Gender Difference, and Pair-Bonding,* Johns Hopkins Univ. Press, 1980

Myers, R. D., *Handbook of Drug and Chemical Stimulation of the Brain,* Medical Economics, 1974

Peele, *Love and Addiction,* Taplinger, 1975

Phillips, *How to Fall Out of Love,* Houghton Mifflin Co., 1978 (popular media)

Physicians' Desk Reference, 35th ed., Medical Economics, 1981

Ralli and Dumm, "Relation of Pantothenic Acid to Adrenal Cortical Function," *Vit. Horm.* 11:133–158, 1953

The Hypothalamus, eds. Reichlin, Baldessarini, and Martin, Raven Press, 1978

Dr. George Rouser, City of Hope Hospital, Duarte, California, [possible mechanism for BHT's disruption of lipid coat surrrounding some viruses], personal communication

Salmon and Geist, "Effect of Androgens Upon Libido in Women," *J. Clin. Endocrinol.* 3:235–238, 1943

Seiden, L. S., and Dykstra, L. A., *Psychopharmacology, A Biochemical and Behavioral Approach,* Van Nostrand Reinhold, 1977

Snipes, et al, "Butylated Hydroxytoluene Inactivates Lipid-containing Viruses," *Science* 187:64–66, 1975

Snipes and Keith, "Hydrophobic Alcohols and di-tert-butyl phenols as Antiviral Agents" in Kabara, ed., *The Pharmacological Effects of Lipids,* the American Oil Chemists' Society, 1978

Brugh, M., Jr., "BHT Protects Chickens Exposed to Newcastle Disease Virus," *Science* 197:1291, 1977

Snyder, S. H., *Biological Aspects of Mental Disorder,* Oxford University Press, 1980

Sorensen, R. C., *Adolescent Sexuality in Contemporary America,* World Publishing, 1973

Tennov, *Love and Limerence, The Experience of Being in Love,* Stein and Day, 1979

Tietze, "New Estimates of Mortality Associated with Fertility Control," *Family Planning Perspectives* 9(2):74–76, March/April 1977 (Dr. Tietze has informed us that he is about to publish an updated version of the fertility risks chart shown in this chapter; however, he says the differences are small.)

VanDeusen, E. L., *Contract Cohabitation—An Alternative to Marriage,* Avon, 1975, 1975 (popular media)

As part of their studies on the psychobiochemical aspects of aging in the neuroendocrine system, Durk and Sandy are engaged in continuing experiments with sexual rejuvenation. Working both independently and in collaboration with each other, they have maintained their sex drives at the teenage to young adult range and explore diverse non-reproductive sexual options. In the course of investigating these areas, we remain our favorite guinea pigs.

Previous human clinical research investigations have generally focused on the anatomical aspects of sex (such as Masters and Johnson's *Human Sexual Response*) or the psychological-psychiatric-emotive aspects (such as Tennov's *Love and Limerence*, and Money's *Love and Love Sickness*). Our interdisciplinary human research will focus on the interaction of genetic behavioral-emotive programs (GROMs, or Genetic Read Only Memories), developmental programs, psychobiochemistry, and sociobiology with personal values, expectations, self image, and fantasy. Readers with similar interests are invited to write to either or both of us: Durk Pearson and/or Sandy Shaw, P.O. Box 758, Redondo Beach, Ca, 90277.

We are scientists, not physicians, so please do NOT waste our time and yours by asking us to diagnose or treat dysfunction or illness. The above address is not for general correspondence; general correspondence sent there will not be processed. (If you wish to write us about other matters, you may do so at P.O. Box 993, Hawthorne, Ca, 90250, but remember that we are able to personally respond to only a very small portion of the immense volume of mail that we receive from our TV audience—over 100,000 letters before the publication of this book.)

Part III Chapter 6: Looking as Young as You Feel

The Salts of PCA and their moisturizing Effects, Technical Bulletin, Ajinomoto Company (with 8 references cited)

Jetten, "Retinoids specifically enhance the number of epidermal growth factor receptors," *Nature* 284:626–631, 17 April 1980

Tanzer, "Cross-Linking of Collagen," *Science* 180:561–566, 1973

Elden, ed. *Biophysical Properties of the Skin,* Wiley Interscience, 1971

Verzar, "The Aging of Collagen," *Sci. Amer.*, April 1963

Laden and Spitzer, "Identification of a natural moisturizing agent in skin," *J. Soc. Cosmet. Chemists* 18:351, 1967

Part III Chapter 7: Male Pattern Baldness and What You Can Do about It

Polysorbate 60 or 80 are available from Atlas Division of ICI America, Inc., Wilmington, DE 19897, (302) 575-3000.

Settel, "Control of Excessive Hair Loss," *Drug & Cosmetic Industry,* Oct. 1977

"A new drug [Minoxidil] stimulates hair growth," *Chem. Eng. News,* pg. 13, May 28, 1973

"New Vasodilator Drugs for Hypertension," *British Med. J.,* pg. 185, 27 Oct. 1973

Dube et al, "In Vivo Effects of Steroid Hormones on the Testosterone 5 alpha-Reductase in Rat Skin," *Endo.* 97(1):211–214, 1975

Hamilton, "Effect of castration in adolescent and young adult males upon further changes in the proportions of bare and hairy scalp," *Jour. Clin. Endocrinol. Metab* 20(10):1309–1318, 1960

Schweikert and Wilson, "Regulation of Human Hair Growth by Steroid Hormones, I. Testosterone Metabolism in Isolated Hairs," *Jour. Clin. Endocrinol. Metab.* 38(5):811–819, 1974

"Is Cholesterol the Cause of Baldness?," *New Scientist,* pg. 639, 1 Mar. 1975

Setalla and Schreck-Purola, *Baldness and Its Cure,* Riverbrook, 1977

Van Deusen, *What You Can Do About Baldness,* Stein and Day, 1978 (popular media)

Robbins, *Chemical and Physical Behavior of Human Hair,* Van Nostrand Reinhold, 1979

Setala et al, "Mechanism of Experimental Tumorigenesis, III. Effect in Mouse Skin of 1,4-Sorbitan and 1,4,3,6-Dianhydrosorbitol Stearates," *Jour. Nat'l Cancer Institute* 23(5):969–974, 1959

Setala et al, "Mechanism of Experimental Tumorigenesis, II. Effect of Mole Ratio Distribution of Span 60 and Span 20 Derivatives on Hyperplasia in Mouse Epidermis," *Jour. Nat. Cancer Inst.* 23(5):953–964, 1959

Setala et al, "Mechanism of Experimental Tumorigenesis. VI. Ultrastructural Alterations in Mouse Epidermis Caused by Locally Applied Carcinogen and Dipole-Type Tumor Promoter," *Jour. Nat. Cancer Inst.* 25(5):1155–1166, 1960

Setala et al, "Mechanism of Experimental Tumorigenesis. V. Ultrastructural Alterations in Mouse Epidermis Caused by Span 60 and Tween 60-Type Agents," *Jour. Nat. Cancer Inst.* 24(2):355–365, 1960

Setala, "Progress in Carcinogenesis, Tumor-Enhancing Factors, A Bio-Assay of Skin Tumor Formation," *Progr. Exp. Tumor Res.* 1: 225–278, 1960

Edmunds and Adams, "Clocked Cell Cycle Clocks," *Science* 211:1002–1013, 1981

Aldridge and Pavlidis, "Clocklike behavior of biological clocks," *Nature* 259:343–344, 1976

Setala et al, *Die Naturewissenschaften* 8:184–185, 1960

Setala et al, *Die Naturewissenschaften* 9:331, 1959

Setala et al, *Die Naturewissenschaften* 9:328, 1959

Setala et al, *Die Naturewissenschaften* 8:187–188, 1960

Takashima and Montagna, "Studies of Common Baldness of the Stump-Tailed Macaque (Macaca speciosa), VI. The Effect of Testosterone on Common Baldness," *Arch. Derm.* 103:527–534, 1971

Happle and Echternacht, "Induction of Hair Growth in Alopecia areata with D.N.C.B.," *The Lancet,* pp. 1002–1003, 1977

Toda et al., eds. *Biology and Disease of the Hair,* University Park Press, 1976

Part III Chapter 8: Exercise

CAUTION: Schizophrenics should use growth hormone (GH) releasers with caution since they <u>may</u> increase the severity of symptoms. GH releasers include L-Dopa, arginine and ornithine (some schizophrenics may experience worsening symptoms, possibly due to the effects of methyl donation by polyamines made from these amino acids in the body), and bromocriptine (in doses over 30 milligrams a day, adverse effects on schizophrenic symptomology may occur in some people). If this occurs, discontinue use of the GH releasers.

"Muscle Loss Occurs in Women with Aging Just as it Does in Men," pg. 13 of Special Report on Aging 1980, U.S. Dept. of Health and Human Services, NIH, NIA [no GH stimulation by exercise in persons over 30 found in Baltimore Longitudinal Study of Aging].

Chapman and Mitchell, "The Physiology of Exercise," *Sci. Amer.* offprint 1011, May 1965

Morehouse, *Total Fitness in 30 Minutes a Week*, Simon and Schuster, 1975

Morehouse & Gross, *Maximum Performance*, Pocket Books, 1977

Prinz et al, "Growth Hormone Levels During Sleep in Elderly males," Presented at the 29th annual Gerontological Society Conference, Oct. 13, 1976

Boyd et al, "Stimulation of Human-Growth-Hormone Secretion by L-Dopa" *New Engl. J. Med.* 183(26):1425–1429, 1970

Johnson et al, "Hormonal responses to exercise in racing cyclists," *Proc. Physiological Soc.*, pp. 23P–24P, April 1974

Part III Chapter 9: Athletics

CAUTION: Schizophrenics should use growth hormone (GH) releasers with caution since they <u>may</u> increase the severity of symptoms. GH releasers include L-Dopa, arginine and ornithine (some schizophrenics may experience worsening symptoms, possibly due to the effects of methyl donation by polyamines made from these amino acids in the body), and bromocriptine (in doses over 30 milligrams a day, adverse effects on schizophrenic symptomology may occur in some people). If this occurs, discontinue use of the GH releasers.

According to Robert A. Swanson, President of Genentech, research studies indicate that bovine growth hormone can enhance meat and milk production without increasing the amount of feed consumed. And since bovine growth hormone is inactive in humans, hormone residues will not be a problem. (*Chemical Engineering*, pg. 11, 6 April 1981)

Morehouse, *Total Fitness in 30 Minutes a Week*, Simon and Schuster, 1975

Camanni et al, "Changes in Plasma Growth Hormone Levels in Normal and Acromegalic Subjects Following Administration of 2-Bromo-alpha-Ergocryptine," *J. Clin. Endocrin. Metab.* 40(3):363–366, 1975

Meites, "Role of Biogenic Amines in the Control of Prolactin and Growth Hormone Secretion," *Psychopharm. Bull.*, Oct. 1976, pp. 120–121

Catt, "Growth Hormone," *The Lancet*, pp. 933–939, 2 May 1970

Leake, "Dimethyl sulfoxide," *Science*, pp. 1646–1649, June 1966

Morehouse & Gross, *Maximum Performance*, Pocket Books, 1977

Barbul et al, "Arginine: A Thymotropic and Wound-Healing Promoting Agent," *Surgical Forum* 28:101–103, 1977

Boyd et al, "Stimulation of Human-Growth-Hormone Secretion by L-Dopa" *New Engl. J. Med.* 183(26):1425–1429, 1970

Ralli and Dumm, "Relation of Pantothenic Acid to Adrenal Cortical Function," *Vit. Horm.* 11:133–158, 1953

Merimee et al, "Arginine-initiated Release of Human Growth Hormone," *New Engl. J. Med.* 280(26):1434–1438, 1969

Marshall and Berrios, "Movement Disorders of Aged Rats: Reversal by Dopamine Receptor Stimulation," *Science* 206:477–479, 1979

Pike and Brown, *Nutrition, an Integrated Approach*, Wiley, 1975

"DMSO cut down to size," *Nature* 247:421, 1974

Pecile and Muller, eds., "Growth and Growth Hormone," *Excerpta Medica*, 1972

Part III Chapter 10: Smoking: Making It Safer With Nutrients

Romano and Goldstein, "Stereospecific Nicotine Receptors on Rat Brain Membranes," *Science* 210:647–650, 1980

Cameron and Pauling, *Vitamin C and Cancer*, Freeman, 1980 (popular media)

Richard Passwater, *Supernutrition*, Dial Press, 1975 (popular media)

Richard Passwater, *Supernutrition for Healthy Hearts*, Dial Press, 1977 (popular media)

Mental Alertness by Shakocius, Pearson, Donsbach, published by Donsbach University, 7422 Mountjoy, PO Box 5550, Huntington Beach, CA 92647 (sold in many health food stores for $1.00) (popular media)

Schrauzer, "Selenium and Cancer: a Review," *Bioinorg. Chem.* 5: 275–281, 1976

Sprince et al, "L-ascorbic acid in alcoholism and smoking: protection against acetaldehyde toxicity as an experimental model," *Int. J. Vit. Nutr. Res.* 47 (Suppl. 1G):185–212, 1977

Fernstrom and Wurtman, "Nutrition and the Brain," *Scientific American*, Feb. 1974

Shamberger et al, "Carcinogen-induced Chromosomal Breakage Decreased by Antioxidants," *Proc. Nat. Acad. Sci.* 70(5):1461–1463, May 1973

Shamberger, "Antioxidants in cereals and in food preservatives and declining gastric cancer mortality," *Cleveland Clinic Quarterly* 39(3):119–124, 1972

Charman et al, "Nicotinic acid in the treatment of hypercholesterolemia," *J. Angiology*, Jan. 1973

Sprince et al, "Protectants Against Acetaldehyde Toxicity: Sulfhydryl Compounds and Ascorbic Acid," *Fed. Proc.* 33(3), pt. 1, March 1974

Hindmarch et al, "The Effects of an Ergot Alkaloid Derivative (Hydergine) on Aspects of Psychomotor Performance, Arousal, and Cognitive Processing Ability," *J. Clin. Pharmacol.* 19 (11–12):726–732, 1979

"Workshop on Advances in Experimental Pharmacology of Hydergine," *Gerontology* 24 (Suppl. 1):1–154, 1978

Bjelke, "Dietary Vitamin A and Human Lung Cancer," *Int. J. Cancer* 15:561–565, 1975

Maugh, "Vitamin A: Potential Protection from Carcinogens," *Science* 186:1198, 1974

Khandwala and Gee, "Linoleic acid hydroperoxide: impaired bacterial uptake by alveolar macrophages, a mechanism of oxidant lung injury," *Science* 182:1364–1365, 1973

Sitaram et al, "Choline: Selective Enhancement of Serial Learning and Encoding of Low Imagery Words in Man," *Life Sci.* 22:1555–1560, 1978

Sporn, "Chemoprevention of Cancer," *Nature* 272:402–403, 1978

Shamberger, "Relationship of Selenium to Cancer: Inhibitory Effect of Selenium on Carcinogenesis," *J. Nat. Cancer Institute* 44(4):931–936, 1970

Sahley and Berntson, "Antinociceptive effects of central and systemic administrations of nicotine in the rat," *Psychopharmacology* (Berlin) 65(3):279–283, 1979

Shakocius and Pearson, "Mind Food," *OMNI* (popular magazine), May 1979 (available as a reprint for $1.00 from OMNI)

"Nonsmokers affected by tobacco smoke," *Science News,* 5 Apr. 1980, pg. 221

Plotkin, Mittermeier, Constable, "Psychotomimetic use of tobacco in Surinam and French Guiana," *J. Ethnopharm.* 2:295–297, 1980

Larry Frederick, "Nicorette gum," *Next* magazine (popular magazine), May/June 1980, pp. 106–107

Repace and Lowrey, "Indoor Air Pollution, Tobacco Smoke, and Public Health," *Science* 208:464–472, 2 May 1980

Battig, "Smoking and the Behavioral Effects of Nicotine," *Trends in Pharmacol Sci,* pp. 145–147, June 1981

Brown, Heitkamp, Song, "Niacin Reduces Paraquat Toxicity in Rats," *Science* 212:1510–1512, 26 June 1981

[Earlier work indicated that paraquat poisoning damaged by similar mechanisms to hyperbaric oxygen, in other words by free radical damage. Both niacin and thiamin (vitamin B-1) were able to help the growth of E. Coli poisoned by either paraquat or hyperbaric oxygen. The authors propose the protective effect of niacin is related to its ability to get around the poisoning effect on the enzyme that is required for the synthesis of nicotinamide adenine dinucleotide (NAD). A derivative, NADPH, is an extremely important reducing agent in cellular metabolism. Another possibility they didn't mention is that niacin itself acts as a spin trap for free radicals. Rats were poisoned with paraquat and either given niacin or not. The rats treated with paraquat and niacin had only a 55 percent death rate compared to a 74 percent death rate for those treated only with paraquat. Powerful antioxidant combinations such as vitamin C, B-1, and the amino acid cysteine could provide much greater protection.]

Shekelle et al, "Dietary Vitamin A and Risk of Cancer in the Western Electric Study," *The Lancet* pp. 1185–1190, 28 Nov. 1981

A 19 year prospective epidemiological study of about 3,000 middle aged men has provided evidence that carotenoids such as beta carotene have a remarkable ability to prevent lung cancer in both smokers and non-smokers. The non-smokers in the lowest quartile of carotenoid intake had about seven times the risk of lung cancer as the non-smokers in the highest quartile. (A quartile is a segment of the study population containing one quarter of the study population.) For smokers, the lowest carotenoid quartile had about eight times the lung cancer risk of the highest quartile. This protective effect is so strong that smokers of up to 30 years' duration in the highest carotenoid quartile had about the same risk of lung cancer as the non-smokers who were below average in carotenoid intake! (The highest quartile was probably averaging *very roughly* 10,000 IU of beta carotene per day.) This does *not* mean that it is safe to smoke cigarettes if you take enough beta carotene; the lethal cardiovascular effects of smoking were *not* affected. Note, too, that fiber and natural antioxidants contained in the vegetables and fruits (the principle carotenoid sources) may have a role in this lung cancer preventive effect. This effect is apparently *not* due to vitamin A.

B. Modan et al, "Retinol, Carotene, and Cancer," *Internatl. J. Cancer* 28:421–424, 1981

This is an epidemiological study on 406 patients with gastrointestinal cancer and 812 matched controls that showed a highly significant correlation between increased carotenoid intake and decreased gastrointestinal cancer. This decreased risk did not appear to be due to vitamin A, but may have also been related to the increased fiber and natural antioxidants that are found in most high carotenoid (high vegetable and fruit) diets.

Myers et al, "Selenium Yeast Studies" in *Selenium in Biology and Medicine,* Spallholz et al, editors, AVI, 1981

Schrauzer and McGinness, "Observations on Human Selenium Supplementation," in *Trace Substances in Environmental Health* 13:64–67, 1979

Most organic sources of selenium, such as selenomethionine, are less effective than selenite in elevating deficient levels of glutathione peroxidase. An exception is a selenized yeast (commercially available from Nutrition 21, Box 390, La Jolla, CA 92038) which exhibits good results in this test. The selenium in this yeast is mostly *not* the seleno amino acids and is not inorganic either. It may involve a seleno-trisulfide organic compound.

Klayman and Gunther, eds., *Organic Selenium Compounds: Their Chemistry and Biology,* Wiley-Interscience, 1973

WHERE TO PURCHASE AN AIR CLEANER

HEPA filter type: Alpaire, Inc., 4880 Havana St., Denver, Colo. 80239 (sizes available for both homes and businesses) electrostatic precipitator type:
    for homes: Sears, Montgomery Ward
    for businesses: Minneapolis Honeywell Co., Minneapolis, Minnesota

Part III Chapter 11: Pollution

Bjelke, "Dietary Vitamin A and Human Lung Cancer," *Int. J. Cancer,* 15:561–565 (1975)

Deitz, editor, *Removal of Trace Contaminants from the Air,* ACS Symposium Series 17, American Chemical Society, Washington, DC, 1975

Demopoulos and Mehlman, eds., [causes of cancer], *J. Environ. Pathology and Toxicology,* vol. 3, March 1980

"Ozone reactions produce singlet oxygen," *Chem. Eng. News,* 18 March 1974, pg. 16

Goldstein et al, "PABA as a protective agent in ozone toxicity," *Arch. Environ. Health* 24:243–247, 1972

Rieley, Cohen, and Lieberman, "Ethane Evolution: A New Index of Lipid Peroxidation," *Science* 183:208–210, 1974

Basu et al, "Plasma Vitamin A in Patients with Bronchial Carcinoma," *Br. J. Cancer* 33:119–121 (1976)

Repace and Lowrey, "Indoor Air Pollution, Tobacco Smoke, and Public Health," *Science* 208:464–472, 2 May 1980

Kitamura, "The treatment of asthmatic patients using an alpha-adrenergic receptor agent, co-dergocrine mesylate (Hydergine)," *Pharmatherapeutics* 2:330–336 (1980)

Sporn, et al, "Prevention of chemical carcinogenesis by Vitamin A and its synthetic analogs (retinoids)," *Fed. Proc.* 35(6)1332–1338, 1 May 1976

"High Anxiety over Flights Through Ozone," *Science* 205:767, 1979

Hindmarch, et al, "The Effects of an Ergot Alkaloid Derivative (Hydergine) on Aspects of Psychomotor Performance, Arousal, and Cognitive Processing Ability," *J. Clin. Pharmacol.* 19 (11–12):726–732, 1979

Khandwala and Gee, "Linoleic acid hydroperoxide: impaired bacterial uptake by alveolar macrophages, a mechanism of oxidant lung injury," *Science* 182:1364–65, 1973

Tappel, "Biological Antioxidant Protection Against Lipid Peroxidation Damage," *Amer. J. Clin. Nutr.* 23(8):1137–1139, 1970

Goldstein et al, "Ozone and Vitamin E," *Science,* 7 Aug. 1970, pg. 605

Chvapil et al, "Effect of Zinc on Lipid Peroxidation in Liver Microsomes and Mitochondria," *Proc. Soc. Exp. Biol. Med.* 141:150–153, 1972

Roehm et al, "The influence of vitamin E on the lung fatty acids of rats exposed to ozone," *Arch. Environ. Health* 24:April 1972

Pryor, "Free Radicals in Biological Systems," *Sci. Amer.,* August 1970

Black and Chan, "Suppression of Ultraviolet Light induced Tumor formation by dietary antioxidants," *J. Inv. Derm.* 65:412–414, 1975

Tappel, "Selenium-glutathione peroxidase and Vitamin E," *Amer. J. Clin. Nutr.* 27:960–965, Sept. 1974

Sprince et al, "Protective action of ascorbic acid and sulfur compounds against acetaldehyde toxicity: implications in alcoholism and smoking," *Agents and Actions* 5(2):164–173, 1975

Roehm et al, "Antioxidants vs. Lung Disease," *Arch. Intern. Med.* 128:88–93, 1971

Lentz and Di Luzio, "Peroxidation of Lipids in Alveolar Macrophages," *Arch. Environ. Health* 28:279–282, May 1974

Harman, "Role of Free Radicals in Mutation, Cancer, Aging, and the Maintenance of Life," *Rad. Res.* 16:753–764, 1962

Weitzman and Stossel, "Mutation Caused by Human Phagocytes," *Science* 212:546–547, 1 May 1981 [These scientists report finding that production of reactive oxygen metabolites could explain the capacity of phagocytes to induce mutation. This is probably the mechanism of asbestos carcinogenesis.]

Demopoulos and Gutman, "Cancer in New Jersey and Other Complex Urban/Industrial Areas," *J. Environ Pathol Toxicol* 3(4):219–235, 1980

WHERE TO PURCHASE AN AIR CLEANER

HEPA filter type: Alpaire, Inc., 4880 Havana St., Denver, Colo. 80239 (sizes available for both homes and businesses) electrostatic precipitator type:
    for homes: Sears & Roebuck, Montgomery Ward
    for businesses: Minneapolis Honeywell Co., Minneapolis, Minnesota

Part III Chapter 12: Alcohol: Making It Safer with Nutrients

Lieber, "The Metabolism of Alcohol," *Scientific American*, Mar. 1976 (available as offprint 1336 from W. H. Freeman, 660 Market St., San Francisco, CA 94104)

Drug Interactions, Medical Economics Co., 1976

Weissman and Myers, "Clinical Depression in Alcoholism," *Am. J. Psychiatry* 137:372–373, 1980

Austin, *Research Issues 24: Perspectives on the History of Psychoactive Substance Use,* National Institute on Drug Abuse, 1978

"Data link alcoholism and opiate addiction," *Chem. Eng. News,* pg. 44, Feb. 16, 1970

Nestoros, "Ethanol Specifically Potentiates GABA-Mediated Neurotransmission in Feline Cerebral Cortex," *Science* 209:708–710, 1980

Streissguth et al, "Teratogenic Effects of Alcohol in Humans and Laboratory Animals," *Science* 209:353–361, 1980

[Catapres®'s effects on Korsakoff's Psychosis], *Annals of Neurology* 7(5):466–469, May 1980

Cadoret et al, [adoptee study indicates alcoholism genetic], *Archives of Gen. Psych.* 37(5):561, 1980

Diaz and Samson, "Impaired brain growth in neonatal rats exposed to ethanol," *Science* 208:751–753, 1980

Samorajski et al, "Dihydroergotoxine (Hydergine®) and alcohol-induced variations in young and old mice," *J. Geront.* 32(2):145–152, 1977

Tanzer, "Crosslinking of Collagen," *Science* 180:561–566, 1973

Sprince et al, "Protectants Against Acetaldehyde Toxicity: Sulfhydryl Compounds and Ascorbic Acid," *Fed. Proc.* 33(3), pt. 1, March 1974

Borison et al, "Metabolism of an Antidepressant Amino Acid," presented in poster session at April 9–14 1978 FASEB meeting in Atlantic City, New Jersey [L-phenylalanine as an antidepressant]

Legros et al, "Influence of Vasopressin on Memory and Learning," *Lancet,* pg. 41, 7 Jan. 1978

Oliveros et al, "Vasopressin in Amnesia," *Lancet,* pg. 42, 7 Jan. 1978

Wurtman and Wurtman, eds., *Nutrition and the Brain, vol. 4, Toxic Effects of Food Constituents on the Brain,* Raven Press, 1979

Swidler, *Handbook of Drug Interactions,* pg. 8, Wiley-Interscience, 1971

Mental Alertness by Sandy Shakocius (now Shaw), Durk Pearson, Kurt W. Donsbach, published by Donsbach University, PO Box 5550, Huntington Beach, CA 92647 and sold in many health food stores—contains some of the material in Part III Chapter 2.

Good News for Smokers by Durk Pearson and Sandy Shaw, published by Donsbach University (address above), sold in many health food stores (contains almost the same material as Part III, Chapter 10).

Schuckit and Rayses, "Ethanol Ingestion: Differences in Blood Acetaldehyde Concentrations in Relatives of Alcoholics and Controls," *Science* 203(5):54–55, 1979

Song and Rubin, "Ethanol Produces Muscle Damage in Human Volunteers," *Science* 175:327–328, 1972

Deitrich and McLearn, "Neurobiological and genetic aspects of the etiology of alcoholism," *Fed. Proc.* 40(2):2051–2055, Feb. 1981

Peters, "The case for vitamin-fortified booze?" *Food Prod Development,*" Sept. 1980

Myers et al, "Selenium Yeast Studies" in *Selenium in Biology and Medicine,* Spallholz et al, editors, AVI, 1981

Schrauzer and McGinness, "Observations on Human Selenium Supplementation," in *Trace Substances in Environmental Health* 13:64–67, 1979

Most organic sources of selenium, such as selenomethionine, are less effective than selenite in elevating deficient levels of glutathione peroxidase. An exception is a selenized yeast (commercially available from Nutrition 21, Box 390, La Jolla, CA 92038) which exhibits good results in this test. The selenium in this yeast is mostly *not* the seleno-amino acids and is not inorganic either. It may involve a seleno-trisulfide organic compound.

Klayman and Gunther, eds., *Organic Selenium Compounds: Their Chemistry and Biology*, Wiley-Interscience, 1973

Part III Chapter 13: Controlling Your Weight

Meites, "Role of Biogenic Amines in the Control of Prolactin and Growth Hormone (GH) Secretion," *Psychopharmacology Bull.*, pp. 20–21, Oct. 1976

Marshall & Lauda, "Purification and Properties of Phaseolamin, an inhibitor of alpha-amylase, from the kidney bean, Phaseolus vulgaris," *J. Biol. Chem.* 250(20):8030–8037, 1975

[Clonidine HCl reduces heroin withdrawal symptoms], *J. Amer. Med. Assoc.* 243(4):343, 25 Jan. 1980

Beller, *Fat and Thin: A Natural History of Obesity*, Farrar, Straus, Giroux, New York, 1977

Sloan and Weir, "Nomograms for prediction of body density and total body fat from skinfold measurements," *J. Appl. Physiol.* 28(2):221, 1970

Morehouse and Gross, *Total Fitness in 30 Minutes a Week*, Simon and Schuster, 1975

"Nobelist ties gut hormone to appetite control by brain," *Medical World News*, 5 Feb. 1979, pg. 18

Barbul et al, "Arginine: A Thymotropic and Wound-Healing Promoting Agent," *Surgical Forum* 28:101–103, 1977

Borison et al, "Metabolism of an antidepressant amino acid," presented in poster session at April 9–14, 1978 FASEB, Atlantic City NJ (about use of L-phenylalanine in depression)

Merimee et al, "Arginine-initiated Release of Human Growth Hormone," *New Engl. J. Med.* 280(26):1434–1438, 1969

Smith, Gibbs, Young, "Cholecystokinin and Intestinal Satiety in the Rat," *Fed. Proc.* 33(5):1146–1149, May 1974

Behavioral Treatments of Obesity, edited by John Paul Foreyt, Pergamon Press, 1977

Morley and Levine, "Stress-induced Eating is Mediated Through Endogenous Opiates," *Science* 209:1259–1260, 1980

Hansen, "Serum Growth Hormone Response to Exercise in Non-Obese and Obese Normal Subjects," *Scand. J. Clin. Lab. Invest.* 31(2):175–178, 1973

Rader, *Dr. Rader's No-Diet Program for Permanent Weight Loss*, Tarcher, 1981 (popular media)

"Opiate antagonist counters obesity," pg. 103, *Science News,* 14 February 1981

We have already seen a weight control clinic (Weight Reduction Medical Clinics in Southern California) advertising (in two of the December 1981 issues of the Los Angeles area *TV Guide*) that it administers an alpha amylase inhibitor (AMYLEX™) to block starch digestion as an aid to weight reduction. Great Earth vitamin stores offer a similar product, Calorase.

Shansky, "Vitamin B-3 in the Alleviation of Hypoglycemia," *Drug and Cosmetic Industry,* Oct. 1981

Part III Chapter 14:
Arming Your Immune System against Arthritis

Walford, "Immunologic theory of aging: Current Status," *Fed. Proc.* 33(9):2020–2027, 1974

Brown, D. H. et al, "Anti-inflammatory Effects of Some Copper Complexes," *J. Med. Chem.* 23:729, 1980

Spallholz et al, "Immunologic Responses of Mice Fed Diets Supplemented with Selenite Selenium," *Proc. Soc. Exp. Med. Biol.* 143:685–689, 1973

Hochschild, "Lysosomes, membranes, and aging," *Exp. Geront.* 6:153–166, 1971

Hochschild, "Effect of membrane stabilizing drugs on mortality in Drosophila Melanogaster," *Exp. Geront.* 6:133–151, 1971

Tappel, "Vitamin E as the biological lipid antioxidant," *Vit. Horm.* 20:493–510, 1962

Cort, "Antioxidant activity of tocopherols, ascorbyl palmitate, and ascorbic acid and their mode of action," *J. Amer. Oil Chem. Soc.* 51(7):321–325, 1974

Oxygen Free Radicals and Tissue Damage, CIBA Foundation Symposium 65, Excerpta Medica, 1979, pg. 55 [artificial superoxide dismutases, such as copper salicylate complexes, etc.]

Leake, "Dimethyl sulfoxide," *Science*, pp. 1646–1649, June 1966

McCord, "Superoxide radical may play a role in arthritis," paper presented at the Third Biennial Conference on Chemical Education, Pennsylvania State Univ., Aug. 1, 1974

Part III Chapter 15:
A Brief Note on Allergies and Asthma

Chapter 19, in Stone, *The Healing Factor: Vitamin C Against Disease*, Grosset & Dunlap, 1972 (popular media)

"Leukotrienes act on human bronchi," *Chem. Eng. News*, 15 Dec. 1980

Kitamura, "The treatment of asthmatic patients using an alpha-adrenergic receptor agent, co-dergocrine mesylate (Hydergine)," *Pharmatherapeutics* 2:330–336, 1980

Borgeat, "Leukotrienes: A major step in understanding of immediate hypersensitivity reactions," *J. Med. Chem.* 24(2): 121–126, Feb. 1981

Hanna, Bach, Pare, Schellenberg, "Slow-reacting substances (leukotrienes) contract human airway and pulmonary vascular smooth muscle in vitro," *Nature* 290:343–344, 1981

Part III Chapter 16: Atherosclerosis

McCully, "Homocysteinemia and Arteriosclerosis," *Amer. Heart J.* 83(4):571–573, April 1972

"Pyridoxine-Responsive Homocystinuria," *Nutr. Rev.* 39 (1):16–18, 1981

Nightingale et al, "Effect of Vitamin C and high Cholesterol Diet on Aortic Atherosclerosis in Dutch Belted Rabbits," paper delivered at FASEB, 62nd Annual Meeting, Atlantic City, NJ, April 9–14, 1978

Bjorksten, "Possibilities and Limitations of Chelation as a Means for Life Extension," *Rejuvenation* 8(3):67–72, 1980

Benditt, "Implications of the Monoclonal Character of Human Artherosclerotic Plaques," *Am. J. of Pathol* 86(3):693–702, March 1977

Robbins, "Effect of Flavonoids on Survival Time of Rats Fed Thrombogenic or Atherogenic Regimens," *J. Athero. Res.,* 7:3–10, 1967

Laughlin, Fisher, and Sherrard, "Blood Pressure Reductions During Self-Recording of Home Blood Pressure," *Amer. Heart J.* 98(5):629–634, Nov. 1979

Mudd, et al, "Homocystinuria: An Enzymatic Defect," *Science* 143:1443–1445, 1964

Edward Gruberg & Stephen Raymond, "Beyond Cholesterol," *Atlantic Monthly,* May 1978 (popular magazine)

Schneiderman and Goldstick, "Carbon Monoxide-induced arterial wall hypoxia and atherosclerosis," *Atherosclerosis* 30:1–15, 1978

Hume et al, "Leucocyte ascorbic acid levels after acute myocardial infarction," *Brit. Heart J.* 34:238–243, 1972

Passwater, *Supernutrition for Healthy Hearts,* Dial Press, 1977 (popular media)

Shute, *Vitamin E for Ailing and Healthy Hearts,* Pyramid, 1972 (popular media)

Bailey, *Vitamin E: Your Key to a Healthy Heart,* Arco, 1971 (popular media)

Sokoloff et al, "Aging, atherosclerosis and ascorbic acid metabolism," *J. Am. Geriat. Soc.* 14(12):1239–1260, 1966

Spittle, "The Action of Vitamin C on Blood Vessels," *Amer. Heart Jour.* 88(3):387–388, Sept. 1974

Verzar, "The Aging of Collagen," *Sci. Amer.*, April 1963

Bjorksten, "The Crosslinkage Theory of Aging," *J. Am. Geriatr. Soc.* 16:408–427, 1968

Ross and Glomset, "Atherosclerosis and the Arterial Smooth Muscle Cell," *Science* 180:1332–1339, 1973

The Notebooks of Leonardo da Vinci, Vol. II, edited by Jean Paul Richter, Dover Publications, 1970

Steve Faber, "It's Not a Big Miracle," *Interface Age*, pp. 70–73, Dec. 1978 (This program is written to run on the Radio Shack TRS-80. A copy of this article and program can be obtained from the author (we don't know his price, but don't assume its free); send a stamped, self-addressed envelope for information: Steve Faber, PO Box 69200, Los Angeles, CA 90069

A version of this program for the Commodore PET computer is also available (again, we don't know the price); send a stamped, self-addressed envelope to: Frank Henn, 4811 Verona Dr. N.W., Calgary, Alberta T3A OP5

We have not personally tested these programs because, although we have many computers, we have neither the TRS-80 nor the Commodore PET.

The basic idea for this program is very simple: administer only the amount of insulin that is really necessary, no more and no less. Although this sounds simple, a diabetic's insulin requirement varies with diet, exercise, state of health, stress, time of day, etc. This program uses the above data in conjunction with urine sugar measurements. You make these measurements yourself by dipping Clinitest urine sugar test strips into your urine and comparing the resulting color with a color chart on the bottle. Be sure to discuss this with your physician. Diabetes mellitus is a serious disease which requires professional management.)

Part III Chapter 17: Stroke

McCully, "Homocysteinemia and Arteriosclerosis," *Amer. Heart J.* 83(4):571–573, April 1972

Fabricant et al, "Virus induced Atherosclerosis," *J. Exp. Med.*, 335–340, 1978

Robbins, "Effect of Flavonoids on Survival Time of Rats Fed Thrombogenic or Atherogenic Regimens," *J. Athero. Res.*, 7:3–10, 1967

Ambrose and DeEds, "Effect of Rutin on Permeability of Cutaneous Capillaries," presented before the Soc. Exp. Biol. and Med, Feb 12, 1947

Laughlin, Fisher, and Sherrard, "Blood Pressure Reductions During Self Recording of Home Blood Pressure," *Amer. Heart J.* 98(5):629–634, Nov. 1979

Edward Gruberg & Stephen Raymond, "Beyond Cholesterol," *Atlantic Monthly*, May 1978 (popular magazine)

Vane and Bergstrom, eds., *Prostacyclin*, Raven Press, 1979

Steiner & Anastasi, "Vitamin E: An inhibitor of the Platelet Release Reaction," *J. Clin. Invest.* 57:732–737, 1976

Hindmarch, et al, "The Effects of an Ergot Alkaloid Derivative (Hydergine) on Aspects of Psychomotor Performance, Arousal, and Cognitive Processing Ability," *J. Clin. Pharmacol.* 19(11–12):726–732, 1979

Sokoloff et al, "Aging, atherosclerosis and ascorbic acid metabolism" *J. Am. Geriat. Soc.* 14(12):1239–1260, 1966

Sprince, Parker, Smith, "L-ascorbic acid in alcoholism and smoking: protection against acetaldehyde toxicity as an experimental model," *Int. J. Vit. Nutr. Res.* 47 (Suppl. 1G):185–212, Nov. 1977

Spittle, "The Action of vitamin C on Blood Vessels," *Amer. Heart Jour.* 88(3):387–388, Sept. 1974

Emmenegger and Meier-Ruge, "The Actions of Hydergine on the Brain," *Pharmacology* 1:65–78, 1968

Zierler et al, "On the antithrombic and antiproteolytic activity of alpha tocopheryl phosphate," *Am. J. Physiol.* 153:127–132, 1948

"Workshop on Advances in Experimental Pharmacology of Hydergine," *Gerontology* 24 (Suppl. 1):1–154, 1978

Legros et al, "Influence of Vasopressin on Memory and Learning," *Lancet*, 7 Jan. 1978, pg. 41

Oliveros et al, "Vasopressin in Amnesia," *Lancet*, 7 Jan. 1978

Bjorksten, "The Crosslinkage Theory of Aging," *J. Am. Geriatr. Soc.* 16:408–427, 1968

Sprince et al, "Protective action of ascorbic acid and sulfur compounds against acetaldehyde toxicity: implications in alcoholism and smoking," *Agents and Actions* 5(2):164–173, 1975

Ross and Glomset, "Atherosclerosis and the Arterial Smooth Muscle Cell," *Science* 180:1332–1339, 1973

Part III Chapter 18: Cardiovascular Disease, Its Prevention or Amelioration: Heart Attacks

According to the February 1981 *Drug & Cosmetic Industry*, a trade publication: "Despite the Food & Drug Administration's refusal last spring to approve a new indication for Ciba-Geigy's gout drug Anturane—that of preventing sudden death in the months following a heart attack—sales of Anturane are up by a factor of five. . . . About 90 percent of current Anturane prescriptions are for heart patients or for use in surgery rather than for its approved use in the treatment of gout, according to market surveys. Meanwhile, Ciba-Geigy is sponsoring clinical tests in Italy, South Africa, and the U.K. [England] in an effort to convince the FDA to reverse its position."

"FDA Says NO to Anturane," *Science* 208:1130–1132, 1980

Turlapaty and Altura, "Magnesium Deficiency Produces Spasms of Coronary Arteries: Relationship to Etiology of Sudden Death Ischemic Heart Disease," *Science* 208:198–200, 1980

Benditt, "Implications of the Monoclonal Character of Human Atherosclerotic Plaques," *Am. J. of Pathol* 86(3):693–702, March 1977

Vane and Bergstrom, eds., *Prostacyclin*, Raven Press, 1979

Ambrose and DeEds, "Effect of Rutin on Permeability of Cutaneous Capillaries," presented before the Soc. Exp. Biol. and Med, Feb 12, 1947

Robbins, "Effect of Flavonoids on Survival Times of Rats Fed Thrombogenic or Atherogenic Regimens," *J. Athero. Res.*, 7:3–10, 1967

McCully, "Homocysteinemia and Arteriosclerosis," *Amer. Heart J.* 83(4):571–573, April 1972

Maeda et al, "Suppression by Thyrotropin-Releasing Hormone (TRH) of Growth Hormone Release Induced by Arginine and Insulin-Induced Hypoglycemia in Man," *J. Clin. Endocrinol. Metab.* 43(2):453–456, 1976

Laughlin, Fisher, and Sherrard, "Blood Pressure Reductions During Self-Recording of Home Blood Pressure," *Amer. Heart J.* 98(5):629–634, Nov. 1979

Mudd, et al, "Homocystinuria: An Enzymatic Defect," *Science* 143:1443–1445, 1964

Edward Gruberg & Stephen Raymond, "Beyond Cholesterol," *Atlantic Monthly,* May 1978 (popular magazine)

Hume, et al, "Leucocyte ascorbic acid levels after acute myocardial infarction," *Brit. Heart J.* 34:238–243, 1972

Steiner & Anastasi, "Vitamin E: An inhibitor of the Platelet Release Reaction," *J. Clin. Invest.* 57:732–737, 1976

Passwater, *Supernutrition for Healthy Hearts,* Dial Press, 1977 (popular media)

Shute, *Vitamin E for Ailing and Healthy Hearts,* Pyramid, 1972 (popular media)

Bailey, *Vitamin E: Your Key to a Healthy Heart,* Arco, 1971 (popular media)

Barnes and Galton, *Hypothyroidism,* Crowell, 1976

Sokoloff et al, "Aging, atherosclerosis and ascorbic acid metabolism," *J. Am. Geriat. Soc.* 14(12):1239–1260, 1966

Tappel, "Biological Antioxidant Protection Against Lipid Peroxidation Damage," *Amer. J. Clin. Nutr.* 23(8):1137–1139, 1970

Tappel, "Vitamin E as the biological lipid antioxidant," *Vit. Horm.* 20:493–510, 1962

Spittle, "The Action of Vitamin C on Blood Vessels," *Amer. Heart Jour.* 88(3):387–388, Sept. 1974

Gordon, et al, "High Density Lipoprotein as a Protective Factor against Coronary Heart Disease; the Framingham Study," *Amer. J. Med.* 62:707–708 May 1977

"Sulfinpyrazone lowers death rate in heart attacks" *New England J. Med.* 298:289–295, 1978

Zierler et al, "On the antithrombic and antiproteolytic activity of alpha tocopheryl phosphate," *Am. J. Physiol.* 153:127–132, 1948

Sprince et al, "Protectants Against Acetaldehyde Toxicity: Sulfhydryl Compounds and Ascorbic Acid," *Fed. Proc.* 33(3), pt. 1, March 1974

Thompson & Bortz, "Significance of High-Density Lipoprotein Cholesterol," *J. Am. Ger. Soc.* 26(10):440–442, 1978

Ginter, "Cholesterol: Vitamin C Controls Its Transformation to Bile Acids," *Science* 179:702–704, 1973

Mehta and Hamby, "Diagonal Ear-Lobe Crease as a Coronary Risk Factor," *New Engl. J. Med.* pg. 260, 1 Aug. 1974

Lichstein et al, "Diagonal Ear-Lobe Crease: Prevalence and Implications as a Coronary Risk Factor," *New Engl. J. Med.* 290(11):615–16, 1974

Frank, "Aural Sign of Coronary-Artery Disease," *New Engl. J. Med.* 289(6):327–328, 1973

Kristensen, "Ear-lobe crease and vascular complications in essential hypertension," *The Lancet*, pg. 265, Feb. 2, 1980

Petrakis and Koo, "Earlobe crease," *The Lancet*, pg. 376, Feb. 16, 1980

Sharrett and Feinleib, "Water constituents and Trace Elements in Relation to Cardiovascular Diseases," *Prev. Med.* 4:20–36, 1975

Barnes, *Solved: The Riddle of Heart Attacks,* Robinson Press, 1976

Slater and Alfin-Slater, "Effect of Dietary Cholesterol on Plasma Cholesterol, HDL cholesterol and Triglycerides in Human Subjects," *Fed. Proc. Abstr.* 2194, 1 Mar 1978

[aspirin and heart attacks], *New Engl. J. Med.*, 13 July 1978

Brown, Kovanen, and Goldstein, "Regulation of Plasma Cholesterol by Lipoprotein Receptors," *Science* 212:628–635, 8 May 1981

Coker et al, "Thromboxane and prostacyclin release from ischaemic myocardium in relation to arrhythmias," *Nature* 291:323–24, 28 May 1981 [Both thromboxane and prostacyclin are released from acutely ischaemic myocardium in dogs with coronary artery ligation. The ratio between these two prostaglandins determines susceptibility to post-infarct arrhythmias.]

Part III Chapter 19: Cancer

Maugh, "Vitamin A: Potential Protection from Carcinogens," *Science* 186:1198, 1974

Bjelke, "Dietary Vitamin A and Human Lung Cancer" *Int. J. Cancer* 15:561–565 (1975)

"The DMBA-induced tumors can also be made to regress in rats treated with 2-bromoergocryptine, a drug which inhibits pituitary prolactin release. Perhaps most significantly of all, T-mediated tumour regression can be reversed by increasing endogenous release of prolactin on treating the tumour-bearing rats with phenothiazines." reported in March 1981 *Trends in Pharmacological Sciences,* pg. x

Novi, "Regression of Aflatoxin B_1-Induced Hepatocellular Carcinomas by Reduced Glutathione," Science 212: 541–542, 1 May 1981 [abstract of paper: "Reduced glutathione administered to rats bearing aflatoxin B_1-induced liver tumors caused regression of tumor growth and resulted in survival of the animals. Since glutathione is a harmless natural product, it merits further investigation as a potential antitumor drug for humans." The author notes that, to her knowledge, the growth of fully transformed malignant cells being reversed by administration of a chemical compound has not been reported previously.]

Basu et al, "Plasma Vitamin A in Patients with Bronchial Carcinoma," *Br. J. Cancer* 33:119–121 (1976)

Anderson, et al, "The Effects of Increasing Weekly doses of ascorbate on certain cellular and humoral immune functions in normal volunteers," *Am. J. Clin. Nutr.* 33:71–76, Jan 1980

Demopoulos and Mehlman, eds., [importance of various causes of human cancer], *J. Environmental Path & Tox.*, vol. 3, March 1980

[increasing consumption of antioxidants leads to lower rate of stomach cancer], *Preventive Medicine* 9:189–196, March 1980

Sporn, et al, "Prevention of chemical carcinogenesis by Vitamin A and its synthetic analogs (retinoids)," *Fed. Proc.* 35(6):1332–1338, 1 May 1976

Spallholz et al, "Immunologic Responses of Mice Fed Diets Supplemented with Selenite Selenium," *Proc. Soc. Exp. Med. Biol.* 143:685–689, 1973

Passwater, *Cancer and Its Nutritional Therapies*, Pivot, 1978 (popular media)

Braun, "The Reversal of Tumor Growth," *Sci. Amer.*, Nov. 1965, pp. 3–9

Snipes et al, "BHT Inactivates Lipid-containing Viruses," *Science*, 188:64–66, 1975

Richardson, "A two year oral study with Hydergine in rats," *Action on Ageing*, Proceedings of a Symposium held at Basle, 20th–21st May 1976, published by MCS Consultants, England, for Sandoz (development of breast cancer suppressed by Hydergine®)

Wattenburg et al, "Dietary Constituents Altering the Responses to Chemical Carcinogens," *Fed. Proc.* 35(6):1327–1331, 1976

Franklyn, "BHT in Sarcoma-prone Dogs," *Lancet*, pg. 1296, 12 June 1976

Kappas and Alvares, "How the Liver Metabolizes Foreign Substances," *Sci. Amer. offprint 1322*, June 1975

Cameron & Pauling, *Vitamin C and Cancer*, Freeman, 1980 (popular media)

Freudenthal and Jones, editors, *Polynuclear Aromatic Hydrocarbons: Chemistry, Metabolism, & Carcinogenesis*, Raven Press, 1976

Greeder and Milner, "Factors Influencing the Inhibitory Effect of Selenium on Mice Inoculated with Ehrlich Ascites Tumor Cells," *Science* 209:825–827, 1980

Sporn, "Combination Chemoprevention of Cancer," *Nature* 287:107–108, 1980

Burnet, *Immunology, Aging, and Cancer*, Freeman, 1976

Whelan, *Preventing Cancer: What You Can Do to Cut Your Risks by Up to 50 Percent*, New York: Norton, 1977 (popular media)

Georgieff, "Free radical inhibitory effect of some anticancer compounds," *Science* 173:537–39, 1971

Schrauzer, "Selenium and Cancer: A review," *Bioinorg. Chem.* 5:275–281, 1976

Mukai and Goldstein, "Mutagencity of Malonaldehyde, a decomposition product of peroxidized polyunsaturated fatty acids," *Science* 191:868–869, 1976

Nockels, "Protective Effects of Supplemental Vitamin E Against Infection," paper presented at 62nd annual meeting (Apr. 9–14, 1978) of FASEB

Shamberger et al, "Carcinogen-induced Chromosomal breakage decreased by antioxidants," *Proc. Nat. Acad. Sci.* 70(5):1461–1463, May 1973

Cameron and Pauling, "Supplemental Ascorbate in the Supportive Treatment of cancer: Prolongation of Survival Times in Terminal Human Cancer," *Proc. Nat. Acad. Sci.* 73(10):3685–89, Oct. 1976

Irwin Stone, "Scurvy and the Cancer Problem," *Amer. Lab.* 8(9):21–29, Sept. 1976

Sporn, "Chemoprevention of Cancer," *Nature* 272:402–403, 1978

Goldstein, "Thymosin: Basic Properties and Clinical Potential in the Treatment of Patients with Immunodeficiency Diseases and Cancer," *Appl. Cancer Chemother. Antiobiot. Chemother.* 24:47–59, 1978

Shamberger, "Relationship of Selenium to Cancer: Inhibitory Effect of Selenium on Carcinogenesis," *J. Nat. Cancer Instit.* 44(4):931–936, 1970

Shamberger, "Antioxidants in cereals and in food preservatives and declining gastric cancer mortality," *Cleveland Clinic Quarterly* 39(3):119–124, 1972

Wattenberg, "Potential Inhibitors of Colon Carcinogenesis," *Dig. Dis.* 19(10):947–953, 1974

Black and Chan, "Suppression of ultraviolet Light induced Tumor formation by dietary antioxidants," *J. Inv. Derm.* 65:412–414, 1975

Jean L. Marx, "Thymic hormones: Inducers of T Cell Maturation," *Science* 187:1183, 1975

Davignon et al, "B.C.G. Vaccination and Leukemia Mortality," *The Lancet,* pg. 638, Sept. 26, 1970

Campbell, Reade, Radden, "Effect of cysteine on the survival of mice with transplanted malignant thymoma," *Nature* 251:158–159, 1974

Wattenburg, "Inhibitors of Chemical Carcinogens," *J. Environ. Pathol. Toxicol* 3(4):35–52, 1980

Honn, Cicone, Skoff, "Prostacyclin: A Potent Antimetastatic Agent," *Science* 212:1270–1272, 12 June 1981 [Prostacyclin is here reported to be a powerful antimetastatic agent against B16 amelanotic melanoma cells, an effect potentiated by a phosphodiesterase inhibitor. The effect may be due to prevention of platelet aggregation around these cancer cells.]

Demopoulos and Gutman, "Cancer in New Jersey and Other Complex Urban/Industrial Areas," *J. Environ Pathol Toxicol* 3(4):219–235, 1980

Demopoulos, Pietronigro, Flamm, Seligman, "The Possible Role of Free Radical Reactions in Carcinogenesis," *J. Environ Pathol Toxicol* 3(4):273–303, 1980

Riley, Vernon, "Psychoneuroendocrine Influences on Immunocompetence and Neoplasia," *Science* 212:1100–1109, 5 June 1981 [Emotional, psychosocial, or anxiety-caused stresses increase plasma concentration of adrenal corticoids and other hormones. A direct result of this is impairment of some parts of the immune system.]

Rettura, Levenson, Seifter, "Anti-tumor and anti-stress actions of L-ornithine," *Fed Proc Abstr,* (72nd Annual Meeting Amer. Soc. Biol. Chem., St. Louis, MO, 31 May–4 June, 1981) 40 (6): abstract #840, 1981

Shekelle et al, "Dietary Vitamin A and Risk of Cancer in the Western Electric Study," *The Lancet* pp. 1185–1190, 28 Nov. 1981
     A 19 year prospective epidemiological study of about 3,000 middle aged men has provided evidence that carotenoids such as beta carotene have a remarkable ability to prevent lung cancer in both smokers and non-smokers. The non-smokers in the lowest quartile of carotenoid intake had about seven times the risk of lung cancer as the non-smokers in the highest quartile. (A quartile is a segment of the study population containing one quarter of the study population.) For smokers, the lowest carotenoid quartile had about eight times the lung cancer risk of the highest quartile. This protective effect is so strong that smokers for up to 30 years in the highest carotenoid quartile had about the same risk of lung cancer as the non-smokers who were below average in carotenoid intake! (The highest quartile was probably averaging *very roughly* 10,000 IU of beta carotene per day.) This does *not* mean that it is safe to smoke cigarettes if you take enough beta carotene; the lethal cardiovascular effects of smoking were *not* affected. Note, too, that fiber and natural antioxidants contained in the vegetables and fruits (the principal carotenoid sources) may have a role in this lung cancer preventive effect. This effect is apparently *not* due to vitamin A.

B. Modan et al, "Retinol, Carotene, and Cancer," *Internatl. J. Cancer* 28:421–424, 1981
     This is an epidemiological study on 406 patients with gastrointestinal cancer and 812 matched controls that showed a highly significant correlation between increased carotenoid intake and decreased gastrointestinal cancer. This decreased risk did not appear to be due to vitamin A, but may have also been related to the increased fiber and natural antioxidants that are found in most high carotenoid (high vegetable and fruit) diets.

Myers et al, "Selenium Yeast Studies" in *Selenium in Biology and Medicine,* Spallholz et al, editors, AVI, 1981

Schrauzer and McGinness, "Observations on Human Selenium Supplementation," in *Trace Substances in Environmental Health* 13:64–67, 1979

Most organic sources of selenium, such as selenomethionine, are less effective than selenite in elevating deficient levels of glutathione peroxidase. An exception is a selenized yeast (commercially available from Nutrition 21, Box 390, La Jolla, CA 92038) which exhibits good results in this test. The selenium in this yeast is mostly *not* the seleno amino acids and is not inorganic either. It may involve a seleno-trisulfide organic compound.

Klayman and Gunther, eds., *Organic Selenium Compounds: Their Chemistry and Biology,* Wiley-Interscience, 1973

The American Cancer Society is to be congratulated on awarding a $900,000 grant to Dr. Paul Talalay and Dr. Ernest Bueding (at Johns Hopkins University Hospital) for research on the anti-cancer properties of BHA (butylated hydroxyanisole), a very close relative of BHT. Both BHA and BHT are powerful free radical scavenging antioxidant food additives. Both BHA and BHT can prevent cancer and extend the life spans of experimental animals. Free radical pathology is finally gaining the prominence that it deserves.

Part III Chapter 20: First Aid

Rosenthal, "Wound Shock," *Sci. Amer.,* Dec. 1958

Cardiopulmonary resuscitation, American National Red Cross, 1974

Ungar, "Experimental traumatic 'shock'," *The Lancet,* April 3, 1943, pp. 421–24

Hilton and Wells, "Nicotinic acid reduction of plasma volume loss after thermal trauma," *Science* 191:861–862, 1976

Barbul et al, "Arginine: A Thymotropic and Wound-Healing Promoting Agent," *Surgical Forum* 28:101–103, 1977

"Workshop on Advances in Experimental Pharmacology of Hydergine," *Gerontology* 24 (Suppl. 1):1–154, 1978

Ralli and Dumm, "Relation of Pantothenic Acid to Adrenal Cortical Function," *Vit. Horm.* 11:133–158, 1953

Leake, "Dimethyl sulfoxide," *Science,* pp. 1646–1649, June 1966

Siebke et al, "Survival After 40 Minutes Submersion Without Cerebral Sequelae," *The Lancet,* June 7, 1975

"New research on CPR questions mechanism," *Science News,* pg. 359, 6 Dec. 1980

Faden, Jacobs, Holaday, "Opiate Antagonist Improves Neurologic Recovery After Spinal Injury," *Science* 211:493–494, 1981

Glogar et al, "Fluorocarbons Reduce Myocardial Ischemic Damage After Coronary Occlusion," *Science* 211:1439–1441, 1981 [the authors attribute the protective effects of the fluorocarbons to their high affinity for oxygen and ability to deliver oxygen to tissue; another factor may be free radical spin trapping by F-tributylamine, a component of the fluorocarbon mixture]

Part III Chapter 21: Your Child's Immune System

Davignon et al, "B.C.G. vaccination and leukemia mortality," *The Lancet,* 26 Sept. 1970, pg. 638

Parent's Guide to Childhood Immunization, U.S. Dept. HEW Public Health Service, DHEW Public # (OS)77-50058, Oct. 1977

WARNING: Immunization of a sick or vitamin deficient infant can result in sudden infant death. These immunizations are recommended only for healthy, well-nourished infants and children. Immunizations and natural infections markedly increase the consumption of the antioxidant nutrients, particularly vitamin C. See Kalokerinos, *Every Second Child,* Thomas Nelson (Australia) Limited, 1974; also published in paperback by Keats Publishing, Inc., New Canaan, Connecticut, 1981 (popular media)

Part IV Chapter 1: Who's Afraid of Cholesterol?

Edward Gruberg & Stephen Raymond, "Beyond Cholesterol," *Atlantic Monthly,* May 1978 (popular magazine)

Passwater, *Supernutrition for Healthy Hearts,* Dial Press, 1977 (popular book)

Gordon, et al, "High Density Lipoprotein as a Protective Factor Against Coronary heart Disease: The Framingham Study," *Amer. J. Med.* 62:707–708 May 1977

Thompson & Bortz, "Significance of High-Density Lipoprotein Cholesterol," *J. Am. Ger. Soc.* 26(10):440–442, 1978

Ginter, "Cholesterol: Vitamin C Controls Its Transformation to Bile Acids," *Science* 179:702–704, 1973

Branen, "Lipid and enzyme changes to organs of monkeys fed BHA and BHT," *Food Product Development,* April 1973

Green, "The Synthesis of Fat," *Sci. Amer.* offprint 67, Feb. 1960

Nightingale et al, "Effect of Vitamin C and High Cholesterol Diet on Aortic Atherosclerosis in Dutch Belted Rabbits," paper delivered at FASEB, 62nd Annual Meeting, Atlantic City, NJ, April 9–14, 1978

Slater and Alfin-Slater, "Effect of Dietary Cholesterol on Plasma Cholesterol, HDL Cholesterol, and Triglycerides in Human Subjects," *Fed. Proc.* Abstr. 2194, 1 Mar. 1978

Pinckney & Pinckney, *The Cholesterol Controversy,* Sherbourne Press, 1973 (popular book)

Brown, Kovanen, Goldstein, "Regulation of Plasma Cholesterol by Lipoprotein Receptors," *Science* 212:628–635, 1981

A fraction of blood lipoproteins called beta-very-low-density lipoprotein (beta-VLDL) delivers cholesterol in the blood to cells in arteries around the heart, according to Dr. Robert W. Mahley and his co-workers. They found that when dietary fat intake rose, the concentration in the blood of the beta-VLDL increased. Conversely, when dietary intake of fat and cholesterol was low, the beta-VLDL was absent. (This was reported in the June 22, 1981 Chem. Eng. News.) Goodman and

Gilman discuss the ability of niacin to reduce VLDL and tri-glycerides on page 768 of the fourth edition of *The Pharma-cological Basis of Therapeutics.* We eat a rather high fat diet but have very low levels of VLDL. When these levels were measured in October of 1978, Sandy had a VLDL lower than 94 percent of women in her age group; Durk had a VLDL lower than 92 percent of men in his age group.

Part IV Chapter 2: Sugar, Diet, and Longevity

The use of microwave ovens for cooking foods is more healthful than the use of ordinary ovens. Foods retain more of their nutrient content, and microwave ovens produce far less of the carcinogens created during fuel combustion and the high temperature oxidation of fat in a regular oven. The only type of cooking which produces a smaller quantity of car-cinogens in the cooking of meat is boiling, which unfortunate-ly destroys most vitamins and other temperature sensitive, water soluble nutrients, along with most of the taste.

Steve Faber, "It's Not a Big Miracle," *Interface Age,* pp. 70–73, December 1978 (This program is written to run on the Ra-dio Shack TRS-80. A copy of this article and program can be obtained from the author (we don't know his price, but do not assume it's free). Send a stamped, self-addressed envelope to:
Steve Faber, PO Box 69200, Los Angeles, CA 90069

A version of this program for the Commodore PET com-puter is available. Send a stamped, self-addressed envelope to the author: Frank Henn, 4811 Verona Dr. N.W., Calgary, Al-berta T3A OP5

We have not personally tested these programs because, although we have many computers, we have neither the TRS-80 or the Commodore PET.

The basic idea for this program is very simple: administer only the amount of insulin that is really necessary, no more and no less. Although this sounds simple, a diabetic's insulin requirement varies with diet, exercise, state of health, time of day, stress, etc. This program uses the above data in conjunc-tion with urine sugar measurements. You can make these measurements yourself by dipping Clinitest® or C-STRIPS®

urine sugar test strips into your urine and comparing the resulting color with a color chart on the bottle. It's very simple. Be sure to discuss this with your physician. Diabetes mellitus is a serious disease and requires professional attention to its management.

Rizzino, Rizzino, Sato, "Defined Media and the Determination of Nutritional & Hormonal Requirements of Mammalian Cells in Culture," *Nutr. Rev.* 37(12):369–378, 1979

Hayashi, Larner, and Sato, "Hormonal Growth Control of Cells in Culture," *In Vitro* 14(1):23–30, 1978

Jeanes and Hodge, *Physiological Effects of Food Carbohydrates,* ACS Symposium Series #15, American Chemical Society, 1975

Levine [sodium fluoride and calcium phosphate mouthwash], *J. R. Soc. Med.* 73:876–881, 1980

Part IV Chapter 3: Spices and Other Food Preservatives

Branen, et al, "Antimicrobial Properties of Phenolic Antioxidants and Lipids," *Food Technology* 34(5):42–53, May 1980 [antiviral properties of BHT]

Today's Food and Additives, General Foods Corp. (For a free copy, write to General Foods Consumer Center, 250 North St., White Plains, NY 10605) (written for laymen)

Lundberg, ed, *Autoxidation and Antioxidants, Vols. I and II,* Wiley Interscience, 1961

Mukai and Goldstein, "Mutagenicity of Malonaldehyde, a decomposition product of peroxidized polyunsaturated fatty acids," *Science* 191:868–869, 1976

Sato and Herring, "Chemistry of warmed-over flavor in cooked meats," *Food Product Development,* Nov. 1973

Harman and Mattick, "Association of lipid oxidation with seed aging and death," *Nature* 260: 323–324, 1976

"Santoquin antioxidant: can it actually slow the process of aging," (advertisement), Monsanto Report No. 6 on Current Technology

Sherwin, "Antioxidants for food fats and oils," *JAOCS* 49(8):468–472, 1972

Cort, "Antioxidant activity of tocopherols, ascorbyl palmitate, and ascorbic acid and their mode of action," *JAOCS* 51(7):321–325, 1974

Shamberger, "Antioxidants in cereals and in food preservatives and declining gastric cancer mortality," *Cleveland Clinic Quarterly* 39(3):119–124, 1972

Thompson and Sherwin, "Investigation of antioxidants for polyunsaturated edible oils," *JAOCS* 43(12):683–686, 1965

Pryor et al, "Autoxidation of Polyunsaturated Fatty Acids," *Arch. Environ. Health,* pp. 201–210, July/August 1976

Harman et al, "Free Radical Theory of Aging: Effect of Dietary Fat on Central Nervous System Function," *J. Am. Geriat. Soc.* 24(7):301–307, 1976

Simic and Karel, *Autoxidation in Food and Biological Systems,* Plenum Press, 1980

Bracco, Loliger, Viret, "Production and Use of Natural Antioxidants," *JAOCS* 58(6):686–690, 1981

Part IV Chapter 4: Life Extension Experiments in Your Home

Cort, "Antioxidant activity of tocopherols, ascorbyl palmitate and ascorbic acid and their mode of action," *JAOCS* 51:321–325, 1974

Koppers Co., Inc., Technical Bulletin on DBPC [BHT] Antioxidant: *Final Report: High Stability Military Automotive Combat Gasoline Desert Storage.*

Part IV Chapter 5: FDA's RDAs

*"My concern is not the cancer rate. My concern is
protection of individual freedom. Each step of protection
brings its own threat. And the increase in that threat with
each decision is geometric not arithmetic. People have to
decide how far they want to go with this protection."*
—*Dr. Sanford Miller, FDA Director of the Bureau of Foods*

One pressure group currently pushing to convince the FDA to ban fortification of snack foods is the self-styled consumer advocate Center for "Science" in the "Public Interest." We hope that the FDA can withstand these pressures for unwise and authoritarian limitations on freedom of choice for both consumers and food manufacturers. There is absolutely no evidence that prohibiting nutritional fortification of snack foods will either reduce their consumption or improve public nutrition. We consider this proposed ban to be very poor public policy.

"FDA's Goyan: Bury the Hatchet," *Chemical Marketing Reporter,* 7 April 1980

Peltzman, *Regulation of Pharmaceutical Innovation,* American Enterprise Institute, 1974

Pauling, "Are Recommended Daily Allowances for Vitamin C Adequate?", *Proc. Nat. Acad. Sci. USA* 71(11):4442–4446, Nov. 1974

Nutrient Requirements of Laboratory Animals, No. 10, The National Research Council, 1978

Nutrient Requirements of Nonhuman Primates, No. 14, The National Research Council, 1978

Ricardo-Campbell, *Food Safety Regulations,* The American Enterprise Institute for Public Policy Research and The Hoover Institution, 1974 (a study of the use and limitations of cost-benefit analysis)

Part IV Chapter 6: Vitamin E

Kornbrust and Mavis, "Relative Susceptibility of Microsomes from Lung, Heart, Liver, Kidney, Brain and Testes to Lipid Peroxidation: Correlation with Vitamin E Content," *Lipids* 15(5):315–322, 1979

Tappel, "Biological Antioxidant Protection Against Lipid Peroxidation Damage," *Amer. J. Clin. Nutr.* 23(8):1137–1139, 1970

Steiner & Anastasi, "Vitamin E: An inhibitor of the Platelet Release Reaction," *J. Clin. Invest.* 57:732–737, 1976

Sundaram et al, "alpha-Tocopherol and Serum Lipoproteins," *Lipids* 16(4):223–227, April 1981 [alpha tocopherol caused objective and subjective remission from benign breast disease in 85 percent of 26 patients given 600 milligrams per day; furthermore, HDL increased and ester cholesterol associated with LDL decreased]

Shute, *Vitamin E for Ailing and Healthy Hearts*, Pyramid, 1972 (popular book)

Bailey, *Vitamin E: Your Key to a Healthy Heart*, Arco, 1971 (popular book)

Goldstein, et al, "Ozone and Vitamin E," *Science*, 7 Aug. 1970, pg. 605

Roehm et al, "The influence of vitamin E on the lung fatty acids of rats exposed to ozone," *Arch. Environ. Health* 24: April 1972

Tappel, "Vitamin E as the biological lipid antioxidant," *Vit. Horm.* 20:493–510, 1962

Cort, "Antioxidant activity of tocopherols, ascorbyl palmitate, and ascorbic acid and their mode of action" *JAOCS* 51 (7):321–325, 1974

Tappel, "Selenium-glutathione peroxidase and Vitamin E," *Amer. J. Clin. Nutr.* 27:960–965, Sept. 1974

Reichel, "Lipid Pigment Formation as a Function of Age, Disease, and Vitamin E Deficiency," International Symposium on Vitamin E, Hakone 1970

Roehm et al, "Antioxidants vs. Lung Disease," *Arch. Intern. Med.* 12:88–93, 1971

Harman, "Role of Free Radicals in Mutation, Cancer, Aging, and the Maintenance of Life," *Rad. Res.* 16:753–764, 1962

Miquel et al, "Effects of dl-alpha tocopherol on the lifespan of Drosophila melanogaster," (paper presented to the 26th Annual Scientific Meeting of the Gerontological Society, Miami Beach, Florida, Nov. 5–9, 1973)

Harman and Mattick, "Association of lipid oxidation with seed ageing and death," *Nature* 260:323–324, 1976

Tappel and Dillard, "In vivo lipid peroxidation: Measurement via exhaled pentane and protection by Vitamin E," *Fed. Proc.* 40(2):174–182, Feb. 1981

Part IV Chapter 7: Vitamin C

Anderson, et al, "The effects of increasing weekly doses of ascorbate on certain cellular and humoral immune functions in normal volunteers," *Am. J. Clin. Nutr.* 33:71–76, Jan 1980

Chope and Breslow, "Nutritional Status of the Aging," *Am. J. Publ. Health* 46:61–67, 1956

Stone, "Hypoascorbemia, the genetic disease causing human requirement for exogenous ascorbic acid," *Perspec. in Biol. and Med.* 10(1):133–34, 1966

Pelletier & Keith, "Bioavailability of Synthetic and natural Ascorbic Acid," *J. Am. Dietetic Assoc.* 64:271–275, 1974

Hume, et al, "Leucocyte ascorbic acid levels after acute myocardial infarction," *Brit. Heart. J* 34:238–243, 1972

Shamberger et al, "Carcinogen-induced Chromosomal Breakage Decreased by Antioxidants," *Proc. Nat. Acad. Sci* 70 (5):1461–63, May 1973

Cameron and Pauling, *Vitamin C and Cancer,* Freeman, 1980 (popular book)

Bjorksten, "The Theoretical Base for the Anti-infective Function of Ascorbic Acid," *Rejuvenation* 7(2):33–36, 1979

Sherry Lewin, *Vitamin C, Its Molecular Biology and Medical Potential,* Academic Press, 1976

Linus Pauling, *Vitamin C, the Common Cold, and the Flu,* Freeman, 1976 (popular book)

Stone, *The Healing Factor: Vitamin C Against Disease,* Grosset and Dunlap, 1972 (popular book)

Nutrient Requirements of Nonhuman Primates, Pub. No. 10, The National Research Council, 1978

Sokoloff et al, "Aging, atherosclerosis and ascorbic acid metabolism," *J. Am. Geriat. Soc* 14(12):1239–1260, 1966

Klenner, "Observations on the dose and administration of ascorbic acid when employed beyond the range of a vitamin in human pathology," *J. Appl. Nutr* Winter 1971, pp. 61–87

Ungar, "Experimental traumatic 'shock'," *Lancet,* April 3, 1943, pp. 421–24

Sprince, Parker, Smith, "L-ascorbic acid in alcoholism and smoking: protection against acetaldehyde toxicity as an experimental model," *Int. J. Vit. Nutr. Res* 47 (Suppl. 1G):185–212, Nov. 1977

Goetzl et al, "Enhancement of random migration and chemotactic response of human leukocytes by ascorbic acid," *J. Clin. Invest* 5:813–818, 1974

Cameron and Pauling, "Supplemental Ascorbate in the Supportive Treatment of cancer: prolongation of Survival Times in Terminal Human Cancer," *Proc. Nat. Acad. Sci. USA* 73(10):3685–89, Oct. 1976

Spittle, "The Action of vitamin C on Blood Vessels," *Amer. Heart Jour* 88(3):387–388, Sept. 1974

Field and Rekers, "Studies of the Effects of Flavonoids on Roentgen Irradiation Disease. II Comparison of the Protective Influence of Some Flavonoids and Vitamin C in Dogs," *J. Clin. Invest* 28:746, 1949

Stone, "Scurvy and the Cancer Problem," *Amer. Lab* 8(9):21–29, Sept. 1976

Bourne, "The Effect of Vitamin C on the Healing of Wounds," *Proc. Nutr. Soc* 4:205–209, 1946

Sprince, et al, "Protectants Against Acetaldehyde Toxicity: Sulfhydryl Compounds and Ascorbic Acid," *Fed. Proc* 33(3), pt. 1 March 1974

Ginter, "Cholesterol: Vitamin C Controls Its Transformation to Bile Acids," *Science* 179:702–704, 1973

Banic, "Prevention of rabies by vitamin C," *Nature* 258:153–154, 1975

Pauling, "Are Recommended Daily Allowances for Vitamin C Adequate?" *Proc. Nat. Acad. Sci. USA* 71(11):4442–4446, Nov. 1974

Part IV Chapter 8: Vitamin A

Jetten, "Retinoids specifically enhance the number of epidermal growth factor receptors," *Nature* 284:626–631, 17 April 1980

Maugh, "Vitamin A: Potential Protection from Carcinogens," *Science* 186:1198, 1974

Bjelke, "Dietary Vitamin A and Human Lung Cancer," *Int. J. Cancer* 15:561–565 (1975)

Basu, et al, "Plasma Vitamin A in Patients with Bronchial Carcinoma," *Br. J. Cancer* 33:119–121 (1976)

Sporn, et al, "Prevention of chemical carcinogenesis by Vitamin A and its synthetic analogs (retinoids)," *Fed. Proc.* 35 (6):1332–1338, 1 May 1976

Smithells et al, "Possible Prevention of Neural-tube Defects by Periconceptional Vitamin Supplementation," *Lancet* pp. 339–340, 16 February 1980

Peto, Doll, Buckley, Sporn, "Can dietary beta-carotene materially reduce human cancer rates?", *Nature* 290:201–208, 1981

Part IV Chapter 9: Niacin

Hilton and Wells, "Nicotinic acid reduction of plasma volume loss after thermal trauma," *Science* 191:861–862, 1976

Charman et al, "Nicotinic acid in the treatment of hypercholesterolemia," *J. Angiology*, Jan. 1973

"The Effect of Nicotinic Acid on the Plasma Free Fatty Acids," *Acta Medica Scandinavica* 172 fasc. 6, 1962

Orthomolecular Psychiatry, edited by Hawkins and Pauling, Freeman, 1973

Miettinen et al, [decrease in serum cholesterol by 25 percent and triglycerides by 30 percent in human subjects after two weeks on 3 grams of niacin per day], *Acta Med. Scand.* 186:247–253, 1969

Goodman and Gilman, *The Pharmacological Basis of Therapeutics*, 4th ed., MacMillan, 1970, pg. 768

A fraction of blood lipoproteins called beta-very-low-density lipoprotein (beta-VLDL) delivers cholesterol in the blood to cells in arteries around the heart, according to Dr. Robert

W. Mahley and his co-workers. They found that when dietary fat intake rose, the concentration in the blood of the beta-VLDL increased. Conversely, when dietary intake of fat and cholesterol was low, the beta-VLDL was absent. (This was reported in the June 22, 1982 *Chem. Eng. News.*) Goodman and Gilman discuss the ability of niacin to reduce VLDL and triglycerides on page 768 of the fourth edition of *The Pharmacological Basis of Therapeutics.* We eat a rather high fat diet but have very low levels of VLDL. When these levels were measured in October of 1978, Sandy had a VLDL lower than 94 percent of women in her age group; Durk had a VLDL lower than 92 percent of men in his age group.

Brown, Heitkamp, Song, "Niacin Reduces Paraquat Toxicity in Rats," *Science* 212:1510–1512, 26 June 1981
    [Earlier work indicated that paraquat poisoning damaged by similar mechanisms to hyperbaric oxygen, in other words by free radical damage. Both niacin and thiamin (vitamin B-1) were able to help the growth of E. Coli poisoned by either paraquat or hyperbaric oxygen. The authors propose the protective effect of niacin is related to its ability to get around the poisoning effect on the enzyme that is required for the synthesis of nicotinamide adenine dinucleotide (NAD). Another possibility they didn't mention is that niacin itself acts as a spin trap for free radicals. Rats were poisoned with paraquat and either given niacin or not. The rats treated with paraquat and niacin had only a 55 percent death rate compared to a 75 percent death rate for those treated only with paraquat. Powerful antioxidant combinations such as vitamin C, B-1, and the amino acid cysteine could provide much greater protection.]

Shansky, "Vitamin B-3 in the Alleviation of Hypoglycemia," *Drug and Cosmetic Industry,* Oct. 1981

Part V Chapter 1: Biochemical Individuality

Briggs & Briggs, "Vitamin C Requirements and Oral Contraceptives," *Nature* 238: 277, 1972

Roger J. Williams, *Biochemical Individuality,* U. of Tex. Press, 1969 (popular book)

Adelman and Britton, "The Impaired Capability for Biochemical Adaptation During Aging," *Bioscience* 25(10):639–643, Oct. 1975

Smithells et al, "Possible prevention of neural-tube defects by periconceptional vitamin supplementation," *The Lancet,* pg. 339, Feb. 16, 1980

Part V Chapter 4: Clinical Laboratory Tests

Laughlin, Fisher, and Sherrard, "Blood Pressure Reductions During Self Recording of Home Blood Pressure," *Amer. Heart J.* 98(5):629–634, Nov. 1979

Merck Manual of Diagnosis and Therapy, Merck & Co., Inc., Rahway, New Jersey, 1972

Garb, *Laboratory Tests in Common Use,* 5th ed., Springer 1971

Pinckney and Pinckney, *The Encyclopedia of Medical Tests,* Pocket Books, 1978

Klein, *Medical Tests & You,* Grosset & Dunlap, 1977

Part V Chapter 5: How to Ask for a Prescription

Physician's Desk Reference, Medical Economics Co., Oradell, NJ 07649

Dorland's Illustrated Medical Dictionary, Saunders Co., 25th edition, 1974.

Part V Chapter 6: Keeping a File of Your Own Medical Records

Privacy Journal, published by Robert Ellis Smith, PO Box 8844, Washington, DC 20003, $65/12 monthly issues; tells how to maintain confidentiality of your medical records and laws that apply

Part V Chapter 7: Our Current Personal Experimental Life Extension Formula

Maugh, "Vitamin A: Potential Protection from Carcinogens," *Science* 186:1198, 1974

Odens, "RNA Effects on Memory," Lecture read at the 16th Convention on Civilisation Diseases, Nutrition and Living conditions, 14–20 Sept. 1970, in Treves and Luxembourg

Ambrose and DeEds, "Effect of Rutin on Permeability of Cutaneous Capillaries," presented before the Soc. Exp. Biol. and Med., Feb. 12, 1947

Schrauzer, "Selenium and Cancer: A review," *Bioinorg. Chem.* 5:275–281, 1976

Chvapil et al, "Effect of Zinc on Lipid Peroxidation in Liver Microsomes and Mitochondria," *Proc. Soc. Exp. Biol. Med.* 141:150–153, 1972

Boyd et al, "Stimulation of Human-Growth-Hormone Secretion by L-Dopa," *New Engl. J. Med.* 283(26):1425–1429, 1970

Zierler et al, "On the antithrombic and antiproteolytic activity of alpha tocopheryl phosphate," *Am. J. Physiol.* 153:127–132, 1948

Goldstein et al, "PABA as a protective agent in ozone toxicity," *Arch. Environ. Health* 24:243–247, 1972

Tappel, "Selenium-glutathione peroxidase and Vitamin E," *Amer. J. Clin. Nutr.* 27:960–965, Sept. 1974

Hawkins and Pauling, eds., *Orthomolecular Psychiatry*, Freeman, 1973

Rotruck et al, "Selenium: biochemical role as a component of glutathione peroxidase," *Science* 179:588–590, 1973

Shamberger, "Relationship of Selenium to Cancer: Inhibitory Effect of Selenium on Carcinogenesis," *J. Nat. Cancer Institute* 44(4):931–936, 1970

Odens, "Prolongation of the Life Span in Rats," *J. Amer. Geriatr. Soc.* 21(10):450–451, 1973

Field and Rekers, "Studies of the Effects of Flavonoids on Roentgen Irradiation Disease. II Comparison of the Protective Influence of Some Flavonoids and Vitamin C in Dogs," *J. Clin. Invest.* 28:746, 1949

Cotzias et al, "Prolongation of the Life-span in Mice Adapted to Large Amounts of L-Dopa," *Proc. Nat. Acad. Sci. USA* 71(6):2466–2469, June 1974

Selenium in Nutrition, National Academy of Sciences, 1971

Anderson, et al, "The Effects of Increasing Weekly doses of ascorbate on certain cellular and humoral immune functions in normal volunteers," *Am. J. Clin. Nutr.* 33:71–76, Jan 1980

Hindmarch et al, "The effects of an ergot alkaloid derivative (Hydergine) on aspects of psychomotor performance, arousal, and cognitive processing ability," *J. Clin. Pharmacol.* 19(11–12):726–732, 1979

Robbins, "Effects of Flavonoids on Survival Time of Rats Fed Thrombogenic or Atherogenic Regimens," *J. Athero. Res.,* 7:3–10, 1967

Sporn, et al, "Prevention of chemical carcinogenesis by Vitamin A and its synthetic analogs (retinoids)," *Fed. Proc.* 35(6):1332–1338, 1 May 1976

Steiner & Anastasi, "Vitamin E: An inhibitor of the Platelet Release Reaction," *J. Clin. Invest.* 57:732–737, 1976

Spallhoz et al, "Immunologic Responses of Mice Fed Diets Supplemented with Selenite Selenium," *Proc. Soc. Exp. Med. Biol.* 143:685–689, 1973

Sherry Lewin, *Vitamin C, Its Molecular Biology and medical Potential,* Academic Press, 1976

Linus Pauling, *Vitamin C, the Common Cold, and the Flu,* Freeman, 1976

Roberts, Adelman, Cristofalo, eds. *Pharmacological Intervention in the Aging Process,* Plenum, 1978

Finch, Hayflick, eds. *Handbook of the Biology of Aging,* Van Nostrand Reinhold, 1977

Carl C. Pfeiffer, *Zinc and other micro-nutrients,* Pivot, 1978

Khandwala and Gee, "Linoleic acid hydroperoxide: impaired bacterial uptake by alveolar macrophages, a mechanism of oxidant lung injury," *Science* 182:1364–65, 1973

Hochschild, "Lysosomes, membranes, and aging," *Exp. Geront.* 6:153–166, 1971

Schwartz, "Correlation between species life span and capacity to activate 7, 12-dimethylbenz(a)anthracene to a form mutagenic to a mammalian cell," *Expt. Cell Res.* 94:445–447, 1975

Schubert et al, "Alterations in the surface properties of cells responsive to nerve growth factor," *Nature* 273:718–723, 1978

Goldstein et al, "Ozone and Vitamin E," *Science*, 7 Aug. 1970, pg. 605

Pelton and Williams, "Effect of panthothenic acid on the longevity of mice," *Soc. Exp. Biol. Med.* 99:632–33, 1958

Nockels, "Protective Effects of Supplemental vitamin E Against Infection,: paper presented at 62nd annual meeting (Apr. 9–14, 1978) of FASEB

Cort, "Antioxidant activity of tocopherols, ascorbyl palmitate, and ascorbic acid and their mode of action," *JAOCS* 51(7):321–325, 1974

Harman, "Free Radical Theory of Aging: Nutritional Implications," *AGE* 1(4):145–152, 1978

Barbul et al, "Arginine: A Thymotropic and Wound-Healing Promoting Agent," *Surgical Forum* 28:101–103, 1977

Charman et al "Nicotinic acid in the treatment of hypercholesterolemia," *J. Angiology,* Jan 1973

Hochschild, "Effect of Dimethylaminoethanol on the Life Span of Senile Male A/J Mice," *Exp. Geront.* 8:181–185, 1973

Hochschild, "Effect of Dimethylaminoethyl p-Chlorophenoxyacetate on the Life Span of Male Swiss Webster Albino Mice," *Exp. Geront.* 8:177–183, 1973

Sprince et al, "Protectants Against Acetaldehyde Toxicity: Sulfhydryl Compounds and Ascorbic Acid," *Fed. Proc.* 33(3), pt. 1, March 1974

Oeriu and Vochitu, "The Effect of the Administration of Compounds Which Contain Sulfhydryl Groups on the Survival Rates of Mice, Rats, and Guinea Pigs," *J. Gerontol.* 20:417, 1965

Robertson, "On the influence of nucleic acids on various origins upon the growth and longevity of the white mouse," *Austr. J. Exptl. Biol. Med. Sci.* 5:47–67, 1928

Gardner, "The Effect of yeast nucleic acid on the survival time of 600 day old albino mice," *J. Geront.* 1:445–452, 1946

Kormendy and Bender, "Chemical Interference with Aging," *Gerontologia* 17:52–64, 1971

"Workshop on Advances in Experimental Pharmacology of Hydergine," *Gerontology* 24 (Suppl. 1):1–154, 1978

Borison et al, "Metabolism of an Antidepressant Amino Acid [L-phenylalanine]," presented in poster session at April 9–14, 1978 FASEB, Atlantic City, NJ

Legros et al, "Influence of Vasopressin on Memory and Learning," *Lancet,* 7 Jan. 1978, pg. 41

Oliveros et al, "Vasopressin in Amnesia," *Lancet,* 7 Jan. 1978 pg. 42

Ginter, "Cholesterol: Vitamin C Controls Its Transformation to Bile Acids," *Science* 179:702–704, 1973

Franklyn, "BHT in Sarcoma-prone Dogs," *Lancet,* pg. 1296, 12 June 1976

Marshall and Berrios, "Movement Disorders of Aged Rats: Reversal by Dopamine Receptor Stimulation," *Science* 206:477–479, 1979

Snipes et al, "Butylated Hydroxytoluene Inactivates Lipid-containing Viruses," *Science* 18: 64–66, 1975

Harman, "Role of Free Radicals in Mutation, Cancer, Aging, and the Maintenance of Life," *Rad. Res.* 16:753–764, 1962

Merimee et al, "Arginine-initiated Release of Human Growth Hormone," *New Engl. J. Med.* 280(26):1434–1438, 1969

Nandy and Schneider, "Effects of dihydroergotoxine mesylate on aging neurons in vitro," *Gerontology* 24 (suppl. 1): 66–70, 1978

Thiodipropionate Antioxidants, 47 refs, Evans Chemetics, Inc., 9 Tokeneke Road, Darien, Conn. 06820

Harman, "Free Radical Theory of Aging: Effect of Free Radical Reaction Inhibitors on the Mortality Rate of Male LAF₁ Mice," *J. Geront.* 23 (4), 1968

Peto, Doll, Buckley, Sporn, "Can dietary beta-carotene materially reduce human cancer rates?" *Nature* 290:201–208, 1981

Richardson, "A two year oral study with Hydergine in rats," *Action on Ageing,* Proceedings of a symposium held at Basle, 20–21 May 1976, published by MCS Consultants, England for Sandoz Corp. (suppression of breast cancer by Hydergine®)

"The DMBA-induced tumours can also be made to regress in rats treated with 2-bromoergocryptine, a drug which inhibits pituitary prolactin release. Perhaps most significantly of all, T-mediated tumour regression can be reversed by increasing endogenous release of prolactin on treating the tumour-bearing rats with phenothiazines." (page x, March 1981 *Trends in Pharmacological Sciences*)

Snipes and Keith, "Hydrophobic Alcohols and Di-tert-butyl Phenols as Antiviral Agents" in Kabara, ed., *The Pharmacological Effect of Lipids,* The American Oil Chemists' Society, 1978

Latshaw and Biggert, "Incorporation of Selenium into Egg Proteins After Feeding Selenomethionine or Sodium Selenite," *Poultry Science* 60(6):1309–1313, June 1981
[Selenium in egg white proteins and yolk fractions increased when chickens were fed a diet supplemented in selenium, whether the source of selenium was sodium selenite (inorganic) or selenomethionine (organic). The increase in selenium in egg white proteins after feeding selenomethionine was parallel to their methionine content, indicating that there was a lack of discrimination between methionine and selenomethionine for protein synthesis as suggested by Ochoa-Solano and Gitler in 1968. Selenomethionine feeding increased selenium more in the white than in the yolk, whereas selenite did the opposite. Fairly large increases in the selenium content of HDL and the protein livetin occurred when the chicken diet was supplemented with sodium selenite. The egg lipids are found in the yolk rather than the white, hence, increasing selenium in the yolk is particularly desirable.]

Shekelle et al, "Dietary Vitamin A and Risk of Cancer in the Western Electric Study," *The Lancet* pp. 1185–1190, 28 Nov. 1981

A 19 .year prospective epidemiological study of about 3,000 middle aged men has provided evidence that carotenoids such as beta carotene have a remarkable ability to prevent lung cancer in both smokers and non-smokers. The non-smokers in the lowest quartile of carotenoid intake had about seven times the risk of lung cancer as the non-smokers in the highest quartile. (A quartile is a segment of the study population containing one quarter of the study population.) For smokers, the lowest carotenoid quartile had about eight times the lung cancer risk of the highest quartile. This protective effect is so strong that smokers of up to 30 years' duration in the highest carotenoid quartile had about the same risk of lung cancer as the non-smokers who were below average in carotenoid intake! (The highest quartile was probably averaging *very roughly* 10,000 IU of beta carotene per day.) This does *not* mean that it is safe to smoke cigarettes if you take enough beta carotene; the lethal cardiovascular effects of smoking were *not* affected. Note, too, that fiber and natural antioxidants contained in the vegetables and fruits (the principal carotenoid sources) may have a role in this lung cancer preventive effect. This effect is apparently *not* due to vitamin A.

B. Modan et al, "Retinol, Carotene, and Cancer," *Internatl. J. Cancer* 28:421–424, 1981

This is an epidemiological study on 406 patients with gastrointestinal cancer and 812 matched controls that showed a highly significant correlation between increased carotenoid intake and decreased gastrointestinal cancer. This decreased risk did not appear to be due to vitamin A, but may have also been related to the increased fiber and natural antioxidants that are found in most high carotenoid (high vegetable and fruit) diets.

Myers et al, "Selenium Yeast Studies" in *Selenium in Biology and Medicine*, Spallholz et al, editors, AVI, 1981

Schrauzer and McGinness, "Observations on Human Selenium Supplementation," in *Trace Substances in Environmental Health* 13:64–67, 1979

Most organic sources of selenium, such as selenomethionine, are less effective than selenite in elevating deficient levels of glutathione peroxidase. An exception is a selenized yeast (commercially available from Nutrition 21, Box 390, La Jolla, CA 92038) which exhibits good results in this test. The selenium in this yeast is mostly *not* the seleno amino acids and is not inorganic either. It may involve a seleno-trisulfide organic compound.

Klayman and Gunther, eds., *Organic Selenium Compounds: Their Chemistry and Biology*, Wiley-Interscience, 1973

Pecile and Muller, eds., "Growth and Growth Hormone," *Excerpta Medica*, 1973

Part V Chapter 8: Is There Anything Perfectly Safe?

Many people, especially those in Washington, suffer from the delusion that things can be made perfectly safe if only they pass enough laws! Unfortunately, nature does not work that way. This approach to safety is apt to strangle the development of new, safer (but always less than perfect) products and processes. See Sam Peltzman's book about the Kefauver Amendment, *Regulation of Pharmaceutical Innovation*.

Another legal delusion can be found in the Delaney Amendment to the FDA act which prohibits the sale of food containing any purposefully or incidentally added man-made carcinogens. Of course, it ignores the much more serious problems of natural carcinogens such as aflatoxins and peroxidized lipids, but its greatest folly is the idea of zero tolerance, which violates the second law of thermodynamics. In a contest between lawyers' laws and nature's laws, nature always wins. The second law of thermodynamics says that everything tends to inexorably mix with everything else. Any glass of water (unless it came from a deep well, a glacier, or Mars) is certain to contain some molecules that were once part of the body of Alexander the Great. With sufficiently sensitive instruments, you can find a little bit of carcinogen in any food, but that does not mean that you should worry about it. Yes, we can find incredibly minute traces of the estrogenic food-to-meat-conversion-stimulation hormone DES in cattle previously treated with it. In our opinion, banning DES in cattle has not significantly increased anyone's safety; but it has significantly increased meat prices, grain prices, and non-human grain consumption. How many poor have starved in Bangladesh because of DES-ban-elevated grain prices?

Another good example of the Delaney delusion can be found in chlorinated water. Water chlorination has saved millions, perhaps even hundreds of millions of lives. However, when water is chlorinated, traces of organic material of both natural and human origins are converted into chlorinated organics, some of which are carcinogens. Under the Delaney amendment, it is a felony to use chlorinated tap water to produce food for sale. It's a good thing for us that laws are not always enforced. It would be better for us if such laws were repealed. Some Congressmen are acutely aware that the Delaney amendment is unscientific nonsense, but they don't dare vote to repeal it because they fear their opponents will charge that they are "procancer irresponsible lackeys bought off by dirty big business." If you want to end the baleful effects of the Kefauver and Delaney Amendments, you will have to let your Congressman know.

Finally, safety regulations should deal with relative risks of alternatives, and stop comparing proposed systems to nonexistent perfection. The risks of nuclear power should be compared to the risks of alternate power systems, as well as to the risks involved in power shortages. For example, the risks of hydroelectric power are substantially greater than nuclear power. The historical failure rate for major dams is between 1 percent and 0.1 percent per year, and such failures can kill as many people as the maximum credible failure (which has never even been approached) of a large power reactor. There are many natural radioisotopes (uranium, thorium, radium, radon, etc.) in coal, and in fact, coal burning power plants release more hazardous radiation into the air and water per kilowatt hour than nuclear power plants, to say nothing of the much more dangerous carcinogenic coal combustion products. Oil has considerably less of the natural radioisotopes and burns cleaner as well, but is it perfectly safe to depend on Mideast oil?

For further information on risk assessment see: David Okrent, "Comment on Societal Risk," *Science:* 208, 25 April 1980.

James L. Repace and Alfred H. Lowery, "Indoor Air Pollution, Tobacco Smoke, and Public Health," *Science* 208:464–472, 2 May 1980

Gio Batta Gori, "The Regulation of Carcinogenic Hazards," *Science* 208:256–260, 18 April 1980

Chris Whipple, "The Energy Impacts of Solar Heating," *Science* 208:262–266, 18 April 1980
(This article does not directly address safety but shows how complex real systems are; a rapid shift to solar heating will increase the use of coal and nuclear energy for at least the next twenty years. The more rapid the shift to solar heating, the greater the necessary increased use of coal and nuclear energy.)

Peltzman, *Regulation of Pharmaceutical Innovation,* American Enterprise Institute, 1974

Schwing and Albers, eds., *Societal Risk Assessment: How Safe is Safe Enough,* Plenum, 1980

Here is another example of how nothing is perfectly safe: "Excess Water Dangerous for Infants," reported in the 5 April 1981 *Medical Hotline* [published by Medical News Service, 119 West 57 St., New York, NY 10019]; Excess water intake by infants can induce hyponatremia, an abnormal concentration of sodium in the blood, which can result in irritability, confusion, lethargy, followed by coma, convulsions, and even death.

Bruce-Briggs, *The War Against the Automobile,* Dutton, 1977

Part V Chapter 11: Caveat Emptor

Kodak Publication No. N-3, *Clinical Photography,* Eastman Kodak Co., Rochester, NY 14650

Approved Drug Products with Proposed Therapeutic Equivalence Evaluations, US DHEW, Pub. Health Serv., FDA, January 1979 (on page 13 of this publication it says,

"Dihydroergotoxine mesylate [Hydergine] is composed of three alkaloids consisting of equal parts (one third each) of dihydroergocornine, dihydroergocristine, and dihydroergocryptine mesylates. Subsequent to completing clinical trials on its product, and as a result of advances in analytical methodology, the original application holder [Sandoz Corporation] discovered its product contains two forms of dihydroergocryptine mesylate, alpha and beta, in the ratio of 2 to 1 respectively. Other marketed products are chemically similar except for different alpha/beta ratios of dihydroergocryptine mesylate.

While there is no information to indicate that differences in the alpha/beta ratio make a clinical difference, products differing in this respect are not considered pharmaceutical equivalents. The Agency [FDA] is aware that dihydroergotoxine mesylate tablets are being reformulated by a number of manufacturers to meet the same specifications. It appears that the problem will be resolved shortly, but until then, those products are coded BS.")

The definition of BS (as described on page 12) is: "If the drug standards for an active ingredient in a particular dosage are judged to be inadequate to determine whether the products subject to that standard are pharmaceutical equivalents, all drug products containing that active ingredient in that dosage form are coded BS."

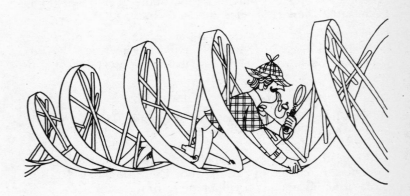

Part V Chapter 12: Epilogue: What Is Coming?

"Three Mice 'Cloned' in Switzerland," *Science* 211:375–376, 1981

Streisinger et al, "Production of clones of homozygous diploid zebra fish *(Brachydanio rerio), Nature* 291:293–96, 28 May 1981

Access to Energy, a pro-science, pro-technology, pro-free enterprise monthly newsletter about energy resources, written by Dr. Petr Beckmann, Box 2298, Boulder, CO 80306, $18/12 monthly issues (popular magazine)

Bronowski, *The Ascent of Man,* Little, Brown and Company, 1973 (popular book)

Gerard K. O'Neill, *The High Frontier,* Bantam, 1976 (popular book)

Osborne, Adam, *Running Wild, The Next Industrial Revolution,* Osborne/McGraw Hill Inc., 1979 (the microelectronics revolution)

Toffler, *The Third Wave,* Morrow, 1980 (popular book)

McKinnell, *Cloning,* Univ. of Minnesota Press, 1978

Vajk, *Doomsday Has Been Cancelled,* Peace Press, 1978 (popular book)

Simon, "Resources, Population, Environment: An Oversupply of False Bad News," *Science* 208:1431–1437, 1980

The Peptider, a manual solid-phase peptide synthesizer, ready to use, $2,450 (Peninsula Laboratories, Inc., PO Box 1111, San Carlos, CA 94070—write for free catalog of supplies)

Cox, *Planning of Experiments,* Wiley, 1958

"Black Holes, Monsters That Eat Space and Time," (½ hour television special), hosted by Durk, written by Durk and Sandy, scientific consultation by Durk and Sandy, special effects consultation by Sandy and Durk, stunt designs by Sandy and Durk, produced by Walt Disney Educational Media, Burbank, Calif. (available on videotape or film for rent)

Hicks, *Fundamental Concepts in the Design of Experiments,* 2nd ed.," Holt, Rinehart, and Winston, 1973

Peng, *The Design and Analysis of Scientific Experiments,* Addison Wesley, 1967

Edmunds and Adams, "Clocked Cell Cycle Clocks," *Science* 211:1002–1013, 1981
    [Here is a testable hypothesis for the mechanism of action of biological clocks; we must admit that we didn't expect this sort of hypothesis to appear so soon. Below is a figure from this paper, showing a proposed clock structure, including DNA tape loops and moving parts.]

WIENER ANALYSIS REFERENCES

Pearson, Durk J. in *Study of Advanced Techniques for Determining Long-Term Performance of Components,* TRW Final Report No. 16568-6028-R000, prepared for Jet Propulsion Laboratory, Pasadena Cal. 91103, under NASA contract NAS 7-782, pp. 3–10 to 3–23 (March 1973)

Fender, Dr. Derek, "New Eye-Saver," *The California Tech,* October 3, 1975, pp. 2–3 (university newspaper)

"Dimensional Analysis," *Electro Technology Reference Series,* August 1962

Wiener, N., *Nonlinear Problems in Random Theory,* Massachusetts Institute of Technology Press, 1958

Cumming, I. G., and May, R., "Using Correlation to Identify Process Dynamics," *Instruments and Control Systems,* July 1972, pp. 59–61

Lee, Y. W., *Statistical Theory of Communication,* Wiley, New York, 1960

Bose, A. G., *Technical Report 309* (Research Laboratory of Electronics, Massachusetts Institute of Technology, Cambridge, 1956); George D. A., *Technical Report 355* (Research Laboratory of Electronics, Massachusetts Institute of Technology, Cambridge, 1959); Barrett, J. A., *J. Electron Control 15* 567 (1963)

Wiener, N., *Extrapolation, Interpolation, and Smoothing of Stationary Time Series* (textbook)

Anderson, G. C., Perry, M. A., "A Calibrated Real-Time Correlator / Averager / Probability Analyzer," *Hewlett-Packard Journal,* November, 1969

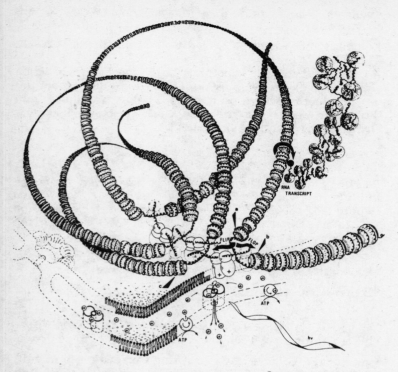

Diagram of a chronogene segment, one possible molecular basis for metering time in longer period cellular oscillations. Transcriptional units of chromosomal DNA, wound around their nucleosomes, loop out from protein complexes that anchor them by their inverted-repeat cruciforms to the nuclear envelope and cross-link them to other units at paired genetic loci. At dawn, light-absorbing pigments in the membrane trigger the opening of ion gates that collapse a membrane potential accumulated by ATP (adenosine triphosphate)-driven pumps; the resulting transient change in electric field reprograms the time-metering transcriptional sequence by switching all the protein links to the flip mode. Upon completion of transcription of the top loop (*a*), transcription is initiated on the adjacent unit (*c*) in response to a (torsional?) signal transmitted across the link rather than on the next unit (*b*) in the tandem sequence (as it would in the flop mode). As the membrane potential restabilizes, the flip mode decays so that the only effective switching is mediated by the link at the end of the transcriptional unit being actively transcribed at the time that the transitions between light and dark occur. In this way, long segments of tandemly arranged units are either inserted into or are deleted from a coupled transcriptional circuit at dusk or dawn to generate the advancing of delaying adjustments that serve to synchronize the clock with the earth's rotation. The genetically programmed siting of the links ensures that the prcise loop lengths required to effect these phase shifts occur at the right places in the multiple-path transcriptional circuit.

Anderson, G. C., Finnie, B. W., Roberts, G.T., "Pseudo-Random and Random Test Signals," *Hewlett-Packard Journal,* September 1967

Marmarelis, P. Z. and Ken-Ichi Naka, "White-Noise Analysis of a Neuron Chain: An Application of the Wiener Theory," *Science* Vol. 175, March 1972, pp. 1276–1278

Lee, Y. W., and Schetzen, M., *Quarterly Progress Report* 60 (Research Laboratory of Electronics, Massachusetts Institute of Technology, Cambridge, 1961)

Shieh, L. S., Navarro, J. M., and Yates, Robert, "Multivariable Systems Identification via Frequency Responses, ' " *Proc. of the IEEE,* August 1974, pp. 1169–1171.

Chandrashekar, M. and Kesavan, H. K., "Network Sensitivity Simplified," *Proc. of the IEEE,* Vol. 62 No. 8, August 1974, pp. 1179–1180

Bussgang, J. J., Ehrman, L., and Graham, J. W., "Analysis of Non-Linear Systems with Multiple Inputs," *Proc. of the IEEE,* Vol. 62, No. 8, August 1974, pp. 1088–1119

Bendat, J. S., *Fundamentals of Time Series Analysis,* published by Time/Data, 1974

Lee, Y. W., and Schetzen, M., "Measurement of the Wiener Kernels of a Nonlinear System by Cross-correlation," *International Journal of Control,* Vol. 2, pp. 237–254, 1965

Schaffner, M. R., "A Procedure for Describing Discrete Processes," Presented at 10th Allerton Conference on Circuit & System Theory, Illinois, October 1972

Bekey, G. A., *System Identification—An Introduction and A Survey,* USC, School of Engineering, CSc-18, 1970.

Buell, J., Kalaba, R., Ruspini, E., & Yakush, A., *A Program for Identification of Linear Systems,* USC, School of Engineering, *Technical Report No. 71-46,* December 1971

Marmarelis, P. Z., "Nonlinear Identification of Bioneuronal Systems Through White-Noise Stimulation," California Institute of Technology, *Paper 6-4*

Marmarelis, P. Z., and Naka, Ken-Ichi, "Identification of Multi-Input Biological Systems," *IEEE Transactions on Biomedical Engineering* Vol. BME-21, No. 2, March 1974, pp. 88–101

Heetderks, W. J. and Williams, W. J., "Partition of Gross Peripheral Nerve Activity into Single Unit Responses by Correlation Techniques," *Science,* Vol. 188, 25 April 1975, pp. 373–375.

Lipson, E. D., "White Noise Analysis of *Phycomyces* Light Growth Response system—
        I. Normal Intensity Range;
       II. Extended Intensity Ranges;
     III. Photomutants Intensity Ranges

Katzenelson, Jacob and Gould, Leonard A., "The Design of Nonlinear Filters and Control Systems, Part I," *Information and Control,* Vol. 5, 1962, pp. 108–143

Katzenelson, Jacob and Gould, Leonard A., "The Design of Nonlinear Filters and Control Systems, Part II," *Information and Control,* Vol. 7, 1964, pp. 117–145

Thomas, E. J., "Some Considerations on the Application of the Volterra Representation of Nonlinear Networks to Adaptive Echo Cancellers," *Bell System Technical Journal,* Vol. 50, no. 8, October 1971, pp. 2797–2805

Swets, John A., "The Relative Operating Characteristic in Psychology," *Science,* vol. 182, December 1973, pp. 990–1000.

Appendix C: Computerized Biomedical Literature Search Service

Kelner, *Searching the Medlars Database: A Practical Guide for Profilers,* (Scotia, N.Y.: Bibliographic Retrieval Services [702 Corporation Park, 12302])

Appendix E: What Is the Government Doing about Aging Research?

SOME COMMENTS AND REFERENCES CONCERNING FREEDOM OF CHOICE FOR PRESCRIPTION DRUGS

The central concepts in our **freedom of choice** proposal include: rechartering the FDA as an advisory—not regulatory—agency with respect to prescription drugs, biomedical devices, and uses; clear marking of non-FDA approved prescription drugs, devices, and uses (on the product's label, package insert, and promotional materials); **split labels,** inserts, and promotional materials for non-FDA approved drugs, devices, and uses wherein both the pharmaceutical firm and the FDA state their own separate opinions; an **opt-out** form, waiving the FDA's protection, which an adult must sign before he or she may purchase FDA unapproved drugs; and another **opt-out** form with which an adult may waive civil lawsuit recourse, except in cases of criminal fraud.

NOTE THAT AN INDIVIDUAL WOULD AUTOMATICALLY CONTINUE TO RECEIVE FDA PROTECTION UNTIL HE OR SHE OPTED-OUT OF THIS PROTECTION IN WRITING.

DID YOU KNOW THAT CONSUMERS HAD FREEDOM OF CHOICE IN DRUG PURCHASES UNTIL 1938?

Before 1938, consumers had nearly complete freedom of choice in their drug purchases. Anyone could simply walk into a drug store and purchase any desired drug (except certain narcotics specified under the Harrison Anti-Narcotics Act of 1914)—no prescriptions were required. In fact, prescription sales in pharmacies accounted for only about ¼ of the drugs sold there.

Consumers obtained only about 5 percent of their drugs through doctors before the Depression. In accord with that economic fact, drug advertising in the 1920s appeared in popular magazines and newspapers aimed at <u>consumers,</u> not doctors (about 5 percent of ads were run for doctors). Consumers, not doctors or regulators, chose the drugs they bought and used. Drug laws at that time were designed to provide protection against fraud, not to control drug purchases by consumers.

One of the pressures for reform of the laws governing the drug industry was the change in attitude by New Deal regulators toward consumer protection. These regulators had little confidence in the marketplace to provide safety to drug consumers and proposed to substitute regulatory force for the voluntary processes of the market. In fact, the 1938 drug law passed Congress following a drug disaster in which about 75 people died from ingesting a toxic solvent containing the sulfa drug, sulfanilamide. As happens so often with governmental "reform," the final impetus to the new drug law was more a matter of emotional hysterical reaction than of dispassionate thinking about the problem.

The 1938 Federal Food, Drug, and Cosmetic Act creating the FDA required prescriptions for some drugs which could be freely purchased prior to the new law, required that labels provide specific information about offered drugs, and gave the FDA the power to prevent the marketing of any drug not meeting the FDA's safety criteria. Even though the FDA was committed to assuring the safety of drugs and required that information about them be supplied to consumers, drug purchasers were no longer free to choose the drugs they wanted to buy. The FDA decided that consumers should not be allowed to choose some drugs, even with full information and even though this was a break with a long prior tradition. As a result, consumers would have to obtain a prescription from a physician before they could obtain some drugs. "The shift from assuming a capable consumer to assuming an incompetent consumer was made within the FDA within six months of the Federal Food, Drug, and Cosmetic Act's passage." (Temin, 1979) Thus, we see the philosophical basis for greatly restricting the freedom of choice and information of drug consumers, a trend that was to continue to the present, particularly accelerated with the passage of the 1962 Kefauver Amendments.

Before 1914 and the Harrison Act which placed very strict federal regulations on opiates (heroin, morphine, opium, etc.), anyone could walk into any drugstore and purchase all the heroin (or morphine, opium, etc.) he or she desired for about $10 an ounce. No prescription or identification was required, and there were no legal age limits. Opiates were cheap and ubiquitous; they were carried in many grocery and dry goods stores and sold by thousands of mail order firms. The best estimate of the number of opiate addicts in the U.S. at this time is about 215,000. (Remember that there was no reason to smuggle opiates into the U.S. so the import records are quite accurate.) (Kolb and Du Mez, "The Prevalence and Trend of Drug Addiction in the United States and Factors Influencing It," U.S. Public Health Service, *Reprint No. 924, 1924.*) With ultra-cheap $10 per ounce heroin universally available, about 0.2 percent of the U.S. population were opiate addicts. Of course, with these free market conditions, there was no addict crime problem. Heroin was used for pain, not as a criminal way of life. Back in the bad old days, medicine could help much less than now; for example, if you had a bad case of arthritis or inoperable cancer, you either accepted the terrible incurable pain or you used opiates.

As of June 1981, legal uncut (pure) heroin costs about $50 per ounce, while black market uncut heroin costs about $7,000 to $12,000 per ounce. Of course, opiate addiction is now so expensive that it is the cause of most violent crime in the streets. According to the BNDD (Bureau of Narcotics and Dangerous Drugs) and the NIMH (National Institute of Mental Health) there were about 250,000 to 345,000 opiate addicts in 1971, or about 0.1 to 0.16 percent of the U.S. population, compared to about 0.2 percent with no laws whatsoever! Of course, there are no reliable figures for black market heroin imports; these figures are strictly for the addicts who repeatedly get in trouble with the law. The actual number of opiate addicts might easily be twice as large, or about 0.2 to 0.3 percent—just about what it was when heroin was a free market drug. The legal prohibition has not protected nonaddicts, though it has greatly increased their chances of becoming victims of violent crime, and it has not helped the opiate addicts either. It has, however, made billions of dollars for organized crime and for crooked narcotics agents. See The Consumers Union book *Licit and Illicit Drugs* for a real eye opener—we honest folk would be better off with heroin back on the free market. If heroin should be available on the free market, what excuse is there for prohibiting thymosin?

We would like to thank Professor of Economics Dr. David Friedman for his extensive constructive criticisms of Appendix E: What Is the Government Doing About Aging Research? His comments have greatly improved this section. Of course, any errors are our own responsibility.

We would like to thank Professor of Economics Dr. Sam Peltzman for his extensive econometric analysis of the costs and benefits of FDA regulations. The results of this analysis were a hell of a shock to everyone, including Dr. Peltzman. Let us hope that the FDA will never be the same.

We would like to thank Nobel laureate Professor of Economics Dr. Milton Friedman and Professor of Economics Dr. Rose Friedman for doing so much to make it possible to talk in public about freedom of choice and free markets without being considered nuts.

We would like to thank Economics Professor Dr. Harold Demsetz for his magnificent address to the 1969 YAF National Convention where he introduced us to the concept of the bureaucrat as a bad wizard rather than a bad man.

Brecher, Edward, and Editors of *Consumer Reports, Licit & Illicit Drugs,* Little, Brown, and Company, 1972

"FDA's Goyan: Bury the Hatchet," *Chemical Marketing Reporter,* 7 April 1980

Senator Alan Cranston, "Coming: Longer Lifespans," *Reader's Digest,* Jan. 1979 (popular media)

Peltzman, Sam, *Regulation of Pharmaceutical Innovation,* American Enterprise Institute, 1974, Washington DC, $3.00 pb.

Peltzman, Sam, "An Evaluation of Consumer Protection Legislation: The 1962 Drug Amendments," *J. Political Econ.,* pp. 1049–91, Sept.–Oct. 1973

Landau, Richard, (Ed.) *Regulating New Drugs,* University of Chicago Center for Policy Study, 1973, $5.25 pb, see particularly pp. 113–211 by Peltzman

Temin, Peter, "The Origin of Compulsory Drug Prescriptions," *The Journ. of Law & Econ.* 22(1):91–105, April 1979

Consumers Union (publishers of *Consumer Reports*) is a private consumer safety and efficacy testing organization supported by consumers who purchase their information, 256 Washington St., Mt. Vernon, NY 10550

"Behind the UL Label," *IEEE Spectrum,* pp. 65–66, January 1973. The Underwriters' Laboratories as a model of market protection—UL is a private organization set up by insurance companies to perform safety and effectiveness testing of a huge number of items from safes and fire alarms to TV sets and toasters.

"Sulfinpyrazone lowers death rate in heart attacks," *New England J. Med.* 298:289–295, 1978

Rand, Ayn, *Atlas Shrugged,* Random House, 1957 (This is a book about the individual versus the collective. The book is still compelling and its predictions remain chillingly realistic. If you read it, you may find that it changes your philosophical outlook.) (popular book)

Ross, Irwin, "Why the Underground Economy is Booming," *Fortune,* 9 October, 1978 (popular magazine)

Bucher, "Government regulations—an area to shirk responsibility in," *Trends in Pharmacological Sciences* 1(7):1–2, 1980

Grant, Richard, *The Incredible Bread Machine,* Bray, 1966 (popular book)

Friedman, David, *The Machinery of Freedom,* Arlington House, 1978, (popular book)

Friedman, Milton, (Nobel laureate, economics) and Friedman, Rose, *Free To Choose,* Harcourt Brace Jovanovich, 1980 (popular book)

> *"Experience should teach us to be most on our guard to protect liberty when the government's purposes are beneficial. Men born to freedom are naturally alert to repel invasion of their liberty by evil-minded rulers. The greatest dangers to liberty lurk in insidious encroachment by men of zeal, well-meaning but without understanding."*
> —*Justice Louis Brandeis (1928),*
> *as quoted in the Friedmans'* Free To Choose

Hayek, Friedrich A. (Nobel laureate, economics), *The Road to Serfdom,* University of Chicago Press, 1944 (popular book)

"No Time to Confuse, A Critique of the Final Report of the Energy Policy Project of the Ford Foundation: *A Time to Choose* America's Energy Future," Institute for Contemporary Studies, 1975

Alchian, Armen A., *Economic Forces At Work*, Liberty Press, 1977

Szasz, Thomas, *Ceremonial Chemistry: The Ritual Persecution of Drugs, Addicts, & Pushers*, Doubleday, 1974

von Mises, Ludwig, *The Anti-Capitalistic Mentality*, Van Nostrand, 1956

von Mises, Ludwig, *Bureaucracy*, Yale University Press, 1962

von Mises, Ludwig, *Human Action: A Treatise on Economics*, Contemporary Books, 1966 (see especially the section on socialism, where von Mises proves that it is impossible to rationally allocate resources under socialism in the absence of a marketplace to establish price relationships)

Manne and Miller, *Auto Safety Regulation: The Cure or the Problem?*, Thomas Horton & Daughters, 1976

Dawkins, *The Selfish Gene*, Oxford Univ. Press, 1976

Darwin, Charles, *Origin of the Species*, University Library, 1972

Gilliland, Alexis, *The Iron Law of Bureaucracy*, (cartoons), Loompanics Unlimited, 1979

"The Prisoner," a TV series starring Patrick McGoohan; about the individual versus the collective, highly recommended

Hofmann, Albert, *LSD: My Problem Child*, McGraw-Hill, 1980 (see the July 1981 issue of *OMNI* for an interview with Dr. Hofmann)

DEVO, "Freedom of Choice" (rock album), Warner Bros. Records, Inc., 1980

Anderson, Poul, *Trader to the Stars*, Berkeley Medallion, 1964 (meet the twenty-first century stellar trader Nicholas Van Rijn)

Russell, Eric Frank, *The Great Explosion*, Panther, 1962 (what happens when a star drive is invented and half the population leaves old bureaucrat-ridden Earth)

Posner, Richard A., *Taxation by Regulation*, Reprint 218, The Brookings Institution, 1971

Wilson, E. O., *Sociobiology: The New Synthesis*, Harvard Univ. Press, 1975

Quote by Walter Oi in his "Economics of Product Safety," *The Bell Journal of Economics and Management Science,* Spring 1973, pg. 27

"Illness, injury rates of chemical workers . . .", *Chemical Engineering,* pg. 19, 29 June 1981

"Chemical Safety Study . . . ," *Chemical Marketing Reporter* 219:3, 50; 29 June 1981

Ricardo-Campbell, Rita, *Food Safety Regulation: A Study of the Use and Limitations of Cost-Benefit Analysis,* American Enterprise Institute for Public Policy Research, Washington, DC, 1974

Goodman, John, *National Health Insurance and the Aged Population,* Center for Health Policy Studies, University of Dallas, Irving, Texas 75061 [This working paper suggests that there is a greater systematic bias against extensive medical care for the aged in countries which have relatively larger governmental support for medical care. In other words, if you are aged, national health "insurance" appears to be bad for your health, and is clearly associated with increased mortality rates among the old.]

Milgram, Stanley, *Obedience to Authority: An Experimental View,* Harper & Row, 1974 [". . . ordinary people, simply doing their jobs, and without any particular hostility on their part, can become agents in a terrible destructive process. Moreover, even when the destructive effects of their work become patently clear, and they are asked to carry out actions incompatible with fundamental standards of morality, relatively few people have the resources needed to resist authority."]

"Consensus on CAT Scans," news item by G. Kolata, *Science* 214:1327–8, 18 Dec. 1981
    A National Institute of Health panel concluded that there are too few—not too many—CAT brain scanners, and that CAT scanners reduce medical costs, not increase them. Furthermore, the legal costs of getting a permit to purchase a CAT scanner may cost as much as the CAT scanner itself and there is no guarantee that these huge legal expenditures will succeed in obtaining the necessary permit.

"Cleaning up the Clean Air Act," news item by Elliot Marshal, *Science* 214:1328–9, 18 Dec. 1981

According to a Brookings Institution report by L. B. Lave and G. S. Oman, good luck, not good regulation, reduced pollution in the 1970s. Current regulations are extremely costly, arbitrary, misdirected, and inefficient.

"Public Willing to Take Some Cancer Risks," a Lou Harris poll reported in the October 1980 issue of *FDA Consumer*

In this poll, 46 percent of the public surveyed thought people should be allowed to decide for themselves whether to use food substances with possible cancer risks. Only 10 percent thought all food substances linked with cancer should be banned.

Appendix F: Cryonics

Smith, *Current Trends in Cryobiology,* Plenum Press, 1970

Ashwood-Smith & Farrant, eds., *Low Temperature Preservation in Medicine and Biology,* University Park Press, 1980

Rinfret and LaSalle, editors, *Cryogenic Preservation of Cell Cultures,* National Academy of Sciences, 1975

Cryonics organizations:

Trans Time, Inc., 1122 Spruce St., Berkeley, CA 94707
(415) 525-7114, Arthur Quaife, President

The Alcor Society for Solid State Hypothermia, Box 312, Glendale, CA 91209,
(213) 956-6042, Allen McDaniels, President

The Cryonics Association, 24041 Stratford, Oak Park, MI 48237
(313) 398-6624, Robert C. W. Ettinger, President

Appendix H: How Long Do Humans and Other Animals Live?

Mazess and Forman, "Longevity and Age Exaggeration in Vilcabamba, Ecuador," *J. Geront.* 34(1);94–98 (1979)

Bada, racemization of L-aspartic acid measurements, Scripps Institute, La Jolla, Calif.

M. L. Jones, *Life Span in Mammals*, Zoological Society of San Diego, P.O. Box 551, San Diego, CA 92112, 1978

Appendix L: Some Case Histories

Kielholz, editor, *A Therapeutic Approach to the Psyche Via the Beta-adrenergic System*, University Park Press, 1978

Sloan and Weir, "Nomograms for Prediction of Body Density and Total Body Fat from Skinfold Measurements," *J. Appl. Physiol.* 28(2):221–222, (1970)

Barnes and Galton, *Hypothyroidism*, Crowell, 1976 (popular book)

Kinsey, Pomeroy, Martin, and Gebhard, *Sexual Behavior in the Human Female*, Saunders, 1953

Kinsey, Pomeroy, Martin, and Gebhard, *Sexual Behavior in the Human Male*, Saunders, 1948

Hirshleifer, Jack, "Economics from a Biological Viewpoint," *The Journal of Law & Economics* XX (1):1–52, April 1977 [As the author says, the study of biology can be regarded as "Nature's economy." "Fundamental concepts like scarcity, competition, equilibrium, and specialization play similar roles in both spheres of inquiry." Highly recommended.]

Wheeler, Jack, *The Adventurer's Guide*, David McKay Co, Inc, New York, New York [How you, too, can experience a real adventure.]

Money, John, *Love & Love Sickness*, Johns Hopkins University Press, 1980

Tennov, Dorothy, *Love and Limerence*, Stein and Day, 1979

A VERY SPECIAL THANK YOU

We want to offer credit where credit is due; without our trusty triple-brained silicon servant word processor, we would never have been able to finish this book. Even if somehow we had managed to complete it, it would have been three years out of date, a very serious deficiency when knowledge in this field is doubling every five years or so. Thanks to three Z-80 based microcomputers, our book has been regularly updated up to our final deadline for completion (July 1981).

Why did we go to all this expense and trouble to have a word processor system, anyway? Our first reason for getting one was to help us write the book, which we had started earlier (aaargh) without one. Anyone who has ever written anything longer than a postcard knows how inconvenient using a typewriter can be. If you make a mistake, it's a hassle. If you want to reorganize your writing, insert a sentence, change the margins, increase the number of lines per inch on the page, or substitute a better word for one you used throughout your writing, you'll just have to retype the whole thing. Not so with a word processor. Its special software turns our computer terminal into a very talented typewriter that can be easily made to jump through hoops. The use of such a sophisticated device is not confined to professional writers, however. We use ours to write all our letters as well, a task at which it produces far more satisfactory results than ordinary typing. We compose the letters right at the terminal, using Word-Star® to change, add, delete, embellish, reorganize, and otherwise make our letters and publications say exactly what we want them to say. We often even change a single word that wasn't quite right. We thought, when we ordered our computer system, that we would be able to write more rapidly than before. That has indeed turned out to be the case. Of even more importance (and to our surprise), the quality of our writing has substantially improved as well. A word processor is the writing perfectionist's dream.

Our word processor system is configured as follows. We recommend it without reservation. We wouldn't write a thousand word magazine column without it. Three of our friends are professional writers; once they tried our system for about fifteen minutes apiece, they couldn't conceive of going back to the old way—so they each promptly purchased a clone of our word processing system. The total cost of the system below is about $7,000. If you earn your living as a professional writer, the economic payback period (from improved quality and quantity of output) will probably be under six months.

SYSTEM CONFIGURATION

Northstar® computer with 64 K byte Northstar® static memory with parity error detect and with two double sided double density quad capacity minifloppy disc drives—an S-100 bus Z-80 CPU system.

Spare minifloppy disc drive (these are mechanical gadgets—they have to be sent in for realignment every now and then so a professional user should have a spare).

Televideo® 920C terminal (with a keyboard laid out like the IBM Selectric® and an additional row of user-defined keys and its own Z-80 CPU smarts).

NEC-5520 Spinwriter®. This is a 55 character per second office electric typewriter quality, heavy duty, very reliable computer printer. It prints bidirectionally and has both horizontal and vertical microspace motion for microspaced justification, subscripts, superscripts, etc. It, too, has its own Z-80 CPU so that the Z-80 CPU (microprocessor central processing unit, the heart of the computer, on a single silicon chip) of the Northstar® can spend its time doing elaborate print formatting instead of having to attend to the picky little details of running the printer. Our three friends purchased the NEC-5510, which has no keyboard and, therefore, is a few hundred dollars less expensive. This is a good idea; we never have used the NEC-5520's keyboard.

Our operating system software is CP/M 2.2®. This program takes care of the nitty gritty of creating and accessing files on the magnetic mini-floppy discs. Make sure that your vendor is willing to teach you how to use the features called STAT, PIP, DIR, LIST, and COPY. Although there are many other features, you do not need to use them for word processing. Beware of the CP/M® manuals; they were written for programmers, not for writers.

Our word processing software is Wordstar® (Micropro). What you see on the TV screen of the TVI-920C smart terminal is what you will see on the printed page; the display is formatted as you edit it, unlike most other word processor programs, where editing and print layout and control are done separately in two stages. Wordstar® is amazingly self-instructing and self-prompting, yet these aids and prompts can be made to go away as you learn to use it by using it.

IMPORTANT: Unless you are a real computer hacker, be sure to purchase everything from one computer store and have them guarantee in writing that they will integrate the system, get it up and running in the word processor mode, and check its function. You want what is called a "turnkey" system—one you simply plug in and turn on. You don't want to have to learn about the rest of CP/M. . . .

Although we have quite a few computers already, each of us has just bought another, an Osborne-1® Z-80 portable microcomputer system. It comes with CP/M 2.2®, Wordstar®, and lots of other software, all integrated and ready to go for $1,795, printer extra. An NEC 5510 formed character (like an office typewriter) printer will cost about $2,500. The Epson MX-80® dot matrix printer at about $500 is less expensive, portable, and a very good buy, but it does not have the outstanding type quality of the NEC-5510. The Osborne-1® has smaller disc drive capacity and a much smaller video screen (for the sake of portability) than our current system, though larger disc drives and big video screens can be purchased as options. We personally recommend a 12 inch screen on a monitor having at least 20 megahertz bandwidth. The screen should be black and white or black and green, not multicolored.

May all these firms and the designers of their fine products live long and prosper. And may you live long and prosper, too!

> Durk Pearson
> Sandy Shaw
> July 1981
> Los Angeles

APPENDIX L:
Some Case Histories

The case histories we describe here do not involve people living to extended life spans because there has not been enough time yet for that to happen. Animal experiments provide our best evidence for the increased life span which some people alive today may achieve. These case histories are about people who used nutrients and prescription drugs to alter some aspect of their biochemistry to make their body functions and biochemistry more like those of healthy young people.

Case histories by themselves do not prove anything because they are not statistically representative, and because they are subject to human bias. Don't forget that a placebo (inactive substance) can temporarily produce the same effects as morphine for about 40 percent of subjects in pain who are told that the substance is morphine. In addition, responses to nutrients and drugs are individual due to biochemical differences between people. Case histories are anecdotal evidence and, therefore, should be used only as supplementary material to animal experiments and double blind controlled clinical studies (see "How Do You Know Who's Right?").

Within these limitations, however, case histories can provide valuable leads. The tradition of self-experimentation is a noble one, but also one in which caution should be excercised, both in regards to what you do to yourself and in the interpretation of results.

As you read these case histories, keep the following in mind:

1.) Each person chose his or her own supplements, his own dose level, and frequency of use.

2.) The persons involved in these self-experiments do not necessarily endorse anything beyond whatever endorsement may be explicitly attributed to them in the description of their case history.

3.) These are self-reports, some of which are supplemented with clinical laboratory test data.

4.) The case histories often refer to a single substance of interest, but subjects may also have been taking other supplements at the same time.

5.) Do not assume that because one of these case histories sounds like a condition you have, that you have the same thing, or that it should be treated in the same way. Do not be careless with your health. Be sure to consult with your physician. An incorrect self diagnosis could kill you.

6.) These are not complete medical case histories; the only items reported here are those that have particular relevance to this book. All of the people discussed here have had many requirements for ordinary medical care. Do not permit these anecdotal reports to convince you that vitamins, minerals, amino acids, other nutrients, antioxidants, or whatever, are panaceas. Nearly all of the medical problems of these self selected experimental subjects were dealt with satisfactorily by "conventional" medicine, and are not reported here. We believe that the information in this book can help you to maintain your health, but it is not a substitute for a physician's care.

THE CASE OF SANDY'S HEARING AND HYDERGINE®

Sandy's hearing suffered severe damage as a result of 6600 rads of radiation through her aural-oral region following the removal of a malignant salivary gland (parotid) tumor in 1971. Severe tinnitus (noises) developed in both ears, and was particularly bad in the right ear (on the side where the tumor had developed and which received the higher dose of radiation). Sandy's ability to hear high frequencies was severely damaged in both ears, but especially in the right one. (Incidentally, her radiologist did not advise her of this severe side effect of her radiation treatment.)

Sandy had been using moderate doses of a few antioxidants on an irregular basis for about two years before she discovered the tumor (which both her surgeon and the case's pathologist told her was a very slow growing type, a mucoepidermoid carcinoma, that she had probably had for at least 12 years and possibly from birth). The tumor showed up (became noticeable as a palpable lump) following a year of deep depression Sandy experienced because of unemployment and limerence problems. When Sandy found out about the tumor, she immediately began taking several grams of vitamin C and 3000 I.U. of vitamin E each day.

The first step of the treatment was to locate a surgeon specializing in cancer who had extensive experience in facial surgery and parotid tumors. Prompt surgery by an expert is of great importance in most solid cancers. Since many cancers are immunosuppressive, it is important to get rid of as much of the tumor as possible, even if all the neoplastic tissue can not be removed. In Sandy's case, the cancer was highly invasive and had penetrated her nervous system. The surgeon carefully dissected out the facial nerves on the right side of Sandy's face, separating them from the cancer as much as possible, and folding them aside while removing the underlying cancerous tissue. This was where the surgeon's experience and skill were vital. He knew that the cancer had penetrated too deeply along the nerve tracts for him to be likely to get all of it, even if he removed as much tissue as possible. Moreover, he realized that if he went too far in trying to dissect the cancer from the facial nerves, that the nerves would be destroyed, resulting in the permanent paralysis of the right side of Sandy's face, impairing her speech and freezing the right side of her face into a grotesque immobile mask. (This sort of outcome is extremely depressing to a patient, and of course such depression further impairs the immune system.) His judgment and skill were both splendid; Sandy's face regained much of its mobility within a week, and all of it within about a month, considerably faster than expected, and he removed most, and probably nearly all, but definitely not quite all of the cancer.

The pathologist, an expert in diagnosing cancers via tissue samples which were sent to him a bit at a time throughout the operation, had provided prompt real time guidance to the surgeon as the operation progressed. The extent of the surgical procedure was guided by the pathologist's prompt microscopic observations of these tissue samples. The success of the treatment depended on the skills of both the surgeon and the pathologist; if you have cancer, it will be well worth your while to seek out a particularly experienced pathologist with the help of your surgeon. The pathologist concurred that a small portion of the cancer was inoperable, and he stated that it was of a type that had a good chance of responding to radiation therapy.

In 1971, parotid cancer victims were generally treated by either surgery or radiation, but relatively few people had been treated with both. Sandy agreed to undergo what at that time was considered an experimental therapy of combined surgery and radiation.

She continued using the doses of antioxidants mentioned above, as well as smaller doses of some other antioxidants during radiation therapy (**CAUTION:** using large doses of antioxidants during radiation treatment can reduce the amount of damage done by the radiation to both normal and cancer cells. Such usage is not recommended to anyone undergoing radiation therapy; it is still strictly experimental. We had found some evidence in the scientific literature that these antioxidants had a greater radioprotective effect on normal cells than cancer cells, and the radiologist had initially told us that x-ray treatment would be continued until the x-ray burn became intolerable, rather than to a fixed total dose. Frankly, our course of action was a gamble made on far less data than we would normally find acceptable, due to the prognosis. Sandy's surgeon said that the tumor was highly invasive, that it had infiltrated her nervous system, that significant portions of the tumor were inoperable, and hence the prognosis was "poor." The pathologist gave a prognosis of "very poor." A literature search made at this time on this condition indicated a 0 to 15 percent 5 year survival rate.)

The radiologist didn't think that a torso shield to protect the thymus gland was necessary or useful, had no idea whatsoever what the thymic radiation dose would be, and refused either to calculate or to measure it on a phantom (a radiologically equivalent dummy), although we offered to pay whatever he wanted for this extra work. He thought the thymus to be unimportant, wouldn't provide a film badge dosimeter, and wouldn't provide a thymus shield. So Sandy took along an old lead radiation shield apron (from Durk's MIT days) and the radiologist permitted her to use it ("Well, it won't hurt you."), although he made it clear how little he thought of our medical knowledge. We knew how little he knew of the immune system. He did not have a good understanding of the basic biochemical mechanisms of his therapy, and he had surprisingly little knowledge of free radicals and substances modulating their effects. He did, however, know how to calculate and deliver the proper x-ray dose, and we had the perspective to realize that <u>that</u> was the professional service that we contracted for. In other areas, his advice was welcomed and considered, but not accepted as gospel. We also sought our own second opinions, as well as those of other scientists and physicians. Most of these additional medical opinions were found by computerized literature searches of MEDLARS, some by manual literature searches, and a few obtained by personal interviews with medical specialists.

Sandy's radiologist warned her beforehand that after 7 to 10 days (about 2200 rads) of radiation, she would experience a complete loss of ability to taste which would slowly return after the completion of the radiation treatments. This loss of taste perception didn't actually take place for 23 days and was less than a complete loss, much to the amazement of the radiologist and oncologist. The radiologist also told Sandy that after about 2200 rads, she would definitely develop a painful bright red radiation burn on the right side of her face. The radiation burn never appeared, not even after 6600 rads, much to his amazement. (He had told Sandy that she could take megavitamins if she wished, but that they would do nothing whatsoever. In fact, he snickered. In spite of his snicker, the laws of physics worked anyway, and his x-rays inflicted their free radical damage on the cancer, further reducing the tumor mass.) We think this delay and reduction in radiation effects is most likely due to the radioprotectant properties of the antioxidants. This factor of about three increase in x-ray radiation protection to normal cells (as measured by loss of taste and resistance to radiation burn) is similar in magnitude to the increased resistance Sandy, Durk, and several other experimental subjects have to burns from solar ultraviolet light.

We realized that solid tumors usually have a poor response to chemotherapy, that chemotherapy would be likely to seriously impair Sandy's immune system, and that her immune system would have to destroy every remaining cancer cell if she was to survive. (Chemotherapy can cure certain types of cancers, such as Hodgkin's disease, but in most cases, it slows the growth but does not completely destroy the cancer. If this is the case, chemotherapy can guarantee some extra time—usually a few months to a couple of years—often at the expense of an impaired immune system which seriously compromises whatever chances you have for long-term survival.)

After we had had the tumor mass reduced as much as possible by surgery and radiation therapy, we proceeded to stimulate Sandy's immune system. In addition to the immunostimulant vitamins, Sandy was inoculated with a wide variety of commercial vaccines designed for immunization against contagious diseases, including smallpox, polio, yellow fever, typhoid, tetanus, whooping cough, and others—just as if she were planning to tour the jungles, outbacks, and boondocks of the world. (**CAUTION**: Although there are some reports in the literature of positive effects from this approach, there are also a few reports of particular immunizations, such as smallpox, causing occasional increases in tumor growth rate. We were in a position where our normal standards of safety and efficacy were inappropriate, to say nothing of the FDA's standards. This is a good example of why any particular safety and efficacy criterion cannot be applied to all cases, as the FDA insists upon doing.)

We had hoped that within two or three months we would be able to provoke an immunological response against the remaining tumor tissue. Although about five weeks after these inoculations, there was a possible reaction (fever, malaise, aches and pains, and redness, swelling, and tenderness at the site of the tumor), we had no ready access to clinical laboratory tests to measure immune responses and, hence, no proof that this was in fact an immunological response provoked by these vaccinations. Nevertheless, Sandy is alive and well, with no indications of tumor survival ten years after its initial discovery. **Do not use this case history as a model for your own cancer therapy, even if you have exactly the same type of tumor. We did this work in 1971, and now consider this approach to be crude, more hazardous, and less effective than what we would do now. The basic concepts remain the same, however: reduce the tumor mass with surgery and, when appropriate, radiation, followed by immunostimulation. Our** current approach to immunostimulation can be found elsewhere in this book. Any such therapy should be closely monitored by clinical laboratory tests and supervised by a clinical research-oriented physician.

Sandy had difficulty understanding speech after the development of the radiation damage. She purchased three hearing aids, which were helpful, but her hearing was still badly impaired. As a professional scientist, she found this particularly detrimental when she attended scientific conferences and found it very difficult to understand what people said. She spent a significant amount of her time at these conferences forming hypotheses about the verbal contents of conversations and lectures. Then Sandy began using Hydergine®. At first, using 3–6 milligrams of Hydergine® per day for several months, Sandy didn't notice any changes in her hearing. Then, Sandy stepped up her dosage of Hydergine® to 12 milligrams per day in response to the reports of Kris Dean concerning his own hearing and Hydergine® use (Kris's case history follows). In a few weeks, she began to notice small sounds, especially high frequency ones, that she hadn't noticed before. At first these new sounds were sometimes alarming, their source being unknown. Sandy soon learned that these were merely normal house noises, the creak and pops of thermal expansion and contraction, sounds from neighboring houses, etc. The level of ear noise (tinnitus) began to decrease. Now, several months later, Sandy's understanding of speech is slightly improved, while her ability to hear isolated sounds is significantly better. Sandy's ability to hear the cooking-completed bell on the Heathkit microwave oven she built is a good example of the latter. After the 6600 rads of x-rays, but before the high dose Hydergine®, Sandy had not been able to hear the bell, even when she was standing right beside the microwave oven in a quiet kitchen. Now, she can reliably hear the bell while she is in the living room, about 35 feet away from the microwave oven and its bell. This represents a high frequency, pure tone threshold detection improvement of at least 20 decibels. Moreover, Sandy can now sometimes hear the oven bell in the living room when the stereo is playing rock and roll at about 90 decibels! Improvements in speech comprehension have not been dramatic to date; a relearning process seems to be involved. Sandy is now using about 20 milligrams of Hydergine® daily and looking for possible further improvements.

Another thing Sandy has noticed since beginning high dose Hydergine® is her acquisition of several new tastes in foods, something which had not happened for years.

THE CASE OF KRIS DEAN AND HIS BAD HEARING

Kris Dean, a 35 year old entrepreneur, suffered an ear infection in his early teens which was never properly treated. He developed a chronic earache, with difficulty in hearing, tinnitus (ear noises) all the time, and intractable pain in his right outer ear (blowing air on it would be quite painful) and sometimes in his left. It hurt to listen to anything at high volume, and he couldn't hear high frequencies (above 4000 Hz) any more.

About three years ago, Kris started taking Hydergine®. The first week, he took 6 milligrams per day. Then he increased his dose to 8 to 10 milligrams per day. Then after a month or so, he began experimenting with daily doses up to about 24–36 milligrams per day, the first time anyone had used such high doses, to our knowledge. The first thing he noticed was how much easier it was for him to hike up and down the San Bernardino mountains. About a year later at those approximate doses, Kris started noticing sounds at higher frequencies (5–8 KHz) that he hadn't been noticing before. Also, the noises in his ears went way down and outer ear pain was much less. He can cope with high intensity sounds now that he says would have driven him up the wall before. In fact, his new hearing acuity forced him to move out of his house. The neighborhood that was quiet when he moved in gradually seemed noisier and noisier (due to improved hearing, not to a real increase in ambient noise level) until he had to go find a quieter place! Kris's frequency range is now above 15 KHz.

In 1969, while Kris was riding his motorcycle, he ended up in a crash with an automobile, and received multiple injuries including a broken and separated left collarbone and a crushed left foot with multiple bone breaks. His surgeon said he'd always have foot problems. Whenever Kris did a lot of walking or hiking, he'd have a dull ache in his foot. But after the use of high doses of Hydergine®, the pain in the foot disappeared. He can now walk up a mountainside without any foot pain. Also, breathing is much easier, with no dizziness or vertigo, and his stamina has been greatly increased.

KRIS DEAN MEETS DR. ALBERT HOFMANN

In 1978, while at the 3rd International Scientific Conference on Native American Shamanism and Sacred Mushrooms, Kris Dean met Dr. Albert Hofmann, the inventor of Hydergine®, and had a most interesting conversation with him (in a group with Durk, Sandy, Dr. Andy Weil, Dr. Alexander Shulgin, and others).

Kris: Dr. Hofmann, I want to thank you for inventing Hydergine®. It helped me regain my hearing; I can't thank you enough.

Dr. H: How many Hydergine® do you take a day, young man?

Kris: I take 24 to 30 or more milligrams a day, Dr. Hofmann.

Dr. H.: Ach, you Americans are all alike, you're all extremists!

Kris: But I can hear again, Dr. Hofmann, and I used to be almost deaf; now I'm not.

*　　　*　　　*

In 1979, Durk and Sandy spoke with Dr. Hofmann at a scientific conference on the Neuropharmacology of Ergot Alkaloids in New York. At that time, Dr. Hofmann inquired about Durk and Sandy's young extremist friend and asked about his health and how he was reacting to the large Hydergine® doses. He indicated that he was interested in the results of the experiments since he had not heard any prior reports of these doses or results.

DR. JACK WHEELER AND HIS MISSING SENSE OF SMELL

Dr. Jack Wheeler is an adventurer who earns his living through his adventurous activities. For example, he wrote a book, "The Adventurer's Guide," about how ordinary people can become involved in exciting adventures. Jack is also an adventurer in more healthful, more youthful living. He became interested in taking Hydergine® because of reports in the scientific literature that we told him about and anecdotal accounts of friends indicating that it could protect the brain from much of aging damage. After taking it (6 to 10 milligrams a day for 2 to 3 months), Jack noticed something remarkable. He could sense the smell of some things around him. This was remarkable because, from the earliest that Jack can remember, he has never been able to sense smells. If someone put ammonia under his nose, he would detect the burning but would smell nothing. But, after use of the high dose Hydergine®, Jack can smell a banana peeled several feet away, and can even distinguish between acetone and isopropyl (rubbing) alcohol, which have rather similar aromas. Although his sense of smell is not normal, it is certainly no longer nonexistent.

SANDY GETS OVER HER PHOBIAS

Phobias are extremely common. Over half the people queried for surveys will admit to having one or more of them. We have long speculated that phobias may be the result of a developmental or aging clock. Phobias seem to occur often in young adulthood and are more frequent among women. It may be that phobias are turned on by an aging clock to inhibit adults of reproductive age, especially women, from engaging in explorative and possibly risky physical activities that involve high places, leaving home (agoraphobia is the commonest phobia), traveling at high speeds, and so on. Curtailing such activities might increase the probability of successful reproduction and raising of children, particularly back in the bad old days before our modern technological civilization. This is a speculation, of course.

In any event, Sandy wanted to get over several severe phobias, particularly fears of flying and public speaking. She was able to do so with little discomfort or will power by using propranolol, an FDA approved medication for the control of high blood pressure which has been used safely and effectively for years for this purpose. In fact, the drop in the death rate from heart attacks in the past decade is thought to be partly a result of the use of propranolol for hypertension.

Under phobic conditions, the body releases adrenaline, while the brain releases its own version of adrenaline, nonradrenalin (which is the same as norepinephrine). This adrenaline-noradrenaline release results in a classic "fight or flight" state in which blood is diverted to the muscles and, in the brain, blood flow is diverted away from the thinking cerebral cortex to the primitive emotional so-called reptile brain. This is great for running away from a sabertooth tiger, but is quite deleterious whenever fighting or fleeing are inappropriate. In this phobic state, the thinking brain is shut down and the body experiences unpleasant symptoms such as shaking, sweating, heart palpitations, queasy stomach, and so on.

Propranolol is one of a class of drugs that block the beta adrenergic receptors, blocking the above-mentioned effects of adrenaline and noradrenaline by preventing them from binding to these receptors. Sandy took 30 to 40 milligrams of propranolol about an hour before giving a lecture or being interviewed on television and experienced none of her previous phobic reactions. At these dose levels, the propranolol had no detectable negative effects on intellectual abilities. And, best of all, after a few successful public speaking experiences, Sandy found she had gotten over this phobia, apparently for good, and didn't need to use the drug any more. Sandy has also used propranolol successfully on her roller coaster and flying phobias, and now actually enjoys both experiences.

SANDY'S BROKEN FOOT AND
AN EXPERIMENTAL BODYBUILDING TECHNIQUE

In January of 1979, Sandy fell and broke her foot at the Gordon Research Conference on the Biology of Aging. She was taken to a local hospital, the foot was x-rayed, and Sandy received a pair of crutches. Not wishing to hobble about on crutches any longer than necessary, Sandy began taking several grams a day of nutrients which are known to promote wound healing and bone repair, especially vitamin C and the amino acid arginine. Arginine stimulates the release of growth hormone by the pituitary gland in the brain. Growth hormone is necessary for growth and repair. Sandy took 10 grams per day of arginine. An unexpected side effect of the large doses of arginine was that Sandy lost about 25 pounds of fat and put on an estimated 5 pounds of muscle while on the arginine, even though she did not engage in strenuous exercise. Her exercises were measured, and the energy required should have used up about one ounce of fat! Growth hormone causes the body to burn up fat and put on muscle, so we had expected some weight loss but we were amazed at the magnitude of the actual results. Sandy wore a size 9/10 jeans before using the growth hormone stimulants in large doses; now she wears a size 5 pair of jeans and looks more like a teenager than she has since she was a teenager! Sandy continues to use about twenty grams a day of arginine (divided into four daily doses of approximately five grams each) and 2 or 3 minutes a week of exercise for bodybuilding and has developed a remarkable set of muscles, particularly her shoulders and biceps. See the following photos of Sandy and her other three photos in Part III, Chapter 9, "Athletics."

PHENYLALANINE AND THE END OF THE BLAHS

Sandy used to have a hard time finishing many projects. She would work on a project enthusiastically for a time and then poop out. Then, about a year ago, Sandy began taking phenylalanine (1 gram at bedtime) and found that this problem no longer bothered her. In addition to helping her get out of bed promptly upon awakening and enabling her to engage in longer term projects, she feels that the phenylalanine has given her greater confidence in herself and has promoted more aggressive and assertive behavior, the latter being very beneficial in her professional career. Phenylalanine has been very helpful when Sandy has suffered from writer's block, too!

As we have mentioned many times in this book, chronic use of high doses of phenylalanine have not been studied for long-term toxicity. Its use in this manner is strictly experimental. People with high blood pressure should be extremely cautious, and must refer to the caution given in Part III, Chapter 3. Doses must be individualized, and in our experience may vary from 50 milligrams per day to 2 grams per day.

"MR. SMITH'S" CASE HISTORY

About 1½ years ago, we met one of our heroes, "Mr. Smith," at a dinner arranged by Merv Griffin. Since then, we have spent many enjoyable hours visiting with "Mr. Smith."

"Mr. Smith" is a professional movie actor, well known for his physically vigorous roles. "Mr. Smith" has taken a strong interest in some of the nutritional and life extension concepts we and others have developed. He has put together his own experimental life extension formula and has explored various nutrients and prescription drugs for this purpose. While experimenting with these materials, "Mr. Smith" has been careful to have clinical laboratory tests and consultations with a research-oriented physician. Here we report on some of the results he has observed. ("Mr. Smith" did not want his real name used here because of his concern that irresponsible tabloids might take quotes out-of-context and otherwise distort the contents.)

CHOLINE AND ALERTNESS

"Mr. Smith" started out taking 2 to 3 "000" gelatin capsules full (about 3 to 4 grams) of choline per day and is currently using about the same; he was also taking 100 to 200 micrograms of selenium in yeast per day (he now uses 300 micrograms of sodium selenite). He says that when using this, he feels good and alert.

IMPROVEMENT IN SPEAKING ABILITY

"Mr. Smith" says that 2 to 3 grams of choline per day, along with about 250 milligrams of Deanol or Deaner® a day, had a beneficial effect on his speaking ability, verbal facility, and recall, so that he could remember to say things during an interview instead of afterward when it was too late. Once, he spoke effortlessly for two hours at an event, whereas ordinarily he would speak for only a short time like ten minutes. One time, he told us, "I couldn't shut myself up!" "Mr. Smith" used to be a man of few words in his public appearances, but the elevated levels of brain acetylcholine have brought him a new facility with the spoken word.

He did experience slight neck stiffness at first with Deaner®, but this symptom soon vanished (he developed tolerance to it).

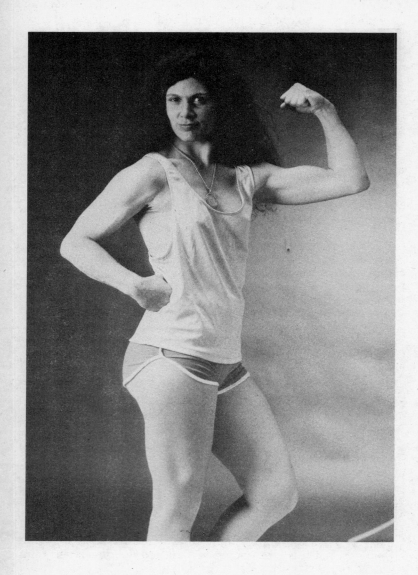

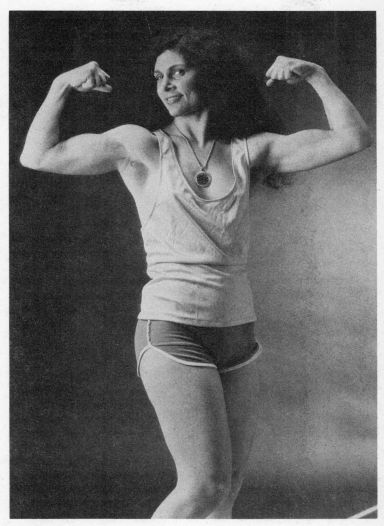

Want to arm wrestle?

HYDERGINE®

"Mr. Smith" has been using Hydergine® as well, about 6 milligrams a day. He reports that during the past 1½ years he has had no colds or flu as long as he takes Hydergine®. He also experiences an increase in mental alertness with Hydergine®. Hydergine®'s effects on "Mr. Smith's" illnesses are most likely due to its powerful antioxidant effects. Many antioxidant nutrients, such as vitamins C, E, and A, the amino acid cysteine, and the minerals zinc and selenium, are able to stimulate the immune system. One major way they do this is by acting as free radical scavengers, which prevents the free radical caused formation of organic peroxides. These organic peroxides can severely inhibit macrophages, important white blood cells which are supposed to roam about looking for bacteria, viruses, and cancer cells to kill and eat. In the presence of the organic peroxides, the macrophages' ability to attack these enemies can be seriously impaired.

The brain contains a huge amount of highly unsaturated fats. These unsaturated fats are easily peroxidized via a free radical route and, consequently, it is especially important to have plenty of antioxidants around. In fact, the brain and spinal cord have special vitamin C pumps, one in the blood-brain barrier (a membrane around the brain which is very picky about what it lets in) and one in each nerve cell itself, which increase the concentration of vitamin C inside of the nerves of the brain and spinal cord to 100 times that in the bloodstream. These pumps use up a great deal of energy in doing this, but the brain requires the antioxidant protection of vitamin C. Hydergine® is a powerful antioxidant which provides substantial protection in the brain against free radical damage to the brain's unsaturated fats. A substantial part of the age related decline of the immune system is due to free radical damage to the hypothalamus and pituitary glands in the brain.

DMSO

"Mr. Smith" is physically active and engages in demanding sports such as skiing where minor injuries are inevitable. He says that he has had very good luck using DMSO for skiing bruises, but he has not had the dramatic experiences with it that some others have had, probably due to his tougher skin and capillaries. See the case history of "Miss Jones."

KEEPING SKIN MOIST

"Mr. Smith" uses a homemade formula containing NaPCA (the sodium salt of pyrollidone carboxylic acid), the primary natural moisturizer in human skin. He finds it great for an aftershave, for going out in the evening, for skiing, shooting on location, and in other drying environments. He particularly likes its nonoily character. Although we have suggested that people look for premium quality cosmetics which contain this substance, our own searches have not been very fruitful. Apparently, the cosmetics industry has not caught on to this outstanding material yet. For a supplier of NaPCA, see Appendix I.

GETTING THE MOST OUT OF EXERCISE

"Mr. Smith" works out to keep in good condition. He is in excellent shape. We told him that he could get much more out of his exercise by using certain nutrients which cause the brain's pituitary gland to release growth hormone. Growth hormone is required for the building of muscle and also causes the body to burn fat for energy. In addition, growth hormone stimulates the thymus gland, resulting in better immune system performance. "Mr. Smith" has been using the growth hormone releasers L-arginine and L-Dopa in conjunction with exercise, usually taking L-Dopa an hour before and L-arginine about twenty minutes before. He reports that, when using L-Dopa, he has <u>much</u> greater stamina. For example, once he started his exercise routine planning to spend about ½ hour; 2½ hours later he was still going strong. This prompt effect is due to increased levels of the neurotransmitter dopamine in the motor areas of the brain. He uses 250 milligrams of L-Dopa and 4 grams of arginine for the exercise.

"Mr. Smith," now 50 years old, says that he can run longer and faster now than he could five years ago, even though he was exercising and taking good care of himself then. He also says that he feels "better than ten years ago maybe."

The increased stamina with L-Dopa is consistent with recent animal experiments. For example, when old rats were put into water and forced to swim, they swam with inefficient motions and for a much shorter time than the young rats. But when the old rats were given L-Dopa and forced to swim, they could not be distinguished from the young rats in their swimming, either in efficiency or in stamina.

TAKING CARE OF FLU

"Mr. Smith" has found the combination of L-arginine and vitamin C effective against flu. He has used a combination of 8 grams per day of arginine the first day, then 6 grams the next day, along with 2 to 3 grams of vitamin C every two hours (24–30 grams a day). This is an excellent combination since these two substances stimulate the immune system by different mechanisms. The L-arginine causes the pituitary gland to release growth hormone, while the vitamin C stimulates the activity of some white blood cells, provides antioxidant protection to the immune system, increases the body's production of interferon, and works in several other ways. See Part IV, Chapter 7 on vitamin C.

IMPROVED APPEARANCE

Old friends of "Mr. Smith" have commented on his improved appearance, especially of his skin and hair, compared to his appearance in a movie about 2½ years ago. Overall appearance depends on the health of a number of biochemical systems, many of which can be seriously damaged by free radicals. For example, the skin is the organ in the body with the third most unsaturated fats, after the brain and spinal cord. These unsaturated fats are highly susceptible to free radical attack. "Mr. Smith's" personal experimental antioxidant formula of nutrients and prescription drugs is a very powerful scavenger of these free radicals and provides substantial protection from them to skin and hair follicles. (For more about hair, see "The Case of Miss Jones' Reluctant Hair" and Part III, Chapter 7 on balding.)

"MR. SMITH'S" NUTRIENT MIX

"Mr. Smith" has a nutrient mix of antioxidants that he devised with our help and which he is using. Each day, he generally takes these substances and total quantities, taken in 3 or 4 divided doses:

10,000 I.U. of vitamin A, 200 milligrams of vitamin B-2, 3 grams of vitamin B-3 (niacin), 3 grams of vitamin B-5 (pantothenate), 1 gram of vitamin B-6, 1 milligram of vitamin B-

12, 6 to 7 grams of vitamin C, 3000 I.U. of vitamin E, 1 to 2 grams of PABA, small amounts of biotin and folate, 2 grams of cysteine, 300 micrograms of selenium (as sodium selenite), 200 milligrams of 10 percent beta carotene, and about 1 gram each of the bioflavonoids rutin and hesperidin complex.

In addition, he takes extra quantities of C (3 to 4 grams a day), L-arginine (for workouts, 6 grams a day), and L-Dopa (¼ gram per day).

PROTECTION AGAINST SUNBURN

"Mr. Smith" says that there was a "real dramatic" effect on his skin's resistance to sunburn when he used canthaxanthin, a carotenoid (chemically related to the yellow coloring matter in carrots, beta carotene). His skin is relatively light and sensitive to sunlight, especially his nose. He began using about 120 milligrams of canthaxanthin per day, then went to the same dose every other day. He looks as if he has a beautiful golden-bronze sun tan and he says his resistance to sunburn is dramatically improved. Recently, when he forgot to use a sunblock on his nose, it received only a minor sunburn compared to what would be expected from earlier experiences.

The other antioxidants in "Mr. Smith's" mix also provide some protection against damage by the sun's ultraviolet light. They do this by interacting with the ultraviolet light, being converted into excited species themselves in the process. By a chain process in which one antioxidant interacts with another one, the excess energy originally derived from the ultraviolet light is eventually released harmlessly via numerous small steps.

In addition to canthaxanthin, beta carotene also provides excellent protection against ultraviolet light from the sun. In his nutrient mix, he gets about 20 milligrams of beta carotene a day. In a recent research report, beta carotene was shown to provide substantial ultraviolet light protection. Hematoporphyrin sensitizes animals to ultraviolet light. When hematoporphyrin was injected into mice, 21 out of 27 died when exposed to sunlight. The injected mice which were also given beta carotene did not die. Humans on beta carotene therapy for erythropoietic protoporphyria (a type of hypersensitivity to sunlight) reported that with beta carotene they could even develop a suntan, whereas before they could not go into the sun at all! The scientist who did this research (Micheline M. Mathews-Roth) says she uses the Hoffmann La-Roche "beadlet" form of beta carotene because these are absorbed better than the crystalline form. (Reference: "Photochemical Toxicity," 7th Annual FDA Science Symposium, March 16–17 1981, Uniformed Service University for Health Sciences, Bethesda, MD). Beta carotene is also fairly effective in protecting victims of xeroderma pigmentosum (a serious genetic disease involving faulty repair of ultra violet light induced DNA damage) from the extremely serious sunburns that they can get from even a short exposure to sunlight. For this protection, XP patients must take enough carotenoids to color their skin. In a recent issue of *Nature*, scientists reported a possible prophylactic anti-cancer effect of beta carotene.

RNA AND SMOOTH SKIN

Using about 1 gram of RNA per day, "Mr. Smith" says his skin has become smoother, contributing to his improved appearance. RNA is an antioxidant and an important information-carrying macromolecule (large molecule) inside of cells. Since skin cells are constantly dividing, their demand for RNA is likely to be rather large compared to many cells which don't divide or divide slowly.

ALLERGIES

Throughout his childhood, "Mr. Smith" had frequent contact with animals without noticeable allergic response. He first detected the development of animal hair (dandruff? microorganisms?) allergies in his mid to late 30s. (This is an all too common development around this age in scientists who work with laboratory animals.) At first, it was cat hair, then dog hair, then the hair of other animals—including horses. It started with stinging, reddened, itchy eyes, then sneezing and even itchy skin. If "Mr. Smith" were extremely tired and overworked, there was sometimes a little bit of asthmatic respiratory impairment. In recent years, he has used antihistamines and other allergy remedies when working professionally with animals. For quite a few years, he would promptly notice allergic eye irritation upon entering a room frequented by a cat or occasionally even a dog.

"Mr. Smith's" use of the antioxidant nutrients and prescription drugs has almost completely eliminated these allergies. He can now comfortably occupy a room with a cat or ride a horse without eye or skin irritation, antihistamines, or other allergy medications. Indeed, he can now play with cats and even rub cat hair into the sensitive skin on the inside of the elbow without skin itching. Since some eye sensitivity still exists to direct eye contact with concentrated allergens, he generally washes his hands after petting cats, but the overall allergy improvement has been quite dramatic.

There are a number of plausible mechanisms by which allergies might be controlled or corrected with the life extension materials that "Mr. Smith" takes. See Durk's case history in this appendix and Part III, Chapter 15, "A Brief Note on Allergies and Asthma" for further information.

THE CASE OF THE DEPRESSED SKYDIVER

A young professional adventurer who skydives and hang glides for a living had a long-term problem of experiencing a period of a day or so of depression every month. We told him about the use of the amino acid phenylalanine for depression. He tried it and told us he has experienced complete relief from his periodic depressions.

THE TRANSFORMATION OF MISS CEE

Miss Cee, a moderately successful young Hollywood screenwriter, used to be so tired. Sometimes she just couldn't get out of bed in the morning. There was a pervasive oppressive feeling of depression. By 8:00 PM, Miss Cee would be falling asleep. To do something like exercise was beyond her. She was a heavy user of cocaine, which depletes brain stores of norepinephrine and vasopressin when used to excess.

Then we told Miss Cee about phenylalanine and she decided to try it. The results were very good. Miss Cee told us that she had much more energy for both work and play. She stayed awake till about 1 AM. She enjoyed taking bike rides. In our most recent conversation, Miss Cee said she was using about 1 gram of DL-phenylalanine per day, taken either in the morning or in the evening. (**NOTE: the right dose of phenylalanine must be individualized. Because this dose works for Miss Cee, don't assume that it will do the same for you. It may be too much or too little for you**). Because we are no longer in contact with Miss Cee, we do not know whether she still uses cocaine to the same extent that she did before taking phenylalanine.

THE CASE OF THE VERY BAD BAD BACK

A businessman friend of ours, let's call him Mr. V, at the age of 50 could no longer participate in the strenuous physical activities he had enjoyed all his life, including snow and water skiing. He had injured his back several years before we met him, in a skiing accident, with the result that his physical activities had to be sharply curtailed. The pain was ever-present. When he drove his car, he could not do so for more than 20 minutes at a time without developing intolerable back pain. So Mr. V purchased a station wagon and, when he traveled over 20 minutes or so, he would have to be chauffeured about lying on a foam rubber pad in the back of the station wagon. The six different doctors Mr. V consulted all told him that he would be disabled for the rest of his life.

We told Mr. V about the beneficial effects of large doses of vitamins A, C and E for life extension purposes, but said nothing to him about possible effects on his back. He immediately began taking 15,000 I.U. of vitamin A, several grams of vitamin C and a couple of thousand units of E each day. About two months later, Mr. V telephoned to tell us that suddenly one day he had noticed that his back didn't hurt anymore! Then he began skiing again. He promptly reinjured his back in a skiing mishap, but more vitamins A, C, and E took care of his back again, and he was skiing again within a week. He was now able to frequently engage in snow and water skiing and travel without having to lie down. The pain would return within a week or two if he stopped taking the vitamins, but his back would be fine so long as he took them.

THE CASE OF THE ARTIST WITH THE ARTHRITIC HANDS

Kelly Freas is an artist and a good one. He designed the Skylab shoulder patch for NASA and is a recognized and honored award winning artist of fantasy and science fiction posters and book covers. We own several original works of his art. Mr. Freas is in his 50s.

In 1969, he was withdrawn (due to adverse side effects) from the cortisone that he had been using for years for the control of a severe allergic rash. The joints in Mr. Freas's hands began rapidly stiffening and swelling. The arthritis quickly became very severe. He could not move his extremely painful, swollen fingers. The arthritis spread to other joints, particularly his toes. For 1½ years, he could not drive a car because he could not hold the steering wheel. He could paint, but had to develop a new style not requiring finger movement. This was a terrible fate for him because he had been justly famed for his finely detailed work. He even had to call his children into his studio to remove the caps from his tubes of paint.

Mr. Freas decided to try vitamin E because he had heard that it could help in arthritis. He took 1000 units of vitamin E a day. It did not help. Then he increased his dose to 5000 units of E a day. His hands began to improve a little. Mr. Freas went up to 10,000 units of vitamin E and a shot glass of cod liver oil (which contains at least 20,000 IU of vitamin A) each day before breakfast. At this dose, his hands slowly regained their normal function, the pain vanished, and the joints returned to normal size. Eight to ten months after starting this regimen, he was able to start driving again, though for a while he had to wear heavy padded gloves. Mr. Freas has found that 10,000 units per day of vitamin E plus a shot glass of cod liver oil (containing at least 20,000 I.U. of vitamin A) maintains the flexibility of his fingers. He has tried reducing the dose, but even at 5000 I.U. of vitamin E per day, the arthritis returns after a few weeks. His arthritis is now practically all gone; he has only occasional minor twinges, and his artistic career is now unimpaired. (See Part IV, Chapter 8.)

MRS. T'S ARTHRITIS AND A SOD-LIKE
COPPER-SALICYLATE COMPLEX

SOD (superoxide dismutase) is a very important natural intracellular (inside cells) enzyme in our bodies which destroys the damaging superoxide free radical. This superoxide radical plays an important role in the damage to joint membranes and lubricating fluids that occurs in rheumatoid arthritis. Unfortunately for the arthritis sufferer, there is relatively little extracellular (outside of cells) SOD, which is what is needed in the joints to destroy the damaging superoxide radicals found there. Taken orally, over 99.99 percent of an SOD dose is destroyed in the digestive tract. (Although an injectable form of SOD is available for racehorses, no such medication is available for human use due to the difficulty of obtaining FDA approval.)

It was recently discovered that copper-salicylate complexes have biochemical properties very much like the enzyme SOD (in fact, in some papers these complexes were described as artificial superoxide dismutases); and these complexes are active when taken orally. Of great practical importance, the ingredients for these complexes are available without prescription in drugstores and health food stores. Moreover, you do not need a laboratory to make your own SOD-like copper-salicylate complex; you simply swallow a tablet of sodium salicylate (bought at a drugstore) along with a tablet of chelated copper from a health food store. That's all there is to it. The copper-salicylate complex forms in your stomach. Although a copper-acetylsalicylic acid (copper-aspirin) complex will work, the complex formed between sodium salicylate (a nonprescription aspirin-like drug) and chelated copper is both more effective and less irritating.

Here is a case where arthritis has been successfully controlled with a SOD-like copper-salicylate complex.

Mrs. T, 63 years old, first developed arthritis in her fingers 4 or 5 years ago. It started with tingling, then pain, then arthritic knobs developed on her finger joints. After this happened, she tried vitamin E at the suggestion of her son. She took 1000 I.U. of vitamin E two to three times a day. This kept the arthritis under control, with no further development of arthritic joint knobs or finger pains. If she discontinued the vitamin E, however, the arthritis would return in a few days.

Unfortunately, as one grows older arthritis tends to become more severe and to spread to more joints.

About six months ago, Mrs. T developed pains in her knees. At her last physical examination, her physician diagnosed these pains as arthritis, too. Several weeks later, after a day spent on her feet, she developed severe back pains which persisted for days and which neither rest nor aspirin corrected.

About a month ago, Mrs. T's son told her about the SOD-like copper salicylate complexes. She started by taking a 650 milligram tablet of sodium salicylate along with two tablets, each containing 2.5 milligrams of copper in the form of an amino acid chelate. (The common copper gluconate chelate will work just as well.) The arthritic pains felt better after several hours and vanished after a few days.

Mrs. T now remains free of arthritic pain with the following regimen: On awakening, one 350 milligram tablet of sodium salicylate plus one 2.5 milligram copper chelate tablet. This dosage is repeated once or twice more later in the day. (The largest dose that she has taken at one time is two 650 milligram sodium salicylate tablets plus two 2.5 milligram copper chelate tablets.)

Mrs. T continues to take 2000 to 3000 I.U. of vitamin E per day plus one tablet each of commercial B-complex, A, and chelated minerals.

DR. B AT SEVENTY ACQUIRES ADDITIONAL ENERGY

Dr. B, a 71 year old retired department head of a physical sciences department at a large university, who is now a science lecturer, consultant, researcher, and entrepreneur, has had interesting experiences in his search for improved health and mental performance. Since using a relatively simple selection of nutrients and prescription drugs, Dr. B has experienced an increase in energy, a greater sex drive, and a sense of well being. In the morning, Dr. B takes about 300 milligrams of Deaner® (Riker), a chelated zinc tablet (containing about 30 milligrams of chelated zinc), ⅓ teaspoon (about one gram) of vitamin C crystals, and a glassful of freshly squeezed orange juice. At bedtime, he takes a 250 milligram tablet of L-Dopa, a 500 microgram (½ milligram) tablet of Hydergine®, and ⅓ teaspoon of vitamin C crystals. Dr. B reports that the Deaner® increased his sex drive (in fact, he calls it "horny juice").

When we first met Dr. B in 1977, he had extensive yellow-brown lipofuscin (age pigment or "liver spots") deposits in his skin. (We verified that these were lipofuscin rather than melanin by their long wave ultra violet induced fluorescence.) He started to take the above formula at this time. These age pigment spots had become noticeably lighter after 6 months, much lighter after a year, and were almost entirely gone after 2 years. At present, Dr. B reports only one spot remaining, though we have not performed a long wave ultraviolet fluorescence test to determine whether this spot is actually age pigment or ordinary melanin. (Melanin is the brown pigment found in suntans, naturally dark skin, freckles, and birthmarks.) This formula, particularly the Deaner®, removes lipofuscin age pigment, but not melanin; it is not a bleach. Dr. B has received many compliments on the smooth, moist, youthful, relatively unwrinkled appearance of his skin, which now looks like that of someone a decade or more younger, whereas in 1977, he looked his age. Dr. B is currently increasing his Hydergine® dose and has added vitamin E and 250 micrograms per day of sodium selenite.

THE CASE OF THE SEDENTARY GOURMET

Mr. J is a 58 year old sedentary lawyer, a bachelor who really enjoys food and eats out regularly at the finest of restaurants. About three years ago, Mr. J's weight was 158 lbs. and both his cholesterol and blood pressure were in the 140+ range. In a recent physical examination, his weight was 138 lbs., cholesterol was 111, and blood pressure 110/70. Mr. J has been using our nutrient mix at about ¼ of our dose levels. Mr. J tells us that he has received many comments on the improvement in his appearance, including his skin. His energy levels are "tremendously higher." The most interesting feature of these changes is that Mr. J has not gone on any special diets. As he says, "I consider myself a gourmet and continue to enjoy foods without regard to their content." Last year after his regular physical checkup and a fairly extensive series of clinical laboratory tests, his physician of many years told him that his checkup was the best he had seen that year for anyone, regardless of age.

THE CASE OF THE BHT EATER

Erwin S. Strauss is a 38 year old sedentary and overweight physicist (MIT graduate) and computer programmer. In early 1969, he read scientific papers about the life extending effects of BHT in animal feeding experiments (performed by Dr. Denham Harman) having initially read about them in the *Wall Street Journal* and in *Playboy* magazine. He decided to take it himself. Beginning in spring 1969, he took 6 grams of BHT daily. After four years at this dose, he discontinued use of the BHT for four years due to doubts he had at the time concerning possible side effects. He resumed using BHT at 6 grams per day about 3½ years ago and still takes it. This is the highest dose that we have heard of being used on a regular basis and over a fairly long period of time. Erwin Strauss has not noticed any immediate benefits as a result of his use of the BHT; his reason for using it is for long-term benefits as a life extension material. He sent us a copy of a series of clinical tests he underwent about 3 years ago (at that time he had not used BHT for the prior three months). He weighed 224 lbs. at 6 feet 3 inches. All tests were normal except that his triglycerides were slightly elevated (normal range is 50 to 200; Erwin Strauss's triglycerides were 212).

BHT AND THE FREE RADICAL THEORY OF HANGOVERS

Mr. H, a 49 year old attorney, was, in his words, a heavy drinker. Each evening, he would consume about a third of a bottle of scotch in a short period of time. By morning, he would have to go to his office with a hangover. We told Mr. H about the free radical theory of aging and about a variety of antioxidants. One of the antioxidants that we mentioned was BHT. Mr. H obtained some BHT for its general free radical scavenging effects but soon discovered an unexpected use. He found that BHT could cure a hangover! Mr. H would take a few grams of BHT when he woke up, and the hangover headache would be gone in about an hour, leaving him relatively refreshed and energetic. Since then, Mr. H has found an even better hangover cure—he has stopped drinking.

We do not suggest the use of BHT for curing hangovers. (**WARNING:** If large doses of BHT and alcohol are taken <u>together</u>, the BHT can temporarily reduce the rate of liver alcohol clearance, thus greatly increasing the effects of the alcohol, so don't try it.) We have included this incident as an example of the wide-ranging applicability of free radical pathology concepts. Most alcohol-induced damage, including hangovers, is caused by free radicals produced by the autoxidation of acetaldehyde, which is made from alcohol via the enzyme alcohol dehydrogenase. BHT is a powerful free radical scavenger. So the surprising finding that a food preservative can cure hangovers turns out to be just what one would expect—if one knows something about free radical pathology. We do suggest several ways of dealing with alcohol, hangovers, and its other hazards, by the use of other free radical scavengers in Part III, Chapter 12.

MR. M AND HIS GENITAL HERPES PROBLEM

Mr. M, a professional computer programmer, has had mouth sores (herpes type I) every few months throughout his life. He also contracted genital herpes (herpes type II), which did not produce any overt symptoms, but he wanted to avoid giving the genital herpes to his girl friends, which he thought would probably be very unpleasant for them. After getting the genital herpes, Mr. M's sexual activity was reduced for about a year. Even a small amount of sexual activity would bring forth a tingle, and then a sore which lasted about a week. We told Mr. M about the use of BHT against herpes infections and he then read a paper on this subject in the September 1975 *Science*. He has taken $\frac{1}{4}$ gram of BHT at bedtime nearly on a daily basis and finds that, at this dose and frequency, he gets no herpes attacks. Or, he can wait for the first tingle and then start the BHT; on this schedule, the tingle disappears overnight and no sore develops or, if it does, it fades within a day or two. This use of BHT is experimental.

Mr. M used phenylalanine and arginine for weight loss and was able to lose 25 pounds. He lost his urge to be constantly snacking.

"THE RIGHT STUFF" FOR ORAL HERPES: BHT

Mr. D is an astronaut, test pilot, high technology R & D consultant, and entrepreneur. His problems with type 1 (oral) herpes started after a severe sunburn that he received on a summer archaeology dig in Mexico. (The solar ultraviolet light causes genetic damage to the skin cells, permitting the expression of herpes virus information previously inserted into the DNA of the skin cells and suppressed by protective mechanisms in these cells.) Since then, he has had sporadic oral herpes lesions. The sores on his lips or their outer edges generally appear within a few days after he is exposed to a lot of sunlight. He flies incessantly, for pleasure, business, and in air races, and he spends a lot of time at military air bases in the desert; hence, he is exposed to a great deal of ultraviolet light damage, with the resulting herpes lesions.

Although both an over-the-counter drug and a drug prescribed by a NASA physician helped somewhat, neither did the job well and the latter destroyed a lot of healthy tissue too. In 1979, we met professionally and told him about our experiences with BHT and its antiherpes effects. Mr. D started taking $1/8$ teaspoon of BHT per day initially, soon increasing it to $1/4$ teaspoon per day. ($1/4$ teaspoon of BHT is about 800 milligrams.) So long as he took it, the herpes was dormant and there were no lesions, even after extensive exposure to sunlight. Mr. D found that 6 to 8 weeks after discontinuing the BHT, herpes lesions would develop one after another, subsequent to solar exposure. At this dose, the half life of BHT (the time it takes for the concentration of BHT in the body to drop to half the initial amount) is very roughly two weeks in humans, so 6 to 8 weeks is 3 to 4 half-lives; tissue BHT residues dropped by roughly a factor of 8 to 16 before the herpes lesions returned. This time period is typical, in our own experience and that of several other self-experimental subjects as well. The problem continued until BHT use was resumed, after which the herpes lesions vanished within a few days.

In 1980, Mr. D spent the summer flying about the world in his jet aircraft. He forgot to take his BHT with him and, about 6 to 8 weeks later (with the harsh solar ultraviolet of the stratosphere pouring through his jet's canopy), herpes hit again. The lesions bothered him incessantly for the last half of the trip until he flew home to his BHT supply. Since then, Mr. D has told his test pilot friends with herpes problems about how, for him, BHT is the right stuff. This use of BHT is experimental.

THE STALLION THAT COULDN'T COME

Imagine being a stud horse that cannot reach an orgasm! A valuable thoroughbred stallion with just such a problem was brought to our attention. One very common mechanism that can cause difficulty in reaching orgasms in both humans and other mammals is inadequate release of supplies of histamine. Histamine release is required for orgasm. We suggested that the horse be given supplements of niacin, which causes histamine release. The horse's handlers told us later that the niacin worked beautifully for a few days but then he began having trouble again. We pointed out that the horse might not be making enough histamine and suggested they supplement his diet with histidine (which is made into histamine) and vitamin B-6 (required for this conversion). They gave the horse supplements of vitamin B-6 in addition to the niacin and found that the combination worked great. In fact, they even had to restrain the horse because they were afraid he might injure himself by the frequent masturbation in which the stallion then engaged!

MR. P, HEAVY USER OF VALIUM AND ALCOHOL

Mr. P is a heavy user of both Valium® and alcohol. But just a few months ago, he used even more. This is the story of how he was able to reduce his consumption without reducing the benefits he seeks from these drugs.

Mr. P now takes 35 each 5 milligram Valium® tablets every two weeks! He drinks a pint of distilled liquor each day! He says that he feels good now, better than when he used even more Valium® and was drinking 2 pints of distilled liquor a day, just a few months ago. When Mr. P first asked us about his drug usage, we told him about new findings about Valium® and Librium®. These drugs work in the brain because they fit into a receptor called the benzodiazepine receptor. It was clear to researchers that if a synthetic drug like Librium® or Valium® fit a specific selective brain receptor, that there must be natural substances which fit the receptors, too, that might provide the same type of tranquilizing effect without the sedative, mind-deadening side effects of high doses of Valium® and Librium®. These two drugs, even after a user has stopped taking them, stay in the body for at least several days, resulting in a hung-over effect. (Nevertheless, Valium® and Librium® are great improvements over prior drugs.)

Recently, researchers have found out about some of these natural substances which fit the benzodiazepine receptors. One is niacinamide. The vitamin inositol and the amino acid GABA enhance niacinamide binding to the benzodiazepine receptors. Niacinamide, inositol, and GABA can, therefore, at least partly replace Valium® or Librium® by binding to the same receptors and providing tranquilization. Mr. P has tried this—he is now taking 2–5 grams of niacin per day, 1–2 grams of GABA per day, and about 5 grams of inositol per day. He says that he is less depressed than before, no longer suffering from monthly deep depressions but only occasional shallow ones. His friends have commented on this improvement. He has been able to cut his alcohol use in half. Mr. P says that GABA feels similar to Valium®, but does not quite give him the energy that he gets from Valium®. Finally, Mr. P uses C, B-1, and cysteine at times when he is drinking and has found it makes it easier for him to get up in the morning (after a bad day) to go to his office.

THE EXPERIENCES OF MR. S

Mr. S, a man in his late twenties, has been using vitamin/mineral supplements for quite some time. In 1974, he began taking 1 gram a day of calcium pantothenate (for a month or two before that, his dose of pantothenate was 100 milligrams per day). At the annual arm wrestling contest in which he and his friends had engaged since 1970, Mr. S won three contests in a row, which he considered exceptional. Previously, he would win his first contest but would then poop out. In addition, during this same period, he found that he could easily do 50 push-ups (he only stopped at 50 because he was afraid of hurting himself), whereas 25 or 30 used to leave him weak. He did say that he felt that these results seem to have "worn off" to some extent since that time. Whether this is due to age effects or other factors, we can't say.

Mr. S discovered, much to his discomfort, that taking acidic vitamins in large doses without neutralizing them can produce unpleasant side effects. He had been using megadoses of vitamins, including unneutralized ascorbic acid (6–10 grams a day) for a few months, and suddenly developed bad hemorrhoids. It took several months for his rear end to recover once he substituted mineral (non-acidic) salts of vitamin C.

One final bit that Mr. S wanted to mention was his successful use of vitamin A (50,000 units a day) and 50 milligrams of chelated zinc a day against acne. It took about a week to clear up. He knows others who have also had good results with this combination. He is familiar with the signs of vitamin A overdosage and has not seen any at this dose. Do not assume that you can safely take this dose of vitamin A; see Part IV Chapter 8 for overdosage symptoms and precautions.

ASTHMA RELIEF WITH PABA

Beatrice Rosenfeld, our science editor, has had bronchial asthma for many years, with severe attacks occurring during periods of respiratory infections, when only corticosteroids provided relief. Ordinarily, she had to use a prescription bronchodilator in a nebulizer six times a day. She was surprised when she started taking 200 milligrams of PABA a day that her asthma cleared up entirely, eliminating the need to use the nebulizer. When we checked with her after about six months, she reported that she has not had any serious attacks since going on the PABA, and most of the time she does not need to use her nebulizer.

JACK'S RESISTANCE TO SUNBURN

In the summer of 1980, professional explorer and adventurer Dr. Jack Wheeler was at Perris Valley parachuting center near Riverside, California. He was exposed to the hot sun and 110 degrees Fahrenheit heat for several hours on and off over the day. Jack was concerned that he might become sunburned, especially his naked back. But, to this surprise, no sunburn took place. Jack had been taking a regimen of antioxidants (our nutrient mix) at doses considerably lower than ours. But he hadn't noticed a sunburn protective effect until he added extra vitamin C and the carotenoid canthaxanthin to his supplements. He says that he can remain in the sun about 2 to 3 times as long now as before he took these recent supplements.

NO MORE SUNBURNS FOR SCOTT

In 1974 (when he was 21), Scott Tips, Esq., could not spend very much time in the sun before his fair skin would burn—about an hour would be his limit. At that time, he began using a simple nutrient combination consisting of about 3 grams of BHT, 600 I.U. of vitamin E, 2 grams of C, and small amounts of other vitamins each day. He was very surprised when, following the winter, he was able to spend three continuous hours out in direct sunlight without either burning or tanning. Scott continues to take supplemental nutrients (a more complex mix than before), and this sunburn protection has been maintained.

"MISS JONES'S" CASE HISTORY

THE CASE OF "MISS JONES'S" RELUCTANT HAIR

We had intended to include photographs in this case history to illustrate the changes taking place in "Miss Jones's" hair. However, "Miss Jones" decided not to let her name be used here (and not to use photos of her, of course) because of her concern that the tabloids would distort and exploit such material out of context.

"Miss Jones," an actress whose fine performances you have probably seen several times, has had her share of hair problems. She used to have a lot of unsightly dandruff and a chronically itchy scalp. Her hair was rather thin and grew so slowly that she was very reluctant to have it cut. In photos of her taken in 1977 when she was being filmed for a popular movie, she wore a small hairpiece at the back of her head under her own hair to increase its apparent thickness and length.

In 1978, she first noticed that a portion of her hair was turning white, starting at the forehead hairline on both sides of the part. This localized loss of hair pigment proceeded back along the part until, by September 1979, it extended back about four inches from the forehead on both sides of the part. This blaze of depigmented hair is also clearly visible in the very popular movie in which "Miss Jones" starred in 1979.

"Miss Jones" met us a few months later, and soon embarked on her own personal life extension experiments, complete with clinical laboratory tests, physician supervision, and nutrients and prescription drugs, especially antioxidants. Her daily total intake of antioxidants (in 3 to 4 divided doses) is: 10,000 I.U. of vitamin A, 200 milligrams of vitamin B-2, 3 grams of vitamin B-3 (niacin), 3 grams of vitamin B-5 (pantothenate), 1 gram of vitamin B-6, 1 milligram of vitamin B-12, 6 to 7 grams of vitamin C, 3000 I.U. of vitamin E, 1 to 2 grams of PABA, small amounts of biotin and folate, 2 grams of cysteine, 300 micrograms of selenium (as sodium selenite), 200 milligrams of 10 percent beta carotene, and about 1 gram each of bioflavonoids rutin and hesperidin complex. She also takes 9 milligrams of Hydergine® in 4.5 milligram tablets. "Miss Jones's" dandruff and itchy scalp were rapidly corrected by the antioxidants. Most cases of dandruff and itchy scalp are not caused by scalp infection, allergy, insect infestation, or lack of hygiene. The dandruff that bothered her responded to the free radical scavengers, indicating that it was caused by free radical caused rancidity (autoxidation) of fats and oils (lipids) in the scalp, resulting in the formation of organic peroxides. These organic peroxides are irritants which suppress a messenger chemical inside of cells (cyclic AMP) and elevate levels of another such hormone inside of cells (cyclic GMP) which results in scalp hyperplasia (excessive cell division) with itching and dandruff. The dandruff itself is clumps of rapidly growing scalp skin cells which have flaked off due to excessive growth of the skin cells under them.

The most popular anti-dandruff shampoos helped somewhat but were unable to solve the problem. These shampoos work by the topical application of antioxidants (for example, selenium sulfide in the case of Selsun Blue® and zinc pyrithione in Head and Shoulders®), not by mere cleaning. The powerful combination of nutrient and prescription antioxidants that "Miss Jones" takes orally has apparently prevented the troublesome scalp lipid autoxidation and, thereby, eliminated the dandruff and scalp itch.

The age-related loss of hair pigment is due to free radical damage to the melanocytes (pigment-producing cells) in the hair follicles. These melanocytes are subject to free radical damage from at least three sources: 1.) Free radicals produced internally during the free radical polymerization (stringing chains or networks of molecules together by chemical means) of L-Dopa and L-tyrosine to form the pigment melanin; 2.) Free radicals produced externally by free radical autoxidation of scalp lipids; 3.) Free radicals produced externally by an autoimmune attack by one's own macrophages (a type of white blood cell) on one's own melanocytes (melanin-manufacturing cells). The free radical scavenging antioxidant mix that "Miss Jones" takes can provide some protection against all these. In this case, the white areas of her hair shrank back almost entirely, with the new hair normally pigmented.

"Miss Jones" says her hair grows quite a bit faster now. The inclusion of the antioxidant amino acid cysteine in her experimental formula may be a major factor since hair is 8 percent cysteine, serum cysteine falls with age, and cysteine is not found in large quantities in most diets (eggs are probably the best natural source, containing about 250 milligrams of cysteine per egg). She says, "My hair is twice as thick now."

THE ACTRESS WHO BRUISED TOO EASILY

"Miss Jones" used to get lots of bruises all of the time because she is physically active, yet has delicate skin. Her improved resistance to bruising is almost certainly due to the antioxidant nutrient mix she is using. The damage in a bruise and the colors, too, are caused by free radical damage in the injured area. A bruise is a crushing injury. The broken capillaries in the injury leak red blood cells which hemolyze (break down), releasing copper and iron into the surrounding tissues, where they catalyze (stimulate) the production of free radicals. It's like a bad spot on a banana, which is also caused by free radical damage. Antioxidants scavenge the free radicals, thereby preventing the damage and even the formation of the black, blue, yellow, and other colors you normally see. We told her about the free radical scavenging properties of DMSO and of its value in crushing injuries. DMSO, given by injection shortly after an experimental crushing spinal cord injury in cats, has been shown to provide a degree of protection against the development of paraplegia that would normally occur in unprotected animals.

Once, she had been skiing and ended up with a grapefruit-sized bruise on her leg. It looked ghastly. Two hours after noticing the bruise, "Miss Jones" used DMSO on it and then again the next morning. She says that the bruise faded out overnight and was gone in a week. She estimates that it would have taken at least a few weeks to disappear without the DMSO.

Another time, she fell down fifteen to twenty feet of stairs, receiving a severe blow on her thigh. This time, she put DMSO on the injured area within about twenty minutes—it never turned black and blue but only a little yellow, then disappeared.

DMSO (dimethyl sulfoxide) can be very effective in preventing the further development of injuries by scavenging free radicals involved in the damage process. DMSO is a scavenger of hydroxyl radicals, the most potent type of free radical known. (These radicals are involved in some forms of arthritis, which is why some arthritics find DMSO so effective for improved mobility and relief of pain. DMSO, however, is not a pain killer. Pain is relieved because the hydroxyl radicals are scavenged, preventing them from continuing to damage the lubricating fluids and joint membranes.) For best results, DMSO should be used soon after an injury occurs, within the first two hours if possible. DMSO should also be used only in conjunction with other antioxidants because DMSO is itself turned into a free radical in the process of interacting with hydroxyl radicals. The DMSO free radical is nowhere near as dangerous as the hydroxyl radical, but it is not harmless and other antioxidants should be present to scavenge it. These DMSO free radicals are the reason that rabbits given huge doses of DMSO without other antioxidants have developed cataracts. Another hydroxyl radical scavenger, though not as potent as DMSO, is the sugar inositol, which is a membrane stabilizer.

TAKING HYDERGINE® THE EUROPEAN WAY

"Miss Jones" obtained a supply of 4.5 milligram Hydergine® tablets in Europe. (Too bad they are not available in the United States due to FDA regulations.) She told us that when she feels illness coming on—the appearance of symptoms like hot eyes and aches all over—she uses two of these 4.5 milligram Hydergine® tablets (a total of 9 milligrams a day) along with the usual amount of nutrient mix and these symptoms are gone after about a day. "Miss Jones" says that when she uses Hydergine®, "I feel on top of things more."

INCREASED RESISTANCE TO SUNBURN

"Miss Jones" used to have very sensitive skin which sunburned easily. She stayed out of the sun. Now she has more resistance to sunburns; her skin doesn't get pink even when she is skiing (she uses a little sunblock, just as she did before when her skin was much more sensitive to the sun). This ability of her skin to resist damage by the sun's ultraviolet light is due, we think, to the protective properties of the antioxidant nutrients and prescriptions drugs she is taking. Everybody we know who is taking significant quantities of supplemental antioxidants and who has since been exposed to solar ultraviolet light for an extended period has reported increased resistance of their skin to sunburns.

DURK'S CASE HISTORY

I was born in 1943, and weighed 9 pounds 12½ ounces. At the age of 2½, I nearly died of bacterial pneumonia; a shot of a new wonder drug called penicillin (which at the time was still a crude yellow-tan gook) brought me from delirium to feeling quite good (albeit a bit weak) in just a few hours. This is when I became intensely interested in science; I wanted to know how and why it worked in case I ever got sick like that again.

By the age of 5, some chronic physiological problems had appeared.

DURK'S BAD BACK

My spine is somewhat abnormally curved, and I had rather bad backaches every day. A back specialist was consulted, who said that surgery would probably not help much and might do harm. He recommended at least several years of wearing a back brace that was less comfortable and less acceptable in appearance than a straitjacket. I preferred the backaches to the brace. My parents weren't at all permissive, and I had to make it clear to them that I would run away from home, if necessary, to escape that ghastly brace. These chron-

ic daily backaches (usually worst in the afternoon) remained
with me until 1968. About two months after I started to take
50,000 IU of vitamin A and about 1200 IU of vitamin E and
3 grams of vitamin C per day, I suddenly realized that I had
not had a backache for several days. The backache returned
within a few days each time I discontinued the vitamins, and
vanished within a day after restarting them. Although this
was not a double blind placebo controlled test, I had not
expected the vitamins to do anything for my bad back. I was
taking the vitamins strictly for prophylaxis against free radical
aging damage, which I thought would have only very long
term effects. Indeed, in 1968, I expected no perceptible short
term effects whatsoever, and was initially quite reluctant to
ascribe the results to the vitamins. Moreover, I am not a
strong placebo responder, and placebo effects rarely persist
for long periods of time. Before using these large doses of antioxidant vitamins, I had had a chronic backache for over 20
years; with the vitamins, I have been normally free of backaches for about 13 years. Of course, overexertion can still occasionally lead to brief back pains, and I have had a few
backaches due to acute attacks of gout as well. My back problem may involve both the spinal curvature and genetic factors
related to my mother's rheumatoid arthritis, which developed
when she was only 19 or 20 years old. Autoimmune diseases
such as rheumatoid arthritis are often heritable.

DURK'S PECULIAR PITUITARY, POLYDIPSIA, AND POLYURIA

A second problem noticed before the age of five was
polyuria and polydipsia (excessive urination and fluid consumption). I would wake up every night and have to urinate.
At first, there was concern that this might be due to diabetes
mellitus (sugar-insulin diabetes), since I had an uncle with
both diabetes mellitus and tuberculosis. (The latter is caused
by a poor T-cell immune system response and the former may
be an autoimmune disease involving T suppressor cell inadequacy.) When tests showed that my blood sugar was normal,
my urine sugar-free, and my kidneys and prostate normal, I
was diagnosed as having a mild case of diabetes insipidus,
caused by inadequate release of the hormone vasopressin by

the pituitary gland. Our physician told us that the available vasopressin preparations were expensive, not very effective, and tended to cause the development of an allergy to beef, so he recommended that I simply drink lots of fluids and use plenty of salt (to replace that lost with the urine). This condition has very slowly progressed over the years (though not to a hazardous extent), so that if I do not now use Diapid®nasal spray (vasopressin), I have to get up and urinate two or sometimes even three times in a night. Diapid® is a synthetic vasopressin and does not contain the potentially allergenic beef protein of the old natural beef posterior pituitary powder preparations.

DURK'S ALLERGIES

A third early problem was occasional migraine headaches, which were eventually traced to an allergic origin. Our physician told me that these allergies sometimes vanished after puberty, and indeed mine did. Another change in allergies also occurred after puberty; I became strongly allergic to cats, whereas before puberty I definitely had plenty of feline acquaintances and no feline allergy. This exact sequence also occurred with my father, though a sample size of one does not demonstrate heritability. My symptoms were like my father's, except that I rarely had breathing impairment: extreme conjunctivitis (red eyes) and eye itching, plus strong itching all over my body. Occasionally, hives developed. These symptoms improved substantially after I started taking high dose A, E, and C, and improved further by the time I was taking what is nearly the formula shown in Appendix G (no arginine or ornithine, only 25 milligrams of vitamin B-2 per day). At this time (1980), Dr. Kurt Donsbach (who publishes some of our pamphlets—see Appendix A) suggested that I had a vitamin B-2 deficiency. He did not know what I was taking at the time, and hence I was rather surprised that he mentioned vitamin B-2, since B-2 was one of the few vitamins that I was not taking in extremely large doses. He said that, in his experience, allergic conjunctivitis often responds well to very large doses of vitamin B-2. Although pessimistic, I tried it and it worked. I can now actually spend the night in an apartment shared by resident cats with only mild conjunctivitis and itching, whereas a couple of years previously, my conjunctivitis and itching would have been more annoying if I even stayed a few hours in a room occupied by cats a year before. I found that 100 milligrams of vitamin B-2 taken 4 times per day is adequate for me. **CAUTION:** Excess vitamin B-2, especially without antioxidant nutrient supplements, may cause photosensitization (excess sensitivity to sunlight).

As soon as I was convinced that B-2 worked for me, I tried to find out why it worked. I found a promising clue in less than 5 minutes in our own technical library. I looked up riboflavin (vitamin B-2) in Goodman and Gillman's *The Pharmacological Basis of Therapeutics* (4th ed., pp. 1410–1411), and found a reference (Beutler, E. "Glutathione reductase: stimulation in normal subjects by riboflavin supplementation," *Science*, vol. 165, pp. 613–615 [1969]), which was also in our own library. A deficiency of reduced glutathione can cause these symptoms, as well as premature hemolysis of red blood cells, which had indeed happened to some of my blood samples. My large cysteine dose would be expected to result in high levels of glutathione (a tripeptide, gamma-L-glutamyl-L-cysteinylglycine, which is made from the 3 amino acids glutamic acid, cysteine, and glycine). Oxidized glutathione is a pro-oxidant, whereas reduced glutathione is an extremely important natural protective antioxidant. (Indeed, reduced glutathione can actually cause aflatoxin induced liver cancers in rats to disappear, apparently reverting to normal liver tissue. See: Novi, "Regression of Aflatoxin B_1-Induced Hepatocellular Carcinomas by Reduced Glutathione," *Science*, vol. 212, pp. 541–542, 1 May 1981.) Vitamin B-2 is required for the enzyme glutathione reductase, which recycles oxidized glutathione back into its protective reduced form. I apparently have an abnormally large B-2 requirement, since no other experimental subjects known to us have shown such symptoms. Nevertheless, we have both increased our B-2 doses, Sandy to 100 milligrams 3 times per day, and I to 100 milligrams 4 times per day. (For further information, see also: Beutler, E. "A series of new screening procedures for pyruvate kinase deficiency, glucose-6-phosphate dehydrogenase deficiency, and glutathione reductase deficiency," *Blood*, vol. 28, p. 553, 1966; and Bamji, M. S. "Glutathione reductase deficiency in red blood cells and riboflavin nutritional status in humans," *Clin. Chim. Acta* vol. 26, p. 263, 1965.)

DURK'S PECULIAR PITUITARY REVISITED

By my teens, there were some other indications of unusual pituitary function. (Of course, my pituitary may have simply been following the erroneous orders of an odd hypothalamus. I will soon undertake a series of radioimmunoassays for hypothalamic and pituitary hormone function to find out.) Taken in isolation, they would not be of sufficient interest to report, but they may have some relevance in the context of my definite mild pituitary-hypothalamic dysfunction. My growth was rather rapid (about 6 feet by 12 years of age), and I was sexually precocious. I became interested in girls at the age of 10, and my current preferred frequency is about 4 times the median (Kinsey, Pomeroy, and Martin, *Sexual Behavior in the Human Male*). This behavior intimately involves unusually early gonadotropin release, LH and FSH (luteinizing hormone and follicle stimulating hormone) from the anterior pituitary, and possibly LHRH (luteinizing hormone releasing hormone) from the hypothalamus. The gonadotropins cause testicular production of testosterone.

The anterior pituitary also produces GH (growth hormone), and my height growth was quite rapid for someone born in 1943. (People are now both sexually maturing more rapidly and growing taller and faster than before, due to nutritional improvements.) Another indicator of early high GH release is to be found in the growth of my knuckles and, to a lesser extent, in my elbows and knees. High levels of GH cause no further height increase once the epiphyses (growth areas) at the ends of the long bones close; however, joint diameters can continue to increase. Although my knuckles are less knobby than in persons with acromegaly (pathological giantism due to extremely high levels of GH), they have caused comment by almost every jeweler who has tried to fit me with a ring. Rings that I can pass over my knuckles only when lubricated with soap are very loose once they are in the normal position on my fingers. (In fact, if you use GH releasers, you should get a jeweler's ring size set, or at least a few cheap but sturdy rings which slide over the knuckle joints with some difficulty. A long-term growth in finger joint diameter (not caused by arthritis, gout, infection, edema, or other disease condition—consult with your doctor) may indicate that your augmented GH levels are too high.)

At 17, I was diagnosed as having varicose veins in my legs (correct) and in my testicles (incorrect, but understandable). My testicles were painfully sensitive to slight pressure and did indeed feel varicose. I discovered the real problem about half a dozen years ago: hyperprolactinemia, the excessive excretion of the polypeptide hormone prolactin by the pituitary. This condition developed after my growth was complete. In fact, it occurred around the time that my weight increased from 172 to 192 in about two months, with no change in exercise or food consumption. This weight change suggests a possible drop in GH release. Both GH and prolactin are secreted by the anterior pituitary. GH and prolactin have similar molecular structures (they probably evolved from the same precursor hormone long ago), and have effects that are mostly opposing, though there is also a small degree of overlap of effects in some animal experiments. Most drugs that increase GH decrease prolactin and vice versa. A switch from relatively high GH release to high prolactin release apparently occurred. In most men, hyperprolactinemia causes loss of libido and potency, but fortunately I was in the minority not so affected. This condition does not usually cause male gynecomastia (breast enlargement), and I exhibited none. It does sometimes cause lactation, and indeed occasional traces of nocturnal lactation could be found on my sheets.

Bromocriptine (Parlodel®, Sandoz) is specific for this condition, causing suppression of pituitary prolactin release within 1 or 2 hours. I obtained some bromocriptine from a scientific colleague in Europe, where it is an approved drug widely used for hyperprolactinemia and for Parkinson's disease. I took an initial dose of 600 micrograms and, within two hours, all testicular hypersensitivity had vanished; palpation revealed no apparent testicular varicosity. Several hours later, things were back to their usual state. So long as I take a total of about 3 milligrams of bromocriptine (divided into four doses) per day, the apparent varicosity and painful hypersensitivity of the testicles, and the nocturnal trace lactation remain absent. The testicular symptoms promptly return whenever I miss a dose, and just as promptly vanish once again when I take it. (The nocturnal trace lactation takes longer to return after discontinuing the drug, typically several days.)

By my teens, there was another abnormality that might also involve pituitary function. I had chronically cold extremities, both hands and feet, though there was no indication of regional hypoxia from circulatory inadequacy. My hands were so cold that I had to go to the bathroom and warm them up with hot water before making out with my girl friends—or else!—They were really cold! I took a number of clinical laboratory thyroid function tests, and invariably had normal blood levels of T3 and T4 (forms of thyroid hormone). These tests measure the amount of thyroid hormone, not its biological effectiveness in the body. A person with normal levels of thyroid hormone may still have a deficiency of thyroid hormone effects if the thyroid receptor number is low, or if the receptors are insensitive, defective, or blocked. After reading Dr. Broda Barnes' book on hypothyroidism, I measured my armpit temperature on awakening several times as per his instructions, and found that my resting body temperature was 97.2 degrees Fahrenheit, below the normal range as stated by Dr. Barnes (97.8 to 98.2 degrees Fahrenheit). I started by taking $\frac{1}{4}$ grain of thyroid extract per day, increasing the dose slowly until my temperature reached the normal range at 1 grain per day. This has also eliminated the generally very untimely "EEEK! Your hands are like ice!" problem which originally motivated me to look into this situation. **CAUTION:** Do not assume that your cold extremities are a thyroid problem; these symptoms can have many causes, with poor circulation being the most common. Be sure to consult with your physician.

DURK'S VARICOSE VEINS

I did, indeed, have varicose veins in my legs, quite possibly inherited from my mother, who has a fairly bad case which developed in her youth. By 17, the calves of my legs felt mushy (that is how everyone palpating them described the feeling) and a mild squeeze would be quite painful. (Fortunately, I had no difficulty in walking long distances.) This problem vanished along with the backaches about two months after I started taking large doses of vitamins A, E, and C in 1968. Discontinuing the vitamins would bring on a relapse within several days. With the vitamins, a sharp slap on my calf is not painful, whereas without them the pain would be severe, and would usually lead to a very painful leg muscle cramp, commonly called a Charley horse. Since childhood, I

had had such occasional leg muscle cramps, most often starting while I was sleeping. These cramps have been completely
abolished by the megavitamins, though they return in a couple of weeks after discontinuing the vitamins. The mushy feel,
the pain, and the cramps are rather reminiscent of white muscle disease. White muscle disease is found in vitamin E and/or
selenium deficient lambs and swine, and is definitely a result
of free radical pathology. White muscle disease is the major
reason that lambs and swine are generally given several times
as much E and selenium in their diets as most supposedly
well-nourished humans.

DURK'S HAIR RAISING EXPERIENCES

I used to have a blizzard of dandruff, itchy scalp, and
very slow growing hair. That was the good news. Then I started going bald in my twenties. . . . For a happy ending to this
tale of woe, see Part III, Chapter 7, "Male Pattern Baldness
and What You Can Do About It."

DURK IGNORES NUTRITION AND
GETS AN AWFUL STOMACHACHE

In 1964 while at MIT, I neglected my nutrition to the
point where I landed in the infirmary with a very painful
preulcerative stomach condition. (I had been taking about
twice the normal workload—there were so many wonderful
things to learn and so little time—and would often forget to
eat for 24 hours, and once for 36 hours. While I utterly ignored the needs of my body, my stomach tried to digest itself,
and partly succeeded.) Yes, in fact, both my father and grandfather had ulcers, and if I had bothered to think about it, the
warning should have been clear. With the help of a physician's advice, lots of Maalox® antacid, and a regularly consumed bland diet, I was back to normal after a few months of
really nasty continuous stomach pain. This experience very
forcefully impressed on me the fact that I was responsible for
my own health, and that while studies in neuroelectronics
were fascinating, I was chronically ignoring my immediate
and practical nutritional requirements. The problem has not
recurred.

DURK'S GOUT

Gout is caused by excessive levels of uric acid and its salts, which crystallize in one's blood and other tissues, the joints and kidneys being particularly subject to damage. Two basic mechanisms may be involved: inadequate urinary excretion of urate, and/or excessive urate production. The enzyme xanthine oxidase oxidizes compounds such as nucleic acids and caffeine to urate, producing hydrogen peroxide and free radicals in the process. Gout is known to be caused by at least 85 different genetic defects, and is frequently heritable, though it can be acquired through kidney damage. Gout is sex-related (though not generally carried on the Y chromosome) in that 95 percent of its victims are males, generally post-pubertal. My grandfather had gout, my father has gout, and so do I. Note: In spite of the appearance of this case history, most medical problems are not heritable; I did not inherit most of my parents' medical problems, which are not discussed here. Nevertheless, it does illustrate the importance of knowing your medical roots (your family medical histories).

My first gout attack occurred in 1976 as a result of what would normally have been a minor back injury. Instead of rapidly improving, my back rapidly became extremely painful. When the pain spread to my knees and feet, I realized that it was either spinal cord damage or gout. At this point, I was on crutches. A serum urate test showed that it was gout, which promptly responded to conventional treatment with colchicine, phenylbutazone, and sulfinpyrazole (Anturane®, Ciba-Geigy). At the time of my first attack, my urate levels were around 18 milligrams per 100 milliliters of serum, whereas 3 to 7 milligrams per 100 milliliters of serum is normal for adult males, and attacks can be expected at over about 9 milligrams per 100 milliliters of serum. My physician was surprised at the extremely high levels of urate that I had had before the injury induced my first attack. I think it plausible that my high doses of membrane stabilizers and antioxidants may have provided this protection.

For a couple of years, I used Anturane® regularly for my gout, with a few attacks per year (generally subsequent to minor foot injury or severe foot hypothermia, both of which can induce urate crystallization). The Anturane® works by increasing renal (kidney) excretion of urate. By about 1978, I had found that allopurinol (Zyloprim®, Burroughs-Wellcome), an inhibitor of xanthine oxidase, worked better for me (but not necessarily for others). My serum urate is now usually normal, and I rarely have even minor foot pain.

DURK AND SUNBURN

My resistance to sunburn has been markedly improved by our life extension experiments, as would be expected from free radical pathology theory. Ultraviolet (UV) light is the cause of sunburn, as is well known, and is the most common single cause of human skin cancer. The burn and the cancer are both caused by the photochemical production of reactive chemical entities in the skin, including free radicals, excited singlet and triplet oxygen, and lipid peroxides and epoxides, all of which can damage both cell membranes and one's genetic blueprints, the DNA. Since these are major random damage mechanisms in aging, an effective biochemical approach to retarding these damaging aging mechanisms should also retard UV burns.

In fact, this has been the case in all of the self-experimental subjects with whom we have been in contact and who have been out in the sun long enough to normally acquire a sunburn. From childhood until 1968, when Sandy and I began our life extension experiments, my solar UV tolerance was constant. After a winter indoors, my first exposure to the spring sun would range from 1 to 2 hours before I would develop the erythema (redness) and tenderness of a sunburn. (Of course, as I built up a tan, my resistance to burning would gradually increase due to the protective effects of the UV-induced deposition of melanin pigment in my skin.)

Our experimental life extension formula provides very substantial protection from UV burns. Taking this formula has extended my initial spring solar UV exposure tolerance from the prior 1 to 2 hours to 5 or 6 hours. Depending on dosage, the self-experimental subjects who exposed themselves to solar UV have typically noticed a 2 to 3 times increase of exposure time required to produce a burn. This correlates well with Sandy's roughly three times increase in resistance to x-ray burns and x-ray induced neurological damage. Tanning does take about twice as long, however.

In the spring of 1981, I added a carotenoid, canthaxanthin, (Orobronze®) to my formula, primarily for its ability to color human skin a golden bronze color without UV exposure, but also for the very substantial protective effects of the carotenoids. The results have been better than expected.

After a winter indoors glued to a computer writing this book with Sandy, we pulled the plug and went on a micro-vacation. I spent 2½ days in the Mohave high desert clothed as shown in the accompanying photos, without even getting a slight sunburn. (This location was about 80 miles south of Death Valley.) The substantial increase in sunburn resistance over the prior summer was presumably due to the addition of Orobronze® (canthaxanthin) to my personal experimental life extension formula (which differs somewhat from Sandy's; see Appendix G). Carotenoids such as beta carotene and canthaxanthin are excellent deactivators of highly reactive and damaging forms of excited oxygen, singlet and triplet oxygen, which are photochemically produced via ultraviolet light. In addition, they are good free radical scavengers (also ultraviolet light induced), and ultraviolet absorbers. The principal mode of activity was not UV (ultraviolet) absorption, however, because my canthaxanthin tan darkened very noticeably due to uv-stimulated melanin production in my skin. Most of the protective effects are probably due to deactivation of excited oxygen and free radicals.

DURK AND GROWTH HORMONE RELEASERS

I have been interested in GH (growth hormone) for several years because of its potential for improving immune system function and tissue repair in adults. Indeed, in 1976 I wrote a research proposal for private funding called "Toward a Possible Life Extension Technology Involving Human Growth Hormone." This proposal dealt with the use of GH releasers (such as arginine, ornithine, L-Dopa, and bromocriptine) to maintain teenage to young adult levels of GH in adults of any age. Human growth hormone manufactured like penicillin, using genetically engineered microbes, will be available in a few years. In the meantime, GH releasers—substances that cause the pituitary gland to release GH—are the most practical way to go. The growth hormones of domestic animals are completely ineffective in humans.

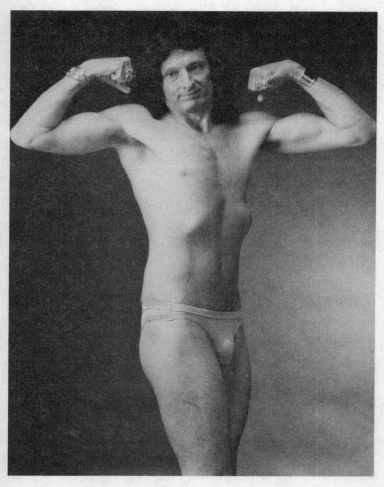

I'd rather eat growth hormone releasing nutrients than exercise. My 13 percent body fat is close to the 12.4 percent average for male athletes who are world class swimmers.

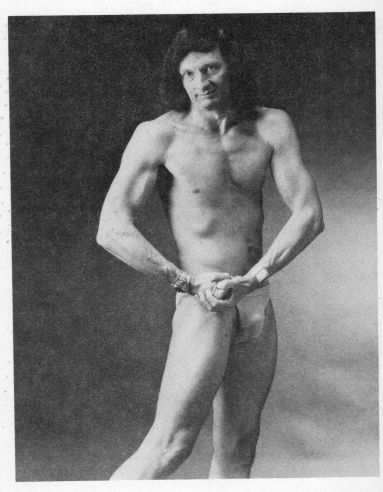

Can life extenders do it longer in the sun? Yes, you can be in the sun longer without burning when you use singlet oxygen quenchers and free radical scavenging antioxidants. Anyone for a romp in the desert?

Sandy's very dramatic muscle growth with GH releasers and mere token exercise had a real impact on my thinking, and when I had to work hard to beat her at arm wrestling. . . . Well, it was simply unacceptable; I have always been strong for my weight, and to have to work hard to beat a woman who weighed 50 pounds less and was over a foot shorter was a bit of a shock. At this time, Sandy was beating quite a few much larger men, including some who exercised regularly. This was when I added the arginine and/or ornithine to my own experimental formula. I reasoned that with my much higher natural levels of testosterone than Sandy, I ought to be able to readily build up a nice set of muscles. All the photos of me in this book were taken at the same session, about two months after I increased my arginine dose from 3 to 8 grams per day. These muscles represent a total investment of about 30 minutes of exercise and a lot of hard thinking. Sandy's GH releaser dose is about three times as large as mine when scaled for our different body weights. Sandy's results have been so outstanding that I have just doubled my arginine and/or ornithine dose. Excessive GH levels can be a health hazard. See the **CAUTION** in Part III Chapter 9, "Athletics." Remember that this is an **experimental** procedure!

PERCENT BODY FAT OF SANDY AND DURK

Sandy and Durk are two sedentary research scientists, but using the techniques described in this book, they have both been able to develop their musculature while also reducing body fat. A simple way to determine percent body fat is to measure the thicknesses of two specified skinfolds, in different places for men and women. Body fat measurements calculated using this system have been correlated with the body density determined by underwater weighing. Muscle is denser than fat; by comparing body weight in air versus submerged in water, density and hence fat percentage can be determined. The paper which gave the instructions for the specific places to measure skinfolds also provided nomograms so that the percent body fat could be determined quickly once the two fatfold measurements have been made. You will need a good medical dictionary (such as *Dorland's Illustrated*) to interpret the instructions concerning where to measure the skinfolds. For further details, see Sloan and Weir, "Nomograms for prediction of body density and total body fat from skinfold measurements," *J. Appl. Physiol.* 28(2):221–222, 1970.

On 21 May, 1981, Sandy and Durk determined their percent body fats using the above technique. The results were:

SANDY'S PERCENT BODY FAT	DURK'S PERCENT BODY FAT
16.4	13

In the July 1980 issue of *The Olympian* (published by the U.S. Olympics Committee), there was an article in which male and female world class (including Olympics) athletes' body fat charts appeared, which were determined by the above skinfold method or underwater weighing. The female athletes, for example, had mean (average) percent body fat ranging from 10.7 (elite athletics 800 meters) to 22.2 (elite canoe and kayak). Female elite Alpine skiers had a mean percent body fat of 17.9%. Sandy's percent body fat is well within the range of these world class female athletes! The male athletes' percent body fat was lower on the average than that of the females, as is to be expected. It ranged from 6.3 (elite athletics 400 meters) to 19.9 (junior ice hockey). The male elite swimmers had a mean percent body fat of 12.4 and male elite canoers and kayakers had 13.0% mean percent body fat. Durk's percent body fat is just within the range of these highly trained world class male athletes. See our photographs in this appendix.

SANDY AND DURK'S CLINICAL LABORATORY TEST FINDINGS

For an explanation of various clinical laboratory tests, see Part V, Chapter 4.

During the past 13 years, we have been taking an experimental life extension formula of increasing complexity. We have both taken hundreds of clinical laboratory tests during this time to monitor for possible toxic effects and for indications of possible beneficial effects. Most of the results of these tests are routine and would be of no interest to the general reader, since they merely confirm the absence of certain possible toxic effects. These test results are available to legitimate research scientists, however. We report here the results of some tests of particular interest.

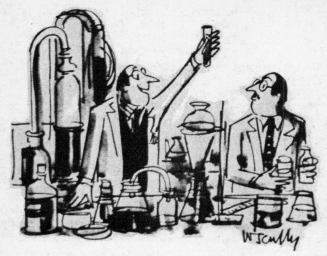

"I've done it! A substitute for health food."

In our first set of clinical laboratory tests after starting our use of large doses of supplemental nutrients (1969), Durk had a cholesterol level of 168, Sandy's was 118. Durk's triglycerides were 198, Sandy's 82. Durk had a uric acid level of 18.3 milligram per 100 milliliters of serum (hazardously high, with gout attacks a real threat), while Sandy's was 9.5 milligrams (also somewhat high). Durk's SGOT and SGPT, measures of liver enzyme activity, were both 70 units. Sandy's SGOT and SGPT were 60 units and 35 units respectively. These levels are somewhat high. We had, however, expected this because BHT, one of the components of our experimental formulation, induces increased levels of some liver enzymes. In fact, when given at very high doses to experimental animals, BHT can induce a reversible liver enlargement. Rhesus monkeys fed 500 milligrams per kilogram or 50 milligrams per kilogram of BHT had lowered cholesterol levels. BHT also lowered the susceptibility of the monkeys' liver lipids (fats) to peroxidation and increased their levels of lipid phosphorus (phospholipids), biological surfactants which help to emulsify and remove fats from the body.

In tests taken in April 1979, Durk and Sandy's potassium levels were apparently hazardously elevated; however, Sandy's high potassium turned out to be due to hemolysis (leakage of potassium from red blood cells damaged in the testing process). Durk's potassium could not be attributed to hemolysis but appears to be an artifact because nobody could survive having such a high potassium level.

Another series of tests taken in May 1979 while attending a gerontology conference were normal (including Durk's potassium) except for moderately elevated SGOT and alkaline phosphatase (liver enzymes) for both Durk and Sandy. These liver enzyme elevations have been stable over the past decade and have not shown a pattern of progressive deterioration. Serum glucose tests using the hexokinase method were normal.

In October 1978, while at another gerontology conference, Durk and Sandy visited Dr. Lundgren's laboratory at Donner Research Laboratories at the University of California at Berkeley to have their HDL and LDL levels measured (see Part III Chapter 18). Dr. Lundgren is the scientist who developed this test of lipoproteins. At that time, Durk had a cholesterol level of only 91.4, while Sandy's was 113.8. The following charts show the HDL, LDL, and ratio of LDL/HDL (the higher the ratio, the greater the risk of heart disease) for Durk and Sandy. Sandy's LDL is in the lowest 1 percent of women; 99 percent have higher LDL's. Durk's LDL is also at the lowest end of the human male range.

A fraction of blood lipoproteins called beta-very-low-density lipoprotein (beta-VLDL) delivers cholesterol in the blood to cells in arteries around the heart, according to Dr. Robert W. Mahley and his co-workers. They found that when dietary fat intake rose, the concentration in the blood of the beta-VLDL increased. Conversely, when dietary intake of fat and cholesterol was low, the beta-VLDL was absent. (This was reported in the June 22, 1981 *Chem. Eng. News.*) Goodman and Gilman discuss the ability of niacin to reduce VLDL and triglycerides on page 768 of the fourth edition of *The Pharmacological Basis of Therapeutics.* We eat a rather high fat diet but have very low levels of VLDL. When these levels were measured in October of 1978, Sandy had a VLDL lower than 94 percent of women in her age group; Durk had a VLDL lower than 92 percent of men in his age group.

SANDY AND DURK'S TEST DATA
6 October 1978

BLOOD FATS   Percent of people of their gen-
                              der and age group with higher
                              measured values of blood fats

	SANDY	DURK
HDL	63	81
VLDL	94	92
LDL	99	100
TG	79	48
CHOL	100	100

HDL is high density lipoproteins
VLDL is very low density lipoproteins
LDL is low density lipoproteins
TG is triglycerides
CHOL is cholesterol

CALCULATION OF RISK OF CARDIOVASCULAR DISEASE—LDL CHOL/HDL CHOL

	TOTAL HDL	HDL CHOLESTEROL (total × .18)	LDL TOTAL	LDL CHOL (total × .45)	LDL CHOL/ HDL CHOL
SANDY	285	51.3	197	88.7	1.72
DURK	170	30.6	178	80.1	2.62

CARDIOVASCULAR DISEASE RISK

	RISK	LDL CHOL/HDL CHOL
Men	½ average	1.00
	average	3.55
	2× average	6.25
	3× average	7.99
Women	½ average	1.47
	average	3.22
	2× average	5.03
	3× average	6.14

The above risk calculations were made from a population of people who did not have drastically reduced cholesterol levels like ours. Therefore, the indicated level of risk may not apply to us.

See Part III Chapter 18 for more on HDL and LDL and their relationship to cardiovascular disease.

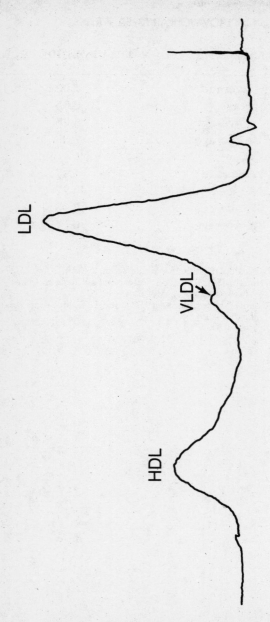

This chart of the distribution of blood fats was prepared from data for a middle-aged smoking man. It is included to show where LDL, VLDL, and HDL peaks are located.

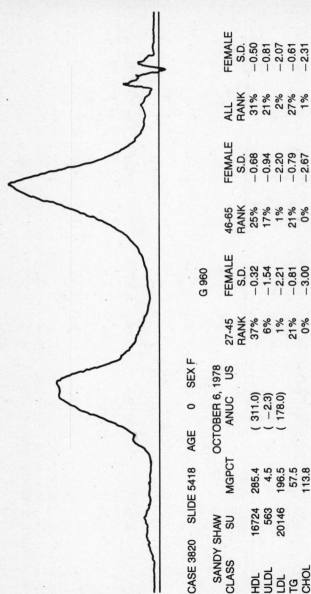

CASE 3820   SLIDE 5418   AGE 0   SEX F   G 960

SANDY SHAW   OCTOBER 6, 1978

CLASS	SU	MGPCT	ANUC US	27-45 RANK	FEMALE S.D.	46-65 RANK	FEMALE S.D.	ALL RANK	FEMALE S.D.
HDL	16724	285.4	(311.0)	37%	−0.32	25%	−0.68	31%	−0.50
ULDL	563	4.5	(−2.3)	6%	−1.54	17%	−0.94	21%	−0.81
LDL	20146	196.5	(178.0)	1%	−2.21	1%	−2.20	2%	−2.07
TG		57.5		21%	−0.81	21%	−0.79	27%	−0.61
CHOL		113.8		0%	−3.00	0%	−2.67	1%	−2.31

BETA PEAK MIGRATED 176 UNITS (27.0 PERCENT OF TOTAL RANGE)

FRACTIONS UTILIZED WS   ALPHA STAINING FACTOR USED IS 1.75
STANDARDIZED USING CHOL

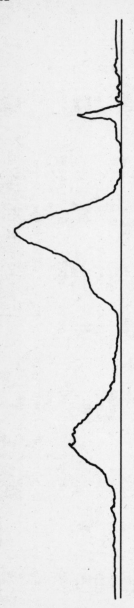

CASE 3819   SLIDE 5417   AGE   0   SEX M

DURK PEARSON   OCTOBER 6, 1978   G 960

CLASS	SU	MGPCT	ANUC	US	27-46 RANK	MALE S.D.	47-66 RANK	MALE S.D.	ALL RANK	MALE S.D.
HDL	8076	170.1	(220.6)		19%	−0.88	22%	−0.79	20%	−0.83
ULDL	2647	26.1	(16.3)		8%	−1.42	8%	−1.42	8%	−1.40
LDL	14824	178.4	(162.1)		0%	−2.86	0%	−3.38	0%	−2.77
TG		116.7			52%	0.06	36%	−0.37	43%	−0.18
CHOL		91.4			0%	−3.67	0%	−4.26	0%	−3.44

BETA PEAK MIGRATED 203 UNITS (29.3 PERCENT OF TOTAL RANGE)

FRACTIONS UTILIZED WS   ALPHA STAINING FACTOR USED IS 1.75
STANDARDIZED USING CHOL

GLOSSARY:
A Layman's Guide to
Word Usage

Note: These are generally not full technical definitions.

acetaldehyde — an aldehyde found in cigarette smoke, auto exhaust, smog, and created in the liver from alcohol. Acetaldehyde autoxidizes (spontaneously oxidizes in the presence of air) to produce the organic peroxide peracetic acid and damaging free radicals, and is a mutagen, carcinogen, and cross-linker.

$$H-\overset{\overset{\displaystyle H}{|}}{\underset{\underset{\displaystyle H}{|}}{C}}-\overset{\overset{\displaystyle }{}}{\underset{\underset{\displaystyle H}{|}}{C}}=O$$

acetaldehyde

acetylcholine — ACh, a natural chemical which is used as a neurotransmitter in the brain (especially for memory and the control of sensory input signals and muscular output signals), and as a neuromuscular transmitter (ACh released by muscle nerves makes muscles contract). It is made by the brain from the precursor nutrient choline.

$$CH_3-\overset{\overset{\displaystyle CH_3}{|}}{\underset{\underset{\displaystyle CH_3}{|}}{N}}-\overset{\overset{\displaystyle H}{|}}{\underset{\underset{\displaystyle H}{|}}{C}}-\overset{\overset{\displaystyle H}{|}}{\underset{\underset{\displaystyle H}{|}}{C}}-O-\overset{\overset{\displaystyle O}{\|}}{C}-CH_3$$

acetylcholine

aerobic — oxygen-requiring metabolic processes and organisms.

aging — the decline of physiological functions which occurs with time, accompanied by a falling probability of survival.

aging clocks — biological clocks which turn physiological processes on or off at specific genetically programmed times. Examples are menopause and male pattern balding.

aldehydes — a class of organic compounds which have an end group with a carbon and oxygen double bonded to each other and with a hydrogen bonded to the same carbon. These compounds, related to formaldehyde, are cross-linkers, mutagens, and carcinogens. Malonaldehyde, created in the breakdown of peroxidized fats, is also carcinogenic and an extremely potent cross-linker. Acetaldehyde is made from alcohol in the liver (the acetaldehyde is a major reason alcoholics have such heavily wrinkled skin) and is found in cigarette smoke and smog. Most aldehydes autoxidize, producing damaging free radicals.

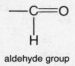

aldehyde group

amino acid — an organic acid containing an amine (ammonia-like) chemical group. Amino acids are connected together in specific ways to form polypeptides and proteins. The simplest amino acid is glycine; its structure is shown under that entry in the glossary.

amyloid — a type of aging pigment which accumulates in nerve cells and is believed to damage nervous tissues by compression and infiltration, and by blocking proper flow of vital nutrients. One type of amyloid is comprised of antibody-antigen complexes and is caused by an autoimmune disease.

anaerobic — metabolic processes and organisms that do not require oxygen. Also means "without oxygen."

androgens — male sex hormones

anecdotal evidence — observations of treatment effects in nonscientific studies, without controls, not blind. These observations cannot prove anything in themselves but sometimes provide leads for useful research.

anoxia — the absence of oxygen

antibody — a large Y shaped protein molecule made by B-cells of the immune system which very selectively binds to other specific protein molecules called antigens. Specific antibodies combine with and inactivate specific viruses, while other specific antibodies mark invading bacteria and cancer cells for destruction by other cells of the immune system.

antigen — a protein which is recognized by antibodies and other parts of the immune system. Different antigens distinguish enemies (such as bacteria, cancer cells, viruses, and foreign tissue) from your own normal cells.

antioxidant — a chemical which combines with free radicals and/or other chemicals that release free radicals that would otherwise attack molecules in the body, and abnormally oxidize them. Susceptible molecules include such vital entities as DNA, RNA, lipids (fats), and proteins. The antioxidant, by reacting with the oxidant, protects these important molecules from being damaged. Examples of antioxidants include vitamins A, C, E, B-1, B-5, B-6, the amino acid cysteine, the food antioxidants BHT and BHA, and the minerals selenium and zinc.

artifact — a peculiar test or experimental result which is due to some unusual detail in the procedure which invalidates the usual interpretation of the test or experiment. Example: our blood sugar appears to be lethally low on the glucose oxidase blood sugar test and lethally high on the orthotoluidine blood sugar test. Both of these results are artifacts because the high levels of antioxidants in our blood interfere with the chemical reactions in these test procedures. (Our blood sugar levels are normal when measured by the hexokinase test, in which high antioxidant levels in the blood do not interfere.)

atherosclerosis — a common degenerative disease of the arteries, caused by free radical damage. Atherosclerotic plaques are tumors which grow into and damage the artery lining. Cholesterol and other fats deposited into the injured area become oxidized, further increasing free radical activity and resulting in adherence of platelets (blood clot-making particles) to plaques. The platelets attract red blood cells which burst (hemolyze), leaking iron and copper, which are powerful free radical autoxidation catalysts. Eventually atherosclerotic arteries narrow and may become blocked by a blood clot, causing a heart attack, stroke, or phlebitis.

ATP — adenosine triphosphate, the universal energy storage molecule. Energy released during the oxidation of foodstuffs to carbon dioxide and water are stored in the high energy phosphate bonds of ATP.

autoantibodies — antibodies which attack other molecules or cells of their own body.

autoimmune — a state in which a person's immune system erroneously attacks some of his or her own cells, damaging them. Rheumatoid arthritis and multiple sclerosis are examples of conditions thought to be autoimmune diseases. As people age, autoimmunity becomes more and more prevalent.

autoxidation — a spontaneous oxidation reaction in which a molecule reacts with oxygen via a free radical, self-catalyzed route. The development of rancidity in fatty foods, the formation of gum in old gasoline, and the spontaneous combustion of rags soaked with oil-base paint are examples of autoxidation.

B-cells — white blood cells which make antibodies, usually under instructions from the white blood cells called T-cells. B-cells are made in your bone marrow, either directly or by division of cells originally made there, and so the name "B-cells."

biological clocks — long-term clocks involving DNA that keep track of time, and which turn on and off various genetic programs which are "set" for various times. Menopause, male pattern balding, and the spawning of salmon are examples of biological aging clocks. A major theory of aging proposes that an aging clock may drastically alter production and use of certain hypothalamic and pituitary gland hormones, thereby causing death. Sleeping and waking take place as a result of a circadian (daily) biological clock, which probably involves somewhat different mechanisms.

carcinogenesis — the process of causing cancer, usually by altering DNA.

carcinogens — cancer causing agents.

carotenoid — a class of very important antioxidants produced by plants which protects them from damage caused by singlet and triplet oxygen and free radicals produced during photosynthesis. Carotenoids also provide protection from UV damage and can prevent the development of cancer in experimental animals. They are usually colored bright yellow, orange, or red. Carotenoids make carrots orange, and fall leaves a beautiful array of colors.

CAT scanner — A modern diagnostic tool for which the inventors have received the Nobel Prize in medicine and physiology. CAT stands for computerized axial tomography. It provides x-ray or gamma ray images of the interior of the body with unprecedented clarity and detail. To make a regular x-ray, one's body is placed between the x-ray source and the x-ray detector which is usually a sheet of x-ray film. The x-ray image is a superimposed set of shadows of everything between source and detector, which can make finding a minute tumor or a tiny blocked artery quite difficult. A CAT scanner scans the x-ray source and electronic x-ray detector completely around the body in a circle. A computer memorizes the radiation detected at every position of the scanner. The computer then performs millions of calculations and synthesizes and displays a series of three dimensional cross sections of the CAT scanned body. From a diagnostic standpoint, it is the next best thing to actually cutting the person up; indeed, much unnecessary surgery has been prevented by the use of CAT scanners.

catalase — an enzyme which catalyzes the breakdown of hydrogen peroxide in the body. Catalase is found in all organisms which require oxygen or can survive in its presence.

catalyst — a chemical which acts to stimulate a particular chemical reaction, usually without itself being permanently chemically changed in the process. Enzymes are a form of biological catalyst. Iron and copper are powerful free radical autoxidation catalysts. The products of free radical autoxidation of lipids (oils and fats) catalyze further autoxidation: hence the process is called autocatalytic. The spontaneous combustion of oil-based paint-soaked rags is autocatalytic autoxidation.

catecholamines — a class of brain neurotransmitters (chemicals which serve to carry communications between nerves) which includes norepinephrine and dopamine. Both of these decline with age, particularly dopamine, with consequent decline of functions dependent on these catecholamines. The autoxidation of dopamine results in 6-OH-dopamine, hydrogen peroxide, and free radicals which damage the receptors for dopamine. 6-OH-dopamine autoxidation is suspected as being responsible for the pathetic "burnt out" schizophrenic and may be involved in producing Parkinsonism.

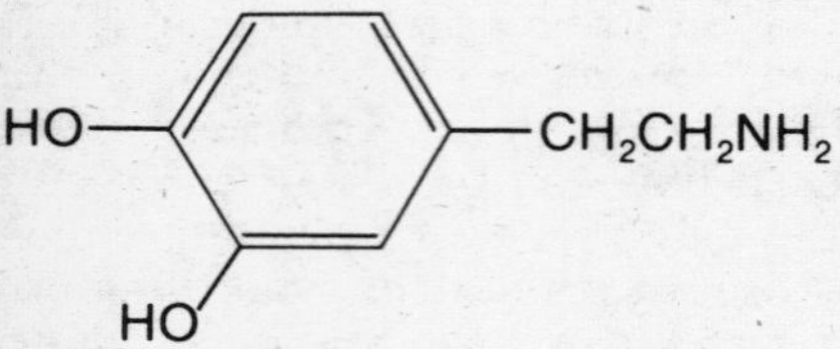

HOCHCH$_2$NH$_2$

HO—⬡—CH$_2$CH$_2$NH$_2$

HO

OH

OH

dopamine 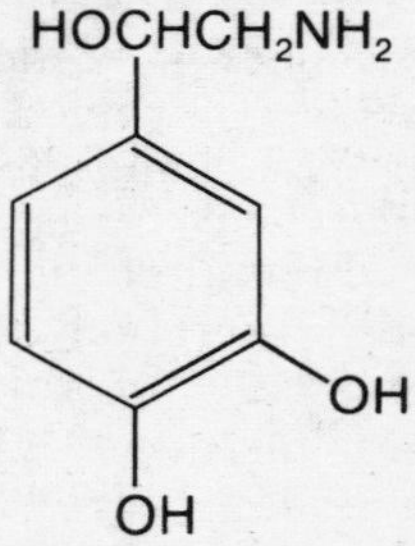   norepinephrine

central nervous system — the brain, spinal cord, optic nerves, retinas, auditory nerves, pituitary and pineal glands, hypothalamus, and other structures enclosed within the special membranes surrounding the brain and spinal cord.

ceroid — an accumulated fluorescent pigment, commonly found in vitamin E deficient animals and humans.

chelation — the process of forming a closely associated complex with a metal in which the metal is surrounded by and multiply bound to part of an organic structure, thereby usually altering both the chemical reactivity and transport properties of the metal.

cholinergic — those parts of the nervous system, both peripheral and in the brain, using acetylcholine as a neurotransmitter. Acetylcholine released at the synapse (junction) between a motor nerve and a muscle fiber causes the muscle fiber to contract. Acetylcholine is an important brain neurotransmitter, too, being involved in memory, long-term planning, control of mental focus, sexual activity, and other functions. It is made in the body from choline in reactions requiring the availability of adequate vitamin B-5 (as part of the enzyme acetyl co-enzyme A).

chromosomes — double stranded DNA helixes which contain the basic blueprints for physiological activities, including some of their associated control and regulation proteins. The DNA from a human cell would be about 1 meter long if stretched out; it is normally stored in compact supercoiled (coiled coils) packages, the microscopic chromosomes.

Citric Acid Cycle (also called the Kreb's Cycle and the Tricarboxylic Acid Cycle) — this cycle stores energy, released by the oxidation of fats, proteins, and carbohydrates in foodstuffs, in high energy phosphate bonds of ATP. About 90 percent of the energy released from food occurs in this Citric Acid Cycle. In the process, a series of acids (see figure in Part II Chapter 4) are oxidized to release the energy used in forming high-energy ATP phosphate bonds, plus carbon dioxide and water. ATP is life's universal energy supply.

clone — an identical twin of another cell or animal, with the same genetic instructions (DNA). Nowadays, this term is sometimes also used to refer to mass produced copies of a DNA strand, as in cloned DNA.

collagen — a connective tissue protein, the most abundant protein in the human body, about 30 percent of total body protein.

complement — a system of protein molecules produced by the immune system which kills antibody-tagged foreign cells by making holes in their cell membranes.

controls — a technique used to evaluate experimental treatments by having two groups of experimental subjects, one to receive treatment, and one subjected to the same conditions but not given the treatment. This way, scientists can find out whether effects they are seeing are due to treatment or some other experimental condition. Non-controlled experiments are considered very difficult to evaluate because of the absence of controls with which to compare treated subjects.

cross-linking — an oxidation reaction in which undesirable bonds form between nucleic acids (RNA and DNA, the genetic blueprint material) or between proteins, often as links between sulfur atoms called disulfide bonds, or between lipids or any combination thereof. The links may be between different proteins or nucleic acids or lipids or between parts of the same protein or nucleic acid or lipid. The result is that the molecule cannot assume the correct shape for proper functioning. Some cross-links are required in proteins for rigidity and structural strength. However, cross-links of an inappropriate, undesired nature form throughout life, resulting in such conditions as artery rigidity, skin wrinkling, and loss of eye focus accommodation due to aging. The hardening and fluid loss ("weeping") of an old gelatin dessert and the deterioration of your automobile's windshield wiper blades and rubber hoses is caused by cross-linking. Free radicals, aldehydes, ozone, ultraviolet light, and x-rays are powerful cross-linkers. The vulcanization which converts soft latex gum into a hard rubber comb involves disulfide bond cross-linking.

de-differentiation — loss by mature cells of some of their specialized properties and reversion to a less developed state. De-differentiation is a normal part of healing and regeneration. De-differentiation is also often a part of the early development of tumors.

dehydroascorbic acid — toxic oxidized form of vitamin C (ascorbic acid); it is a pro-oxidant rather than antioxidant.

differentiation — a genetic clock program of cellular development with time. Cells begin with the ability to turn into many different tissue types; through the process of differentiation, they become more and more specialized in function and generally retain the properties of cells of a specific type of tissue.

diffusion — a passive form of random movement, in which areas of high chemical concentration gradually spread throughout an entire system, equalizing the chemical concentration over the system. For example, the exchange of gases in the lungs occurs by simple diffusion across capillary walls.

disulfide — a sulfur to sulfur bond found in both normal and abnormal cross-linked proteins, bonding a protein to parts of the same molecule or to other molecules. These bonds provide the three dimensional structure of molecules containing them. Latex is vulcanized to form rubber by the controlled formation of disulfide bonds.

disulfide bond

DMSO — dimethyl sulfoxide, a hydroxyl radical-scavenging solvent that rapidly penetrates the skin.

$$H_3C—S—CH_3$$

$$\parallel$$

$$O$$

DMSO

DNA — deoxyribonucleic acid, the genetic material, encoding full plans for how living organisms are constructed and how they function. Damage to DNA is believed to be a central feature of both aging and cancer.

dopamine — an important brain neurotransmitter (chemical which enables nerve cells to communicate with each other) which plays a role in body movement, motivation, primitive drives and emotions including sexual behavior, and immune system function. See molecular structure under "catecholamines."

dopaminergic — those parts of the nervous system in the brain which use dopamine as neurotransmitter.

dosimeter — a device for measuring accumulated exposure to x-rays, gamma rays, or other hazardous radiation.

double blind — a technique used in modern scientific research to separate facts from the hopes and wishes of both scientists and experimental subjects. A treatment which is to be tested is administered by scientists who do not know whether they are using the active treatment or the inactive placebo. The experimental subjects don't know which is which, either. The test results are evaluated by scientists who also do not know which group received the active treatment and which the placebo. At the end of the experiment, the secret code is broken, and the responses of the subjects to the real experimental treatment are compared with their responses to the placebo.

EEG — electroencephalogram, the brain's electrical output as measured on the scalp.

EKG — electrocardiogram, the heart's electrical output as measured by electrodes placed on the skin of the torso.

endorphins — natural polypeptide opiate-like substances recently discovered in the brain; one function is the control of pain.

enkephalins — natural small polypeptide opiate-like substances found in the brain which have a much shorter duration of action than the endorphins.

enzyme — a protein which acts as a catalyst in certain metabolic reactions, usually specifically acting on a particular substance or class of substances. Enzymes are generally not themselves destroyed in these reactions. Proper enzyme function depends on the three dimensional configuration of the enzyme molecule, and often requires that the enzyme be properly integrated into a cell membrane.

epidemiology — study of the frequency of occurrence of diseases in natural human or animal populations outside the laboratory.

epistemology — the study of the sources of knowledge; that is, the principles by which one may distinguish what is true from what is not true.

epoxide — a very reactive oxidized form of organic compound, in which two carbon atoms are bonded both to each other and to a single oxygen atom in an organic molecule (see figure). For example, polynuclear aromatic hydrocarbon epoxides and cholesterol epoxides are carcinogenic and mutagenic. Epoxides are excellent cross-linkers, and this reaction is catalyzed by free radicals; this is what happens when you mix epoxy resin and catalyst—the pastes or liquids cross-link to form a hard solid.

epoxide group

esters — The class of organic compounds formed in the reaction of an alcohol and an acid, by the elimination of water. Amyl acetate, the principal aroma note in bananas, is an ester, as are many fruity and floral scents.

estrogens — female sex hormones.

fibroblasts — connective tissue cells.

film badge dosimeter — a dosimeter using photographic film which is sensitive to hazardous high energy radiation, such as x-rays. It is about the size of a badge and is worn in a similar manner by x-ray technicians, nuclear plant workers, and others exposed to these hazards.

free radical — an atom or molecule with an unpaired electron. These chemically reactive entities are produced in the course of normal metabolism, in the breakdown of peroxidized fats in the body, by radiation (radiation sickness is a free radical disease), in ozone interactions with lipids, in the attack of oxidizing agents on fatty acids, particularly those that are unsaturated, and so on. Free radicals are major sources of damage that cause aging, cardiovascular disease, and cancer. Free radical scavengers, molecules which can block free radical chain reactions, have extended experimental animals' life spans and reduced cardiovascular disease and cancer incidence.

GABA — gamma aminobutyric acid. GABA is an amino acid which functions as an inhibitory neurotransmitter in the central nervous system.

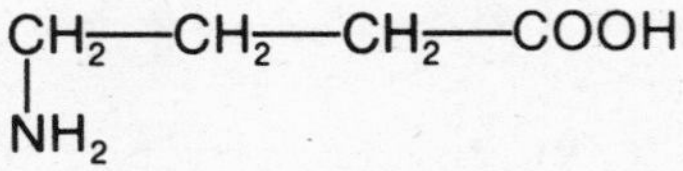

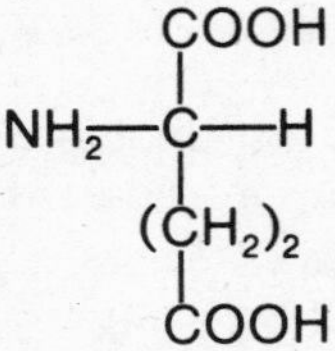

$$CH_2\!-\!CH_2\!-\!CH_2\!-\!COOH$$
$$|$$
$$NH_2$$

GABA

gene — the basic unit of DNA in chromosomes which codes for a protein or affects the expression of genetic information.

glutamate or **glutamic acid** — an excitatory animo acid neurotransmitter in the central neı vous system.

$$COOH$$
$$|$$
$$NH_2\!-\!C\!-\!H$$
$$|$$
$$(CH_2)_2$$
$$|$$
$$COOH$$

glutamic acid

glutathione peroxidase — selenium-and-cysteine-containing enzyme which catalyzes the breakdown of peroxides, while controlling the potentially dangerous free radicals. It also directly scavenges free radicals.

glycine — aminoacetic acid, the simplest amino acid. It is an inhibitory neurotransmitter in the central nervous system.

$$H—CH—COOH$$
$$\underset{NH_2}{|}$$

glycine

glycoprotein — a molecule containing both carbohydrate and protein parts. Many antigens are glycoproteins.

Gompertz Law — a mathematical description of the fact that, as the human population ages, the number of survivors drop off, eventually reaching zero.

It is expressed mathematically as:

$$R_m = -\,1/n \times dn/dt = R_o \times e^{alpha \times t}$$

where n = population size at time t
      dn/dt = death rate
      R_o = a constant, the mortality rate at t = 0
      alpha = a constant
      t = age
      R_m = mortality rate

growth hormone — a polypeptide hormone secreted by the anterior lobe of the pituitary gland in the brain. Growth hormone (GH) plays a crucial role in growth and repair, as well as stimulating the immune system. The GH peaks during sleep which are typical of young people are frequently absent or small in older people, and in those who are obese.

HDL — high density lipoproteins, a fat-transporting fraction of blood which is believed to be associated with a reduced risk of heart disease. See Part III chapter 18.

hemolysis — bursting (lysis) of red blood cells. One way of measuring vitamin E deficiency is by finding out how easily the red blood cells burst when subjected to lysing agents such as hydrogen peroxide. Higher serum levels of vitamin E protect the red blood cells against hemolysis, unless they are then exposed to even higher concentrations of the oxidant hydrogen peroxide.

histamine — an amine which is released during traumas and under stressful conditions. Histamine is necessary for growth and healing, is a capillary dilator (widens these small blood vessels), stimulates stomach acid secretion, and is required for orgasm. Excess histamine release can be toxic. Vitamin C can help detoxify histamine in the body.

histamine structure

histone — a basic protein associated with nucleic acids. Histones are important parts of the DNA control system, suppressing the expression of or causing the expression of specific parts of the DNA blueprints in conjunction with other nucleoproteins.

hormone — a chemical messenger that is transported (often by the bloodstream) a relatively long distance from its source to the cells it affects. Insulin, vasopressin, testosterone, and cortisone are all examples.

hydroxyl radicals — a particularly reactive, damaging type of free radical, formed when superoxide radicals react with hydrogen peroxide. Hydroxyl radicals are thought to be the principal damaging agent to joint membranes in arthritis. X-rays do most of their damage via hydroxyl radicals. Hydroxyl radicals can attack and damage any molecule in your body.

hypercholesterolemia — a class of often hereditary conditions in which the cholesterol levels in the blood are extremely high.

hypothalamus — the master gland of neuroendocrine (hormone) control in the brain. It controls the pituitary's production and release of its own hormones. Appetite and body temperature control centers are located in the hypothalamus. It releases many hormones including LHRH, a natural aphrodisiac. An aging clock or clocks may be located in the hypothalamus.

hypoxia — a condition of oxygen deficiency (but not total absence) in part or all of the body. Under conditions of hypoxia, free radical production is greatly stimulated.

immune system — specialized cells, organs, glycoproteins, and polypeptides which protect the body by locating, killing, and eating foreign invaders (bacteria, parasites, viruses), atherosclerotic plaques, and cancer cells. Includes white blood cells, thymus gland, lymphatic system, spleen, bone marrow, antibodies, complement, and interferon.

infarct — tissue which has died due to lack of oxygen resulting from a blood clot blocking an artery.

inhibitory neurotransmitter — decreases the activity of neurons; examples are GABA (gamma aminobutyric acid), serotonin, and glycine.

interferon — a class of protective proteins produced by the white cells and fibroblasts which prevent viruses from penetrating body cells and which may also help to regulate cell development.

involution — atrophy, shrinking in volume and mass.

LDL — low density lipoproteins, a fraction of blood associated with an increased risk of heart disease and, possibly, cancer.

L-Dopa — a natural amino acid precursor to the neurotransmitter dopamine.

lipids — fats and oils. Fats are solid at body temperature, while oils are liquid at that temperature. Especially important are lipids found in the cellular membranes. Lipids, especially polyunsaturated, are sensitive to damage by oxidants and free radicals.

lipid soluble — dissolves in fats or oils.

lipofuscin — a yellow-brown pigmented waste material deposited in many nerve and skin cells, where it is believed to interfere with cellular metabolism. Lipofuscin is made up of cross-linked, peroxidized lipids and cross-linked proteins. Lipofuscin deposits in skin are colloquially called "age spots" or "liver spots."

lipopigments — aging pigments: lipofuscin, ceroid, and amyloid. See Part II chapter 8.

lymphocyte — type of white blood cell which arises in lymph glands.

lysosomes — special digestive structures in cells, containing powerful tissue-dissolving enzymes. Damage to lysosomes can result in leakage of these enzymes and subsequent tissue damage.

macrophage — a type of white blood cell, which kills and eats bacteria, viruses, and cancer cells.

malonaldehyde — an aldehyde formed as a breakdown product of peroxidized polyunsaturated lipids in the body. Malonaldehyde is a mutagen, carcinogen, and cross-linker.

malonaldehyde

membrane stabilizers — compounds which can protect cellular membranes from damage. Some examples are vitamin E, PABA, inositol, Deaner®, and hydrocortisone.

mitochondria — structures in cells that act as power plants. Mitochondria oxidize food to water, carbon dioxide, and energy. This energy is used by the mitochondria to convert low energy ADP (adenosine diphosphate) to high energy ATP (adenosine triphosphate), the cell's universal energy molecule. Mitochondria, especially those in liver cells, oxidize many drugs and toxins, too. This usually reduces their toxicity, but in some cases can increase it (e.g., metabolically activating PAH to its carcinogenic epoxide form). Free radicals are a normal and essential part of mitochondrial oxidation, but dangerous if they escape from the protective control systems in the mitochondria.

mixed function oxidase — an enzyme system in the liver mitochondria (and to a lesser extent in mitochondria in other cells) which detoxifies many poisons by altering them chemically. Some foods, such as brussels sprouts, activate this system.

monamine oxidase (MAO) — an enzyme which, in the brain, degrades certain neurotransmitters (such as serotonin, dopamine, and norepinephrine). In aging brains, these neurotransmitters may decline in concentration or receptors may be lost or develop insensitivity to them. Monamine oxidase inhibitors are sometimes used as anti-depressants. By reducing the degradation of neurotransmitters, their concentrations can be increased. Examples of monamine oxidase (MAO) inhibitors are isocarboxazid, phenelzine, and tranylcypromine. GH-3 is a mild MAO inhibitor.

mutagen — a chemical which causes alterations in DNA structure, usually resulting in faulty cell function and sometimes in cancer.

neurites — thin tendrils growing from each neuron in the brain in large numbers, through which the neurons communicate with each other. There may be over 100,000 neurites growing from a single neuron. The natural hormone nerve growth factor stimulates growth of neurites (required for learning). Hydergine® (Sandoz) may also stimulate neurite growth via the same mechanism as nerve growth factor.

neurochemical — a chemical found in and active in the nervous system.

neurons — nerve cells.

neurotransmitter — a chemical which serves to carry messages between neurons in the brain. Dopamine, norepinephrine, acetylcholine, serotonin, and GABA are several important known neurotransmitters; there are many others under investigation.

niacin — vitamin B-3, also called nicotinic acid. See Part IV Chapter 9.

niacin structure

nitrosamines — cancer causing chemicals formed by the chemical combination of nitrites and amines (found in proteins and many other organic molecules). Some bacteria make nitrites in the gut, even in the absence of dietary nitrite or nitrate. The formation of nitrosamines can be blocked by vitamin C.

norepinephrine — an important brain neurotransmitter (chemical which enables brain cells to communicate with each other) which plays a role in primitive drives and emotions such as motivation, aggression, and acquisition of food and sex, and body movement. It is sometimes called noradrenaline and is, in fact, the brain's version of adrenaline.

oxidation — a type of chemical reaction in which an electron is attracted away from the oxidized entity. Oxygen is the most familiar oxidizer.

ozone — an excited, highly oxidized form of oxygen; its formula is O_3. It attacks a wide variety of organic molecules, particularly lipids, often producing free radicals in the process.

perfuse — to pour over or through.

peroxidase — an enzyme which catalyzes the breakdown of peroxides in the body.

peroxides — highly oxidized compounds like hydrogen peroxide (H-O-O-H), which not only oxidize lipids directly but in so doing create free radicals which spread in a chain reaction until stopped (quenched) by enzymes like peroxidases, catalases, and superoxide dismutase or by antioxidants like vitamin E and BHT.

peroxidized — a chemical which has been oxidized, so that a peroxide (relative of hydrogen peroxide, H-O-O-H) forms. Unsaturated fats (lipids) in the body are particularly susceptible to peroxidation.

PGI$_2$ — see prostacyclin.

phenylpropanolamine — a chemical closely resembling amphetamine which is used in some over-the-counter appetite control products. Although it has milder side effects than amphetamine, phenylpropanolamine can, after prolonged use, cause depletion of brain norepinephrine (NE) and possible depression. Phenylalanine is a natural precursor to NE, and its use as an appetite inhibitor does not result in NE depletion.

pituitary gland — a gland in the brain which produces and releases several hormones, including growth hormone, LH, FSH, TSH, vasopressin, ACTH, and others. An aging clock may be located in the pituitary.

placebo — a non-active substance used in an experiment to find out the purely psychological effects of the experimental design, and distinguish these from physiological drug effects. When pain patients are given a placebo which they are told is morphine, for example, about 40 percent of these patients obtain pain relief, though this percentage rapidly drops with repeated doses of placebo.

plaques — tumors which form in arteries, damaging the lining and resulting in deposition of platelets, red blood cells, cholesterol and other lipids which are subsequently autoxidized, swelling the wall and subsequently narrowing the artery.

plasma — the watery part of the blood, from which corpuscles have been removed.

polycyclic aromatic hydrocarbons (PAH) — compounds found in combustion tars, created in the burning of nearly all fuels, which are metabolically activated (especially in the liver) to a mutagenic and carcinogenic form. These are the most important human chemical carcinogens and are suspected of being responsible for up to as much as 80 percent of human cancers other than skin cancers. Tobacco smoke is by far the most important source for humans.

polynuclear aromatic hydrocarbons — PAH, same as polycyclic aromatic hydrocarbons.

polypeptides — small proteins, such as hormones. The bond between adjacent amino acids in a protein is called a peptide bond.

polyunsaturated fats — fats containing two or more double bonds between some of their carbon atoms; these bonds are susceptible to autoxidation attack by oxygen and free radicals, which converts polyunsaturated fats to carcinogenic, immune suppressive, clot promoting, cross-linking peroxidized fats. Antioxidants can protect these polyunsaturated fats from such chemical attacks. The more unsaturated (the more double bonds), the more readily autoxidized.

precursor — a chemical which can be converted to another is a precursor of the latter.

primary antioxidant — an antioxidant which blocks formation of peroxides by scavenging free radicals. Examples are vitamins A, C, E, B-1, B-5, B-6, cysteine, zinc, and selenium.

progeria — a group of inherited conditions resembling accelerated aging. Victims generally die before their teens of strokes or heart attack, looking like little old men or women, bald, bent over, with wrinkled faces, and so on.

prophylactic — as a preventive.

prostacyclin — the prostaglandin hormone PGI_2, a natural hormone made by normal artery wall lining cells (intima) to inhibit the formation of abnormal blood clots. Peroxidized lipids can block prostacyclin manufacture, thus fostering the development of blood clots.

proteases — enzymes which break down proteins. An example is bromelain, found in raw pineapple. Some proteases have been found to stimulate the immune system.

quench — to terminate a chemical reaction, as in quenching a fire, or to return an excited energetic reactive molecule to its most stable lowest energy state.

receptors — special biological structures found on cells where active molecules such as hormones, enzymes, and neurotransmitters are attached to the cell surface. The cell then responds to the presence of the chemical in the receptors. Loss of and/or damage to receptors is one important event in aging.

reduction — a chemical reaction in which an electron is donated to the reduced entity.

refereed journals — scientific journals in which a committee of scientists review papers before they are published, checking for adequate experimental design and whether the experimental results support the conclusions reached.

regeneration — regrowth of lost body cells, tissues, organs, and limbs. See Part II chapter 12.

retinoid — a substance closely related chemically to vitamin A. (Vitamin A is retinoic acid and its esters, or retinyl alcohol.) Retinoids regulate growth of epithelial cells (skin, lung, and gut) and are often powerful antioxidants and cancer preventing agents. The early stages of some epithelial cancers can be converted back into normal tissue by some retinoids. Retinoids are also chemically closely related to and made from carotenoids.

RNA — ribonucleic acid, which carries instructions from DNA (deoxyribonucleic acid) in the nucleus to cell polyribosomes, where proteins are made according to the RNA instructions copied from the DNA master version of the cell's blueprints.

saturated fats — fats containing no carbon-to-carbon double bonds; these fats are less susceptible to autoxidation (conversion to a peroxidized, immune-suppressive, clot promoting, carcinogenic form) than are polyunsaturated fats.

secondary antioxidant — an antioxidant which can break down already formed peroxides, and can also block their formation. An example is the food additive thiodipropionic acid.

serotonin — an inhibitory neurotransmitter required for sleep; its natural precursor is the essential amino acid tryptophan, found in relatively large quantities in bananas and milk.

serotonin structure

singlet oxygen — an activated energetic reactive form of oxygen, which is produced by the reaction of ultraviolet light with oxygen in the skin, as well as in other chemical reactions. Singlet oxygen can damage important macromolecules such as DNA. Singlet oxygen quenchers include beta-carotene (gives carrots their yellow color), which is pro-vitamin A, converted in the body to vitamin A on demand.

stem cells — cells which remain in an immature state of development until needed to replace cells that have died. They can then develop (differentiate) into mature cells. Examples are bone marrow cells and the cells lining the gastrointestinal tract.

stimulatory neurotransmitter — increases activity of neurons; examples are norepinephrine and glutamate.

stimulus barrier — a mental state or drug state in which a person's brain can more readily filter out unwanted sensory stimuli. Examples include some of the most commonly used drugs: nicotine, alcohol, tranquilizers, caffeine. After regular use of these chemical stimulus barriers, discontinuing their use can result in the opposite effect, an increased sensitivity to sensory stimuli (as in withdrawal from cigarettes or alcohol).

sulfhydryl — a sulfur atom bonded to a hydrogen atom is a sulfhydryl group. A sulfhydryl compound contains one or more sulfhydryl groups. Examples include vitamin B-1 and the amino acid cysteine.

superoxide dismutase (SOD) — a zinc and copper or manganese containing enzyme which reacts with superoxide radicals to convert them to less dangerous chemical entities. It is the fifth most common protein in the human body. All organisms not killed by air contain SOD. Intracellular cytoplasmic SOD generally contains zinc and copper, while mitochondrial SOD contains zinc and manganese.

superoxide radical — a free radical thought to play a central role in arthritis and cataract formation. Our major intracellular (inside of cells) defense against them is the enzyme superoxide dismutase.

synapse — the gap between nerve cells. One nerve cell stimulates another one to fire an electric pulse by secreting special chemicals called neurotransmitters into the synapse between the cells.

synergy — when chemicals or drugs are used together, they may show negative or positive synergy. Positive synergy occurs when the sum of the effects of chemicals acting together is greater than the additive effects of the individual chemicals. Negative synergy occurs when the sum of effects of the mixture is less than that of the individual components of the mix. Antioxidant mixtures commonly exhibit positive synergy, although negative synergy can also occur.

systemic — throughout the body.

T-cells — thymus-derived white blood cells which kill and eat foreign invaders (bacteria, viruses, and cancer cells), or control the production or attack of other T-cells or the antibody-making B-cells.

thiol — a sulfhydryl compound. An example is vitamin B-1 (thiamine).

thrombosis — blood clot blocking a blood vessel.

thymocyte — white blood cell arising in or processed in the thymus.

thymus — the master gland of the immune system, located behind the breastbone. The thymus "instructs" T-cells when to mature or reproduce, and what targets to go after. This gland shrinks in young adulthood, and immune system decline follows. The shrinkage and decline can be prevented or reversed by several methods and materials. See Part II chapter 5.

tissue culture — the growth of cells as tissue in a special medium. While the properties of tissue in culture differs in some ways from tissues in the body, particularly in lacking many of the protective mechanisms of the whole animal, tissue culture research can provide valuable data at relatively low cost.

topical — applied externally.

toxic — poisonous. Toxic effects of a substance are dependent on the dose. At sufficiently high doses, anything—even the inert gas helium—is toxic. (High pressure helium causes convulsions even when adequate oxygen is present.)

transformation — the process whereby a normal cell turns into a cancer cell. This process involves cellular de-differentiation. See Part II chapter 12 on regeneration.

triglycerides — a class of fats found in the bloodstream.

triplet oxygen — oxygen in an excited electronic state in which the oxygen atom has two single electrons in two high energy orbitals with their spins in the same direction. Because of the unpaired electrons, triplet oxygen is even more highly reactive than singlet oxygen, and can cause biological damage. Under physiological conditions, triplet oxygen very rapidly decays to somewhat less energetic singlet oxygen. Beta-carotene and other carotenoids quench both triplet and singlet oxygen. Regular atmospheric oxygen is in an unexcited triplet state (it has two unpaired electrons), which is why it is both a good free radical initiator and scavenger.

uric acid — a chemical formed in the body during the metabolic breakdown of RNA, caffeine, and related substances by the enzyme xanthine oxidase. Uric acid or sodium hydrogen urate crystals precipitating into joints and kidneys can cause gout, with severe pain and possibly even permanent damage.

uric acid

water soluble — dissolves in water.

INDEX

A (vitamin), 419–23, 483, 694–95
for acne, 756; for age pigment removal,
175; antioxidant, 55; for arthritis, 162,
298, 300, 747; and atherosclerosis, 313–
16, 324; authors' dosage, 612; for back
pain, 746–47, 762; and beta carotene,
420, 422, 476, 802; and cancer prevention, 87, 332, 666, 684, 703; and cod liver
oil allergy, 305, 485, 747; and cross-link
formation, 93, 98; and cystic fibrosis, 339;
dosage, 420–21, 436, *in authors' formula,*
612, *for drinkers,* 280, *excessive,* 87, 93,
420, 476, *in experimental formula,* 468,
in "Miss Jones" formula, 758, *in "Mr.
Smith" formula,* 742, *for smokers,* 245;
Durk and, 762–63, 767; and epithelial
cell normalization, 151, 421; esters and
stability, 492; fat solubility, 77–78; free
radical protection, 102, 107, 110, 112,
273, 278, 280; immune system improvement, 86–87, 89, 308, 740; for nonsmokers, 252; overdosage **caution,** 420–21,
756; overweight persons and, 250; oxidation of, 421; peroxidized fat prevention,
367, 371; precursors to and ozone protection, 261, 476; and retinoids, 801; for sexual capacity, 196; and singlet oxygen,
476; for skin, 93, 163, 165, 210; for smokers, 162, 241, 246–47; and stroke prevention, 318, 320; temperature sensitivity,
313; thymus gland size and, 82, 87; zinc
and, 470. **Cautions and Warnings,** 87, 93,
overdosage symptoms, 420–21, 756
Abhazia villagers, 65, 615
Accidents and emergency situations, 344–55
amnesia victims, 128, 164, 173; barbiturate overdose, 354; choking victim, 355;
CPR and, 305–52, *illus.* 353; first aid
techniques, 345–48; Hydergine® for, 177,
257, 350, 525; and naloxone, 354; nutrients for, 345, 347–48; paramedic medical
kits, 350–52, 354, 525; poisoning, 354,
524; synthetic blood and, 351, 524; vasopressin release, 128, 173
Acerola berries, 55
Acetaldehyde, 92, 783
alcohol and, 24, 92, 209, 242, 265, 269–
71, 273, 276, 279, 282, 563, 752, 783; alcoholics' heredity and, 270–71; B-1, C,
and cysteine for, 24, 92, 162, 242, 265,
272, 326, 341, 413, 475, 481, *research on,*
525; cigarette smoke and, 92, 162, 242,
256, 265; and cross-linking, 92, 242, 325–
26; Hydergine® as protection, 178; and
oxidation of fats, 250, 273, 279; SOD as
protection, 147
Acetaldehyde dehydrogenase, 271
Acetic acid, 53
Acetylcholine (ACh), 126, 128, 129, 131, 274,
798
defined, 783, 788–89; and depression,
186–87; for memory, 126, 129, 131, 170,
274; for muscles, 129, 131, 229; nutrients
and drugs for, 126, 135, 187, 193, 274,
431, 484; and sexual activity, 126, 131,

197–98, 274; side effects for excess stimulation, 187; stimulus barrier effect, 126,
131, 250; synthesis and degradation, diagram, 130; and vasopressin, 129, 131.
Warning: used with manic-depressive
psychosis, 187
See also Choline; Deaner® (Riker).
Acetyl co-enzyme A, 187, 227, 447, 451, 789
Aches and pains, 25, 47
Acid hydrolases, 106
Acidic vitamins, 487–89
and hemorrhoids, 756; neutralization of,
244, 246–47, 249, 281, 415, 426, 435–36,
462, 755–56; pH of, 491; ulcers and, xxiv,
426; supplier, 620; vitamin C intravenous
solutions, 345. **Caution and Warnings,**
xxiv, 244, 246–47, 249, 281, 415, 426,
436, 462, 755–56
Acid indigestion, 414, 426, 464, 487–89
Acid phosphatase test, 448, 451
Acne, 756
Acromegaly, 136, 765
ACTH 4-10 (adrenocorticotropic hormone),
168, 180, 799
Active Oxygen Method test (AOM), 378–79
Acyl radicals, 279
Adaptability rate, 430
Adelman, Dr. Richard, 71–72, 430
ADH (antidiuretic hormone). *See* Vasopressin.
Adipose tissues and insulin, 372
Adrenal gland, 121, 140, 420
Adrenaline, 328, 734–35, 799
Adult-onset diabetes, 84, 373
Advanced Research Health Products Corpo-
ration, 619
Adventurers' Guide, The (Wheeler), 733
Advertisements, 493, 495–99
for drugs before 1938, 713–14; for vita-
min supplements and California law,
597–98
Aerobic energy, 227
defined, 784
Aflatoxin organisms, 31, 383–84, 570, 764
AGE News, 535
Age differential and nutrient program, 430–
31
Aging, 5–6, 11, 58–59, 63–74
attacking agents, targets and results,
chart, 154–55; definition, 8–9; DNA damage and, 791; effects of, 8, 70–74; and
FDA, 4–5; of foods, 375–84; Hydergine®
retardation of, 651; intervention benefits
vs. costs, 26–29, 458; intervention techniques, 23–25; lay health periodicals and,
495–96, 499; life extension program and,
161–66; plastic surgery and, 499, 501;
process interaction and feedback loops,
diagram, 156; programmed *vs.* random
agents of, 18–19, 67–71; random damage
and repair, 67–74, 770; rates of, 9, 65, 70,
74, 429; reversal of, xxix–xxxi, 15, 23–25,
32–33; and sex, 196–207; stroke causa-
tion, 319; theories of, 44–51, 56, 153–57
See also Aging clocks; Aging pigment accumulation; Cross-linking; Free radicals;

Chicken: arginine/ornithine found in, 192;
cooked, shelf-storage life of, 388–89;
cooking of, 382
See also Poultry.
Childbearing, 39
See also Pregnancy; Reproduction.
Children, 20, 39
Vitamin A overdosage **caution**, 420; and
atherosclerosis, 312–13; experimental formula **warning**, xxiv, 431, 468, 611; immunizations and, 356–60; NGF/neurite
levels, 176; regeneration capacity, 149;
vitamin deficiency, immunizations and
SIDS, **Warning**, 358, 686; vitamin tablet
fillers and reactions, 305, 485. **Caution: A**
vitamin overdose, 420. **Warnings:** immu-
nization of vitamin-deficient children
and SIDS, 358, 686; life extension pro-
gram not for, xxiv, 431, 468, 611
Chimpanzees, 18, 20, 146, 614, 616
Chinchilla, mountain, life span, 616
Chio, Dr., 121
Chloramphenicol, 583–85
Chlorination, 570
Chlorine, 259–60, 315, 705
Chlorohydrins, 279
Chloromycetin®, 583
p-Chlorophenoxyacetic acid, 123
Chlorphenteramine, *illus.*, 295
Chocolate, 292
Choking (accidental), 344
first aid for, 355
Cholecystokinin (CCK), 286, 291–92
Cholesterol, 53
excretion of, 366
See also Antioxidants; Serum cholesterol.
Choline: and acetylcholine production, 126,
228, 250–51, 274, 783, 788; for alcohol
drinkers, 274, *daily dose*, 280; for alertness, 737; with B-5, 187; dosage, 187,
247, 469; intestinal bacteria and fishy
smell, side effect, 164; and manic-depres-
sives, **caution**, 187; for membrane stabilization, 250, 483; for memory and
learning, 126, 163–64, 168, 186, 250–51,
483, 788; nicotine substitute, 256; for
"rheumatism," 300; and serum cholesterol level, 483; and sex drive, 198, 788; side
effects, 164, 187, 441; and sleep, 190,
193; for smokers, dosage, 245, 247. **Warning:** in manic-depressive psychosis, 187
See also Acetylcholine.
Choline bitartrate: diarrhea side effect, 135,
164, 171
Choline chloride (hydrochloride), 135, 164,
171
authors' life extension formula dosage,
613; experimental formula dosage, 468
Cholinergic system, 134–35, 250, 788–89
Chromosomes, 84–85, 506–07, 789
Ciba-Geigy Company, 575
See also Anturane®
Cicero, 70
Cigarette smoke: acetaldehyde in, 92, 96,
162, 242–43, 265, 340, 413, 475, 783; and

cancer, 784, 800; carbon monoxide and
nitrogen oxide in, 244, 257; heavy metals
in, 244; macrophages and, 481–82; nicotine in, 243; odors from, 239, 252–53;
sidestream *cf.* inhaled, 252; skin wrinkling, 247
See also Cancer; Cardiovascular disease;
Smoking and smokers.
Cigarettes: Hydergine® protection, 257; nico-
tine-fortification of, 255, 563–64; nico-
tine-tar ratios of brands, 255; nutrient
protection for nonsmokers, 252–55; tar,
5, 241, 252, *and cancer deaths,* 265
Circadian (daily) clock, 786
Circulation: in brain, 351; and cold extremities, **caution,** 767; and vitamin E, 405–
06; in legs, **Warning,** 316; and thyroid
function, 766–67. **Caution:** cold extremities symptoms, 767. **Warning:** antioxi-
dants not a substitute treatment for poor
leg circulation, 316
See also Cardiovascular disease.
Cities: and air pollution, 146–47, 261, *cancer
rates,* 104, 147; lead pollution, 261
Citric acid, 227, 368–69
Citric acid (Krebs) cycle, 78, 187, 227–28,
435, 475, 479
athletic performance and, 227–28; definition of, 789; *diagram* of, 79
Clarke, Arthur C., 208
Claudication, 406
Claustrophobia magazine, 534
Clean Air Act, 720
Cleveland, Ohio, 104, 147, 561
Cline, Dr. Martin J., 21, 506
Clinical Guide to Undesirable Drug Interactions and Interferences (Garb), 444
Clinical laboratory tests, 441–466
with authors' life extension formula must
be extensive and frequent, **warning,** 611;
C vitamin effect on findings, **precaution,**
459; case histories and, 737, 750–51, 757–
58; HDL/LDL ratio, 325, *Durk and
Sandy, test results,* 775–79; before immune system stimulation, 90; with life
extension nutrient program, **caution and
warning,** xxiii–xxiv, 166, 430, 442, 458,
462, 466–67; normal values and reasons
for tests, *charts,* 450–53; records of, 434,
438–39, 458–59; regularity of, **caution
and warning,** xxiii–xxiv, 166, 430, 442,
458, 462, 466–67; results to physician,
xxiv; short screen for toxic effects, 447;
for thyroid function, 323, 767; toxic and
metabolic effects of life-extension nutrients, 29, 448–49; **Precaution:** C vitamin
possible effect on, 459. **Cautions and
Warnings:** importance of life extension
nutrient program regularity, xxiii–xxiv,
166, 430, 442, 458, 462, 466–67; authors'
formula and, 611
See also Hexokinase blood sugar test.
Clinistix®, 315
Clinistrips®, 446
Clinitest® urine sugar test, 675, 688–89

Index

authors have no interest in becoming cult leaders, xxiii

authors are not infallible, xxiii

authors have no control over foundations nor receive any grants therefrom, 619, 621

authors' suggestions no substitute for physicians' treatment of serious disorders such as heart disease, high blood pressure, cancer, kidney disease, etc., xxiv

authors have no control over life extension associations or institutions, and receive no support therefrom, 535

authors' *caveat* re limited knowledge of aging processes, xxiv–xxv

clinical laboratory test importance, xxiii–xxiv; results sent to physician, xxiv

experimental formulas *not* for children or pregnant women, xxiv, 431, 468, 611

FDA nonapproval of nutrients and drugs for life extension, xxiv

Megadoses of vitamins and serious illnesses, xxiv

Physicians: and megadose vitamins, xxiv; and lab test results, xxiv; and consultation with regarding experimental program, xxiv

prescription drugs and nutrients used for life extension are experimental, xxiii–xxiv

principles governing reasonable use of this book, xxiii–xxiv

readers' responsibilities and values, xxiii

See also Cautions; Warnings.

Diseases: aging and resistance to, 8, 25, 28, 72, 83; degenerative, 6, 11, 74, 129, 334; and FDA, 4–5, 7; genetic differences and, 429, 435; and immune system, 81–83; and infections, 356–57; study of occurence of, 792; venereal, 199; and vitamin megadoses, caution and warning, xxiv. **Warning:** for serious disorders, patient must remain under physician's care, xxiv, 316, 341, 675, 689

See also names of diseases; Infections.

Disulfide bonds, 95

DL-alpha tocopherol (vitamin E), 31, 261, 407

acetate, 619, *authors' formula dosage,* 611

D-leucine, 293

DL-phenylalanine, 136, 185–86, 288, 293, 746

DMAE (dimethylaminoethanol), 122, 495

authors' life extension formula dosage, 613

DMBA, 144, 333, 339

concentrations, binding to DNA and species' life spans, *figures,* 145; -induced tumors and 2-bromoergocriptine, 680, 702

DMSO (dimethyl sulfoxide), 348–49, 791

antioxidants needed with, 298, 348–49, 760; for brain and spinal cord trauma, 238, 348, 525; free radical scavenger, 347–48, 477; hormone esters and scalp

treatment, 214–15; for injuries, 237–38, 347, 477, 740, 759–60; rabbits and cataracts, 760. **Caution:** 298, 348–49, 760

DNA (deoxyribonucleic acid), 71, 75–76, 791

aging clocks in, 137–39, 141–42, 786; alcohol damage to, 269; antioxidant protection for, 785; control system damage and cancer, 331–32; and carcinogens, 787; and chromosomes, 789; cloned, 789; and cross-linking, 91–92, 98, 789; DMBA and PAH binding to, 144–46, 241, 264, 451, *illus.,* 145; double helix, *illus.,* 76, *discovery of,* 550; vitamin E for, 404–05; free radical damage, 101–06, 153, 157, 244, 246, 250, 265, 280, 297, 402–04, *chart,* 154–55; future developments in human genome sequencing, 21, 506, 514–15; genes and, 18–21, 793; herpes viruses and, 206, 753; histones, 795; hormonal changes and developmental clock, 286; mutagens and selenium, 24, 88, 798; regeneration of organs and limbs, 148–49; repair mechanisms, 20, 68, 138–39; RNA and, 76, 472, 802; skin cells and herpes, 753; singlet oxygen and, 422, 476, 802; ultraviolet light damage, 146, 770, 802, *figure,* 147; and xeroderma pigmentosum, 744

Docosahexanoic acid, 111, 413

Doctors. *See* Physicians.

Dogs, 405.

and vitamin C, 409, 412; cooling experiments, 608–09; hair allergy, 744–45; heart attacks and vagus nerve, 326

See also Pets.

Dolomite, 249, 436, 488

Dolphins, 508, 616

Donne, John, 41

Donner Research Laboratories, 777

Donsbach, Dr. Kurt, 763

L-Dopa. *See* L-Dopa in L column.

Dopamine, 127, 131–36, 479, 798

B-6 effect when taking L-Dopa for Parkinsonism, caution, 431, 474; and vitamin C, 414; definition, 791; and GH release, 229; lipofuscin accumulation, 126, 221; L-phenylalanine as precursor, 185; and MAO inhibitors, 797; and schizophrenia, 134; and sex drive increase, 127, 197. **Warning:** in Parkinson's disease, B-6 not to be taken with L-Dopa, xxiv, 134, 431, 474–75

See also Catecholamines.

Dopaminergic nervous system, 129, 139, 176, 791, *chart,* 155

Hydergine* for, 176; and L-Dopa, 133, 197–98, 481; low levels and sleep disorders, 131, 190, 192, *and Parkinsonism,* 132–33; menstrual recycling and stimulation, 139–40, 197, 471; stimulants for, 139–40, 229, 236, 471; stimulation of hypothalamus, 290

Dorland's Illustrated Medical Dictionary, 431, 774

Dosages of nutrients and drugs

(**Warning:** *Be sure to read carefully all*

Index

Neurological damage, 354
Neuronophages, 125
Neurons, 796, 798, 802
  See also Nerve cells.
Neuropharmacology of Ergot Alkaloids, Conference, 733
Neurotransmitters, 125–36, 169, 803
  and autoxidation, 131–35; B-6 for, 474;
  vitamin C for, 409, 413–14; decline and
  destruction of, 153, 157, *chart,* 154–55;
  definition, 798; and depression, 181–87;
  diagrams, 130, 131, 132; glutamate, 793;
  glycine, 794; and free radicals, 153, 157;
  inhibitory, 796; L-Dopa for, 481; and
  MAO inhibitors, 797–98; and sexual activity, 126–27, 129, 131, 197–98; and sleep
  disorders, 135, 189–94; synaptic terminals, 184, 186, *figures,* 130–32
  See also catecholamines.
Newark, New Jersey, 104, 146, 515–16, 561
New chemical entities (NCEs), 580, 587
New Drug Application, 573–75
New England Journal of Medicine, 329
Newton, 526
New York Academy of Science, 224
New York City, 261
NGF. *See* Nerve growth factor (NGF).
Niacin (vitamin B-3) (nicotinic acid), 424–26
  and alcohol, 193–94; for arthritis, 162;
  and biotin cream for hair loss, 218; burns
  and fluid loss, 347; definition, 798; dosages, *authors' formula,* 425–26, 463, *experimental formula,* 469, *frequency of,*
  458–59; for drinkers, 280–82; and drowsiness, 193, 426; flushing and tingling effects, 244, 247, 282–83, 426, 434–35, 463,
  470, **Caution:** *gradual dosage increase,*
  247, 249, 283, 426, 435; and free radicals,
  665, 696; for histamine release, 754; molecule structure, *diagram,* 243; neutralization of acidity, **precaution,** 247, 249, 426,
  435–36, 487–88; paraquat toxicity and,
  243; and psychedelic drugs, 426; for
  schizophrenics, 426, 466; lowering of serum cholesterol, 24, 243, 327, 365, 424–
  25, 434, 463, 483, *dosage,* 425; sexual excitation and, 204–05, 282; for smokers,
  245–47, 424–25; and stamina, 227; as
  tranquilizer substitute, 282, 426, 755; vasodilation effect, 243, 247, 327, 424–26;
  and VLDL lowering, 327, 688, 695–96,
  777. **Caution:** gradual dosage increase on
  full stomach, 247, 249, 283, 426.
  See also Niacinamide.
Niacinamide (nicotinamide), 193–94, 426, 463
  for calm and tranquility, 282, 426; and
  stamina, 227; substitute for tranquilizers,
  755
Nicolle, Charles, 490
Nicorette chewing gum, 256
Nicotinamide. *See* Niacinamide.
Nicotinamide adenine dinucleotode. *See*
  NADP; NADPH.
Nicotine, 413
  and cigarette fortification, 255, 563–64;
  chewing gum with, 256; choline substi-

tute for, 251; Hydergine® protection
  from, 257; molecular structure, *diagram,*
  243; *cf.* niacin, 243, 424–25; stimulus barrier effect, 240, 250–51, 256; and tar ratio in cigarettes, 255
Nicotinic acid. *See* Niacin.
Nijinsky, Vaslav, 653
Nitrogen gas, 403
Nitrogen oxides, 147, 244, 250, 349
  and free radicals, 332
Nitrates, 31, 244, 261, 336, 383–84, 410, 798
Nitrites, 31, 244, 261, 336, 383–84, 410, 798
Nitrosamines, 31, 244, 261, 336, 383–84, 410
  definition, 798
N-nitroso compounds, 339, 413
Nockels, Dr. Cheryl F., 86
No-Diet Program for Permanent Weight Loss
  (Rader), 293
Nomograms, 774
Nonsmokers, 252–54
  carotenoids and, 666, 684, 703; and lung
  cancer, 258, 266
Nootropyl® (UCB), 168
Noradrenaline, 734–35, 799
Noradrenergic nervous system, 176
Norepinephrine (NE), 126–28, 176, 734, 798,
  802
  and vitamin C, 413–14; cocaine and depletion of, 745; definition, 799; and Hydergine®, 136; and L-Dopa, 132, 288,
  479; for learning and memory, 126, 171;
  loss of and effects, 129, 171–72, 185–86,
  251, 287–91; and MAO inhibitors, 797;
  phenylpropanolanine and depletion, 498,
  799; and sex drive, 126, 129, 197; side effects from excess of, 136
  See also Catecholamines.
Nose growth, 501
NOVA television show, 537
NOx, 413
Nuclear power plants, 106, 264, 518, 705
Nucleases, 206
Nucleic acids, 92–93, 98, 169, 242, 769, 795
  See also DNA; RNA.
Nucleic acid analogs, *chart,* 154
Nucleo-proteins, 219
Nugent, Ted, 653
Nureyev, Rudolf, 509, 515, 653
Nutrient life extension program. *See* Life extension experimental nutrient program.
"Nutrient Requirements of Nonhuman Primates" (Nat'l Research Council), 398
"Nutrient Requirements of Laboratory Animals" (Nat'l Research Council), 398
Nutrients, manufacturers and suppliers, 618–
  21
Nutrition, 44, 46–51
  Congressional legislation, 399–401; cooking methods and, 369; cult leaders, xxiii,
  49–51; false claims and misinformation,
  495–99; improved, and effect on aging
  curve, 10; RDAs and, 392–99; unidentified cofactors of vitamins, 53–54
Nutrition and the Brain (Wurtman and Wurtman), 164
Nuts, 383

Obesity, 284–95
adult-onset diabetes and, 373; alcohol drinkers and, 279; antioxidant nutrients for, 250; artificial sweetener ban and, 570–71, 595; cancer and cardiovascular disease risk, 108, 249–50, 284–85; cholesterol levels and, 338; choline as nicotine replacement, 250; dehydroepiandrosterone experiments, 524; evolutionary mechanisms, 285–86; food addiction and, 293; and GH decline, 794; HDL/LDL ratio and, 324–25; high blood pressure and heart disease, 294; phenylalanine for, 251; smokers who quit, and weight gain, 250–51; and starch digestion, 294; and sugar, 370; weight loss methods, 286–94. **Caution:** overweight persons with high blood pressure and/or heart disease must consult with physician, 294; and sodium restrictions, 294
See also Calories; Weight control.
Obsolescence. *See* Programmed obsolescence.
Occam, William of, 45
Occam's Razor, 45
Occult blood urine test, 447, 449
Occupational Safety and Health Administration (OSHA), 266, 561–62
Octopuses, 141
Ocular herpes, 573
Odens, Dr. Clifford, 430
Odors, 239, 252–53, 261–63
Offspring, 18–20
future DNA developments and heredity, 506; high mutation rates and aging clocks, 147; of mice, and antioxidants, 112
Oi, Dr. Walter, 567
Oils. *See* Fats and oils (dietary); Lipids; Peroxidized fats; Polyunsaturated fats; Unsaturated fats.
Old people, 11, 15–17, 111
broken-hip problem, 152; lack of concentration and forgetfulness, 131; and depression, 129, 468; and GH decline, 794; and national health insurance, 719; neurotransmitter insufficiency, 125–29, 131; nutrient program and, xxviii, 430–31; skin moisture, 162–63, 165; sleep disturbances, 131, 134–35, 189–94
See also Memory; Senility.
Olympic athletes, 93
body fat percentage, 775; future scandals, 508–09
Oman, G. S., 720
OMNI magazine, 533, 535
Opiates, 354, 714–15
Oncologist, 729
Optic nerve, 788
Opt-out procedure, 569, 573–74, 591–92, 713
Oral anticoagulants, 283
Caution: use with alcohol, 283
Oral contraceptives. *See* Birth control pills.
Orange juice, 272
Organic peroxides, 24, 758
abnormal clotting and PGI₂ inhibition,

70, 320; acetaldehyde autoxidation and, 279; antioxidant protection, 740, 758; from cooked meat and fat, 314; protective enzymes and, 280, 425, 515–16; protective antioxidants and, 371; targets attacked and results, *chart*, 154–55
Organoleptic panel, 387
Organs and regeneration, 148
Orgasm, 173, 196, 204–05, 282, 484, 754, 795
L-ornithine. *See* L-ornithine in L-column.
Orobronze® (Rorer), 97–98, 211, 422–23
authors' life extension formula, 612; Durk and, 771. **Caution:** overdose danger, 423
Ortho-Novum®, 201
Orthotoluidine blood sugar test, 416, 443, 785
Osborne Computer Corporation, 625
OTC (over-the-counter) drugs, 348
Ovaries, 197–99
aging clocks in, 71, 197
Ovalbumin, 53
Overeating, 23
addictive, 293
Overweight people. *See* Obesity.
Ovomucoid, 53
Oxalate urine test, 447, 449, 453
Oxidase enzyme system, 259–60, 334
Oxidants, 115, 154–55
See also Free radicals; Hydrogen peroxides; Organic peroxide; PAH.
Oxidation, 24, 31, 115–16
in animals and plants, 402–03; and brain aging, 111; control of, 378; definition, 799; and vitamin E, 402; source of free radicals, 101, 269–70; of lipids, 66, 68, 103, 106, 115–16, 123; singlet oxygen, 422, 476; smoking and obesity, 249–51
See also Cross-linking; Free radicals; Oxygen; Peroxidized fats.
Oxidation and reduction reactions, 95
vitamin C and, 414
Oxidation of organic compounds by molecular oxygen, 107
Oxidation products. *See* Mutagens; Carcinogens; Epoxides; Hydroperoxides; Hydroxyl free radicals.
Oxidative degradation, 103, 476
of dopaminergic system, 133, 139
Oxidative polymerization, 103
Oxygen, 376
aerobic energy and, 227, 784; anaerobic processes, 784; atherosclerosis and low levels, 299, 314; to brain, and free radicals, 101–02, 265, 275, 318; vitamin C exposure to, 491; and free radical formation, 102–19, 318; hyperbaric, use **precaution**, 119; low levels and vitamin E, 405–06; low levels and old people, 111, 187, 318; singlet and beta carotene, 422–23; stability of dietary fats and oils, 378–79. **Caution:** levels of and free radical activity, 119
See also Hypoxia; Oxidation; Singlet oxygen.
Oxytocin, 131, 469, 484
Ozone, 31, 147, 250, 799

and cross-linking, 790; and free radicals, 332, 793; protection from, 260–61; toxicity, *and vitamin E*, 404, *and PABA*, 248, 473

Ozone analyzer and generator, 516

P, Mr., case history, 754–55

PABA (p-aminobenzoic acid), 55, 77, 473–74
in anti-aging creams, 495; for arthritis and rheumatism, 162, 298, 300; in authors' life extension formula, 612; for bronchial asthma, 756; for slowing cross-linking, 93, 97; esters *cf.* plain, 209, 263–64; experimental formula dosage, 469; for hair, 217, 473; membrane stabilizer, 797; in "Miss Jones" formula, 758; in "Mr. Smith" formula, 743; protection from nitrogen oxides, 246; for nonsmokers, 252; protection for obese persons, 250; protection against ozone damage, 248, 261, 473; for skin, 165; for smokers, 245–46, 248; as UV light screen, 209, 263, 422, 474. **Precautions:** acidity must be neutralized, 435–36; should be discontinued when taking sulfa drugs, 248, 469, 474

PAH (polynuclear or polycyclic aromatic hydrocarbons), 241, 264, 279, 797
and cancer, 264, 339; conversion to epoxides, 279, 341, 413, 792; definition, 800; and LDL, 325, 364; and longevity, 144–46; nutrients for, 144–46, 264, 337–38; targets in body, *chart*, 154; in tobacco smoke, 241, 256, 279, 337, 340

Painkillers, 349
for arthritis, 747–49, 760; for back pain, 746; D-phenylalanine, 136, 186, 289; endorphins, 293, 791; enkephalins, 186, 414, 792; Hydergine® for, 732; and placebo effect, 800; for varicose veins and cramps, 767–68

Pancreas, 372
cancer of, 337; serum amylase test, 451

Pantothenic acid, 31, 227–28, 430, 436
See also Calcium pantothenate (B-5).

Pap smear test and estrogens, 200–01

Papain, 87, 89, 163, 237, 384

Papaya, 99, 163, 237, 384
side effect, sore mouth, 99, 237. **Caution:** do not eat when ulcer present, 99, 237

"Parable of the Blind Men and the Elephant, The" (Saxe), 63–64

Paralysis, 354, 356–57

Paramedics, 344
cost-effectiveness of programs, 562; and emergency medical kit drugs, 350–54, 525

Paraplegia, 759

Paraquat-contaminated cannabis: poisoning by and niacin 243, 665, 696. **Caution:** health hazard, 242–43

Parasites, 796

Parenchymal cancer, 266

Parents' Guide to Childhood Immunization (HEW), 357

Parkinsonism, 127, 132–34, 414, 522

L-Dopa and bromocriptine for, 127, 132–35, 236, 766; 6-OH-dopamine autoxidation and, 788. **Caution:** L-Dopa without antioxidants, 133. **Warning:** do not use B-6 supplements with L-Dopa, xxiv, 134, 431–32, 474–75

Parlodel®. *See* Bromocriptine.

Parotid cancer, 726–30
Warning: Sandy's cancer therapy should not be used as model, 730

Parrots, 518

Pathologists and cancer surgery, 727–28

Patents on drugs, 336
Anturane® and, 575–76; and FDA delays, 564
See also names of prescription drugs.

Pauling, Dr. Linus, 53–54, 56, 408, 464, 531
terminal cancer patients and vitamin C study, 336–37, 411

Pauling Institute of Science and Medicine, 536

PBI, 448, 452

PCP, 426

PDR. *See Physician's Desk Reference.*

P-chlorophenoxyacetic acid, 123

Peak output (exercise), 223–26
and jogging, 229

Peanuts, 570

Pearson, Durk, 761–71
allergy, 763–64; backaches, 761–62; body fat percentage, 774–75; cardiovascular disease risk, 778; clinical lab test findings, 775–79; cold extremities and thyroid function, 766–67; GH release, 765–66; gout and, 769–70; HDL/LDL ratio, 777; male pattern baldness, 212, 214, 217–20, 768; muscle buildup, 771, 774; *photographs*, 230–32, 772–73; pituitary dysfunction, 762–63, 765–67; sex drive, 765; sex research, 758; stomach problems and nutrition, 768; sunburn resistance with canthaxanthin, 770–71; testicular sensitivity, 766; varicose veins, 767–68

Pelletier and Keith study, 409

Peltzman, Dr. Sam, 567–68, 704, 716
econometric analysis, 578–89, 594

Pelvic infections, 411

D-Penicillamine, 299

L-Penicillamine: **Caution:** lethal, 299

Penicillin, 350, 761, 771

Peninsula Laboratories, Inc., 180, 624

Penis, 197

Peptide synthesizer, 180, 527, 624
See also Polypeptides.

Peracetic acid, 279, 340

Perfuse, defined, 799

Peristaltic stimulant, 187

Peroxidase, 103, 142, 516, 799

Peroxides, 88, 115–17
definition, 799; degradation of, 476; protection against, 104, 114; value, 378–81

Peroxidized, defined, 799

Peroxidized fats (rancid fats), 88, 102, 106–08, 770
and aging pigments, 112, 121, 174–75;